PARK'S
THE PEDIATRIC
ARDIOLOGY HANDBOOK

PARK'S THE PEDIATRIC CARDIOLOGY HANDBOOK

Myung K. Park, MD, FAAP, FAAC
Professor Emeritus (Department of Pediatrics)
Former Director of Pediatric Cardiology
Former Director of Preventive Cardiology and Weight Management Clinics
University of Texas Health Science Center
San Antonio, Texas

Mehrdad Salamat, MD, FAAP, FACC
Clinical Associate Professor of Pediatrics
Texas A & M University Health Science Center
Bryan, Texas
and
Attending Pediatric Cardiologist
Driscoll Children's Hospital
Corpus Christi, Texas

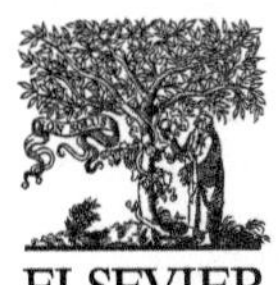

Elsevier
3251 Riverport Lane
St. Louis, Missouri 63043

PARK'S THE PEDIATRIC CARDIOLOGY
HANDBOOK, SIXTH EDITION

ISBN: 978-0-323-7-1866-0

ISBN: 9780323718660

Content Strategist: Marybeth Thiel
Content Development Specialist: Kevin Travers
Content Development Manager: Meghan Andress
Publishing Services Manager: Deepthi Unni
Project Manager: Srividhya Vidhyashankar
Design Direction: Ryan Cook

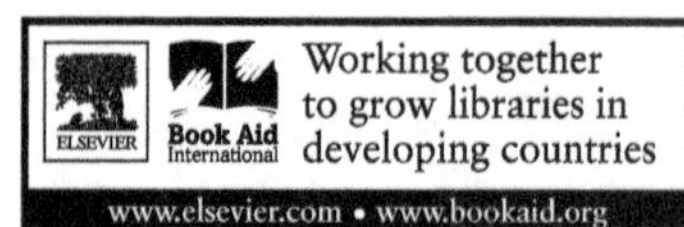

Printed in United States of America
Last digit is the print number: 9 8 7 6 5 4 3 2

DEDICATION

To my wife Issun;
Our sons (Douglas, Christopher, and Warren);
Daughters-in-law (Bomin and Soyeon); and
Grandchildren (Natalie, Audrey, and Madeleine)
—Myung K. Park, MD, FAAP, FAAC

To my wife Nazia;
Our children (Bita and Pedram); and
My beloved mother
—Mehrdad Salamat, MD, FAAP, FACC

Preface to the Fifth Edition

Since the publication of the fifth edition of *The Pediatric Cardiology Handbook*, important advances have been made in both the diagnosis and treatment of children with congenital and acquired heart diseases. These advances make it necessary to update the handbook. Although extensive updating and revisions have been made throughout the book, the handbook maintains its original goal of providing readers with fundamental and practical information in the management of children with cardiac problems.

Although every topic and chapter have been updated, certain topics received more extensive revision. Important revisions were made to noninvasive imaging techniques, device management of certain heart conditions, medical and surgical managements of selected congenital heart defects, infective endocarditis, acute rheumatic fever, cardiomyopathies, cardiac arrhythmias, congestive heart failure, pulmonary hypertension, and ambulatory blood pressure monitoring. More extensive revisions were made in the following topics: neonatal pulse oximetry screening; blood pressure measurement and normal standards in children; Kawasaki disease; long QT syndrome; short QT syndromes; pediatric preventive cardiology, including childhood obesity; and sports participation screening using the new 14-point evaluation.

I believe this handbook will be an important companion to cardiology fellows, pediatricians, family practitioners, house staff, and medical students. This handbook will also serve well any health care providers who deal with children, including physician assistants, nurse practitioners, and nursing students. This handbook may prove to be a very useful compendium even for practicing cardiologists because it makes basic as well as advanced information in the practice of cardiology available instantly.

I am very pleased to report that my longtime friend, Dr. Mehrdad Salamat, has accepted my invitation to become a coauthor of this handbook and to become the primary author of the future editions of the handbook. Dr. Salamat is an ardent teacher of pediatric cardiology, beloved by medical students, residents, pediatricians, and nursing staffs, and respected by his peers. His participation as coauthor has made this revision more objective and balanced. I am certain that Dr. Salamat would continue to maintain the original goal of this handbook in the future. I wish him the best in carrying out the paramount responsibility.

Myung K. Park, MD, FAAP, FAAC
San Antonio, Texas

Contents

PART V Arrhythmias and Atrioventricular Conduction Disturbances

PART VI Special Problems

PART VII Cardiac Surgical Patients

Appendices

Frequently Used Abbreviations

AR	Aortic regurgitation
AS	Aortic stenosis
ASD	Atrial septal defect
AV	Atrioventricular
BAH	Biatrial hypertrophy
BAV	Bicuspid aortic valve
BBB	Bundle branch block
BP	Blood pressure
B-T shunt	Blalock-Taussig shunt
BVH	Biventricular hypertrophy
CA	Coronary artery
CAD	Coronary artery disease
CHD	Congenital heart disease or defect
CHF	Congestive heart failure
COA	Coarctation of the aorta
CPB	Cardiopulmonary bypass
CV	Cardiovascular
CVD	Cardiovascular disease
DORV	Double-outlet right ventricle
ECD	Endocardial cushion defect
Echo	Echocardiography
HCM	Hypertrophic cardiomyopathy
HDL	High-density lipoprotein
HLHS	Hypoplastic left heart syndrome
HOCM	Hypertrophic obstructive cardiomyopathy
HT	Hypertension
IE	Infective endocarditis
IHSS	Idiopathic hypertrophic subaortic stenosis
IRBBB	Incomplete right bundle branch block
IVC	Inferior vena cava
LA	Left atrium or left atrial
LAD	Left axis deviation
LAE	Left atrial enlargement
LAH	Left atrial hypertrophy
LBBB	Left bundle branch block

LDL	Low density lipoprotein
LICS	Left intercostal space
LLN	Lower limit of normal
LLSB	Lower left sternal border
LPA	Left pulmonary artery
LPL	Left precordial lead
L-R shunt	Left-to-right shunt
LRSB	Lower right sternal border
LSB	Left sternal border
LV	Left ventricle or left ventricular
LVH	Left ventricular hypertrophy
LVOT	Left ventricular outflow tract
MLSB	Mid-left sternal border
MPA	Main pulmonary artery
MR	Mitral regurgitation
MRSB	Mid-right sternal border
MS	Mitral stenosis
MVP	Mitral valve prolapse
PA	Pulmonary artery
PAC	Premature atrial contraction
PAPVR	Partial anomalous pulmonary venous return
PAT	Paroxysmal atrial tachycardia
PBF	Pulmonary blood flow
PDA	Patent ductus arteriosus
PFO	Patent foramen ovale
PH	Pulmonary hypertension
PR	Pulmonary regurgitation
PS	Pulmonary stenosis
PV	Pulmonary vein or pulmonary venous
PVC	Premature ventricular contraction
PVM	Pulmonary vascular marking
PVOD	Pulmonary vascular obstructive disease
PVR	Pulmonary vascular resistance
RA	Right atrium or right atrial
RAD	Right axis deviation
RAE	Right atrial enlargement
RAH	Right atrial hypertrophy
RBBB	Right bundle branch block

RICS	Right intercostal space
R-L shunt	Right-to-left shunt
RPA	Right pulmonary artery
RPL	Right precordial lead
RV	Right ventricle or right ventricular
RVE	Right ventricular enlargement
RVH	Right ventricular hypertrophy
RVOT	Right ventricular outflow tract
S1	First heart sound
S2	Second heart sound
S3	Third heart sound
S4	Fourth heart sound
SBE	Subacute bacterial endocarditis
SEM	Systolic ejection murmur
SVC	Superior vena cava
SVR	Systemic vascular resistance
SVT	Supraventricular tachycardia
TAPVR	Total anomalous pulmonary venous return
TG	Triglycerides
TGA	Transposition of the great arteries
TOF	Tetralogy of Fallot
TR	Tricuspid regurgitation
TS	Tricuspid stenosis
ULN	Upper limit of normal
ULSB	Upper left sternal border
URSB	Upper right sternal border
VSD	Ventricular septal defect
VT	Ventricular tachycardia
WPW	Wolff-Parkinson-White (preexcitation or syndrome)

PART I

BASIC TOOLS IN EVALUATION OF CARDIAC PATIENTS

Initial evaluation of children with possible cardiac problems includes (1) history taking, (2) physical examination, (3) electrocardiographic (ECG) evaluation, and (4) chest radiography. Many cardiologists obtain an echocardiogram (echo), instead of a radiograph, for initial complete cardiac evaluation. The weight of information gained from these techniques varies with the type and severity of the disease.

Chapter 1

History and Physical Examination

I. HISTORY TAKING

Prenatal, natal, perinatal, postnatal, past, and family histories should be obtained.

A. GESTATIONAL AND PERINATAL HISTORY

1. Maternal infection: Rubella during the first trimester of pregnancy commonly results in PDA and PA stenosis (rubella syndrome, see Table 1.1). Other viral infections early in pregnancy may be teratogenic. Viral infections (including human immunodeficiency virus) in late pregnancy may cause myocarditis.
2. Maternal medications: The following is a partial list of suspected teratogenic drugs that cause CHDs.
   a. Amphetamines (VSD, PDA, ASD, and TGA), phenytoin (PS, AS, COA, and PDA), trimethadione (fetal trimethadione syndrome: TGA, VSD, TOF, HLHS, see Table 1.1), lithium (Ebstein's anomaly), retinoic acid (conotruncal anomalies), valproic acid (various noncyanotic defects), and progesterone or estrogen (VSD, TOF, and TGA) are highly suspected teratogens.
   b. Warfarin may cause fetal warfarin syndrome (TOF, VSD, and other features, such as ear abnormalities, cleft lip or palate, and hypoplastic vertebrae) (see Table 1.1).
   c. Excessive maternal alcohol intake may cause fetal alcohol syndrome (in which VSD, PDA, ASD, and TOF are common) (see Table 1.1).
   d. Cigarette smoking causes intrauterine growth retardation but not CHD.
3. Maternal conditions:
   a. Maternal diabetes increases the incidence of cardiomyopathy in infants and CHD (TGA, VSD, PDA, ECD, COA, and HLHS) and cardiomyopathy (see Table 1.1).
   b. Maternal lupus erythematosus and mixed connective tissue diseases have been associated with congenital heart block in the offspring.
   c. History of maternal CHD may increase the prevalence of CHD in the offspring to as much as 15%, compared with 1% in the general population (see Appendix, Table A.2).

4. Birth weight:
   a. Small for gestational age may indicate intrauterine infection or use of chemicals or drugs by the mother.
   b. High birth weight is often seen in infants of diabetic mothers.

B. POSTNATAL AND PRESENT HISTORY

1. Poor weight gain and delayed development may be caused by CHF, severe cyanosis, or general dysmorphic conditions. Weight is more affected than height.
2. Cyanosis, squatting, and cyanotic spells suggest TOF or other cyanotic CHD.
3. Tachycardia, tachypnea, and puffy eyelids are signs of CHF.
4. Frequent lower respiratory tract infections may be associated with large L-R shunt lesions.
5. Decreased exercise tolerance may be a sign of significant heart defects or ventricular dysfunction.
6. Heart murmur. The time of its first appearance is important. A heart murmur noted shortly after birth indicates a stenotic lesion (AS, PS). A heart murmur associated with large L-R shunt lesions (such as VSD or PDA) may be delayed. Appearance of a heart murmur in association with fever suggests an innocent heart murmur.
7. Chest pain. Ask if chest pain is exercise-related or nonexertional. Also ask about its duration, nature, and radiation. Nonexertional chest pain is unlikely to have cardiac causes (except for pericarditis). Cardiac causes of chest pain are usually exertional and are very rare in children and adolescents. The three most common causes of noncardiac causes of chest pain in children are costochondritis, trauma to chest wall or muscle strain, and respiratory diseases (see Chest Pain in Chapter 20).
8. Palpitation may be caused by paroxysms of tachycardia, sinus tachycardia, single premature beats; rarely hyperthyroidism or MVP (see Chapter 22).
9. Joint pain. Joints that are involved, presence of redness and swelling, history of trauma, duration of the pain, and migratory or stationary nature of the pain are important. History of recent sore throat and rashes and family history of rheumatic fever are frequent in acute rheumatic fever. History of rheumatoid arthritis is also an important clue to the diagnosis.
10. Neurologic symptoms. Stroke may result from embolization of thrombus from infective endocarditis, polycythemia, or uncorrected or partially corrected cyanotic CHD. Headache may be associated with polycythemia or rarely with hypertension. Choreic movement may result from rheumatic fever. Fainting or syncope may be due to vasovagal responses, arrhythmias, long QT syndrome, epilepsy, or other noncardiac conditions (see Syncope in Chapter 21).

11. Medications, cardiac and noncardiac (name, dosage, timing, route of administration and duration).
12. Syndromes and diseases of other systems with associated cardiovascular abnormalities are summarized in Tables 1.1 and 1.2, respectively.

C. FAMILY HISTORY

1. Certain hereditary diseases may be associated with varying frequency of cardiac anomalies (see Table 1.1).
2. CHD in the family. The following provides some information on the chance of occurrence of CHD in the family when family history is positive for CHD.
   a. The incidence of CHD in the general population is about 1% (8 to 12 per 1000 live births). When one child is affected, the risk of recurrence in siblings is increased to about 3% (see Appendix, Table A.1).
   b. However, the risk of recurrence is related to the incidence of particular defects: lesions with high prevalence (e.g., VSD) tend to have a high risk of recurrence, and those with low prevalence (e.g., tricuspid atresia, persistent truncus arteriosus) have a low risk of recurrence (see Appendix, Table A.1).
   c. The probability of recurrence is substantially higher when the mother, rather than the father, is the affected parent (see Appendix, Table A.2). Tables A.1 and A.2 can be used for counseling.

II. PHYSICAL EXAMINATION

A. INSPECTION

1. General appearance. Happy or cranky, nutritional state, respiratory status such as tachypnea, dyspnea, or retraction (they may be signs of serious CHD), pallor (seen with vasoconstriction from CHF or circulatory shock, or severe anemia), and sweat on the forehead (seen in CHF).
2. Inspection for any known syndromes or conditions (see Table 1.1).
3. Malformations of other systems may be associated with varying frequency of CHD (see Table 1.2).
4. Acanthosis nigricans (a dark pigmentation of skin crease on the neck and/or axillae) is often seen in obese children and those with type 2 diabetes and may signify the presence of hyperinsulinemia.
5. Precordial bulge, with or without actively visible cardiac activity, suggests chronic cardiac enlargement. Pectus excavatum may be a cause of a heart murmur. Pectus carinatum is usually not a result of cardiomegaly.
6. Cyanosis usually signals a serious CHD. A long-standing arterial desaturation (usually more than 6 months), even of a subclinical degree, results in clubbing of the fingers and toes.

TABLE 1.1

MAJOR SYNDROMES ASSOCIATED WITH CARDIOVASCULAR ABNORMALITIES

DISORDERS	CV ABNORMALITIES: FREQUENCY AND TYPES	MAJOR FEATURES	ETIOLOGY
22q11.2 deletion syndrome (overlaps with and includes DiGeorge syndrome and velocardiofacial syndrome)	Frequent (74%); TOF (20%), VSD (14%), interrupted aortic arch (13%), truncus arteriosus (6%), vascular ring (6%), ASD (4%), others (10%).	Wide ranges of abnormalities of multiple organ systems, with each person having different manifestations; characteristic facies ("elfin facies," ptosis, hypertelorism, auricular abnormalities), cleft lip and other palatal abnormalities (69%), feeding problems, learning difficulties (90%), congenital heart defects (74%), hypocalcemia (50%), renal anomalies (31%), autoimmune disorders (77%), hearing loss, laryngoesophageal anomalies, growth hormone deficiency, seizures, autism (20%), psychiatric disorders (25% of adults), behavioral problems, and others	Most cases new mutations; otherwise AD; Microdeletion of 22q11.2
Alagille syndrome (arteriohepatic dysplasia)	Frequent (85%); peripheral PA stenosis with or without complex CV abnormalities.	Peculiar facies (95%) consisting of deep-set eyes; broad forehead; long straight nose with flattened tip; prominent chin; and small, low-set malformed ears Paucity of intrahepatic interlobular bile duct with chronic cholestasis (91%), hypercholesterolemia, butterfly-like vertebral arch defects (87%) Growth retardation (50%) and mild mental retardation (16%)	AD 30%-50%; rest: new mutations; Mostly mutations in 20p12.2 (±)
CHARGE association	Common (65%); TOF, truncus arteriosus, aortic arch anomalies (e.g., vascular ring, interrupted aortic arch)	*C*oloboma, *h*eart defects, choanal *a*tresia, growth or mental *r*etardation, *g*enitourinary anomalies, *e*ar anomalies, genital hypoplasia	Most cases new mutations; 8q12.2
Carpenter syndrome	Frequent (50%); PDA, VSD, PS, TGA	Brachycephaly with variable craniosynostosis, mild facial hypoplasia, polydactyly, and severe syndactyly ("mitten hands")	AR; 6p12.1-p11.2 19q13.2

TABLE 1.1 *(continued)*

MAJOR SYNDROMES ASSOCIATED WITH CARDIOVASCULAR ABNORMALITIES

DISORDERS	CV ABNORMALITIES: FREQUENCY AND TYPES	MAJOR FEATURES	ETIOLOGY
Cockayne syndrome	Accelerated atherosclerosis	Senile-like changes beginning in infancy, dwarfing, microcephaly, prominent nose and sunken eyes, visual loss (retinal degeneration) and hearing loss	AR; 10q11.23 5q12.1
Cornelia de Lange (de Lange's) syndrome	Occasional (30%); VSD	Synophrys and hirsutism, prenatal growth retardation, microcephaly, anteverted nares, downturned mouth, mental retardation	AD; Mutation in 5p13.2 (>50%)
Cri du chat syndrome (deletion 5p syndrome)	Occasional (25%); variable CHD (VSD, PDA, ASD)	Cat-like cry in infancy, microcephaly, downward slant of palpebral fissures	Partial deletion, short arm of chromosome 5
Crouzon disease (craniofacial dysostosis)	Occasional; PDA, COA	Ptosis with shallow orbits, premature craniosynostosis, maxillary hypoplasia	AD; Mutation in 10q26.13
DiGeorge syndrome (part of 22q11.2 deletion syndrome)	Frequent; interrupted aortic arch, truncus arteriosus, VSD, PDA, TOF	Acronymically known as CATCH 22 syndrome: *C*ardiac defects, *A*bnormal facies (hypertelorism, short philtrum, cleft palate, downslanting eye), *T*hymic hypoplasia, *C*left palate, and *H*ypocalcaemia resulting from 22q11 deletions	AD; Microdeletion of 22q11.2
Down syndrome (trisomy 21)	Frequent (40%-50%); ECD, VSD	Hypotonic, flat facies, slanted palpebral fissure, small eyes, mental deficiency, simian crease	Trisomy 21
Ehlers-Danlos syndrome (vascular Ehlers-Danlos syndrome [type 4])	Frequent; ASD, aneurysm of aorta and carotids, intracranial aneurysm, MVP	Hyperextensive joints, hyperelasticity, fragility and bruisability of skin, poor wound healing with thin scar	AD; Mutation in 2q32.2

TABLE 1.1 *(continued)*

MAJOR SYNDROMES ASSOCIATED WITH CARDIOVASCULAR ABNORMALITIES

DISORDERS	CV ABNORMALITIES: FREQUENCY AND TYPES	MAJOR FEATURES	ETIOLOGY
Ellis-van Creveld syndrome (chondroectodermal dysplasia)	Frequent (50%); ASD, single atrium	Short stature of prenatal onset, short distal extremities, narrow thorax with short ribs, polydactyly, nail hypoplasia, neonatal teeth	AR; Mutation in 4p16.2
Fetal alcohol syndrome	Occasional (25%-30%); VSD, PDA, ASD, TOF	Prenatal growth retardation, microcephaly, short palpebral fissure, mental deficiency, irritable infant or hyperactive child	Ethanol or its by-products
Fetal trimethadione syndrome	Occasional (15%-30%); TGA, VSD, TOF	Ear malformation, hypoplastic midface, unusual eyebrow configuration, mental deficiency, speech disorder	Exposure to trimethadione
Fetal warfarin syndrome	Occasional (15%-45%); TOF, VSD	Facial asymmetry and hypoplasia; hypoplasia or aplasia of the pinna with blind or absent external ear canal (microtia); ear tags; cleft lip or palate; epitubular dermoid; hypoplastic vertebrae	Exposure to warfarin
Friedreich ataxia	Frequent; hypertrophic cardiomyopathy progressing to heart failure	Late-onset ataxia, skeletal deformities	AR; Mutation in 9q21.11
Goldenhar syndrome (craniofacial macrosomia)	Frequent (35%); VSD, TOF	Facial asymmetry and hypoplasia, microtia, ear tag, cleft lip or palate, hypoplastic vertebrae	Usually sporadic
Glycogen storage disease II (Pompe disease)	Very common; cardiomyopathy	Large tongue and flabby muscles, cardiomegaly; LVH and short PR interval on ECG, severe ventricular hypertrophy on echocardiogram; normal FBS and GTT	AR; Mutation in 17q25.3

TABLE 1.1 *(continued)*

MAJOR SYNDROMES ASSOCIATED WITH CARDIOVASCULAR ABNORMALITIES

DISORDERS	CV ABNORMALITIES: FREQUENCY AND TYPES	MAJOR FEATURES	ETIOLOGY
Holt-Oram syndrome (cardio-limb syndrome)	Frequent; ASD, VSD	Defects or absence of thumb or radius	AD; Mutations in 12q24.21
Homocystinuria	Frequent; medial degeneration of aorta and carotids, atrial or venous thrombosis	Subluxation of lens (usually by 10 yr), malar flush, osteoporosis, arachnodactyly, pectus excavatum or carinatum, mental defect	AR; Mostly mutation in 21q22.3
Infant of diabetic mother	CHDs (3%-5%); TGA, VSD, COA; cardiomyopathy (10%-20%); PPHN	Macrosomia, hypoglycemia and hypocalcemia, polycythemia, hyperbilirubinemia, other congenital anomalies	Fetal exposure to high glucose levels
Kartagener syndrome (primary ciliary dyskinesia)	Dextrocardia (12%)	Situs inversus, chronic sinusitis and otitis media, bronchiectasis, abnormal respiratory cilia, immotile sperm	AR; Different genes
LEOPARD syndrome (Noonan syndrome with multiple lentigines)	Very common; PS, HOCM, long PR interval on ECG	*L*entiginous skin lesion, *E*CG abnormalities, *o*cular hypertelorism, *p*ulmonary stenosis, *a*bnormal genitalia, *r*etarded growth, *d*eafness	AD; 85% mutation in 12q24.13
Long QT syndrome: Jervell and Lange-Nielsen syndrome (1) Romano-Ward syndrome (2)	Very common; long QT interval on ECG, ventricular tachyarrhythmia	Congenital deafness (not in Romano-Ward syndrome), syncope resulting from ventricular arrhythmias, family history of sudden death (±)	Multiple mutations; AR (1) AD (2)
Marfan syndrome	Frequent; aortic aneurysm, aortic and/or mitral regurgitation; MVP	Arachnodactyly with hyperextensibility, subluxation of lens; pectus deformity, myopia	AD; Mutation in 15q21.1

TABLE 1.1 *(continued)*

MAJOR SYNDROMES ASSOCIATED WITH CARDIOVASCULAR ABNORMALITIES

DISORDERS	CV ABNORMALITIES: FREQUENCY AND TYPES	MAJOR FEATURES	ETIOLOGY
Mucopolysaccharidosis Hurler syndrome (type I) Hunter syndrome (type II) Morquio syndrome (type IV); types A & B	Frequent; aortic and/or mitral regurgitation, coronary artery disease	Coarse features, large tongue, depressed nasal bridge, kyphosis, retarded growth, hepatomegaly, corneal opacity (not in Hunter syndrome), mental retardation; most patients die by 10 to 20 years of age	AR (I) 4p16.3 XR (II) Xq28 AR (IV) 16q24.3 (A) 3p22.3 (B)
Muscular dystrophy (Duchenne type)	Frequent; cardiomyopathy, PVC	Waddling gait, "pseudohypertrophy" of calf muscle	XR; Xp21.2-p21.1
Neurofibromatosis (von Recklinghausen disease; NF type 1)	Occasional; PS, COA, pheochromocytoma	Café-au-lait spots, multiple neurofibroma, acoustic neuroma (type 2), variety of bone lesions	AD; 30%-50% new mutations 17q11.2
Noonan syndrome (Turner-like syndrome)	Frequent; PS (dystrophic pulmonary valve), LVH (or anterior septal hypertrophy)	Similar to Turner syndrome but may occur both in males and females, without chromosomal abnormality	Usually sporadic; AD; 12q24.13 (~50%)
Pierre Robin sequence	Occasional; VSD, PDA; less commonly ASD, COA, TOF	Micrognathia, glossoptosis, cleft soft palate,	Usually sporadic
Osler-Rendu-Weber syndrome (hereditary hemorrhagic telangiectasia)	Occasional; pulmonary arteriovenous fistula	Hepatic involvement, telangiectases, hemangioma or fibrosis	AD
Osteogenesis imperfecta	Occasional; aortic dilatation, aortic regurgitation, MVP	Excessive bone fragility with deformities of skeleton, blue sclera, hyperlaxity of joints	AD or AR
Progeria (Hutchinson-Gilford syndrome)	Accelerated atherosclerosis	Alopecia, atrophy of subcutaneous fat, skeletal hypoplasia and dysplasia	AD; Mutations in 1q22

TABLE 1.1 *(continued)*

MAJOR SYNDROMES ASSOCIATED WITH CARDIOVASCULAR ABNORMALITIES

DISORDERS	CV ABNORMALITIES: FREQUENCY AND TYPES	MAJOR FEATURES	ETIOLOGY
Rubella syndrome	Frequent ($>$ 95%); PDA and PA stenosis	Triad of the syndrome: deafness, cataract, and CHDs; others include intrauterine growth retardation, microcephaly, microphthalmia, hepatitis, neonatal thrombocytopenic purpura	Maternal rubella infection during the first trimester
Rubinstein-Taybi syndrome	Occasional (25%); PDA, VSD, ASD	Broad thumbs or toes; hypoplastic maxilla with narrow palate; beaked nose; short stature; mental retardation,	Sporadic; 16p13.3 deletion
Smith-Lemli-Opitz syndrome	Occasional; VSD, PDA, others	Broad nasal tip with anteverted nostrils; ptosis of eyelids; syndactyly of 2nd and 3rd toes; short stature; mental retardation	AR; Mutations in 11q13.4
Thrombocytopenia-absent radius (TAR) syndrome	Occasional (30%); TOF, ASD, dextrocardia	Thrombocytopenia, absent or hypoplastic radius, normal thumb; "leukemoid" granulocytosis and eosinophilia	AR; Deletion of 1q21.1
Treacher Collins syndrome	Occasional; VSD, PDA, ASD	Underdeveloped lower jaw and zygomatic bone; defects of lower eyelids with downslanting palpebral fissure; malformation of auricle or ear canal defect; cleft palate	AD; 60% new mutation
Trisomy 13 syndrome (Patau syndrome)	Very common (80%); VSD, PDA, dextrocardia	Low birth weight, central facial anomalies, polydactyly, chronic hemangiomas, low-set ears, visceral and genital anomalies	Trisomy 13
Trisomy 18 syndrome (Edwards syndrome)	Very common (90%); VSD, PDA, PS	Low birth weight, microcephaly, micrognathia, rocker-bottom feet, closed fist with overlapping fingers	Trisomy 18

TABLE 1.1 *(continued)*

MAJOR SYNDROMES ASSOCIATED WITH CARDIOVASCULAR ABNORMALITIES

DISORDERS	CV ABNORMALITIES: FREQUENCY AND TYPES	MAJOR FEATURES	ETIOLOGY
Tuberous sclerosis	Frequent; rhabdomyoma	Triad of adenoma sebaceum (2–5 yr of age), seizures, and mental defect; cystlike lesions in phalanges and elsewhere; fibrous-angiomatosus lesions (83%) with varying colors in nasolabial fold, cheeks, and elsewhere.	AD; {2/3} of new mutations
Turner syndrome (XO syndrome)	Frequent (35%); COA, bicuspid aortic valve, AS; hypertension, aortic dissection later in life	Short female; broad chest with widely spaced nipples; congenital lymphedema with residual puffiness over the dorsum of fingers and toes (80%).	XO with 45 chromosomes
VATER association (VATER or VACTERL syndrome)	Common (> 50%); VSD, other defects	*V*ertebral anomalies, *a*nal atresia, *c*ongenital heart defects, *t*racheo*e*sophageal (TE) fistula, *r*enal dysplasia, *l*imb anomalies (e.g., radial dysplasia)	Sporadic
Velocardiofacial syndrome (Sprintzen syndrome) (part of 22q11.2 deletion syndrome)	Very common (85%); truncus arteriosus, TOF, pulmonary atresia with VSD, interrupted aortic arch (type B), VSD, and TGA	Structural or functional palatal abnormalities, unique facial characteristics ("elfin facies" with auricular abnormalities, prominent nose with squared nasal root and narrow alar base, vertical maxillary excess with long face), hypernasal speech, conductive hearing loss, hypotonia, developmental delay and learning disability	AD; Micro-deletion of 22q11.2

TABLE 1.1 *(continued)*

MAJOR SYNDROMES ASSOCIATED WITH CARDIOVASCULAR ABNORMALITIES

DISORDERS	CV ABNORMALITIES: FREQUENCY AND TYPES	MAJOR FEATURES	ETIOLOGY
Williams syndrome	Frequent; supravalvular AS, PA stenosis, renal artery stenosis	Varying degree of mental retardation, so-called elfin facies (consisting of some of the following: upturned nose, flat nasal bridge, long philtrum, flat malar area, wide mouth, full lips, widely spaced teeth, periorbital fullness); hypercalcemia of infancy?	Sporadic; 7q23 deletion
Zellweger syndrome (cerebrohepatorenal syndrome)	Frequent; PDA, VSD or ASD	Hypotonia, high forehead with flat facies, hepatomegaly, albuminemia	AR; Multiple genes

AD, *autosomal dominant;* AR, *autosomal recessive* XR, *sex-linked recessive;* ±, *may or may not be present. Other abbreviations are listed on pp. xi-xii.*

From Park, M. K., & Salamat, M. (2020). *Park's Pediatric cardiology for practitioners* (7th ed.) Philadelphia: Mosby.)

TABLE 1.2

INCIDENCE OF ASSOCIATED CHDS IN PATIENTS WITH OTHER SYSTEMS' MALFORMATIONS

ORGAN SYSTEM AND MALFORMATION	FREQUENCY (%)	SPECIFIC CARDIAC DEFECT
CENTRAL NERVOUS SYSTEM		
Hydrocephalus	6	VSD, ECD, TOF
Dandy-Walker syndrome	3	VSD
Agenesis of corpus callosum	15	No specific defect
Meckel-Gruber syndrome	14	No specific defect
THORACIC CAVITY		
TE fistula, esophageal atresia	21	VSD, ASD, TOF
Diaphragmatic hernia	11	No specific defect
GASTROINTESTINAL SYSTEM		
Duodenal atresia	17	No specific defect
Jejunal atresia	5	No specific defect
Anorectal anomalies	22	No specific defect
Imperforate anus	12	TOF, VSD
VENTRAL WALL		
Omphalocele	21	No specific defect
Gastroschisis	3	No specific defect
GENITOURINARY SYSTEM		
Renal agenesis		
Bilateral	43	No specific defect
Unilateral	17	No specific defect
Horseshoe kidney	39	No specific defect
Renal dysplasia	5	No specific defect

ECD, *endocardial cushion defect;* TE, *tracheoesophageal. Other abbreviations are listed on pp. xi-xii.*

Adapted from Copel, J. A., & Kleinman, C. S. (1986). Congenital heart disease and extracardiac anomalies: Association and indications for fetal echocardiography. *American Journal of Obstetrics and Gynecology*, 154, 1121–1132.

B. PALPATION

1. Precordium
   a. A hyperactive precordium is characteristic of heart diseases with high volume overload, such as L-R shunt lesions or severe valvular regurgitation.

b. A thrill is often of real diagnostic value. The location of the thrill suggests certain cardiac anomalies: upper left sternal border (ULSB), PS; upper right sternal border (URSB), AS; lower left sternal border (LLSB), VSD; suprasternal notch, AS, occasionally PS, PDA, or COA; over the carotid arteries, AS or COA.

2. Peripheral pulses
   a. Check the peripheral pulse for the rate, irregularities (arrhythmias), and volume (bounding, full, or thready).
   b. Strong arm pulses and weak leg pulses or pulse delay suggest COA.
   c. The right brachial artery pulse stronger than the left brachial artery pulse may suggest COA or supravalvular AS.
   d. Bounding pulses are found in aortic runoff lesions (e.g., PDA, AR, large systemic AV fistula).
   e. Weak and thready pulses are found in CHF and circulatory shock.

C. BLOOD PRESSURE

Every child should have blood pressure (BP) measurement as part of the physical examination whenever possible. To determine if obtained BP readings of a child is normal or abnormal, BP readings are compared with reliable BP standards. Unfortunately, there have been multiple problems and confusion regarding the correct method of measuring BP and the reliable normative BP standards for children. Scientifically unsound arm length–based BP cuff selection methods recommended by two earlier NIH Task Forces (1977 and 1987) have dominated the fields and they have been the source of confusion for decades, contributing to the lack of reliable normative BP standards for children. Although the Working Group of the National High Blood Pressure Education Program (NHBPEP) has recently corrected the BP cuff selection method, the majority of their BP data source includes earlier studies using the wrong BP cuff selection method, which resulted in their scientifically and logically unsound BP standards for children (see the following text).

1. The following are currently recommended BP measurement techniques.
   a. The width of the BP cuff should be 40% of the circumference of the arm (or leg) with the cuff long enough to completely or nearly completely encircle the extremity. When a 40% cuff is not available, it is better to choose one size bigger (not smaller) than the ideal one.
   b. The NHBPEP recommends Korotkoff phase 5 (K5) as the diastolic pressure but this is debatable. Earlier studies indicate that K4 agrees better with true diastolic pressure for children ≤ 12 years.
   c. Averaging of two or more readings should be obtained.
   d. The child should be in sitting position with the arm at the heart level.
2. BP Standards Recommended by the NHBPEP

   The normative BP standards recommended by the Working Group are not as good as it was made to believe. Readers should be aware of a few major flaws in the NHBPEP's normative values.
   a. First, BP data presented in the NHBPEP standards are not obtained by using the same methodology as the program has recommended.

The majority of the studies included in their data analysis were conducted using the arm length–based cuff selection method, which has been abandoned because of its unscientific nature. These values are also from single measurement, rather than the averages of multiple readings, as currently recommended. They also are not from a nationally representative population.

b. Expressing children's BP levels by age and height percentiles is statistically and logically unsound. Height has no statistically important role in children's BP levels.
   (1) Partial correlation analysis done in the San Antonio Children's Blood Pressure Study (SACBPS) shows that, when auscultatory BP levels were adjusted for age and weight, the correlation coefficient of systolic BP with height was very small ($r = 0.068$ for boys; $r = 0.072$ for girls), whereas when adjusted for age and height, the correlation of systolic pressure with weight remained high ($r = 0.343$ for boys; $r = 0.294$ for girls). These findings indicate that the contribution of height to BP levels is negligible. The apparent correlation of height to BP levels may be secondary to a close correlation that exists between height and weight ($r = 0.86$).
   (2) A similar conclusion was reached with oscillometric BP levels in the same study. Thus we have recommend children's BP value be expressed as a function of age only, as has been done earlier by National Institutes of Health (NIH) Task Forces.
c. Recommending additional computations and using scientifically unsound complex BP tables on such highly variable office BP readings is unreasonable and counterproductive. Analyzing unscientifically obtained data by additional computation does not improve the worth of the data.
d. The NHBPEP does not point out that the auscultatory and oscillometric BP readings are not interchangeable. SACBPS, in which both auscultatory and oscillometric methods were used, found that oscillometric systolic pressures are significantly higher than auscultatory BP readings (see following text for further details).
e. The NHBPEP does not emphasize the important contribution of the "white coat phenomenon" in office BP readings. White coat phenomenon is probably the most common cause of high BP readings in pediatric practice.

3. Reliable normative BP standards. Which normal BP standards should be used and why?
   a. The NIH Task Force BP standards (of 1987) are no longer acceptable because they were obtained by using the arm length–based BP cuff selection method.
   b. The BP standards of the NHBPEP are riddled with major flaws as outlined in the preceding section. These standards reflect violation of basic scientific principles. Although not acceptable as reliable

pediatric BP standards, the NHBPEP's normative values are presented in Appendix B for the sake of completeness (Tables B.1 and B.2, Appendix B).

c. Normative BP percentile values from the SACBPS are recommended as better BP standards than the NHBPEP standards until nationwide data using the currently recommended methods become available. These are the only available BP standards that have been obtained according to the currently recommended method. In the SACBPS, BP levels were obtained in more than 7000 tri-ethnic (white, Hispanic, and African American) school children enrolled in kindergarten through the 12th grade in the San Antonio, Texas, area. Both the auscultatory and oscillometric (model Dinamap 8100) methods were used in the study. The data are the averages of three readings. Auscultatory BP data were expressed according to age and gender. These BP standards are normally distributed from the mean value, and thus the effect of obesity is not a problem in using the standards (Figs. 1.1 and 1.2). Percentile BP values for these figures are presented in Appendix B (Tables B.3 and B.4).
d. When BP is measured using an oscillometric device, one should use a device-specific normative BP standards. SACBPS found that the readings by auscultatory method and by Dinamap 8100 are significantly different and thus are not interchangeable. Percentile BP values by an oscillometric method (Dinamap model 8100) are presented in Appendix B (Tables B.5 and B.6).

4. Accuracy of oscillometric BP values.
   a. The accuracy of indirect BP measurement by an oscillometric method (Dinamap model 1846) has been demonstrated. One caution is that not all oscillometric devices in clinical use have been validated for their accuracy. Accuracy of oscillometric BP does not mean that BPs obtained by the oscillometric method should agree with those obtained by the auscultatory method. Auscultatory BP method is another indirect BP measurement method using a different detection device; only direct intraarterial BP measurement is the gold standard.
   b. SACBPS found that BP levels obtained by the Dinamap (model 8100) were on the average 10 mm Hg higher than the auscultatory method for the systolic pressure and 5 mm Hg higher for the diastolic pressure. Therefore the auscultatory and the Dinamap BPs are not interchangeable. This does not mean, however, that the oscillometric BP methods are less reliable than the auscultatory method.
   c. Therefore oscillometric specific normative BP standards are needed. One should not use normative auscultatory BP standards when an oscillometric method is used. Dinamap 8100–specific BP standards are presented in Appendix B (see Tables B.5 and B.6).

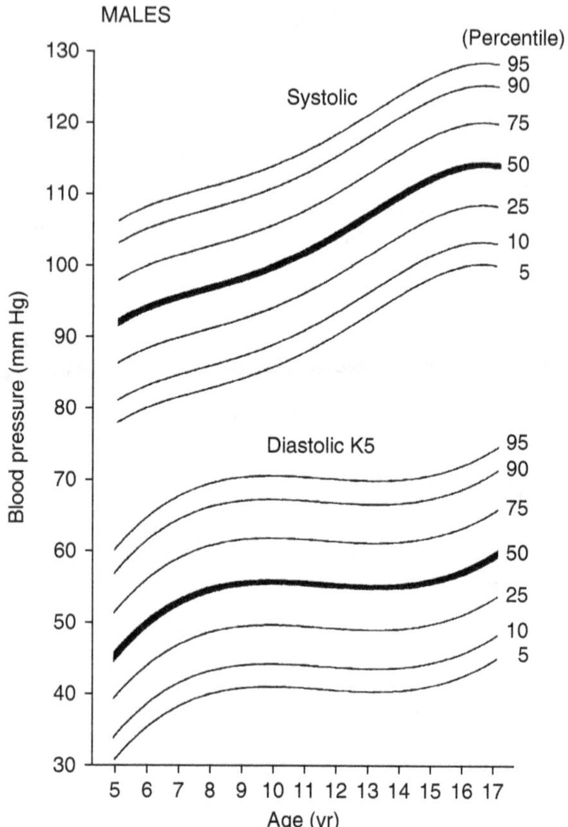

FIG. 1.1

Age-specific percentile curves of auscultatory systolic and diastolic (K5) pressures in boys 5 to 17 years of age. BP values are the averages of three readings. The width of the BP cuff was 40% to 50% of the circumference of the arm. *(From Park, M.K., Menard, S.W., & Yuan C. (2001). Comparison of blood pressure in children from three ethnic groups.* American Journal of Cardiology, *87, 1305–1308.)*

d. The oscillometric method also provides some advantages over the auscultation method.
   (1) It eliminates observer-related variations.
   (2) It can be successfully used in infants and small children. Auscultatory BP measurement in small infants is not only difficult to obtain but is also inaccurate.

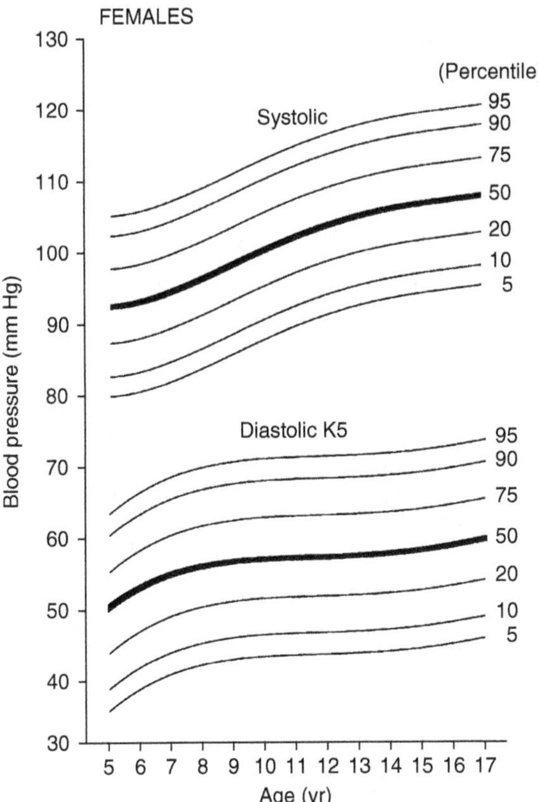

FIG. 1.2

Age-specific percentile curves of auscultatory systolic and diastolic (K5) pressures in girls 5 to 17 years of age. BP values are the averages of three readings. The width of the BP cuff was 40% to 50% of the circumference of the arm. *(From Park, M.K., Menard, S. W., & Yuan, C. (2001). Comparison of blood pressure in children from three ethnic groups.* American Journal of Cardiology, *87, 1305–1308.)*

(3) Percentile values of normative oscillometric BPs in neonates and children up to 5 years of age are presented in Appendix B (Table B.7).

5. Comparison of arm and leg BP values.

Four-extremity BP measurements are often obtained in neonates and children to rule out COA.

a. Even with a considerably wider cuff used for the thigh, the Dinamap systolic pressure in the thigh or calf is about 5 to 10 mm Hg higher than that in the arm. This reflects in part the phenomenon of peripheral amplification of systolic pressure (see following text). If the systolic pressure is lower in the leg, COA may be present.
b. In the newborn, the systolic pressures in the arm and the calf are the same.

6. BP levels in neonates and small children.
   a. BP measurement is important in newborns and small children to diagnose COA, hypertension, or hypotension. In contrast to the recommendations of the NHBEP, the auscultatory method is difficult to apply in newborns and small children because of weak Korotkoff sounds in these age groups, and thus normative auscultatory BP standards are not reliable. Therefore the oscillometric method is frequently used instead. The same BP cuff selection method as used in older children applies to this age group (i.e., the cuff width 40% [up to 50%] of the circumference of the extremity).
   b. Abbreviated normative Dinamap BP standards for newborns and small children (≤5 years) are presented in Table 1.3. Full percentile values are presented in Appendix B (see Table B.7).
7. The important concept of peripheral amplification of systolic pressure.
   Many physicians incorrectly think that peripherally measured BP, such as those measured in the arm, are the same as the central aortic pressure (or the left ventricular pressure). The systolic pressure measured at a peripheral site, by either direct or indirect method, is usually not the same as the central aortic pressure. In fact, arm systolic pressures are in general higher than central aortic pressures and are much higher in certain situations. This phenomenon is called peripheral amplification of systolic pressure (see Fig. 1.3). The systolic amplification increases as the site of BP measurement moves distally. The following list summarizes key points of this important phenomenon.

TABLE 1.3

NORMATIVE BLOOD PRESSURE LEVELS (SYSTOLIC/DIASTOLIC [MEAN] IN MM HG) BY DINAMAP MONITOR (MODEL 1846 SX) IN CHILDREN UP TO AGE 5 YEARS

AGE	MEAN BP LEVELS	90TH PERCENTILE	95TH PERCENTILE
1–3 days	64/41 (50)	75/49 (59)	78/52 (62)
1 mo-2 yr	95/58 (72)	106/68 (83)	110/71 (86)
2–5 yr	101/57 (74)	112/66 (82)	115/68 (85)

Adapted from Park, M. K., & Menard, S. M. (1989). Normative oscillometric blood pressure values in the first five years in an office setting. *American Journal of Diseases of Children, 143,* 860–864.

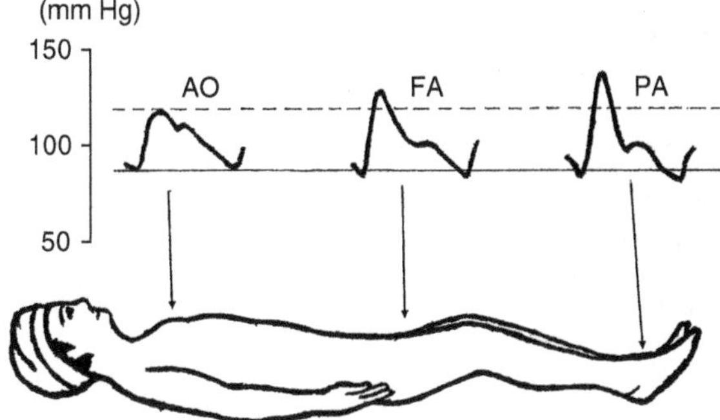

FIG. 1.3
Schematic drawing of pulse wave changes seen at different levels of the systemic arteries. *(From Park, M. K., & Salamat, M. (2020).* Park's pediatric cardiology for practitioners *(7th ed.). Philadelphia: Mosby.)*

a. The amplification is limited to the systolic pressure (not in the diastolic and mean pressures).
b. The systolic amplification is greater in children (with more reactive arteries) than in older adults who may have degenerative arterial disease.
c. Pedal artery systolic pressures are higher than the radial artery pressures.
d. The amplification is more marked in vasoconstricted states.
    (1) Patients in impending circulatory shock (with a high level of circulating catecholamines) may show normal peripheral artery systolic pressure when the central aortic pressure is abnormally low. Early diagnosis of an impending circulatory shock can be missed if one pays attention only to the systolic pressure; monitoring the mean arterial and diastolic pressures should be more useful in this situation.
    (2) Subjects receiving catecholamine infusion or other vasoconstrictors may show much higher peripheral systolic pressure than the central aortic pressure.
    (3) A child in congestive heart failure (in which peripheral vasoconstriction exists) may exhibit an exaggerated systolic amplification.
    (4) Arm systolic pressure in subjects running on treadmills can be markedly higher than the central aortic pressure (see Fig. 5.1).
e. Reduced level of peripheral amplification of systolic pressure is noted in vasodilated states (such as in subjects receiving vasodilators).

8. Need for simplified BP tables

The main reason for measuring BP routinely is to identify those children with hypertension or those at risk of developing hypertension. Even though the BP standards from the San Antonio Study are simple enough to use, it is still time-consuming to check the complete table in a busy practice. In 2009, Kaelber and Picket proposed a simple table of BP levels, without height percentiles, that may require attention or additional investigation being at "elevated blood pressure levels (formerly called prehypertensive levels). Elevated blood pressure is defined as BP levels between the 90th and 95th percentiles for children and 120 to 129 systolic and 80 mm Hg diastolic for adolescent (> 13 years) and adults. We followed suit and developed similar tables of the 90th percentile values for both auscultatory and oscillometric BP for children based on the San Antonio Study (Table 1.4).

TABLE 1.4

THE 90TH PERCENTILES OF BLOOD PRESSURE BY AUSCULTATORY AND OSCILLOMETRIC METHODS FROM THE SAN ANTONIO STUDY

AUSCULTATORY					OSCILLOMETRIC				
AGE (YR)	MALE		FEMALE		AGE (YR)	MALE		FEMALE	
	SP	DP	SP	DP		SP	DP	SP	DP
5	103	60	102	60	5	115	68	114	68
6	105	64	103	63	6	117	68	115	68
7	107	66	104	65	7	118	69	116	69
8	108	68	106	67	8	119	70	118	70
9	109	68	108	67	9	121	70	119	70
10	111	68	110	68	10	122	71	121	71
11	113	68	112	68	11	124	71	122	71
12	116	68	113	68	12	126	71	123	71
13	118	68	115	68	13	129	71	125	71
14	120	68	116	68	14	131	72	125	72
15	120	69	117	69	15	133	72	126	72
16	120	71	117	69	16	134	72	126	72
17	120	73	118	70	17	134	72	126	72
≥18	120	73	120	70					

SP, systolic pressure; DP, diastolic pressure. The 90th percentile of systolic pressure for males ≥ 14 years is higher than 120 mm Hg in the San Antonio study, but 120 is listed to be consistent with the definition of elevated blood pressure in the adult.

Values are from Park, M. K., Menard, S. W., & Yuan, C. (2001). Comparison of blood pressure in children from three ethnic groups. *American Journal of Cardiolology, 87*, 1305–1308.

D. AUSCULTATION

Systematic attention should be given to heart rate and regularity; intensity and quality of the heart sounds, especially the second heart sound; systolic and diastolic sounds (ejection click, midsystolic click, opening snap); and heart murmurs.

1. Heart sounds
   a. The first heart sound (S1) is associated with closure of the mitral and tricuspid valves and is best heard at the apex or LLSB. Splitting of the S_1 is uncommon in normal children. Wide splitting of the S1 may be found in RBBB or Ebstein anomaly.
   b. The second heart sound (S2), which is produced by the closure of the aortic and pulmonary valves, is evaluated in the ULSB (or the pulmonary area) in terms of the degree of splitting and the relative intensity of the P2 (the pulmonary closure sound) in relation to the intensity of the A2 (the aortic closure sound). Although best heard with a diaphragm, both components are readily audible with the bell as well.
      (1) The degree of splitting of the S_2 normally varies with respiration, increasing with inspiration and decreasing or becoming single with expiration (Fig. 1.4).
      (2) Abnormal S2 may take the form of wide splitting, narrow splitting, single S2, abnormal intensity of the P2, or rarely, paradoxical splitting of the S2 (see Box 1.1 for summary of abnormal S2).
   c. The third heart sound (S3) is best heard at the apex or LLSB (Fig. 1.5). It is commonly heard in normal children, young adults, and patients with dilated ventricles and decreased compliance of the ventricles (e.g., large shunt VSD, CHF).

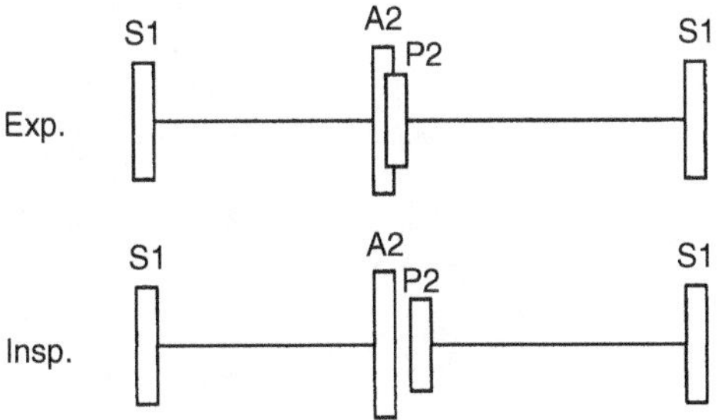

FIG. 1.4

Relative intensity of the A2 and P2 and the respiratory variation in the degree of splitting of the S2 at the ULSB (pulmonary area). *(From Park, M. K., & Salamat, M. (2020).* Park's pediatric cardiology for practitioners *(7th ed.) Philadelphia: Mosby.)*

BOX 1.1

SUMMARY OF ABNORMAL S2

ABNORMAL SPLITTING

1. Widely split and fixed S2
   a. Volume overload (e.g., ASD, PAPVR)
   b. Pressure overload (e.g., PS)
   c. Electrical delay (e.g., RBBB)
   d. Early aortic closure (e.g., MR)
   e. Occasional normal child
2. Narrowly split S2
   a. Pulmonary hypertension
   b. AS
   c. Occasional normal child
3. Single S2
   a. Pulmonary hypertension
   b. One semilunar valve (e.g., pulmonary atresia, aortic atresia, persistent truncus arteriosus)
   c. P2 not audible (e.g., TGA, TOF, severe PS)
   d. Severe AS
   e. Occasional normal child
4. Paradoxically split S2
   a. Severe AS
   b. LBBB, WPW syndrome (type B)

ABNORMAL INTENSITY OF P2

1. Increased P2 (e.g., pulmonary hypertension)
2. Decreased P2 (e.g., severe PS, TOF, TS)

See abbreviations listed on pp xi-xii.

   d. The fourth heart sound (S4) at the apex, which is always pathologic (Fig. 1.5), is audible in conditions with decreased ventricular compliance or CHF.
   e. Gallop rhythm generally implies pathology and results from the combination of a loud S3 or S4 and tachycardia. It is common in CHF.
2. Systolic and diastolic sounds
   a. An ejection click sounds like splitting of the S_1 but is best audible at the base rather than at the LLSB (Fig. 1.5). The ejection click is associated with stenosis of the semilunar valves (e.g., PS at 2 to 3 LICS, AS at 2 RICS or apex) and enlarged great arteries (e.g., systemic hypertension, pulmonary hypertension, and TOF).
   b. A midsystolic click with or without a late systolic murmur is heard near the apex in patients with MVP (Fig. 1.5).

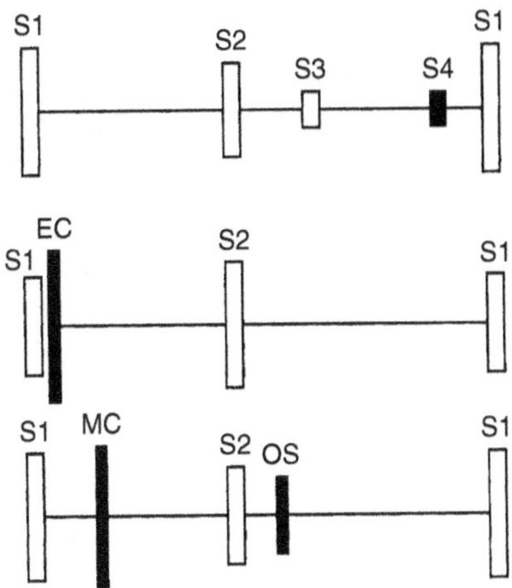

FIG. 1.5
Relative position of the heart sounds, ejection click (*EC*), midsystolic click (*MC*), and diastolic opening snap (*OS*). Filled bars show abnormal sounds. *(From Park, M. K., & Salamat, M. (2020).* Park's pediatric cardiology for practitioners *(7th ed.) Philadelphia: Mosby.)*

   c. Diastolic opening snap is audible at the apex or LLSB in mitral stenosis (MS) (Fig. 1.5).

3. Heart murmurs. Each heart murmur should be analyzed in terms of intensity, timing (systolic or diastolic), location, transmission, and quality (e.g., musical, vibratory, blowing).
   a. Intensity of the murmur is customarily graded from 1 to 6.
      (1) Grade 1, barely audible.
      (2) Grade 2, soft but easily audible.
      (3) Grade 3, moderately loud but not accompanied by a thrill.
      (4) Grade 4, louder and associated with a thrill.
      (5) Grade 5, audible with the stethoscope barely on the chest.
      (6) Grade 6, audible with the stethoscope off the chest.
   b. Classification of heart murmurs. Heart murmurs are classified as systolic, diastolic, or continuous.
4. Systolic murmurs
   a. Classification of systolic murmurs. A systolic murmur occurs between S1 and S2. Systolic murmur was initially classified by Aubrey Leatham in 1958 into two types, ejection or regurgitant, depending on the timing of the onset, not the termination, of the murmur in relation to the S_1. Recently Joseph Perloff proposed a

new classification according to the time of *onset* and *termination* into 4 types: midsystolic (ejection), holosystolic, early systolic, and late systolic.

(1) Ejection systolic murmur (also called stenotic, diamond-shaped or Perloff's midsystolic) has an interval between S1 and the onset of the murmur and is crescendo-decrescendo. The murmur may be short or long (Fig. 1.6A). These murmurs are caused by flow of blood through stenotic or deformed semilunar valves or increased flow through normal semilunar valves and are therefore found at the base or over the midprecordium. These murmurs may be pathologic or innocent.

(2) Regurgitant systolic murmur begins with the S1 (no gap between the S_1 and the onset of the murmur) and usually lasts throughout systole (pansystolic or holosystolic) but may be decrescendo ending in middle or early systole (Fig. 1.6B). Perloff's holosystolic and early systolic murmurs are regurgitant murmurs. These murmurs are always pathologic and are associated with only three conditions: VSD, MR, and TR.

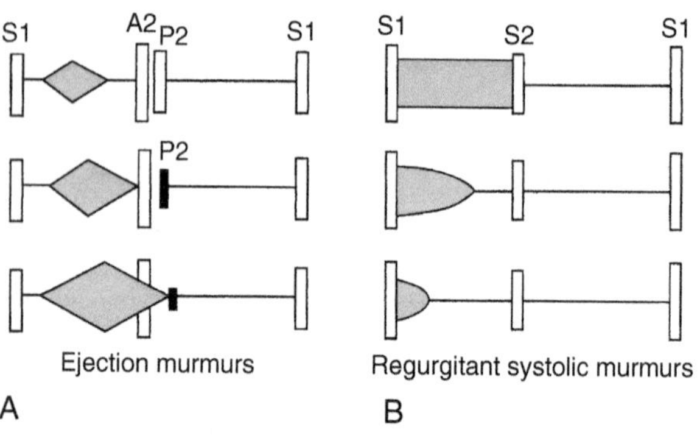

FIG. 1.6

Ejection and regurgitant systolic murmurs. (A) An ejection systolic murmur is audible in pulmonary valve stenosis (and other conditions). With mild stenosis, the apex of the diamond is in the early part of systole (*top*). With increasing severity of obstruction to flow, the murmur becomes louder and longer and its apex moves toward S2 (*middle*). In severe PS, the murmur may last beyond A2 and the P2 is sometimes too soft to be audible (*bottom*). (B) Regurgitant systolic murmur starts with S1. Most regurgitant systolic murmur in children is due to VSD and is holosystolic, extending all the way to S2 (*top*). In some children, especially those with small VSDs, and some neonates with VSD, the regurgitant systolic murmur may be decrescendo and ends in middle or early systole (not holosystolic) (*middle bottom*), but never crescendo-decrescendo.

(3) Late systolic murmur of Perloff is the hallmark of MVP (see Fig. 13.4).

b. Location. In addition to the type of murmur (ejection vs. regurgitant), the location of maximal intensity of the murmur is of great importance in determining the origin of the murmur. Fig. 1.7 illustrates systolic murmurs that are audible maximally at the various locations. Tables 1.5 through 1.8 summarize other clinical findings (e.g., physical examination, chest radiography, and ECG) that may aid diagnosis according to the location of a systolic murmur.

c. Transmission. A systolic ejection murmur at the base that transmits well to the neck is likely to be aortic, and one that transmits well to the sides of the chest and the back is likely to arise in the pulmonary valve or pulmonary artery.

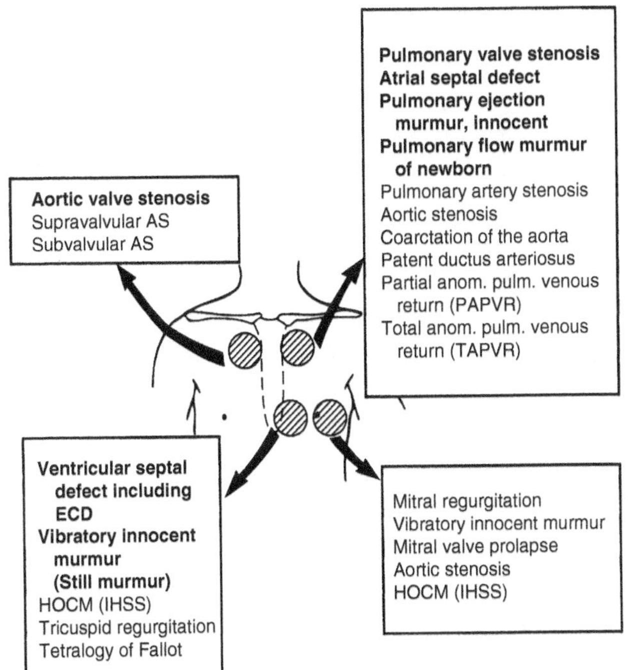

FIG. 1.7

Systolic murmurs audible at various locations. More common conditions are shown in boldface type (see also Tables 1.5 through 1.8). *(From Park, M. K., & Salamat, M. (2020).* Park's pediatric cardiology for practitioners *(7th ed.) Philadelphia: Mosby.)*

TABLE 1.5

DIFFERENTIAL DIAGNOSIS OF SYSTOLIC MURMURS AT THE UPPER LEFT STERNAL BORDER (PULMONARY AREA)

CONDITION	IMPORTANT PHYSICAL FINDINGS	ECG FINDINGS	CHEST RADIOGRAPHY FINGINGS
Pulmonary valve stenosis	SEM, grade 2-5/6 Thrill (±)[a] S2 may be split widely when mild Ejection click (±) at 2LICS[a] Transmit to the back	Normal if mild RAD RVH[a] RAH if severe	Prominent MPA (poststenotic dilatation)[a] Normal PVM
ASD	SEM, grade 2-3/6 Widely split and fixed S_2[a]	RAD RVH RBBB (rsR′ pattern)[a]	Increased PVM[a] RAE, RVE[a]
Pulmonary flow murmur of newborn	SEM, grade 1-2/6 in newborns No thrill Good transmission to the back and axillae[a]	Normal	Normal
Pulmonary flow murmur of older children	SEM, grade 2-3/6 No thrill Poor transmission	Normal	Normal Occasional pectus excavatum or straight back
Pulmonary artery stenosis (PA stenosis)	SEM, grade 2-3/6	RVH or Normal	Prominent hilar vessels (±)

TABLE 1.5 *(continued)*

DIFFERENTIAL DIAGNOSIS OF SYSTOLIC MURMURS AT THE UPPER LEFT STERNAL BORDER (PULMONARY AREA)

CONDITION	IMPORTANT PHYSICAL FINDINGS	ECG FINDINGS	CHEST RADIOGRAPHY FINGINGS
	Occasional continuous murmur in the back, if severe P2 may be loud Transmits well to the back and both lung fields[a]		
AS	SEM, grade 2-5/6 Also audible in 2RICS[a] Thrill (±) at 2RICS and/or SSN[a] Ejection click at apex, 3LICS, or 2RICS (±)[a] Paradoxically split S2 if severe	Normal or LVH	Dilated aorta
TOF	Long SEM, grade 2-4/6, louder at MLSB [a] Thrill (±) Loud, single S2 Cyanosis, clubbing (±)[a]	RAD RVH or BVH[a] RAH (±)	Decreased PVM[a] Normal heart size Boot-shaped heart [a] Right aortic arch (25%)
COA	SEM, grade 1-3/6 Loudest at left interscapular area (back)[a] Weak or absent femoral pulses[a]	LVH in children RBBB (or RVH) in infants	Classic "3" sign on plain film or "E" sign on barium esophagogram[a] Rib notching (±)

1

TABLE 1.5 *(continued)*

DIFFERENTIAL DIAGNOSIS OF SYSTOLIC MURMURS AT THE UPPER LEFT STERNAL BORDER (PULMONARY AREA)

CONDITION	IMPORTANT PHYSICAL FINDINGS	ECG FINDINGS	CHEST RADIOGRAPHY FINGINGS
	Hypertension in arms Frequent associated aortic stenosis, bicuspid aortic valve, or MR		
PDA	Continuous murmur at left infraclavicular area (grade 2-4/6)[a] Occasional crescendic systolic only Bonding pulses, if large [a] Thrill (±)	Normal, LVH, or BVH	Increased PVM[a] LAE, LVE[a]
TAPVR	SEM, grade 2-3/6 Widely split and fixed S2 (±) Quadruple or quintuple rhythm[a] Diastolic rumble at LLSB[a] Mild cyanosis (↓Po_2) and clubbing (±)[a]	RAD RAH *RVH	Increased PVM[a] RAE and RVE Prominent MPA "Snowman" sign
PAPVR	Physical findings similar to those of ASD S_2 not fixed unless associated with ASD	Same as in ASD	Increased PVM[a] RAE and RVE[a] "Scimitar" sign (±)

BVH, *biventricular hypertrophy;* 2LICS, *second left intercostal space;* 3LICS, *third left intercostal space;* LVE, *left ventricular enlargement;* 2RICS, *second right intercostal space;* SSN, *suprasternal notch;* ±, *may or may not be present. Other abbreviations are listed on pp. xi-xii.*

[a]Findings that are characteristic of the condition.

TABLE 1.6

DIFFERENTIAL DIAGNOSIS OF SYSTOLIC MURMURS AT THE UPPER RIGHT STERNAL BORDER (AORTIC AREA)

CONDITION	IMPORTANT PHYSICAL FINDINGS	ECG FINDINGS	CHEST RADIOGRAPHY FINDINGS
Aortic valve stenosis	SEM, grade 2–5/6, at 2RICS, may be louder at 3LICS Thrill (±)[a], URSB, SSN, and carotid arteries Ejection click[a] Transmits well to neck [a] S_2 may be single	Normal or LVH with or without "strain"	Mild LVE (±) Prominent ascending aorta or aortic knob
Subaortic stenosis	SEM, grade 2–4/6 AR murmur may be present in discrete stenosis[a] No ejection click	Normal or LVH	Usually normal
Supravalvular aortic stenosis	SEM, grade 2–3/6 Thrill (±) No ejection click Pulse and BP may be greater in right than left arm (Coanda effect)[a] Peculiar facies and mental deficiency (±) (in Williams syndrome)[a] Murmur may transmit well to the back (PA stenosis)	Normal, LVH or BVH	Unremarkable

BP, *blood pressure;* 3LICS, *third left intercostal space;* 2RICS, *second right intercostal space;* SSN, *suprasternal notch;* URSB, *upper right sternal border;* ± , *may or may not be present. Other abbreviations are listed on pp. xi-xii.*

[a]Findings characteristic and important in the diagnosis of the condition.

1

TABLE 1.7

DIFFERENTIAL DIAGNOSIS OF SYSTOLIC MURMURS AT THE LOWER LEFT STERNAL BORDER

CONDITION	IMPORTANT PHYSICAL FINDINGS	ECG FINDINGS	CHEST RADIOGRAPHY FINDINGS
VSD	Regurgitant systolic, grade 2–5/6[a] May not be holosystolic Well localized at LLSB Thrill often present[a] P2 may be loud	Normal, LVH, or BVH	Increased PVM[a] LAE and LVE (cardiomegaly)[a]
Complete ECD	Similar to findings of VSD Diastolic rumble at LLSB[a] Gallop rhythm common in infants (with CHF)[a]	Superior QRS axis[a] LVH or BVH	Similar to large VSD
Vibratory innocent murmur (Still's)	SEM, grade 2–3/6 Musical or vibratory with midsystolic accentuation[a] Maximum between LLSB and apex[a]	Normal	Normal
Hypertrophic obstructive cardiomyopathy (HOCM)	SEM, medium pitched, grade 2–4/6; murmur is louder when standing Maximum at LLSB or apex Thrill (±) Sharp upstroke of brachial pulses[a] May have murmur of MR	LVH Abnormally deep Q waves in leads V5 and V6	Normal or globular LVE

TABLE 1.7 *(continued)*

DIFFERENTIAL DIAGNOSIS OF SYSTOLIC MURMURS AT THE LOWER LEFT STERNAL BORDER

CONDITION	IMPORTANT PHYSICAL FINDINGS	ECG FINDINGS	CHEST RADIOGRAPHY FINDINGS
TR	Regurgitant systolic, grade 2–3/6[a] Triple or quadruple rhythm (in Ebstein's anomaly)[a] Mild cyanosis (±) Hepatomegaly with pulsatile liver and neck vein distention when severe	RBBB, RAH, and first-degree AV block and/or WPW in Ebstein's	Normal PVM RAE if severe
TOF	Murmurs can be louder at ULSB (Table 1.5)	(see Table 1.5)	(see Table1.5)

BVH, *biventricular hypertrophy;* P2, *pulmonary closure component of the second heart sound;* ± , *may or may not be present. Other abbreviations are listed on pp xi-xii.*

[a]Findings characteristic and important in the diagnosis of the condition.

1

TABLE 1.8

DIFFERENTIAL DIAGNOSIS OF SYSTOLIC MURMURS AT THE APEX

CONDITION	IMPORTANT PHYSICAL FINDINGS	ECG FINDINGS	CHEST RADIOGRAPHY FINDINGS
MR	Regurgitant systolic, may not be holosystolic, grade 2–3/6[a] Transmits to left axilla (less obvious in children) May be loudest in the midprecordium	LAH and LVH	LAE and LVE
MVP	Midsystolic click with or without late systolic murmur[a] High frequency of thoracic skeletal anomalies (pectus excavatum, straight back) (85%)[a]	Inverted T wave in lead aVF (±)	Normal
Aortic valve stenosis	The murmur and ejection click may be best heard at the apex rather than at 2RICS	Normal or LVH with or without "strain"	Mild LVE (±) Prominent ascending aorta or aortic knob
HOCM	The murmur of HOCM may be maximal at the apex (may represent MR)	LVH Abnormally deep Q waves in leads V_5 and V_6	Normal or globular LVE
Vibratory innocent murmur	This innocent heart murmur may be loudest at the apex (than at the left lower sternal border)	Normal	Normal

2RICS, *second right intercostal space;* ±, *may or may not be present. Other abbreviations are listed on pp xi-xii.*

[a]Findings characteristic and important in the diagnosis of the condition.

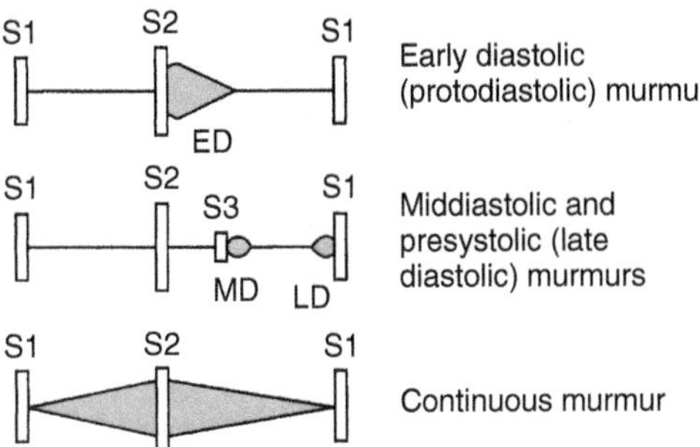

FIG. 1.8

Diastolic murmurs and the continuous murmur. *(From Park, M. K., & Salamat, M. (2020).* Park's pediatric cardiology for practitioners *(7th ed.). Philadelphia: Mosby.)*

   d. Quality. Ejection systolic murmurs of AS or PS have a rough, grating quality. A common innocent murmur in children (Still murmur) has a characteristic vibratory or humming quality.

5. Diastolic murmurs. Diastolic murmurs occur between S_2 and S_1. There are the following three types.
   a. Early diastolic (protodiastolic) decrescendo murmurs are caused by AR or PR (Fig. 1.8). AR murmurs are high pitched, are best heard at the 3 LICS, and radiate to the apex. PR murmurs are usually medium pitched but may be high pitched if pulmonary hypertension is present, best heard at the 2 LICS, and they radiate along the left sternal border.
   b. Middiastolic murmurs are low pitched, starting with a loud S3 (see Fig. 1.8). Best heard with the bell of the stethoscope, these murmurs are caused by anatomic (MS, TS) or relative stenosis of the mitral or tricuspid valve (VSD, ASD). MS murmurs are best heard at the apex (apical rumble), and TS murmurs are heard along the LLSB.
   c. Presystolic, or late diastolic, murmurs are low pitched and occur late in diastole or just before the onset of systole (see Fig. 1.8). They are found with anatomic stenosis of the mitral or tricuspid valve.
6. Continuous murmurs. Continuous murmurs begin in systole and continue without interruption through the S_2 into all or part of diastole (see Fig. 1.8). A combined systolic and diastolic murmur, such as from AS and AR or PS and PR, is called a to-and-fro murmur to distinguish it from a machinery-like continuous murmur. Continuous murmurs are caused by the following:

TABLE 1.9

COMMON INNOCENT HEART MURMURS IN INFANTS AND CHILDREN

TYPE (TIMING)	DESCRIPTION OF MURMUR	AGE GROUP
Classic vibratory murmur (Still's murmur) (systolic)	Maximal at MLSB or between LLSB and apex Grade 2–3/6 Low-frequency vibratory, "twanging string," groaning, squeaking, or musical	3–6 yr Occasionally in infancy
Pulmonary ejection murmur (systolic)	Maximal at ULSB Grade 1–3/6 in intensity, early to mid-systolic Blowing in quality	8–14 yr
Pulmonary flow murmur of newborn (systolic)	Maximal at ULSB Transmits well to the left and right chest, axilla, and back Grade 1–2/6 in intensity	Premature and full-term newborns Usually disappears by 3–6 mo of age
Venous hum (continuous)	Grade 1–3/6 continuous murmur, maximal at right (or left) supraclavicular and infraclavicular areas Inaudible in the supine position (typically heard only in the sitting position) Intensity changes with rotation of the head and compression of the jugular vein	3–6 yr
Carotid bruit (systolic)	Right supraclavicular area and over the carotids Grade 2–3/6 in intensity Occasional thrill over a carotid	Any age

LLSB, *lower left sternal border;* MLSB, *mid-left sternal border;* ULSB, *upper left sternal border*

a. Aortopulmonary or arteriovenous connection (e.g., PDA, arteriovenous [AV] fistula, after B-T shunt surgery, or, rarely, persistent truncus arteriosus).
b. Disturbances of flow patterns in veins (venous hum).
c. Disturbances of flow patterns in arteries (COA, peripheral PA stenosis).

7. Innocent murmurs. Over 80% of children have innocent murmurs of one type or other sometime during childhood, most commonly beginning at about 3 or 4 years of age. All innocent heart murmurs are accentuated or brought out in high-output states, most importantly with fever. Clinical characteristics of these murmurs are summarized in Table 1.9.
8. Pathologic murmurs. When one or more of the following are present, the murmur is likely to be pathologic and require cardiac consultation: (1) symptoms, (2) cyanosis, (3) abnormal chest radiography (heart size and/or silhouette and pulmonary vascularity), (4) abnormal ECG, (5) a systolic murmur that is loud (grade 3/6 or with a thrill) and long in duration, (6) a diastolic murmur, (7) abnormal heart sounds, and (8) abnormally strong or weak pulses.

Chapter 2

Electrocardiography

One normal cardiac cycle is represented by successive waveforms on an ECG tracing: the P wave, the QRS complex, and the T wave (Fig. 2.1A). These waves produce two important intervals, PR and QT, and two segments, PQ and ST.

In normal sinus rhythm the sinoatrial (SA) node is the pacemaker for the entire heart; the SA node impulse depolarizes the right and left atria by a contiguous spread, producing the P wave (Fig. 2.1). When the atrial impulse arrives at the AV node, it passes through the node much more slowly than any other part of the heart, producing the PQ interval. Once the electrical impulse reaches the bundle of His, conduction becomes very fast and spreads simultaneously down the left and right bundle branches to the ventricular muscle through the Purkinje fibers, producing the QRS complex. The repolarization of the ventricle produces the T wave, but the repolarization of the atria is not usually visible on the ECG tracing. The ST segment represents phase 2 (plateau) of the action potential during which no net ionic movement occurs because the outward current (carried by K^+ and Cl^- ions) and inward current (carried by Ca^{2+} ions) are in competition.

A. VECTORIAL APPROACH TO THE ECG

A scalar ECG, which is routinely obtained in clinical practice, shows only the magnitude of the forces against time. The vectorial approach views the standard scalar ECG as three-dimensional vector forces that vary with time. When leads, which represent the frontal and horizontal projection, are combined, one can derive three-dimensional information on the direction of the electromotive force from scalar ECG. The limb leads (i.e., leads I, II, III, aVR, aVL, and aVF) provide information about the frontal projection, while the precordial leads (V4R, and V1 through V6) provide information about the horizontal plane (Fig. 2.2). The vectorial approach clarifies the meaning of the ECG waves and the concept of axes, such as the P axis, QRS axis, and T axis. It is important for the readers to become familiar with the orientation of each scalar ECG lead. Once learned, the vectorial approach lets the readers see the waves of the ECG as three-dimensional figures with the direction and magnitude.

1. The hexaxial reference system.

   The *hexaxial reference system* is composed of six limb leads (leads I, II, III, aVR, aVL, and aVF). It gives information about the left-right and superior-inferior relationships (Fig. 2.2A). The positive pole of each lead is indicated by the lead labels (and + signs). The positive deflection (i.e., the R wave) is the force directed toward the positive pole, and the negative deflection (i.e., the S wave) is the force directed toward the negative pole. Therefore the R wave in lead I represents the leftward

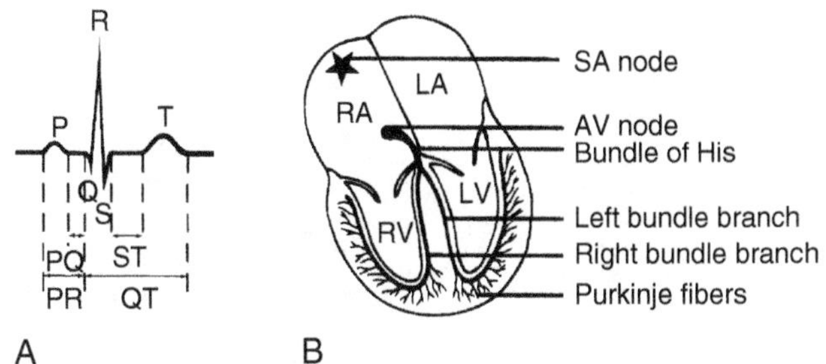

FIG. 2.1

(A) Definition of ECG configuration and (B) diagrammatic representation of the conduction system of the heart. *(From Park, M. K., & Guntheroth, W. G. (2006).* How to read pediatric ECGs *(4th ed.). Philadelphia: Mosby.)*

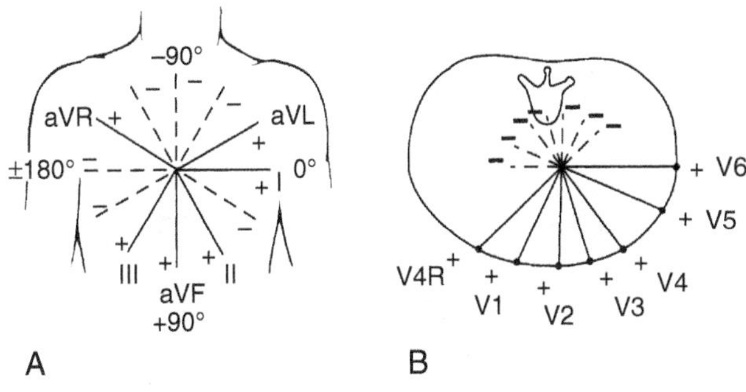

FIG. 2.2

(A) Hexaxial reference system. (B) Horizontal reference system. *(From Park, M. K., & Guntheroth, W. G. (2006).* How to read pediatric ECGs *(4th ed.). Philadelphia: Mosby.)*

force and the S wave in lead I the rightward force. The R wave in aVF is the inferior force, and the S wave in the same lead represents the superior force. The R wave in lead II is the left and inferior force, and the R wave in lead III is the right and inferior force.

An easy way to memorize the hexaxial reference system is shown in Fig. 2.3 by a superimposition of a body with stretched arms and legs on the *x*- and *y*-axes. The hands and feet are the positive poles of certain leads. The left and right hands are the positive poles of leads aVL and aVR, respectively. The left and right feet are the positive poles of leads II

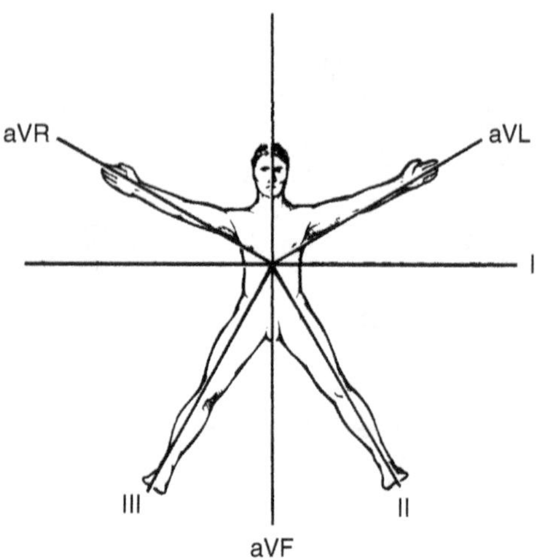

FIG. 2.3
Easy way to memorize the hexaxial reference system.

and III, respectively. The bipolar limb leads I, II, and III are clockwise in sequence for the positive poles.

2. The horizontal reference system.

The *horizontal reference system,* on the other hand, gives information about the anteroposterior and left-right relationships. The horizontal reference system uses precordial leads (e.g., V4R, V1, V2, V5, and V6) (Fig. 2.2B). The positive poles of the precordial leads are marked by the lead labels. The R wave in V2 represents the anterior force and the S wave in the same lead represents the posterior force. The R wave in V_6 is the leftward force and the S wave in the same lead is the rightward force. The R wave in V1 (as well as in V4R) is the right and anterior force and the S wave in this lead is the posterior and leftward force. The V4R lead is very useful in pediatrics; the position of the V4R lead is in the right chest at the mirror image position of the V4 lead.

B. NORMAL PEDIATRIC ELECTROCARDIOGRAMS

1. ECGs of normal infants and children are different from those of normal adults. The RV dominance seen in the ECG of neonates and infants is the result of the fetal circulation. The RV dominance is most marked in the neonate and is gradually replaced by the LV dominance of later childhood and adulthood.

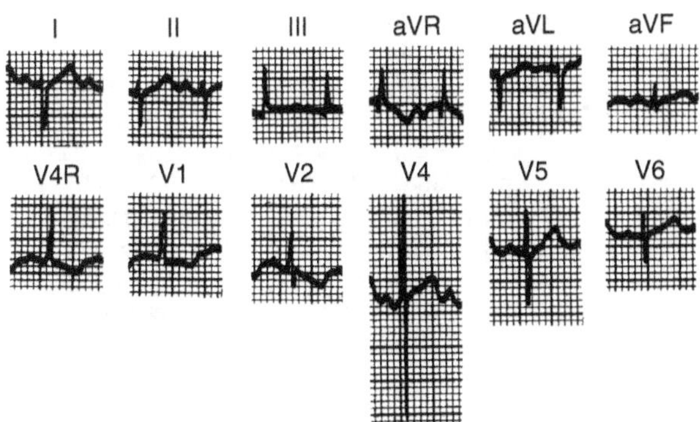

FIG. 2.4

ECG of a normal newborn infant.

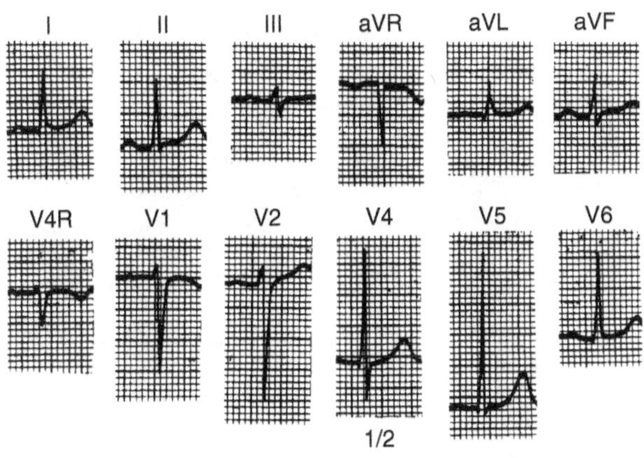

FIG. 2.5

ECG of a normal young adult.

2. By age 3 to 4 years, pediatric ECGs resemble those of the adult. Figs. 2.4 and 2.5 are ECGs from a newborn and an adult, respectively.
3. The pediatric ECG has the following characteristics:
   a. The heart rate is faster than in the adult.
   b. All the durations and intervals (PR interval, QRS duration, and QT interval) are shorter than in the adult.

c. The RV dominance of the neonate and infant is expressed in the ECG by the following:
   (1) RAD is usually present.
   (2) Large rightward forces are seen (with tall R waves in aVR and the RPLs (i.e., V4R, V1, and V2) and deep S waves in lead I and the LPLs (i.e., V5 and V6).
   (3) The R/S ratios in the RPLs are large and those in the LPLs are small. The R/S ratio is the ratio of the R amplitude and the S amplitude in a given lead.

d. The T wave is inverted in V1 in infants and small children with the exception of the first 3 days, when the T waves may be normally upright.

C. ROUTINE INTERPRETATION

The following sequence is one of many approaches that can be used in routine interpretation of an ECG.

- Rhythm (sinus or nonsinus), considering the P axis.
- Heart rate (atrial and ventricular rates, if different).
- The QRS axis, the T axis, and the QRS-T angle.
- Intervals and duration: PR, QRS, and QT.
- The P wave amplitude and duration.
- The QRS amplitude and R/S ratio; also note abnormal Q waves.
- ST-segment and T wave abnormalities.

1. Rhythm
   a. Definition of sinus rhythm. Sinus rhythm is the normal rhythm at any age. It must meet the following two characteristics (Fig. 2.6A).
      (1) A P wave preceding each QRS complex with a regular PR interval. (The PR interval may be prolonged as in first-degree AV block.)
      (2) The P axis between 0 and +90 degrees (with upright P waves in leads I and aVF).
   b. The ECG of sinus rhythm. Because the SA node is located in the right upper part of the atrial mass, the direction of atrial depolarization is from the right upper part toward the left lower part, with the resulting P axis in the left lower quadrant (0 to +90 degrees) (Fig. 2.6A). For the P axis to be between 0 and +90 degrees, P waves must be upright in leads I and aVF (Fig. 2.7A). P waves may be flat but they should not be inverted in these two leads.
   c. Nonsinus rhythm. Even when there are P waves in front of the QRS complexes, if the P axis is not in the left lower quadrant (0 to +90 degrees), the cardiac rhythm is not sinus rhythm. Examples of nonsinus rhythm are shown in Figs. 2.6B and 2.7B. The P axis is in the left upper quadrant in Fig. 2.6B with upright P waves in lead I and inverted P waves in a VF in Fig. 2.7B. The rhythm

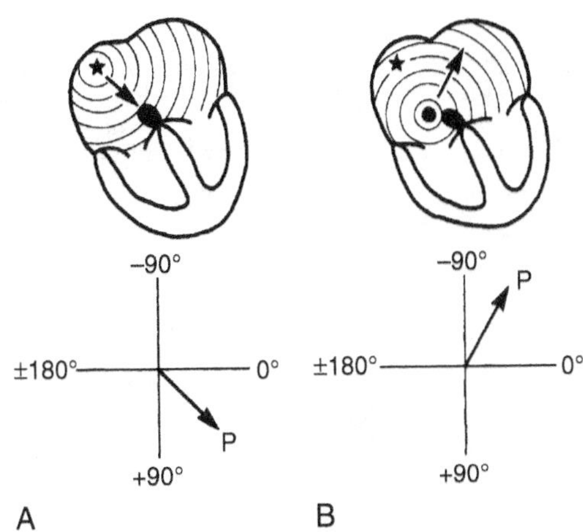

FIG. 2.6
Comparison of P axis in sinus rhythm (A) and nonsinus rhythm or low atrial rhythm (B). In sinus rhythm, the P axis is between 0 and +90 degrees, and in nonsinus rhythm, the P axis is out of the 0 to +90-degree quadrant.

in this case is called "low atrial rhythm" or "coronary sinus rhythm."

2. Heart rate. At the usual paper speed of 25 mm/sec, 1 mm = 0.04 sec and 5 mm = 0.2 sec.
   a. The heart rate may be calculated by dividing 60 (seconds) by the R-R interval in seconds.
   b. For quick estimation, inspect the R-R interval in millimeters and use the following relationship: 5 mm, 300/sec; 10 mm, 150/sec; 15 mm, 100/sec; 20 mm, 75/sec; 25 mm, 60/sec (Fig. 2.8).
   c. Normal resting heart rates per minute according to age are shown in Table 2.1. Tachycardia is a heart rate faster than the upper range of normal, and bradycardia is a heart rate slower than the low range of normal for that age.
3. The QRS axis, the T axis, and the QRS-T angle
   a. **Successive approximation method**. A convenient way of determining the QRS axis is by the use of the hexaxial reference system (see Fig. 2.2A).
      (1) Step 1. Locate a quadrant using leads I and aVF (Fig. 2.9).
      (2) Step 2. Find a lead with equiphasic QRS complex (in which the height of the R wave and the depth of the S wave are equal). The QRS axis is perpendicular to the lead with equiphasic QRS complex in the predetermined quadrant.

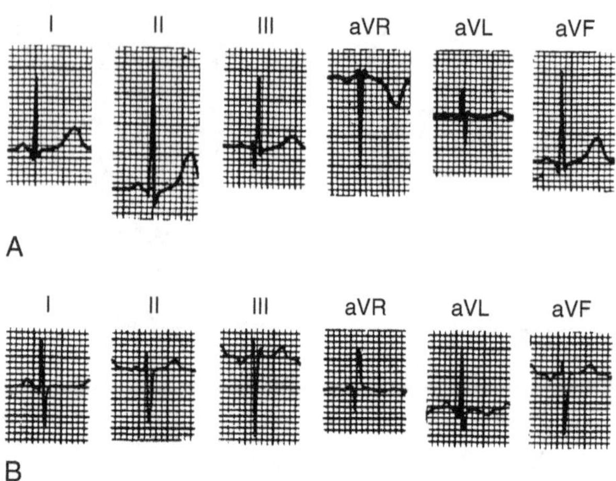

FIG. 2.7

Sinus or nonsinus rhythm determined by the P axis. (A) Sinus rhythm with the P axis between 0 and +90 degrees. (B) A nonsinus rhythm with the P axis in the 0 to −90-degree quadrant.

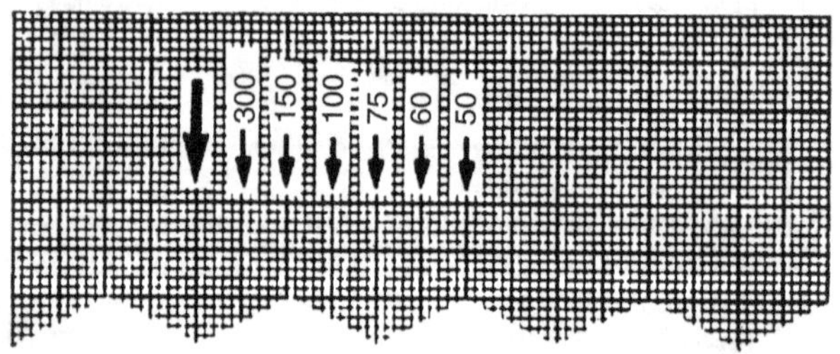

FIG. 2.8

Quick method of estimating heart rate.

(3) **Example 1.** Determine the QRS axis in Fig. 2.10A.
  (a) Step 1. The axis is in the left lower quadrant (0 to +90 degrees), since the R waves are upright in leads I and aVF.
  (b) Step 2. The QRS complex is equiphasic in aVL. Therefore the QRS axis is +60 degrees, which is perpendicular to aVL (Fig. 2.10B).

TABLE 2.1

NORMAL RANGES OF RESTING HEART RATE

AGE	BEATS/MIN
Neonates	110-150
2 yr	85-125
4 yr	75-115
More than 6 yr	60-100

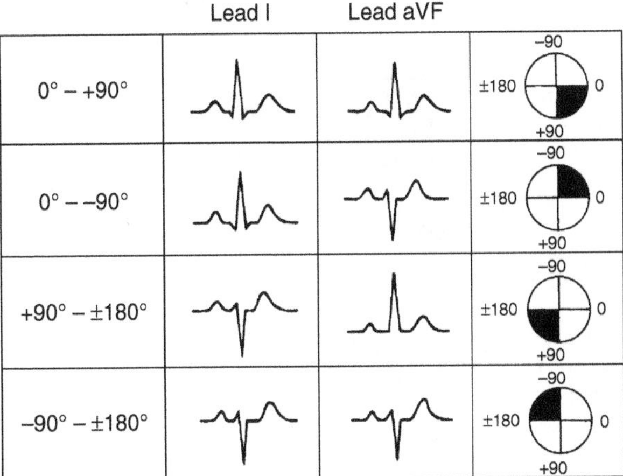

FIG. 2.9
Locating quadrants of the QRS axis using leads I and aVF. This figure is also used in determining the P and T axes. In the *top panel,* the QRS complexes are upright in both leads I and aVF, and thus the axis is in the 0 to +90 degrees quadrant. The P and T waves are also upright in leads I and aVF, and thus, the P and T axes are in the left lower quadrant (0 to +90 degrees) as well. The P axis in this quadrant indicates a sinus rhythm. The normal T axis is always in the left lower quadrant (0 to +90 degrees) at any age. Using the similar approaches, the QRS axis can be located for other panels. *(From Park, M. K., & Guntheroth, W. G. (2006).* How to read pediatric ECGs *(4th ed.). Philadelphia: Mosby.)*

(4) **Example 2.** Determine the QRS axis in Fig. 2.11A.
   (a) Step 1. The QRS complexes are negative in lead I and negative in aVF, placing the axis in the right upper quadrant (−90 to −180 degrees) (see bottom panel of Fig. 2.9).

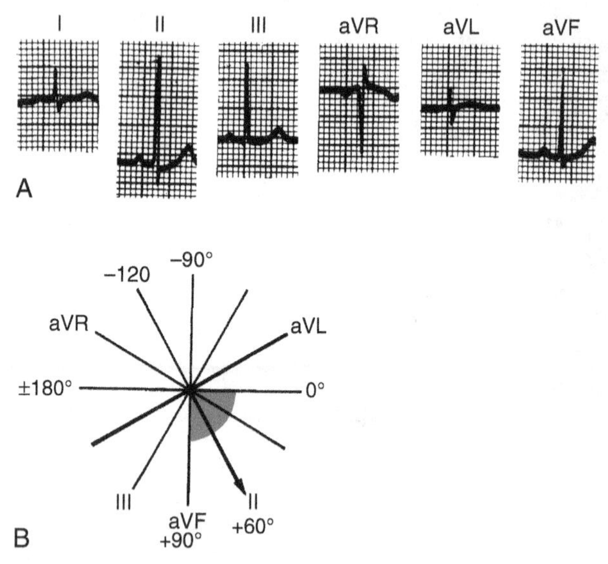

FIG. 2.10
An example of a QRS axis determination using the successive approximation method. The six limb leads shown at the top (A) are from a 6-year-old child. The QRS axis is plotted in a hexaxial reference system *(B)* (see text).

(b) Step 2. It is almost equiphasic in aVL. Therefore the axis is close to −120 degrees. The QRS axis in the right upper quadrant is called *indeterminate*, that is, neither right nor left.

b. The QRS axis.
   (1) The normal QRS axis varies with age (see Table 2.2).
   (2) The abnormal QRS axis has the following significance:
      (a) LAD (with the QRS axis less than the lower limits of normal) is seen in LVH, LBBB, and left anterior hemiblock (or superior QRS axis, characteristically seen with ECD and tricuspid atresia).
      (b) RAD (with the QRS axis greater than the upper limits of normal) is seen in RVH and RBBB.
      (c) A superior QRS axis is present when the S wave is greater than the R wave in aVF. It includes the left anterior hemiblock (in the range of −30 degrees to −90 degrees) and extreme RAD.

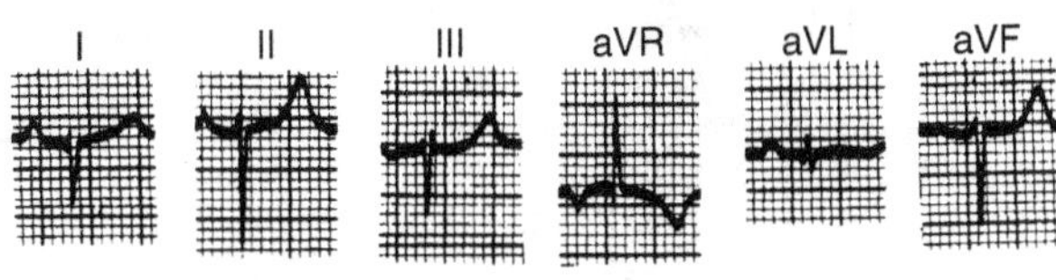

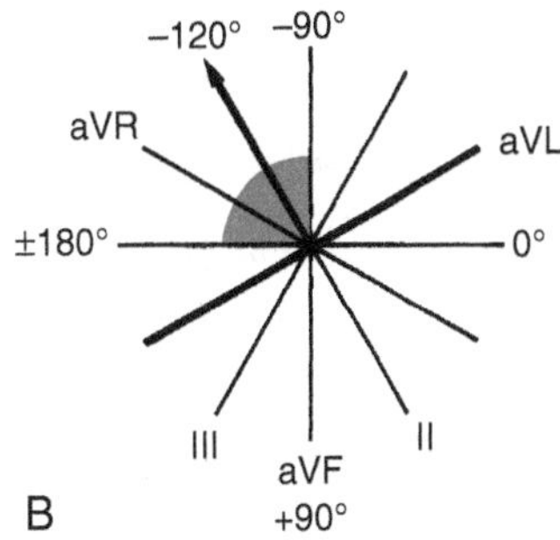

FIG. 2.11

An example of a QRS axis determination using the successive approximation method. The six limb leads shown at the top (A) are from a 2-year-old child with Down syndrome. The QRS axis is plotted in a hexaxial reference system (B) (see text).

TABLE 2.2

MEAN AND RANGE OF NORMAL QRS AXES

AGE	RANGE
1 wk-1 mo	+110 degrees (+30 to +180)
1-3 mo	+ 70 degrees (+10 to +125)
3 mo-3 yr	+ 60 degrees (+10 to +110)
>3 yr	+ 60 degrees (+20 to +120)
Adults	+ 50 degrees (−30 to + 105)

c. The T axis can be determined by the same method as that used to determine the QRS axis.
   (1) **Examples.** Determine the T axis in Fig. 2.11A.
      (a) In Fig. 2.11A, the positive T wave in lead I and the positive T wave in aVF place the T axis in the left lower quadrant (0 to +90 degrees).

(b) The T wave is nearly flat in aVL, and therefore the T axis is perpendicular to this lead, close to +60 degrees (or the positive pole of lead II, which shows the tallest T wave).

(2) The normal T axis is 0 to +90 degrees.

(3) The abnormal T axis (outside the 0 to +90-degree quadrant) is present when the T wave is inverted in lead I or aVF (usually resulting in a wide QRS-T angle). An abnormal T axis suggests conditions with abnormal myocardial repolarization (myocarditis, myocardial ischemia), ventricular hypertrophy with strain, or RBBB.

d. The QRS-T angle is the angle formed by the QRS axis and the T axis.

(1) The normal QRS-T angle is less than 60 degrees except in the newborn period, when it may be more than 60 degrees.

(2) The QRS-T angle of more than 60 degrees is unusual and that of more than 90 degrees is certainly abnormal. The abnormal QRS-T angle (above 90 degrees) is seen in severe ventricular hypertrophy with strain, ventricular conduction disturbances, ventricular arrhythmias, and myocardial dysfunction of a metabolic or ischemic nature.

(3) In Fig. 2.11, the QRS-T angle is about 180 degrees (because the QRS axis is −120 degrees and the T axis is about +60 degrees).

4. Intervals

a. **The PR interval.** The PR interval is measured from the onset of the P wave to the beginning of the QRS complex (see Fig. 2.1A).

(1) The normal PR interval varies with age and heart rate (Table 2.3). The older the person and the slower the heart rate, the longer the PR interval.

(2) A prolonged PR interval (first-degree AV block) may be seen in myocarditis (viral, rheumatic, or diphtheric), digitalis or quinidine toxicity, certain CHDs (ECD, ASD, Ebstein anomaly), hyperkalemia, other myocardial dysfunction, and in otherwise normal hearts.

(3) A short PR interval is present in WPW preexcitation, Lown-Ganong-Levine preexcitation, Duchenne muscular dystrophy (or relatives of these patients), Friedreich ataxia, pheochromocytoma, glycogen storage disease, and otherwise normal children.

(4) Variable PR intervals are seen in wandering atrial pacemaker and Wenckebach (Mobitz type I) second-degree AV block.

b. **The QRS duration.** Normal QRS duration varies with age and is shorter in infants and children than in adults (Table 2.4).

(1) A prolonged QRS is characteristic of ventricular conduction disturbances, which include bundle branch blocks (BBBs),

TABLE 2.3

PR INTERVAL WITH RATE AND AGE (UPPER LIMITS OF NORMAL)

	AGE							
	0-1 MO	**1-6 MO**	**6 MO-1 YR**	**1-3 YR**	**3-8 YR**	**8-12 YR**	**12-16 YR**	**ADULT**
<60						0.16 (0.18)	0.16 (0.19)	0.17 (0.21)
60-80					0.15 (0.17)	0.15 (0.17)	0.15 (0.18)	0.16 (0.21)
80-100	0.10 (0.12)				0.14 (0.16)	0.15 (0.16)	0.15 (0.17)	0.15 (0.20)
100-120	0.10 (0.12)			(0.15)	0.13 (0.16)	0.14 (0.15)	0.15 (0.16)	0.15 (0.19)
120-140	0.10 (0.11)	0.11 (0.14)	0.11 (0.14)	0.12 (0.14)	0.13 (0.15)	0.14 (0.15)		0.15 (0.18)
140-160	0.09 (0.11)	0.10 (0.13)	0.11 (0.13)	0.11 (0.14)	0.12 (0.14)			(0.17)
160-180	0.10 (0.11)	0.10 (0.12)	0.10 (0.12)	0.10 (0.12)				
>180	0.09	0.09 (0.11)	0.10 (0.11)					

From Park, M. K., & Guntheroth, W. G. (2006). *How to read pediatric ECGs* (4th ed.). Philadelphia: Mosby.

TABLE 2.4

QRS DURATION ACCORDING TO AGE: MEAN (UPPER LIMITS OF NORMAL[a]) (IN SECONDS)

	AGE							
	0-1 MO	**1-6 MO**	**6-12 MO**	**1-3 YR**	**3-8 YR**	**8-12 YR**	**12-16 YR**	**ADULTS**
Seconds	0.05 (0.07)	0.055 (0.075)	0.055 (0.075)	0.055 (0.075)	0.06 (0.075)	0.06 (0.085)	0.07 (0.085)	0.08 (0.10)

Derived from percentile charts in charts in

[a]Upper limit of normal refers to the 98th percentile.

Davignon, A., Rautaharju, P., Boisselle, E., Soumis, F., Marguerite Mégélas, M., & Choquette, A. (1980). Normal ECG standards for infants and children. *Pediatric Cardiology, 1,* 123-131.

WPW preexcitation, and intraventricular block. (See later section: "Ventricular Conduction Disturbances").

(2) A slight prolongation of the QRS duration may also be seen in ventricular hypertrophy.

c. **The QT interval.** The QT interval normally varies primarily with heart rate. The heart rate–corrected QT interval (QTc) can be calculated with Bazett formula:

$$QTc = QT/\sqrt{RR\ interval}$$

(1) According to the Bazett formula, the normal QTc interval (mean ± SD) is 0.40 (± 0.014) seconds with the upper limit of normal 0.44 seconds in children 6 months and older.

(2) The QTc interval is slightly longer in the newborn and small infants with the upper limit of normal QTc 0.47 seconds in the first week of life and 0.45 seconds in the first 6 months of life.

(3) Prolonged QT intervals predispose to serious ventricular arrhythmias.

(a) Prolonged QT intervals may be seen in long QT syndrome (e.g., Jervell and Lange-Nielsen syndrome, Romano-Ward syndrome), hypocalcemia, myocarditis, diffuse myocardial diseases (including hypertrophic and dilated cardiomyopathies), head injury, severe malnutrition, and so on.

(b) A number of drugs are also known to prolong the QT interval. Among these are antiarrhythmic agents (especially class IA, IC, and III), antipsychotic phenothiazines (e.g., thioridazine, chlorpromazine), tricyclic antidepressants (e.g., imipramine, amitriptyline), arsenics, organophosphates, antibiotics (e.g., azithromycin, erythromycin, trimethoprim-sulfa, amantadine), and antihistamines (e.g., terfenadine) (see Box 16.1, Acquired Causes of QT Prolongation).

(4) Short QT intervals can also predispose to serious ventricular arrhythmias.

(a) Short QT interval is seen with hypocalcemia or hyperthermia. It is also a sign of a digitalis effect.

(b) Short QT syndrome (in which the QTc is ≤300 milliseconds) is a familial cause of sudden death by ventricular tachycardia.

d. **The JT interval.** The JT interval is useful when the QT interval is prolonged secondary to a prolonged QRS duration. It is measured from the J point (the junction between the S wave and the ST segment) to the end of the T wave. The JT interval is also expressed as a rate-corrected interval (called JTc) using the Bazett formula. A prolonged JT interval has the same significance as the prolonged QTc interval. Normal JTc (mean ± SD) is 0.32 ± 0.02 seconds with the upper limit of normal 0.34 seconds.

5. P wave duration and amplitude. Abnormal amplitude or duration indicates atrial hypertrophy.
   a. Normally the P wave amplitude is less than 3 mm. Tall P waves indicate RAH.
   b. The duration of the P waves is shorter than 0.09 seconds in children and shorter than 0.07 seconds in infants. Long P wave durations are seen in LAH.
6. QRS amplitude, R/S ratio, and abnormal Q waves
   a. QRS amplitude varies with age (Tables 2.5 and 2.6).
      (1) Large QRS amplitudes (either large R waves or deep S waves) are found in ventricular hypertrophy and ventricular conduction disturbances (e.g., BBBs, WPW preexcitation).
      (2) Low QRS voltages are seen in pericarditis, myocarditis, hypothyroidism, and normal neonates.
   b. The R/S ratio in normal infants and small children is large in the right precordial leads (RPLs) and is small in the left precordial

TABLE 2.5

R VOLTAGES ACCORDING TO LEAD AND AGE: MEAN (AND UPPER LIMIT[a]) (IN MM)

	AGE							
LEAD	**0-1 MO**	**1-6 MO**	**6-12 MO**	**1-3 YR**	**3-8 YR**	**8-12 YR**	**12-16 YR**	**ADULTS**
I	4 (8)	7 (13)	8 (16)	8 (16)	7 (15)	7 (15)	6 (13)	6 (13)
II	6 (14)	13 (24)	13 (27)	12 (23)	13 (22)	14 (24)	14 (24)	5 (25)
III	8 (16)	9 (20)	9 (20)	9 (20)	9 (20)	9 (24)	9 (24)	6 (22)
aVR	3 (8)	2 (6)	2 (6)	2 (5)	2 (4)	1 (4)	1 (4)	1 (4)
aVL	2 (7)	4 (8)	5 (10)	5 (10)	3 (10)	3 (10)	3 (12)	3 (9)
aVF	7 (14)	10 (20)	10 (16)	8 (20)	10 (19)	10 (20)	11 (21)	5 (23)
V3R	10 (19)	6 (13)	6 (11)	6 (11)	5 (10)	3 (9)	3 (7)	
V4R	6 (12)	5 (10)	4 (8)	4 (8)	3 (8)	3 (7)	3 (7)	
V1	13 (24)	10 (19)	10 (20)	9 (18)	8 (16)	5 (12)	4 (10)	3 (14)
V2	18 (30)	20 (31)	22 (32)	19 (28)	15 (25)	12 (20)	10 (19)	6 (21)
V5	12 (23)	20 (33)	20 (31)	20 (32)	23 (38)	26 (39)	21 (35)	12 (33)
V6	5 (15)	13 (22)	13 (23)	13 (23)	15 (26)	17 (26)	14 (23)	10 (21)

Voltages measured in millimeters, when 1 mV = 10 mm paper.

[a]Upper limit of normal refers to the 98th percentile.

Data from Park, M. K., & Guntheroth, W. G. (2006). *How to read pediatric ECGs* (4th ed.). Philadelphia: Mosby.

TABLE 2.6

S VOLTAGES ACCORDING TO LEAD AND AGE: MEAN (AND UPPER LIMIT[a]) (IN MM)

	AGE							
LEAD	**0-1 MO**	**1-6 MO**	**6-12 MO**	**1-3 YR**	**3-8 YR**	**8-12 YR**	**12-16 YR**	**ADULTS**
I	5 (10)	4 (9)	4 (9)	3 (8)	2 (8)	2 (8)	2 (8)	1 (6)
V3R	3 (12)	3 (10)	4 (10)	5 (12)	7 (15)	8 (18)	7 (16)	
V4R	4 (9)	4 (12)	5 (12)	5 (12)	5 (14)	6 (20)	6 (20)	
V1	7 (18)	5 (15)	7 (18)	8 (21)	11 (23)	12 (25)	11 (22)	10 (23)
V2	18 (33)	15 (26)	16 (29)	18 (30)	20 (33)	21 (36)	18 (33)	14 (36)
V5	9 (17)	7 (16)	6 (15)	5 (12)	4 (10)	3 (8)	3 (8)	
V6	3 (10)	3 (9)	2 (7)	2 (7)	2 (5)	1 (4)	1 (4)	1 (13)

Voltages measured in millimeters, when 1 mV = 10 mm paper.
[a]Upper limit of normal refers to the 98th percentile.
Data from Park, M. K., & Guntheroth, W. G. (2006). *How to read pediatric ECGs* (4th ed.). Philadelphia: Mosby.

TABLE 2.7

R/S RATIO ACCORDING TO AGE: MEAN, LOWER, AND UPPER LIMITS OF NORMAL

		AGE							
LEAD		**0-1 MO**	**1-6 MO**	**6 MO-1 YR**	**1-3 YR**	**3-8 YR**	**8-12 YR**	**12-16 YR**	**ADULT**
V1	LLN	0.5	0.3	0.3	0.5	0.1	0.15	0.1	0.0
	Mean	1.5	1.5	1.2	0.8	0.65	0.5	0.3	0.3
	ULN	19	S = 0	6	2	2	1	1	1
V2	LLN	0.3	0.3	0.3	0.3	0.05	0.1	0.1	0.1
	Mean	1	1.2	1	0.8	0.5	0.5	0.5	0.2
	ULN	3	4	4	1.5	1.5	1.2	1.2	2.5
V6	LLN	0.1	1.5	2	3	2.5	4	2.5	2.5
	Mean	2	4	6	20	20	20	10	9
	ULN	S = 0	S = 0	S = 0	S = 0	S = 0	S = 0	S = 0	S = 0

LLN, *lower limit of normal;* ULN, *upper limit of normal.*
From Guntheroth, W. G. (1965). *Pediatric electrocardiography.* Philadelphia: WB Saunders.

leads (LPLs) because of the presence of tall R waves in the RPLs and deep S waves in the LPLs (Table 2.7). Abnormal R/S ratios are seen in ventricular hypertrophy and ventricular conduction disturbances.

c. Normal Q waves are narrow (0.02 seconds) and are usually less than 5 mm in LPLs and aVF (Table 2.8). They may be as deep as 8 mm in lead III in children younger than 3 years old.

TABLE 2.8

Q VOLTAGES ACCORDING TO LEAD AND AGE: MEAN (AND UPPER LIMIT[a]) (IN MM)

	AGE							
LEAD	0-1 MO	1-6 MO	6-12 MO	1-3 YR	3-8 YR	8-12 YR	12-16 YR	ADULTS
III	1.5 (5.5)	1.5 (6.0)	2.1 (6.0)	1.5 (5.0)	1.0 (3.5)	0.6 (3.0)	1.0 (3.0)	0.5 (4)
aVF	1.0 (3.5)	1.0 (3.5)	1.0 (3.5)	1.0 (3.0)	0.5 (3.0)	0.5 (2.5)	0.5 (2.0)	0.5 (2)
V5	0.1 (3.5)	0.1 (3.0)	0.1 (3.0)	0.5 (4.5)	1.0 (5.5)	1.0 (3.0)	0.5 (3.0)	0.5 (3.5)
V6	0.5 (3.0)	0.5 (3.0)	0.5 (3.0)	0.5 (3.0)	1.0 (3.5)	0.5 (3.0)	0.5 (3.0)	0.5 (3)

Voltages measured in millimeters, when 1 mV = 10 mm paper.

[a]Upper limit of normal refers to the 98th percentile.

Data from charts in Davignon, A., Rautaharju, P., Boisselle, E., Soumis, F., Mégélas, M., & Choquette, A. (1980). Normal ECG standards for infants and children. *Pediatric Cardiology, 1,* 123-131.

(1) Deep Q waves may be present in the LPLs in LVH of volume overload type.
(2) Deep and wide Q waves are seen in myocardial infarction and myocardial fibrosis.
(3) Q waves are normally absent in RPLs.
  (a) Q waves in V1 may be seen in ventricular inversion (levo TGA [L-TGA]), severe RVH, single ventricle, and occasional neonates.
  (b) Absent Q waves in V6 may be seen in LBBB and ventricular inversion.

7. The ST segment and the T wave
   a. The normal ST segment is isoelectric. Some forms of ST segment shifts are nonpathologic and include J depression and early repolarization. Pathologic ST-segment shift may assume either a downward-sloping or a sustained horizontal depression and is seen with myocarditis, pericarditis, and myocardial ischemia or infarction. A further discussion follows later in this chapter.
   b. The T wave
      (1) Normal T axis should be in the left lower quadrant (0 to +90 degrees).
      (2) Tall peaked T waves may be seen in hyperkalemia, LVH (volume overload), and cerebrovascular accident.
      (3) Flat or low T waves may occur in normal neonates or with such conditions as hypothyroidism, hypokalemia, pericarditis, myocarditis, myocardial ischemia, hyperglycemia, or hypoglycemia.

D. ATRIAL HYPERTROPHY

Abnormalities in the P wave amplitude and/or duration characterize atrial hypertrophy (Fig. 2.12).

1. RAH accompanies tall P waves (at least 3 mm).

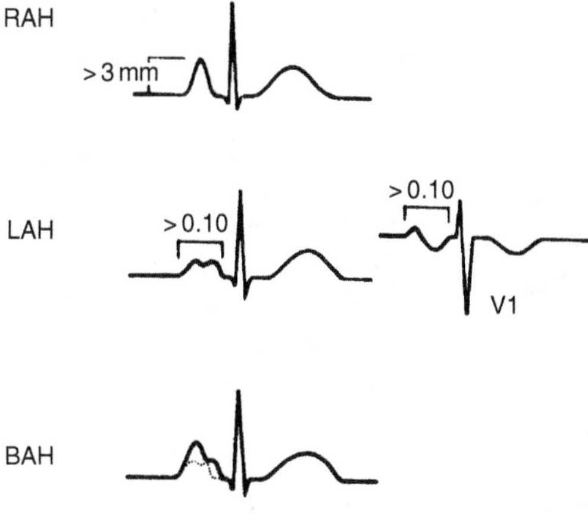

FIG. 2.12

Criteria for atrial hypertrophy. *(From Park, M. K., & Guntheroth, W. G. (2006).* How to read pediatric ECGs *(4th ed.). Philadelphia: Mosby.)*

2. LAH accompanies wide P wave duration (at least 0.1 seconds in children and >0.08 seconds in infants). A biphasic P wave in V1 is not a sign of LAH, unless the P wave duration is greater than 0.08 seconds for infants and greater than 0.1 second for children.
3. BAH accompanies a combination of tall and wide P waves.

E. VENTRICULAR HYPERTROPHY

1. Ventricular hypertrophy produces abnormalities in one or more of the following: the QRS axis, the QRS voltages, the R/S ratio, the T axis, and miscellaneous changes.
   a. The QRS axis is usually directed toward the hypertrophied ventricle (see Table 2.2 for the normal QRS axis).
      (1) RAD is seen with RVH.
      (2) LAD is seen with LVH. However, LAD is rare with LVH caused by pressure overload; in this situation, the QRS axis is more often directed inferiorly.
   b. Changes in QRS voltages. Anatomically, the RV occupies the right and anterior aspect, and the LV occupies the left, inferior, and posterior aspect of the ventricular mass. With ventricular hypertrophy, the voltage of the QRS complex increases in the direction of the respective ventricle (see Tables 2.5 and 2.6 for normal R and S voltages).
      (1) In the frontal plane (Fig. 2.13A)
         (a) LVH shows increased R voltages in leads I, II, aVL, aVF, and sometimes III, especially in small infants.

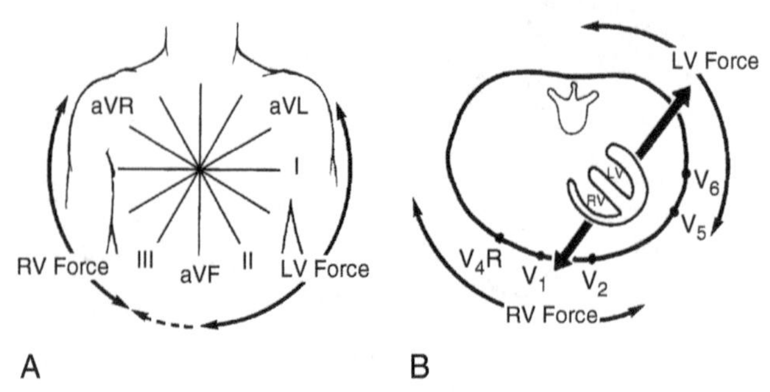

FIG. 2.13

Left and right ventricular forces on the frontal (A) and horizontal (B) projections. (A), Hexaxial reference system. (B) Horizontal plane. *(From Park, M. K., & Guntheroth, W. G. (2006).* How to read pediatric ECGs *(4th ed.). Philadelphia: Mosby.)*

(b) RVH shows increased R voltages in aVR and III and increased S voltages in lead I

(2) In the horizontal plane (Fig. 2.13B)

(a) LVH shows tall R waves in V5 and V6 and/or deep S waves in V4R, V1, and V2.

(b) RVH shows tall R waves in V4R, V1, and V2 and/or deep S waves in V5 and V6.

c. Changes in the R/S ratio. An increase in the R/S ratio in the RPLs suggests RVH, and a decrease in the ratio in these leads suggests LVH. An increase in the R/S ratio in the LPLs suggests LVH and a decrease in the ratio suggests RVH (Table 2.7).

d. The T axis changes in severe ventricular hypertrophy with relative ischemia of the hypertrophied myocardium (resulting in a wide QRS-T angle). In the presence of criteria of ventricular hypertrophy, a wide QRS-T angle (≥90 degrees) with the T axis outside the normal range indicates a strain pattern. When the T axis remains in the normal quadrant (0 to +90 degrees), a wide QRS-T angle indicates a possible strain pattern.

e. Miscellaneous nonspecific changes

(1) RVH

(a) An upright T wave in V1 after 3 days of age is a sign of probable RVH.

(b) A Q wave in V1 (either qR or qRs) suggests RVH, although it may be present in ventricular inversion.

(2) LVH

(a) Deep Q waves (≥5 mm) and/or tall T waves in V5 and V6 are signs of LVH of the volume overload type (often seen with a large-shunt VSD).

(b) Deep Q waves seen in the inferior leads (II, III, and aVF) may also be a sign of LVH (dilated or hypertrophied LV). Normally, the Q wave in lead III may be as deep as 6 mm in small children.

2. Criteria for RVH
   a. RAD for the patient's age (see Table 2.2).
   b. Increased rightward and anterior QRS voltages in the presence of normal QRS duration. Increased QRS voltages in the presence of a prolonged QRS duration indicate a ventricular conduction disturbance, such as BBB or WPW preexcitation, rather than ventricular hypertrophy.
      (1) R in V1, V2, or aVR greater than the upper limits of normal for the patient's age (see Table 2.5).
      (2) S in I and V6 greater than the upper limits of normal for the patient's age (see Table 2.6).
   c. Abnormal R/S ratio (see Table 2.7).
      (1) R/S ratio in V1 and V2 greater than the upper limits of normal for age.
      (2) R/S ratio in V6 less than 1 after 1 month of age.
   d. Upright T wave in V1 in patients more than 3 days of age, provided that the T is upright in the LPLs (V5, V6). Upright T in V1 is not abnormal in patients 6 years or older.
   e. A Q wave in V1 (qR or qRs pattern) may be seen with severe RVH. (It is more likely ventricular inversion.)
   f. In the presence of RVH, a wide QRS-T angle (≥90 degrees) with the T axis outside the normal range (usually in the 0- to −90-degree quadrant) indicates a "strain" pattern.
   g. The more independent criteria for RVH that are satisfied, the more probable RVH is. An abnormal force both rightward and anterior is stronger evidence than one that is anterior only or rightward only. For example, large S waves seen in two leads, I and V6 (rightward forces), are not as strong as a large S wave seen in lead I and a large R wave seen in V2 (reflecting both rightward and anterior forces). An example of RVH with "strain" is shown in Fig. 2.14.
3. RVH in the newborn. The diagnosis of RVH in the neonate is particularly difficult because of the normal dominance of the RV during that period of life. The following clues, however, are helpful.
   a. S waves in lead I ≥12 mm.
   b. R waves in aVR ≥8 mm.
   c. The following abnormalities in V1 also suggest RVH.
      (1) Pure R wave (with no S wave) in V1 greater than 10 mm.
      (2) A qR pattern in V1 (also seen in 10% of healthy newborn infants).
      (3) Upright T waves in V1 in neonates older than 3 days of age (with upright T in V6).
   d. RAD greater than +180 degrees.

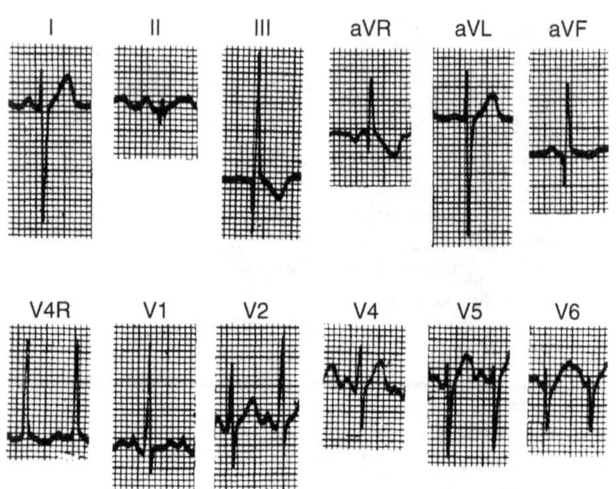

FIG. 2.14

Tracing from a 10-month-old infant with severe TOF. The tracing shows RVH with strain. There is RAD (+150 degrees). The R waves in III (22 mm) and aVR (9 mm) and the S waves in I (19 mm) and V6 (8 mm) are abnormally large, indicating RVH. The R/S ratios in V1 and V2 are abnormally large, and the ratio in V6 is smaller than the LLN (see Table 2.7), also indicating RVH. The S wave is inverted in aVF, with a T axis of −10 degrees and a wide QRS-T angle (160 degrees).

4. Criteria for LVH
   a. LAD for the patient's age (see Table 2.2).
      Increased leftward, inferior, and posterior QRS voltages in the presence of normal QRS duration.
      (1) R in I, II, III, aVL, aVF, V5, or V6 greater than the upper limits of normal for age (see Table 2.5).
      (2) S in V1 or V2 greater than the upper limits of normal for age (see Table 2.6).
   b. Abnormal R/S ratio: An R/S ratio in V1 and V2 less than the lower limits of normal for the patient's age (see Table 2.7).
   c. Q in V5 and V6, 5 mm or more, coupled with tall symmetric T waves in the same leads (volume overload type).
   d. In the presence of LVH, a wide QRS-T angle (≥90 degrees) with the T axis outside the normal quadrant indicates a "strain" pattern. This is manifested by inverted T waves in lead I or aVF.
   e. The more of the preceding independent criteria satisfied, the more probable LVH is. For example, abnormal leftward forces seen in three leads (I, V5, and V6) are not as strong as the situation in which

abnormal leftward force (e.g., deep S in I) is combined with abnormal posterior forces (deep S in V2) or abnormal inferior force (tall R in aVF or tall R in II). With obstructive lesions (e.g., AS), the abnormal force is more likely inferior (not showing LAD). With a volume overload (e.g., VSD), the abnormal force is more likely to the left (showing LAD). An example of LVH is shown in Fig. 2.15.

5. Criteria for biventricular hypertrophy (BVH).

   Diagnosis of BVH is often difficult because the abnormal LV and RV forces are opposite in direction and therefore tend to cancel out, resulting in relatively small (or even normal) QRS voltages.

   a. Positive voltage criteria for RVH and LVH in the absence of increased QRS duration (such as BBB or WPW preexcitation). Many cases of large QRS voltages suggestive of BVH are seen in ventricular conduction disturbances (with increased QRS duration).
   b. Positive voltage criteria for RVH or LVH and large voltages (but within normal limits) for the other ventricle, again in the presence of normal QRS duration.
   c. Large equiphasic QRS complexes in two or more of the limb leads and in the midprecordial leads (V2 through V5), called Katz-Wachtel phenomenon.

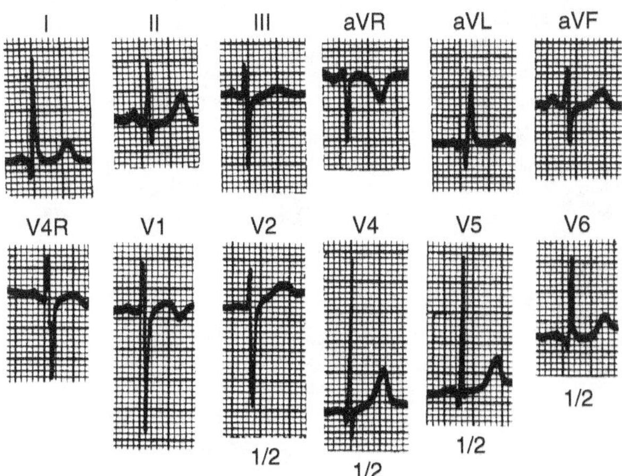

FIG. 2.15
Tracing from a 4-year-old boy with moderate VSD. The tracing shows LVH without strain pattern. The QRS axis is 0 degrees (LAD for age). The R waves in I (17 mm), aVL (12 mm), V5 (44 mm), and V6 (27 mm) are beyond the ULN, indicating abnormal LV force. The T axis (+50 degrees) is in the normal range. Note one-half standardization for some precordial leads.

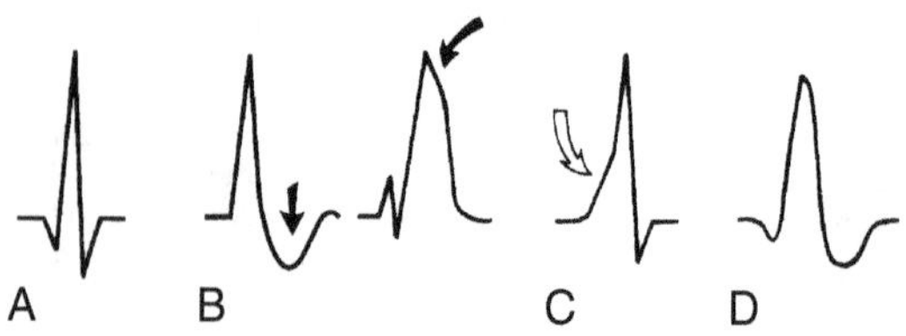

FIG. 2.16

Schematic diagram of three types of ventricular conduction disturbances. (A) Normal QRS complex. (B) QRS complexes in RBBB with terminal slurring (*black arrows*). (C) Preexcitation with delta wave (*initial slurring, open arrow*). (D) Intraventricular block in which the prolongation of the QRS complex is throughout the duration of the QRS complex. *(From Park, M. K., & Guntheroth, W. G. (2006).* How to read pediatric ECGs *(4th ed.). Philadelphia: Mosby.)*

F. VENTRICULAR CONDUCTION DISTURBANCES

Conditions that are grouped together as ventricular conduction disturbances have in common abnormal prolongation of QRS duration (Fig. 2.16). The normal QRS duration varies with age (see Table 2.4). In infants, QRS duration of more than 0.08 seconds (not 0.1, as in adults) meets the requirement for RBBB. Therefore accurate determination of the QRS duration is necessary to diagnose ventricular conduction disturbances. Three types of ventricular conduction disturbances and their characteristic findings are as follows.

- Right and left bundle branch blocks, in which the prolongation of the QRS duration is in the terminal portion of the QRS complex (i.e., "terminal slurring") (Fig. 2.16B).
- WPW preexcitation shows the prolongation in the initial portion of the QRS complex (i.e., initial slurring or delta wave) (Fig. 2.16C).
- Intraventricular block in which the prolongation is throughout the QRS complex (Fig. 2.17D).

1. RBBB
   a. RBBB is the most common form of ventricular conduction disturbance in children.
   b. The RV depolarization is delayed with the terminal slurring of the QRS complex directed toward the RV (e.g., rightward and anteriorly). The RV depolarization is unopposed by the LV depolarization due to asynchronous depolarization of the opposing forces, and therefore the manifest QRS voltages are abnormally large, often a source of misinterpretation of the condition as ventricular hypertrophy. The same is the case with LBBB. Thus larger QRS voltages for both the RV and the LV are seen in RBBB and LBBB. (Only RBBB is presented here because LBBB is extremely rare in pediatric patients.)
   c. The two most common pediatric disorders that present with RBBB are ASD and conduction disturbances following heart

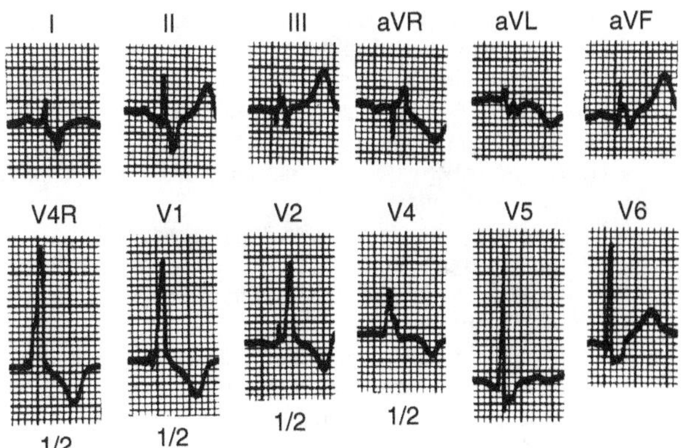

FIG. 2.17

Tracing from a 6-year-old boy who had corrective surgery for TOF that involved right ventriculotomy for repair of VSD and resection of infundibular narrowing. The QRS axis is only minimally rightward (about +115 degrees), but the terminal (slurred) portion of the QRS is clearly rightward. The QRS duration is prolonged (0.13 sec). The T vector remains normal (+10 degrees). Although there are abnormally large R voltages in V4R, V1, and V2, with abnormal R/S ratios, one cannot make the diagnosis of an additional RVH; it may all be due to RBBB.

surgery involving a right ventriculotomy. Other conditions often associated with RBBB include Ebstein anomaly, COA in infants younger than 6 month, ECD, PAPVR, and occasionally in normal children.

d. The significance of RBBB in children is different from that in adults. In several pediatric examples of RBBB, the right bundle is anatomically intact.
   (1) In ASD, the prolonged QRS duration is the result of a longer pathway through a dilated RV, rather than an actual block in the right bundle.
   (2) Right ventriculotomy for repair of VSD or TOF disrupts the RV subendocardial Purkinje network and causes prolongation of the QRS duration without necessarily injuring the right bundle.
e. RSR′ pattern. Although the RSR′ (or rSr′) pattern in V1 is unusual in adults, this pattern is a *normal* finding in infants, toddlers, and small children. Some of them are incorrectly interpreted as *incomplete right bundle branch block (IRBBB)* or RVH by computer readouts and by physicians alike. Looking at it from vectorcardiographic points of view, in order for a newborn ECG

pattern to change to the adult pattern, it has to go through a stage in which the rSr′ or RsR′ pattern appears; it is almost impossible for a newborn ECG to change to the adult pattern without going through the rSr′ (or rsR′) stage. The following clarifies some issues related to the rSr′ pattern in V1.

(1) An rsR′ pattern in V_1 is normal if the QRS duration and QRS voltage are normal.

(2) If the rSr′ pattern is associated with slightly prolonged QRS duration (not to satisfy the criterion of RBBB), it is then incomplete RBBB. In this case, the QRS voltage could be slightly increased.

(3) If the rsR′ pattern is associated with slightly prolonged QRS duration and an abnormally large QRS voltage, it is still IRBBB, not ventricular hypertrophy.

(4) RVH is justified only if an abnormal QRS voltage is present in the presence of normal QRS duration.

f. IRBBB: The pathophysiology and clinical significance of IRBBB are similar to that of RBBB as discussed earlier. Some cardiologists prefer the term “RV conduction delay” rather than a “block” as in IRBBB. The prevalence of IRBBB in the pediatric population is not known, but it may be around 1% among normal children and 5% to 10% in the adult population.

g. Criteria for RBBB (see Fig. 2.17)

(1) RAD at least for the terminal portion of the QRS complex. The initial QRS vector is normal.

(2) QRS duration longer than the upper limits of normal for the patient’s age (see Table 2.4).

(3) Terminal slurring of the QRS complex directed to the right and usually, but not always, anteriorly.

(a) Wide and slurred S in I, V5, and V6.

(b) Terminal, slurred R′ in aVR and the RPLs (i.e., V4R, V1, and V2), with an rsR′ pattern.

(4) ST-segment shift and T-wave inversion are common in adults but not in children.

(5) It is unsafe to make a diagnosis of ventricular hypertrophy in the presence of RBBB, because a greater manifest potential for both ventricles is expected to occur without actual ventricular hypertrophy as a result of asynchronous unopposed forces of the RV and LV (as explained earlier).

2. Intraventricular block. In intraventricular block, the prolongation is throughout the duration of the QRS complex, and does not resemble either RBBB or LBBB (see Fig. 2.16D). It is associated with metabolic disorders (hyperkalemia), myocardial ischemia (e.g., during or after cardiopulmonary resuscitation), drugs (e.g., quinidine, procainamide, tricyclic antidepressants), and diffuse myocardial diseases (myocardial fibrosis and systemic diseases with myocardial

involvement). Conditions seen with the intraventricular block are often more serious than those seen with BBB or WPW preexcitation.

3. WPW preexcitation
   a. In WPW preexcitation, the initial portion of the QRS complex is slurred, with a "delta" wave (see Fig. 2.16C). Fig. 2.18 is an example of WPW preexcitation.
   b. WPW preexcitation results from an anomalous conduction pathway (i.e., bundle of Kent) between the atrium and the ventricle, bypassing the normal delay of conduction in the AV node.
   c. In the presence of this finding, diagnosis of ventricular hypertrophy cannot be made safely for the same reason as with BBB.
   d. Patients with WPW preexcitation are prone to attacks of paroxysmal SVT. When there is a history of SVT, the diagnosis of WPW syndrome is justified.
   e. Criteria for WPW preexcitation
      (1) Short PR interval, less than the lower limits of normal for the patient's age. The lower limits of normal PR interval are as follows:
         (a) <3 years, 0.08 seconds
         (b) 3-16 years, 0.1 seconds
         (c) >16 years, 0.12 seconds

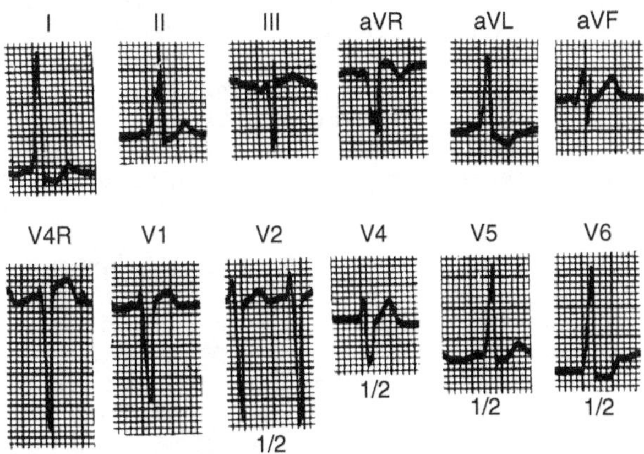

FIG. 2.18

Tracing from a 6-month-old infant with possible glycogen storage disease. The QRS duration is increased to 0.1 seconds (ULN is 0.06 for age). There are delta waves in the initial portion of the QRS complex, which are best seen in I, aVL, and V5. The QRS axis is 0 degree (LAD for age) and the large leftward and posterior QRS voltages are abnormal, but with preexcitation the diagnosis of LVH cannot be made.

(2) Delta wave (initial slurring of the QRS complex).
(3) Wide QRS duration (beyond the ULN).

f. Other rare forms of preexcitation can also result in extreme tachycardia.
(1) Lown-Ganong-Levine preexcitation is characterized by a short PR interval and normal QRS duration (without a delta wave). James fibers (which connect the atrium and the bundle of His) bypass the upper AV node and produce a short PR interval, but the ventricles are depolarized normally through the His-Purkinje system. When there is history of SVT, the condition may be called Lown-Ganong-Levine syndrome; in the absence of such a history, the ECG should be read as "short PR interval."
(2) Mahaim-type preexcitation is characterized by a normal PR interval and long QRS duration with a delta wave. Mahaim fiber connects the AV node (or lateral right atrial wall) and the right ventricle bypassing the bundle of His and "short-circuiting" into the right ventricle, with resulting QRS complexes of LBBB morphology.

4. Ventricular hypertrophy vs. ventricular conduction disturbances

Two common pediatric ECG abnormalities, ventricular hypertrophy and ventricular conduction disturbances, often manifest with increased QRS voltages, and thus are not always easy to differentiate from each other. An accurate measurement of the QRS duration is essential. The following approach may aid in differentiating these two conditions (Fig. 2.19).

a. When the QRS duration is normal, normal QRS voltages indicate a normal ECG, and increased QRS voltages may indicate ventricular hypertrophy.
b. When the QRS duration is clearly prolonged, normal as well as increased QRS voltages indicate ventricular conduction disturbance. In this situation, an increased QRS voltage does not indicate the presence of an additional ventricular hypertrophy.
c. When the QRS duration is only borderline increased, the separation of ventricular hypertrophy and ventricular conduction disturbances is difficult. In general, a borderline increase in the QRS voltage, especially without the terminal or initial slurring, favors ventricular hypertrophy rather than conduction disturbances. When the QRS voltage is normal, the ECG may be interpreted either as normal or as a mild RV or LV conduction delay.

G. PATHOLOGIC ST-SEGMENT AND T-WAVE CHANGES

Not all ST-segment shifts are abnormal. Elevation or depression of up to 1 mm in the limb leads and up to 2 mm in the precordial leads is within normal limits.

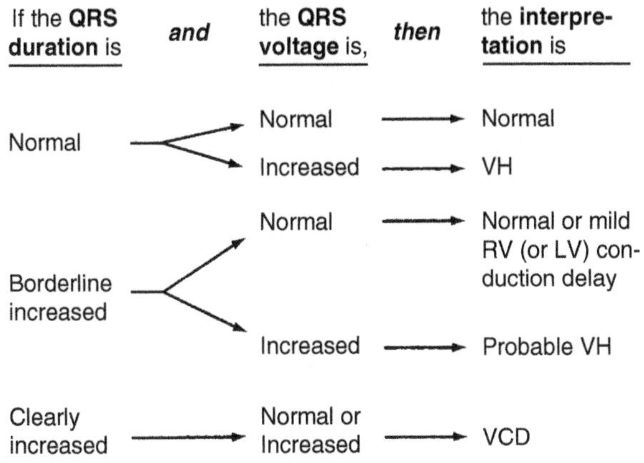

FIG. 2.19
Algorithm for differentiating between ventricular hypertrophy and ventricular conduction disturbances. *VCD,* ventricular conductive disturbance; *VH,* ventricular hypertrophy.

1. **Nonpathologic ST-segment shift.** Two common types of nonpathologic ST segment shifts are J depression and early repolarization. The T vector remains normal in these situations.
   a. **J depression.** J depression is a shift of the junction between the QRS complex and the ST segment (J point) without sustained ST segment depression (Fig. 2.20A).
   b. **Early repolarization.** In early repolarization, all leads with upright T waves have elevated ST segments, and leads with inverted T waves have depressed ST segments. This condition, seen in healthy adolescents and young adults, resembles the ST- segment shift seen in acute pericarditis; in the former, the ST segment is stable, and in the latter, the ST segment returns to the isoelectric line.
2. **Pathologic ST-segment shift**. Abnormal shifts of the ST segment often are accompanied by T wave inversion. A pathologic ST-segment shift assumes one of the following forms.
   - Downward slant followed by a diphasic or inverted T wave (see Fig. 2.20B).
   - Horizontal elevation or depression sustained for >0.08 seconds (see Fig. 2.20C).

   Examples of pathologic ST-segment shifts and T wave changes include LVH or RVH with strain; digitalis effects; pericarditis; myocarditis; and myocardial infarction.

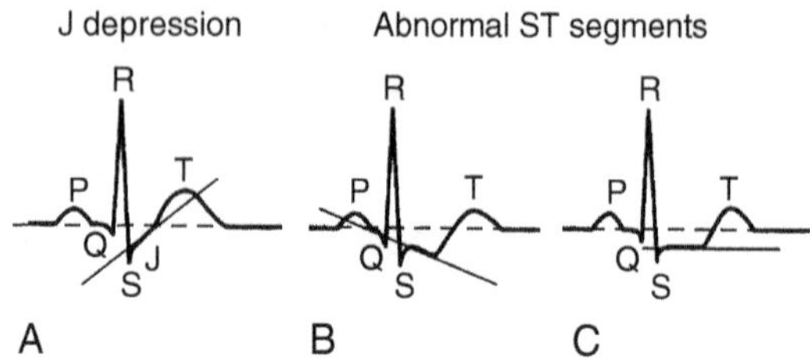

FIG. 2.20
Nonpathologic (nonischemic) and pathologic (ischemic) ST and T changes. (A) Characteristic nonischemic ST-segment alteration called J depression; note that the ST slope is upward. (B) and (C) Ischemic or pathologic ST-segment alterations. Downward slope of the ST segment is shown in (B). Horizontal ST segment is sustained in (C).

a. **Pericarditis:** The ECG changes seen in pericarditis consist of the following.
   (1) Pericardial effusion may produce low QRS voltages (with <5 mm in every one of the limb leads).
   (2) Subepicardial myocardial damage produces the following time-dependent changes in the ST segment and T wave (see Fig. 2.21).
      (a) ST-segment elevation in the leads representing the LV.
      (b) The ST-segment shift returning to normal within 2 or 3 days.
      (c) T wave inversion (with isoelectric ST segment) 2 to 4 weeks after the onset of pericarditis.
b. **Myocarditis:** ECG findings of rheumatic or viral myocarditis are relatively nonspecific and may involve all phases of the cardiac cycle: first- or second-degree AV block, low QRS voltages (5 mm or less in all six limb leads), decreased amplitude of the T wave, QT prolongation, and/or cardiac arrhythmias.
c. **Myocardial infarction (MI):** The ECG findings of myocardial infarction (MI), which are time dependent, are illustrated in Fig. 2.22. Leads that show these abnormalities vary with the location of the infarction. They are summarized in Table 2.9.
   (1) In adult patients with acute MI, the more common ECG findings are those of the early evolving phase, which consists of pathologic Q waves (abnormally wide and deep), ST-segment elevation, and T-wave inversion.
   (2) Frequent ECG findings in children with acute MI include wide Q waves, ST- segment elevation (>2 mm), and QTc prolongation (>0.44 sec) with accompanying abnormal Q waves.

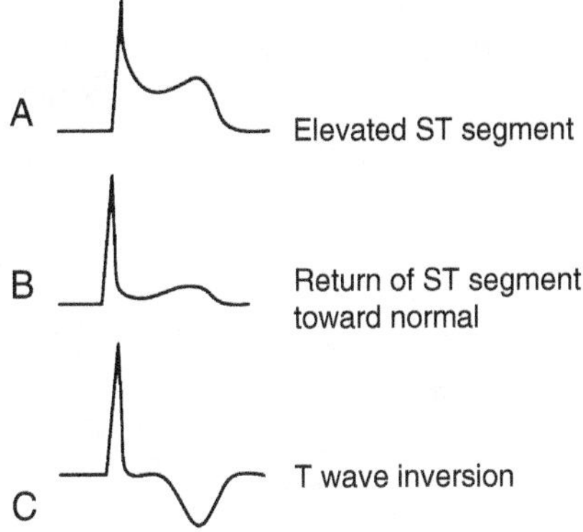

FIG. 2.21
Time-dependent changes of the ST segment and T wave in pericarditis. *(From Park, M. K., & Guntheroth, W. G. (2006).* How to read pediatric ECGs *(4th ed.). Philadelphia: Mosby.)*

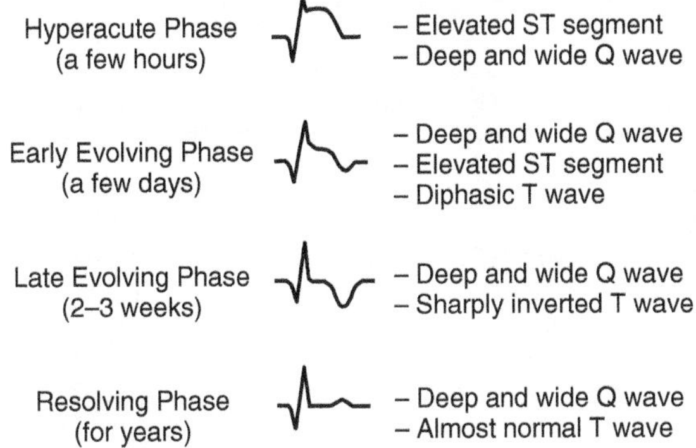

FIG. 2.22
Sequential changes in the ST segment and T wave in myocardial infarction. *(From Park, M. K., & Guntheroth, W. G. (2006).* How to read pediatric ECGs *(4th ed.). Philadelphia: Mosby.)*

(3) The duration of the pathologic Q wave is $\geq$0.04 seconds in adults; it should be at least 0.03 seconds in children.

H. ELECTROLYTE DISTURBANCES

ECG signs of abnormal serum calcium and potassium levels appear in the ST segment and T wave, respectively.

TABLE 2.9

LEADS SHOWING ABNORMAL ECG FINDINGS IN MYOCARDIAL INFARCTION

	LIMB LEADS	PRECORDIAL LEADS
Lateral	I, aVL	V5, V6
Anterior		V1, V2, V3
Anterolateral	I, aVL	V2 through V6
Diaphragmatic	II, III, aVF	
Posterior		V1 through V3[a]

[a]None of the leads is oriented toward the posterior surface of the heart. Therefore ECG changes seen in leads V1 through V3 will be mirror images of expected changes of the infarction (e.g., tall and slightly wide R waves comparable to abnormal Q waves, and tall and wide, symmetric T waves in V1 and V2).

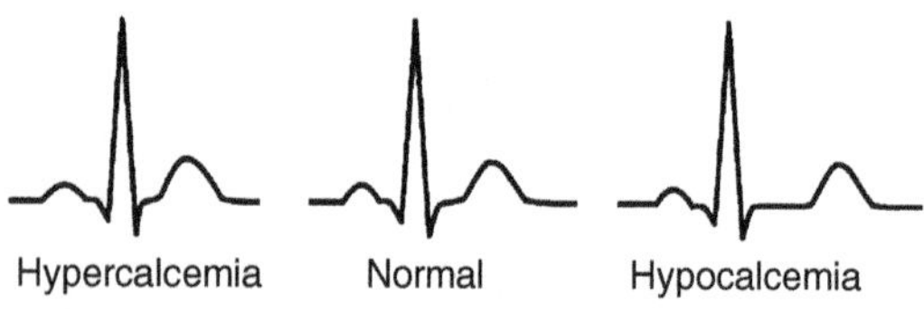

FIG. 2.23

ECG findings of hypercalcemia and hypocalcemia. *(From Park, M. K., & Guntheroth, W. G. (2006).* How to read pediatric ECGs *(4th ed.). Philadelphia: Mosby.)*

1. Calcium
   a. **Hypocalcemia** produces the prolongation of the ST segment, with resulting prolongation of the QTc interval. The T-wave duration remains normal.
   b. **Hypercalcemia** shortens the ST segment without affecting the T wave, with resultant shortening of the QTc interval (Fig. 2.23).
2. Potassium
   a. **Hypokalemia** produces one of the least specific ECG changes.
      (1) When the serum potassium K level is < 2.5 mEq/L, ECG changes consist of a prominent U wave with apparent prolongation of the QTc interval, flat or diphasic T waves, and ST-segment depression (Fig. 2.24).
      (2) With further lowering of serum K, the PR interval becomes prolonged, and sinoatrial block may occur.
   b. **Hyperkalemia.** A progressive hyperkalemia produces the following sequential changes in the ECG (Fig. 2.24). These ECG changes are usually seen best in leads II and III and the left precordial leads.
      (1) Tall, tented T waves, best seen in the precordial leads
      (2) Prolongation of QRS duration

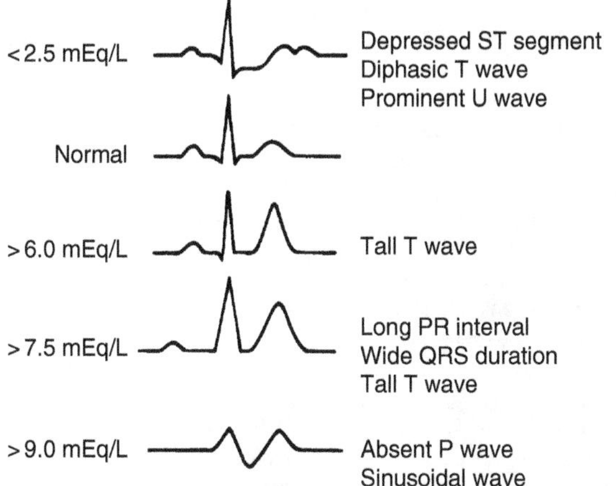

FIG. 2.24

ECG findings of hypokalemia and hyperkalemia. *(From Park, M. K., & Guntheroth, W. G. (2006).* How to read pediatric ECGs *(4th ed.). Philadelphia: Mosby.)*

(3) Prolongation of PR interval
(4) Disappearance of P waves
(5) Wide, bizarre diphasic QRS complexes (sine wave)
(6) Eventual asystole

Chapter 3

Chest Roentgenography

Chest radiography was an essential part of cardiac evaluation before the echocardiographic (echo) studies became widely available to cardiologists. This simple test remains very useful to physicians who do not have access to the echocardiograph. In addition, cardiovascular abnormalities may be incidentally suspected by chest radiographic films.

Information to be gained from chest radiographs includes (1) heart size and silhouette, (2) enlargement of specific cardiac chambers, (3) pulmonary blood flow (PBF) or pulmonary vascular markings (PVM), and (4) other information regarding lung parenchyma, spine, bony thorax, abdominal situs, and so on.

I. HEART SIZE AND SILHOUETTE

1. Heart size: The cardiothoracic (CT) ratio is obtained by dividing the largest transverse diameter of the heart by the widest internal diameter of the chest (Fig. 3.1). The CT ratio is calculated by the following formula.

   $$\text{CT ratio} = (A + B)/C$$

   A CT ratio of more than 0.5 beyond infancy is considered to indicate cardiomegaly. However, the CT ratio cannot be used with any accuracy in neonates and small infants, in whom a good inspiratory chest film is rarely obtained.
2. Normal cardiac silhouette: The structures that form the cardiac borders in the posteroanterior and lateral projections of a chest radiograph are shown in Fig. 3.2. In the neonate, however, a typical normal cardiac silhouette as shown in Fig. 3.2 is rarely seen because of the presence of a large thymus.
3. Abnormal cardiac silhouette: The overall shape of the heart sometimes provides important clues to the type of cardiac defect (Fig. 3.3).
   a. Boot-shaped heart with decreased PVM is seen in infants with cyanotic TOF and in some infants with tricuspid atresia (Fig. 3.3A).
   b. Narrow waist and egg-shaped heart with increased PVM in a cyanotic infant strongly suggest TGA (Fig. 3.3B).
   c. Snowman sign with increased PVM is seen in infants with the supracardiac type of TAPVR (Fig. 3.3C).

II. CARDIAC CHAMBERS AND GREAT ARTERIES

1. Individual chamber enlargement
   a. Left atrial enlargement (LAE): Mild LAE is best recognized in the lateral projection by posterior protrusion of the LA border (Fig. 3.4). An enlargement of the LA may produce a double density on the posteroanterior view of a heavily exposed film. With further

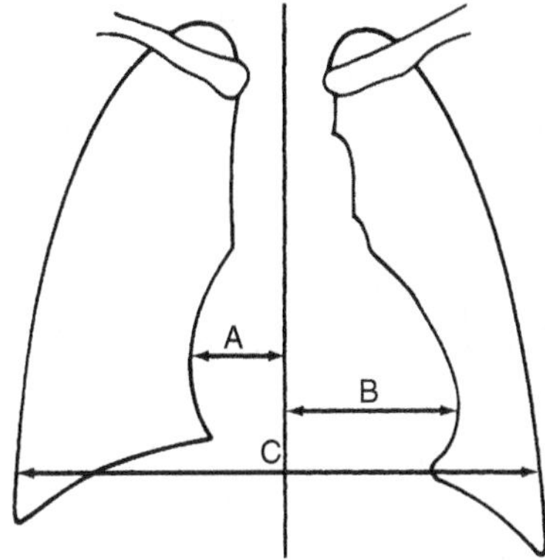

FIG. 3.1

Measurement of the cardiothoracic ratio from the posteroanterior view of a chest radiograph.

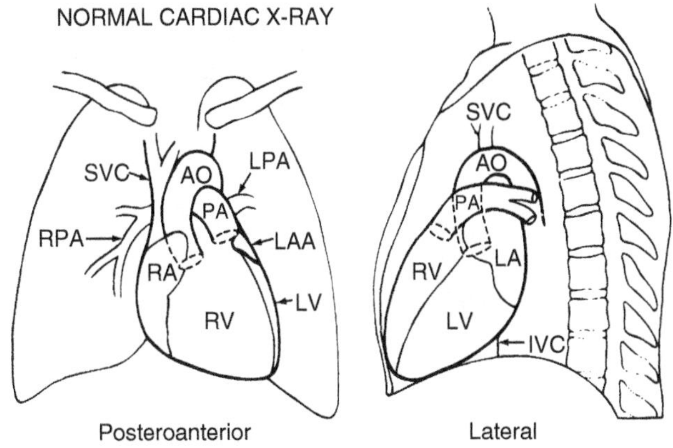

FIG. 3.2

Posteroanterior and lateral projections of normal cardiac silhouette. *(From Park, M. K., & Salamat, M. (2020).* Park's pediatric cardiology for practitioners *(7th ed.). Philadelphia: Mosby.)*

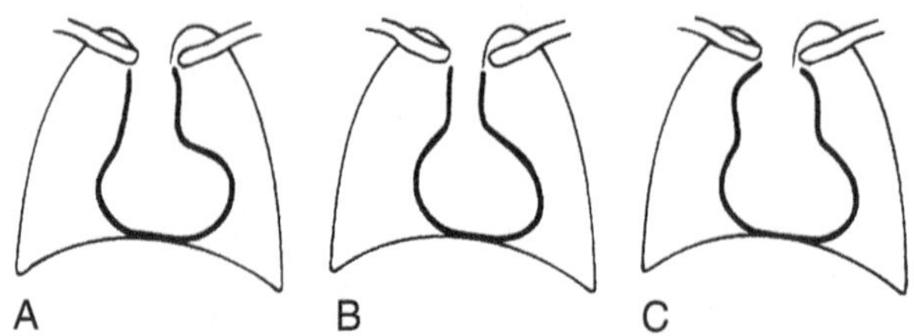

FIG. 3.3
Abnormal cardiac silhouette. (A) Boot-shaped heart. (B) Egg-shaped heart. (C) Snowman sign. *(From Park, M. K., & Salamat, M. (2020).* Park's pediatric cardiology for practitioners *(7th ed.). Philadelphia: Mosby.)*

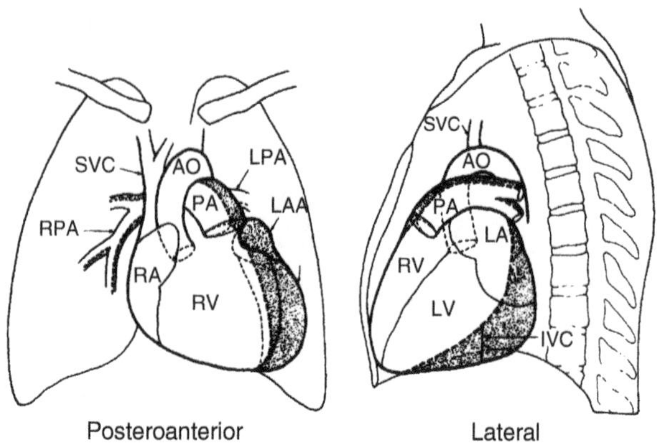

FIG. 3.4
Posteroanterior and lateral view diagrams of chest radiograph demonstrating an enlargement of the LA and LV, as seen in a patient with a moderate VSD. The enlargement of the LA, LV, and main PA and increased pulmonary vascular markings are present.

enlargement, the left atrial appendage becomes prominent on the left cardiac border, and the left main-stem bronchus is elevated.

b. Left ventricular enlargement (LVE): In the posteroanterior view, the apex of the heart is displaced to the left and inferiorly. In the lateral view, the lower posterior cardiac border is displaced further posteriorly (Fig. 3.4).

c. Right atrial enlargement (RAE): In the posteroanterior projection an enlargement of the RA results in an increased prominence of the right lower cardiac border (Fig. 3.5).
d. Right ventricular enlargement (RVE): RVE is best recognized in the lateral view by the filling of the retrosternal space (Fig. 3.5).

2. The size of the great arteries
   a. Prominent main pulmonary artery (MPA) segment in the posteroanterior view is due to one of the following (Fig. 3.6A):
      (1) Poststenotic dilatation (e.g., pulmonary valve stenosis)
      (2) Increased blood flow through the PA (e.g., ASD, VSD)
      (3) Increased pressure in the PA (i.e., pulmonary hypertension)
      (4) Occasional normal adolescence, especially in girls
   b. A concave MPA segment with resulting boot-shaped heart is seen in TOF and tricuspid atresia (Fig. 3.6B).
   c. Dilatation of the aorta. An enlarged ascending aorta (AA) is seen in AS (due to poststenotic dilatation/associated aortopathy) and TOF and less often in PDA, COA, or systemic hypertension. When the ascending aorta and aortic arch are enlarged, the aortic knob (AK) may become prominent on the posteroanterior view (Fig. 3.6C).

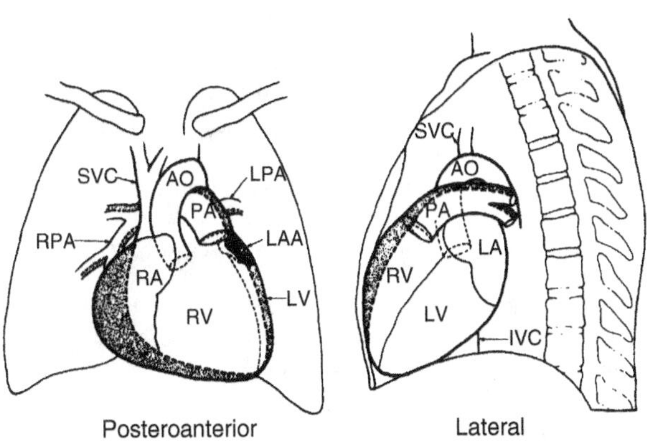

FIG. 3.5
Posteroanterior and lateral view diagrams of chest radiograph demonstrating an enlargement of the RA and RV, as seen in a patient with a large ASD. The pulmonary vascular markings are also increased. The RV enlargement is best seen in the lateral view. *AO,* aorta; *LAA,* left atrial appendage. Other abbreviations are found on pages xi–xiii.

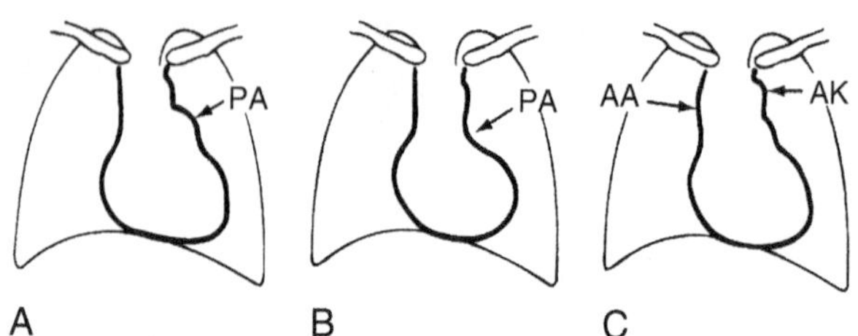

FIG. 3.6

Abnormalities of the great arteries. (A) Prominent main PA segment. (B) Concave PA segment. (C) Dilation of the ascending aorta (*AA*) and prominence of the aortic knob (*AK*). *(From Park, M. K., & Salamat, M. (2020).* Park's pediatric cardiology for practitioners *(7th ed.). Philadelphia: Mosby.)*

III. PULMONARY VASCULAR MARKINGS

One of the major goals of radiologic examination is the assessment of pulmonary blood flow.

1. Increased pulmonary vascular marking (PVM) is present when the pulmonary arteries appear enlarged and extend into the lateral third of the lung field, where they are not usually present, and there is an increased vascularity to the lung apices where the vessels are normally collapsed.
   a. Increased PVM in an acyanotic child suggests a L-R shunt lesion such as ASD, VSD, PDA, ECD, PAPVR, or any combination of these.
   b. In a cyanotic infant, an increased PVM may indicate TGA, TAPVR, HLHS, persistent truncus arteriosus, or single ventricle.
2. A decreased PVM is suspected when the hilum appears small, the remaining lung fields appear black, and the vessels appear small and thin. Ischemic lung fields in cyanotic patients suggest critical stenosis or atresia of the pulmonary or tricuspid valves or TOF.
3. Pulmonary venous congestion, which is characterized by a hazy and indistinct margin of the pulmonary vasculature, is seen with HLHS, MS, TAPVR, cor triatriatum, and so on.
4. Normal pulmonary vasculature is present in patients with mild to moderate PS and in patients with small L-R shunt lesions.

IV. SYSTEMATIC APPROACH

The interpretation of chest radiographs should include a systematic routine to avoid overlooking important anatomic changes relevant to cardiac diagnosis.

1. Location of the liver and stomach gas bubble
   a. The cardiac apex should be on the same side as the stomach or opposite the hepatic shadow.

   b. When there is heterotaxia, with the apex on the right and the stomach on the left, or vice versa, the likelihood of a serious heart defect is great.
   c. A midline liver is associated with asplenia (Ivemark's) syndrome or polysplenia syndrome.

2. Skeletal aspect of chest radiographs
   a. Pectus excavatum may create the false impression of cardiomegaly in the posteroanterior projection.
   b. Thoracic scoliosis and vertebral abnormalities are frequent findings in cardiac patients.
   c. Rib notching is a specific finding of COA in a child usually older than 5 years, generally seen between the fourth and eighth ribs.
3. Identification of the aorta
   a. When the descending aorta is seen on the left of the vertebral column, a left aortic arch is present.
   b. When the descending aorta is seen on the right of the vertebral column, a right arch is present. A right aortic arch is frequently associated with TOF or persistent truncus arteriosus.
   c. A "figure 3" in a heavily exposed film or an E-shaped indentation in a barium esophagogram is seen with COA.
4. Upper mediastinum
   a. The thymus is prominent in healthy infants and may give a false impression of cardiomegaly.
   b. A narrow mediastinal shadow is seen in TGA or DiGeorge syndrome.
   c. A "snowman" sign is seen in infants (usually older than 4 months) with supracardiac type of TAPVR.
5. Pulmonary parenchyma
   a. A long-standing density, particularly in the right lower lung field, suggests bronchopulmonary sequestration.
   b. A vertical vascular shadow along the right lower cardiac border may suggest PAPVR from the lower lobe (the scimitar syndrome).

PART II

SPECIAL TOOLS USED IN CARDIAC EVALUATION

A number of special tools are available to the cardiologist in the evaluation of cardiac patients. Noncardiologists have the opportunity to be exposed to some noninvasive tools, such as echocardiography, exercise stress test, and ambulatory ECG (e.g., Holter monitor). Magnetic resonance imaging (MRI) and computed tomography (CT) are other noninvasive tools that have become popular in recent years. Cardiac catheterization and angiocardiography are invasive tests. Although catheter intervention procedures are not diagnostic, they are included in this section because they are usually performed with cardiac catheterization.

Chapter 4

Noninvasive Imaging Tools

4

I. ECHOCARDIOGRAPHY

Echocardiography (echo) is an extremely useful noninvasive test used in the diagnosis and management of heart disease. An echo study currently begins with real-time two-dimensional echo (2D echo), which produces high-resolution tomographic images of cardiac structures and their movement, and vascular structures leaving and entering the heart. With the support of Doppler and color flow mapping (as described later), echo studies provide reliable anatomic and quantitative information, such as ventricular function, pressure gradients across cardiac valves and blood vessels, and estimation of pressures in the great arteries and ventricles.

A. TWO-DIMENSIONAL ECHOCARDIOGRAPHY

Routine 2D echo is obtained from four transducer locations: parasternal, apical, subcostal, and suprasternal notch positions. Abdominal and subclavicular views are also useful. Figs. 4.1 through 4.9 illustrate selected standard 2D echo images of the heart and great vessels. A brief description of the standard 2D echo views follows.

1. Parasternal long-axis views (Fig. 4.1)
    a. The standard long-axis view (Fig.4.1A).
        (1) This is a very important view in evaluating abnormalities in or near the mitral valve, LA, LV, LVOT, aortic valve, aortic root, ascending aorta, and ventricular septum.
        (2) In the normal heart there is aortic-mitral continuity (i.e., the anterior mitral leaflet is contiguous with the posterior wall of the aorta).
        (3) The right and noncoronary cusps of the aortic valve are imaged but the left coronary sinus (CS) cusp is out of this plane.
        (4) VSDs of TOF and persistent truncus arteriosus are readily seen adjacent to the aortic valve.
        (5) The anterior and posterior leaflets of the mitral valve and their chordal and papillary muscle attachments are imaged. MVP is best evaluated in this view.
        (6) The CS is seen frequently as a small circle in the atrioventricular groove. An enlarged CS may suggest left SVC, TAPVR to CS, coronary AV fistula, and rarely elevated RA pressure.
        (7) Pericardial effusion is readily seen in this view.

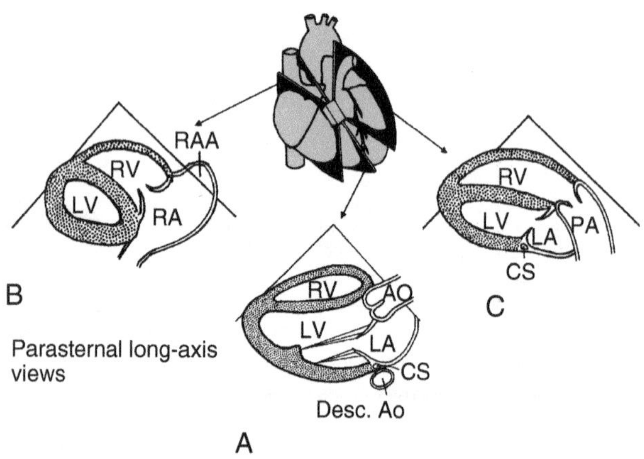

FIG. 4.1

Diagram of important two-dimensional echo views obtained from the parasternal long-axis transducer position. (A) Standard long-axis view. (B) RV inflow view. (C) RV outflow view. *AO,* aorta; *CS,* coronary sinus; *Desc. Ao,* descending aorta; *LA,* left atrium; *LV,* left ventricle; *PA,* pulmonary artery; *RA,* right atrium; *RAA,* right atrial appendage; *RV,* right ventricle. *(From Park, M. K., & Salamat, M. (2020).* Park's pediatric cardiology for practitioners *(7th ed.). Philadelphia: Mosby.)*

b. The RV inflow view (Fig. 4.1B).
   (1) This view shows abnormalities of the RA cavity, RV inflow, and the tricuspid valve.
   (2) Abnormalities in the tricuspid valve (regurgitation, prolapse) are evaluated. It is a good view to record the velocity of the TR jet (to estimate RV systolic pressure).
   (3) The ventricular septum near the tricuspid valve (TV) is the inlet muscular septum; the remainder is the trabecular septum.
   (4) The right atrial appendage (RAA) can also be imaged in this view.
c. The RV outflow view (Fig. 4.1C).
   (1) Abnormalities in the RVOT, pulmonary valve, and main PA are readily imaged and their severity easily estimated.
   (2) The supracristal infundibular (outlet) septum is seen near the pulmonary valve.

2. Parasternal short-axis views: These views evaluate the aortic valve, coronary arteries, mitral valve, and papillary muscles.
   a. The aortic valve level (Fig. 4.2A).
      (1) The normal aortic valve has a circle with a tri-leaflet aortic valve that has the appearance of the letter Y during diastole.

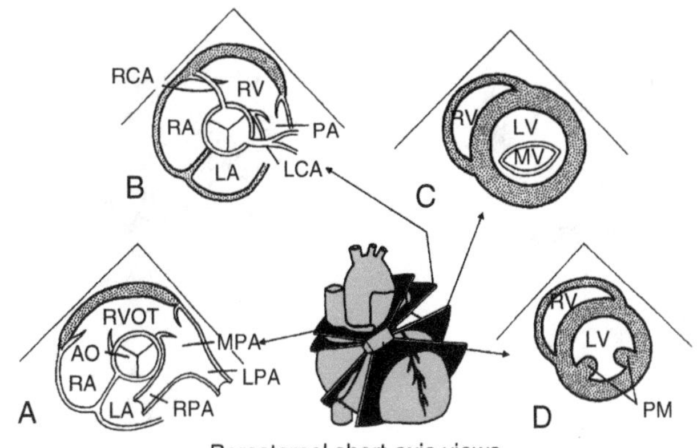

FIG. 4.2

Diagram of a family of parasternal short-axis views. (A) Semilunar valves and great arteries level. (B) Coronary artery level. (C) Mitral valve level. (D) Papillary muscle level. *AO,* aorta; *LA,* left atrium; *LCA,* left coronary artery; *LPA,* left pulmonary artery; *LV,* left ventricle; *MPA,* main pulmonary artery; *MV,* mitral valve; *PA,* pulmonary artery; *PM,* papillary muscle; *RA,* right atrium; *RCA,* right coronary artery; *RPA,* right pulmonary artery; *RV,* right ventricle; *RVOT,* right ventricular outflow tract. *(From Park, M. K., & Salamat, M. (2020).* Park's pediatric cardiology for practitioners *(7th ed.). Philadelphia: Mosby.)*

Abnormalities of the aortic valve (bicuspid, unicuspid, or dysplastic) are evaluated in this view.

(2) Stenoses of the pulmonary valve and PA branches can be evaluated by Doppler and color flow mapping.
(3) PDA is interrogated with color flow imaging and Doppler study.
(4) The membranous VSD is seen just distal to the tricuspid valve (at the 10-o'clock position).
(5) Both the infracristal and supracristal outlet VSDs are imaged anterior to the aortic valve near the pulmonary valve (at the 12- to 2-o'clock position).

b. Coronary arteries (Fig. 4.2B).
   (1) The right coronary artery (CA) arises from the anterior coronary cusp.
   (2) The left main CA arises in the left coronary cusp near the main PA. Its bifurcation into the left anterior descending and circumflex coronary artery is usually imaged.
   (3) The dimension of the coronary arteries is measured in this view (see Table D.6 in Appendix D).

c. The mitral valve. The mitral valve is seen as a "fish mouth" during diastole (Fig. 4.2C).

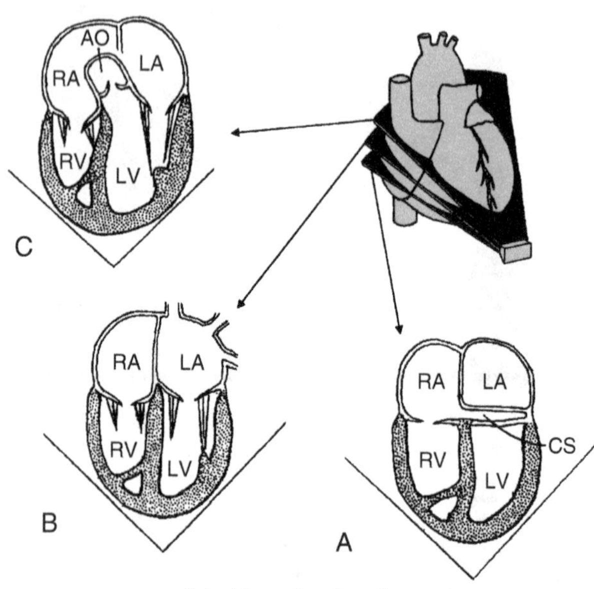

FIG. 4.3

Diagram of two-dimensional echo views obtained with the transducer at the apical position. (A) The posterior plane view. (B) The standard apical four-chamber view. (C) The apical "five-chamber" view. *AO*, aorta; *CS*, coronary sinus; *LA*, left atrium; *LV*, left ventricle; *RA*, right atrium; RV, right ventricle. *(From Park, M. K., & Salamat, M. (2020).* Park's pediatric cardiology for practitioners *(7th ed.). Philadelphia: Mosby.)*

d. Papillary muscles (Fig. 42D).
   (1) Two papillary muscles are normally seen at the 4-o'clock (anterolateral) and 8-o'clock (posteromedial) positions. Occasionally, accessory papillary muscles or left ventricular strands are imaged in the normal heart.
   (2) The ventricular septum seen at this level is the trabecular septum.

3. Apical four-chamber views (Fig. 4.3).
   a. The CS (Fig. 4.3A) is seen in the most posterior plane. The ventricular septum seen in this view is the posterior trabecular septum.
   b. The middle plane of the apical four-chamber view (Fig. 4.3B).
      (1) This view is good to evaluate the atrial and ventricular chambers, such as relative size and contractility of atrial and

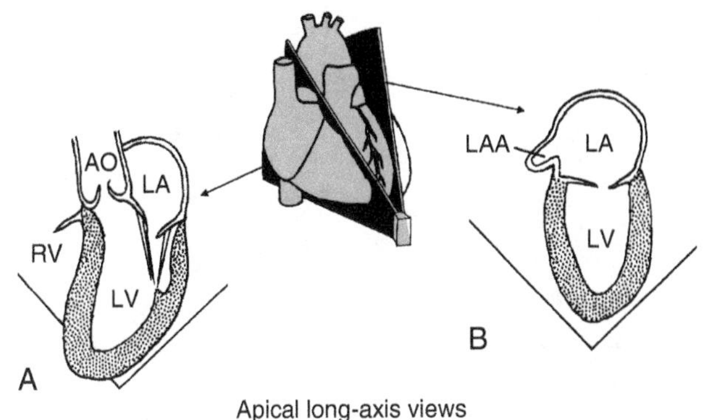

FIG. 4.4

Apical long-axis views. (A) Apical "three-chamber" view. (B) Apical "two-chamber" view. *AO,* aorta; *LA,* left atrium; *LAA,* left atrial appendage; *LV,* left ventricle; *RV,* right ventricle. *(From Park, M. K., & Salamat, M. (2020).* Park's pediatric cardiology for practitioners *(7th ed.). Philadelphia: Mosby.)*

ventricular chambers, AV valve abnormalities, and images of some pulmonary veins.

(2) Anatomic right and left ventricles can be identified in this view.
   (a) Normally the TV insertion to the septum is more apicalward than the mitral valve (5–10 mm in older children and adults). The ventricle attached to the TV is the RV. (The TV insertion is displaced more apically in Ebstein anomaly.)
   (b) The anatomic RV is also heavily trabeculated and has the moderator band, while the LV is smooth walled without prominent muscle bundles.

(3) The inlet ventricular septum (where an ECD occurs) is imaged just under the AV valves; the remainder of the septum is the trabecular septum. (The membranous septum is *not* imaged in this view.)

(4) The presence and severity of regurgitation of both AV valves are evaluated in this view.

(5) The inflow velocities of both the mitral and tricuspid valves are measured here.

(6) The TR jet velocity is measured (to estimate RV systolic pressure).

(7) Abnormal chordal attachment of the atrioventricular valve (straddling) and overriding of the septum are also noted in this view.

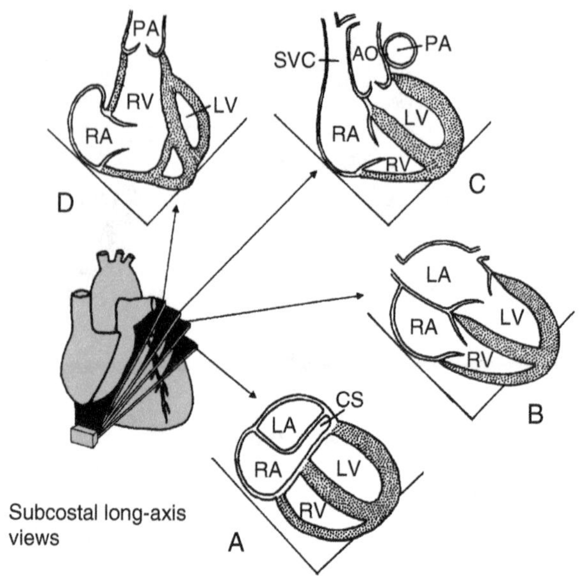

FIG. 4.5

Diagram of subcostal long-axis views. (A) Coronary sinus view posteriorly. (B) Standard subcostal four-chamber view. (C) View showing the LV outflow tract and the proximal aorta. (D) View showing the RV outflow tract and the proximal main pulmonary artery. *AO*, aorta; *CS*, coronary sinus; *LA*, left atrium; *LV*, left ventricle; *PA*, pulmonary artery; *RA*, right atrium; *RV*, right ventricle; *SVC*, superior vena cava. *(From Park, M. K., & Salamat, M. (2020).* Park's pediatric cardiology for practitioners *(7th ed.). Philadelphia: Mosby.)*

c. The apical "five-chamber" view (Fig. 4.3C) is obtained by further anterior angulation of the transducer.
   (1) The LVOT, aortic valve, subaortic area, and proximal ascending aorta are shown in this view.
   (2) Stenosis and regurgitation of the aortic valve and the anatomy of the LV outflow tract (including subaortic membrane) are best evaluated in this view.
   (3) The membranous VSD is visualized just under the aortic valve.

4. Apical long-axis views (Fig. 4.4A)
   a. The apical long-axis view (or apical three-chamber view) shows structures similar to those seen in the parasternal long-axis view.
   b. The apical two-chamber view (Fig. 4.4B).
      (1) The LA, mitral valve, and LV are imaged. The left atrial appendage (LAA) can also be imaged.

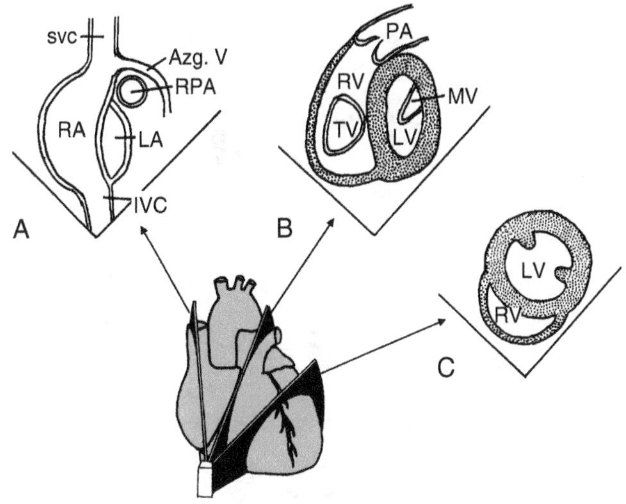

FIG. 4.6

Subcostal short-axis (sagittal) views. (A) Entry of venae cavae with drainage of the azygos vein. (B) View showing the RV, RV outflow tract, and pulmonary artery. (C) Short-axis view of the ventricles. *Azg. V,* azygos vein; *LA,* left atrium; *LV,* left ventricle; *MV,* mitral valve; *PA,* pulmonary artery; *RA,* right atrium; *RPA,* right pulmonary artery; *RV,* right ventricle; *SVC,* superior vena cava; *TV,* tricuspid valve. *(From Park, M. K., & Salamat, M. (2020).* Park's pediatric cardiology for practitioners *(7th ed.). Philadelphia: Mosby.)*

(2) The view of the LV apex provides diagnostic clues for cardiomyopathy, apical thrombus, and aneurysm.

5. Subcostal Long-Axis (Coronal) Views (Fig. 4.5): These views are shown from posterior to anterior direction.
   a. The CS is seen posteriorly (Fig. 4.5A). This plane shows structures similar to those shown in Fig. 4.3A.
   b. The standard subcostal four-chamber view (Fig. 4.5B) is obtained by anterior angulation. This view emphasizes the atrial septum and its morphologic features, including the atrial septal defect and atrial septal aneurysm.
   c. Further anterior angulation (Fig. 4.5C) shows the LV outflow tract, aortic valve, and ascending aorta.
   d. Further anterior angulation (Fig. 4.5D) shows the entire RV (including the inlet, trabecular, and infundibular portions), the pulmonary valve, and the main pulmonary artery. Stenosis of the

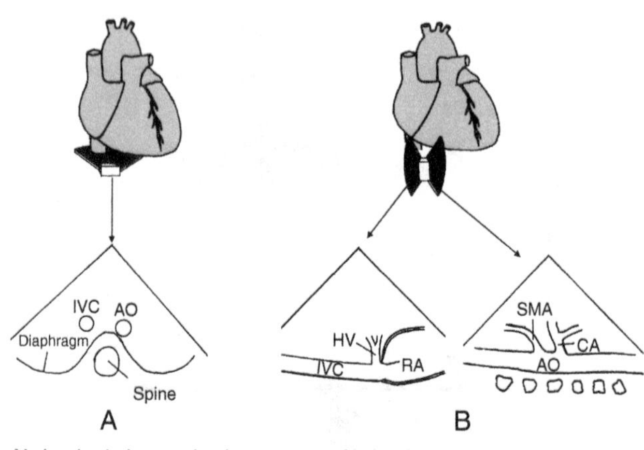

FIG. 4.7

Subcostal abdominal views. Left, abdominal short-axis view. Right, abdominal long-axis view. (A) IVC view. (B) Abdominal descending aorta view. *AO*, aorta; *CA*, celiac axis; *HV*, hepatic vein; *IVC*, inferior vena cava; *RA*, right atrium; *SMA*, superior mesenteric artery. *(From Park, M. K., & Salamat, M. (2020).* Park's pediatric cardiology for practitioners *(7th ed.). Philadelphia: Mosby.)*

pulmonary valve and the anatomy of the RV outflow tract can be evaluated in this view.

e. Four parts of the ventricular septum can be imaged from this transducer position: trabecular (in A), inlet (in B), membranous (in C, under the aortic valve), and subarterial infundibular septum (in D) (see Fig. 7.7 for location of different types of VSD).

6. Subcostal short-axis (or sagittal) views (Fig. 4.6)
   a. Fig. 4.6A:
      (1) Both the SVC and IVC are seen to connect to the RA.
      (2) A small azygos vein and the right PA can also be seen in this view.
      (3) In patients with ASD, the size of the posterosuperior (PS) and postero-inferior (PI) rims of atrial septal defect is measured in this view.
   b. A leftward angulation (Fig. 4.6B) shows the RV outflow tract, pulmonary valve, and pulmonary artery. The tricuspid valve is seen on end.
   c. Further leftward angulation (Fig. 4.6C) shows views similar to the parasternal short-axis view (Fig. 4.2D).

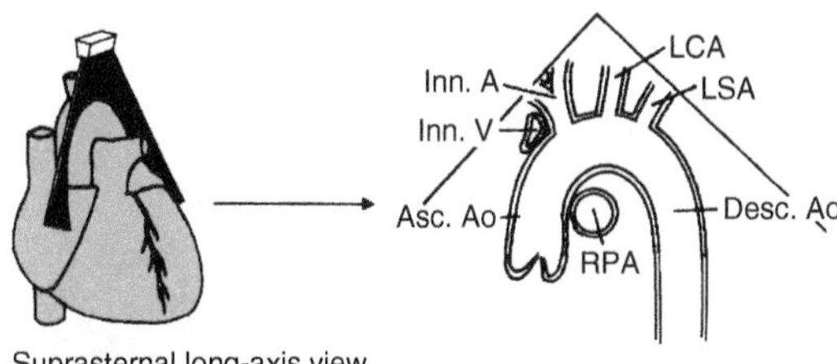

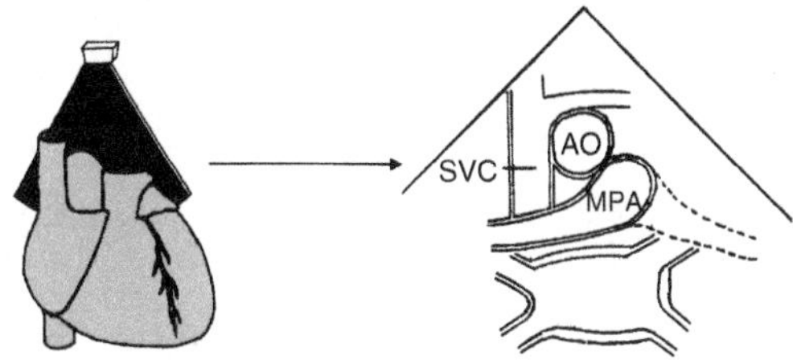

FIG. 4.8

Diagram of suprasternal notch two-dimensional echo views. *Upper panel:* Long-axis view. *Lower panel:* Short-axis view. *AO,* aorta; *Asc. Ao,* ascending aorta; *Desc. Ao,* descending aorta; *Inn. A,* innominate artery; *Inn. V,* innominate vein; *LA,* left atrium; *LCA,* left carotid artery; *LSA,* left subclavian artery; *MPA,* main pulmonary artery; *PA,* pulmonary artery; RPA, right pulmonary artery; *SVC,* superior vena cava. *(From Park, M. K., & Salamat, M. (2020).* Park's pediatric cardiology for practitioners *(7th ed.). Philadelphia: Mosby.)*

7. Subcostal views of the abdomen
   a. Abdominal short-axis view (left panel of Fig. 4.7A).
      (1) This view shows the descending aorta on the left and the IVC on the right of the spine. The aorta should pulsate.
      (2) Both hemidiaphragms are seen, which move symmetrically with respiration. (Asymmetric or paradoxical movement of the diaphragm is seen with paralysis of the hemidiaphragm).
   b. Abdominal long-axis views (right panel of Fig. 4.7B).
      (1) Left panel of Fig. 4.7B
         (a) The IVC is imaged longitudinally to the right of the spine.
         (b) The IVC collects the hepatic vein (HV) before draining into the RA. The failure of the IVC to join the RA indicates interruption of the IVC (with azygous continuation), which is seen in polysplenia syndrome.
         (c) The eustachian valve may be seen at the junction of the IVC and the RA.

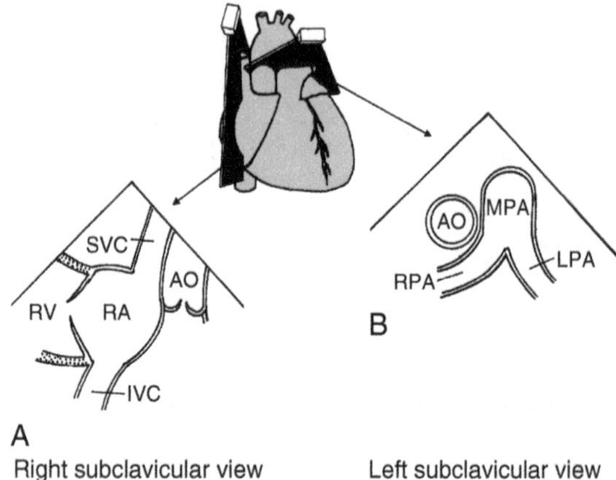

FIG. 4.9

Diagram of subclavicular views. (A) Right subclavicular view. (B) Left subclavicular view. *AO,* aorta; *IVC,* inferior vena cava; *LPA,* left pulmonary artery; *MPA,* main pulmonary artery; *RA,* right atrium; *RPA,* right pulmonary artery; *RV,* right ventricle; *SVC,* superior vena cava. *(From Park, M. K., & Salamat, M. (2020).* Park's pediatric cardiology for practitioners *(7th ed.). Philadelphia: Mosby.)*

(2) Right panel of Fig. 4.7B
   (a) The descending aorta is imaged longitudinally to the left of the spine.
   (b) The celiac artery (CA) and the superior mesenteric artery (SMA) are easily imaged.
   (c) A pulsed wave Doppler examination of the abdominal aorta in this view is helpful in identifying the coarctation by demonstrating delayed rate of systolic upstroke and persistent diastolic flow.

8. Suprasternal long-axis view (upper panel of Fig. 4.8)
   a. This view images the entire (left) aortic arch. Failure to visualize the aortic arch in the usual manner may suggest the presence of a right aortic arch.
   b. Three arteries arising from the aortic arch are the innominate (or brachiocephalic), left carotid, and left subclavian arteries.
   c. The innominate vein is seen in front of and the right PA is seen behind the ascending aorta.
   d. Good images of the isthmus and upper descending aorta are very important to diagnose coarctation of the aorta.
   e. Doppler studies with the cursor placed proximal and distal to the coarctation are important in estimating the severity of the narrowing.

9. Suprasternal short-axis view (lower panel of Fig. 4.8)
   a. The SVC is seen to the right of the circular transverse aorta. The innominate vein is seen superior to the circular aorta.
   b. The right PA is seen in its length under the circular aorta.
   c. The left innominate vein can be imaged, which arises from the SVC and traverses superior to the circular aorta.
   d. Beneath the right PA is the LA. Four pulmonary veins are imaged with a slight posterior angulation.
10. The subclavicular views
    a. The right subclavicular view (Fig. 4.9A). This view is useful in the assessment of the SVC and the RA junction as well as the ascending aorta.
    b. The left subclavicular view (Fig. 4.9B). This view is useful for examination of the branch pulmonary arteries.
11. *Quantitative dimension of cardiovascular structures from 2D echo studies:* Selected normal dimensions of cardiac structures and the great arteries are presented in Appendix D. These tables are frequently used in practice of pediatric cardiology. They include M-mode measurements of the LV (Table D.1); stand-alone M-mode measurements of the RV, aorta, and LA (Table D.4); two-dimensional measurements of aortic root and aorta (Table D.5). Normal dimensions of coronary arteries are shown in Table D.6.

B. M-MODE ECHOCARDIOGRAPHY

The M-mode echo provides an "ice pick" view of the heart. It has limited capability in demonstrating the spatial relationship of structures but remains an important tool in the evaluation of certain cardiac conditions and functions, particularly by measurements of dimensions and timing. It is usually performed as part of 2D echo studies.

1. M-mode echo recording (Fig. 4.10)
   a. Line 1 passes through the aorta (AO) and LA, where the dimensions of these structures are measured.
   b. Line 2 traverses the mitral valve. Anterior and posterior mitral valve motion is recorded for analysis.
   c. Line 3 goes through the main body of the RV and LV. Along line 3, the dimensions of the RV and LV and the thickness of the interventricular septum and LV posterior wall are measured during systole and diastole. Pericardial effusion is best detected on line 3.
2. **Cardiac Chamber Dimensions.** Most dimensions are measured during diastole, coincident with the onset of the QRS complex; the LA dimension and LV systolic dimension are exceptions (see Fig. 4.10). Normal values are shown as a function of growth (see Appendix D).
3. **Left Ventricular Systolic Function.** LV systolic function is evaluated by the fractional shortening (or shortening fraction) or ejection fraction.

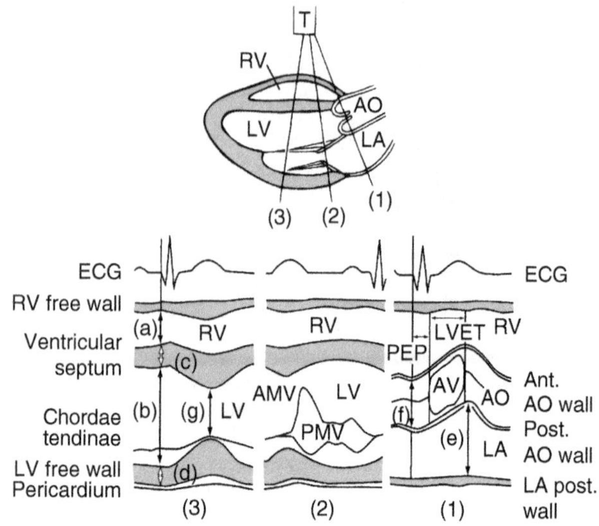

FIG. 4.10

Examples of M-mode recording and measurement of cardiac dimensions. The dimension of the aorta (*AO*) and left atrium (*LA*) is measured along line (1). Line (2) passes through the mitral valve and records the movement of the anterior and posterior mitral leaflets. Measurement of chamber dimensions and wall thickness of right and left ventricles is made along line (3). The following measurements are shown in this figure: (a), right ventricular (RV) dimension; (b), left ventricular (*LV*) diastolic dimension; (c), interventricular septal thickness; (d), LV posterior wall thickness; (e), LA dimension; (f), aortic dimension; (g), LV systolic dimension. *AMV*, anterior mitral valve; *Ant.*, anterior; *ECG*, electrocardiogram; *LVET*, left ventricular ejection time; *PMV*, posterior mitral valve; *Post.*, posterior; *T*, transducer. *(From Park, M. K., & Salamat, M. (2020).* Park's pediatric cardiology for practitioners *(7th ed.). Philadelphia: Mosby.)*

a. **Fractional shortening** (or shortening fraction) is derived by the following formula:

$$FS\ (\%) = Dd - Ds/Dd \times 100$$

where FS is fractional shortening, Dd is end-diastolic dimension of the LV, and Ds is end-systolic dimension of the LV. This is a reliable and reproducible index of LV function, provided there is no regional wall-motion abnormality and there is concentric contractility of the LV.

(1) Mean normal value of FS is 36%, with 95% prediction limits of 28% to 44%.

(2) Fractional shortening is decreased in a poorly compensated LV regardless of cause (e.g., pressure overload, volume overload, primary myocardial disorders, and doxorubicin cardiotoxicity).

(3) FS is increased in some volume-overloaded ventricles (e.g., VSD, PDA, AR, and MR) and HCM.

(4) If the interventricular septal motion is flat or paradoxical, the shortening fraction will not accurately reflect ventricular ejection.

b. **Ejection fraction** relates to the change in volume of the LV with cardiac contraction. It is obtained by the following formula:

$$EF\ (\%) = (Dd)^3 - (Ds)^3/(Dd)^3 \times 100,$$

where EF is the ejection fraction and Dd and Ds are end-diastolic and end-systolic dimensions, respectively, of the LV.

(1) Normal mean ejection fraction is 66% with ranges of 56% to 78%.

(2) The ejection fraction is a derivative of the fractional shortening and offers no advantages over the fractional shortening. In the previous formula, the minor axis is assumed to be half of the major axis of the LV; this assumption is incorrect in children.

C. COLOR FLOW MAPPING

A color-coded Doppler provides images of the direction and disturbances of blood flow superimposed on the echo structural image. In general, red is used to indicate flow toward the transducer and blue is used to indicate flow away from the transducer. A turbulent flow appears as light green. This is useful in the detection of shunt or valvular lesions. Color may not appear when the direction of flow is perpendicular to the ultrasound beam.

D. DOPPLER ECHOCARDIOGRAPHY

A Doppler echo combines the study of cardiac structure and blood flow profiles. Doppler ultrasound equipment detects frequency shifts and thus determines the direction and velocity of blood flow with respect to the ultrasound beam. By convention, velocities of red blood cells moving toward the transducer are displayed above a zero baseline; those moving away from the transducer are displayed below the baseline. The Doppler echo is usually used with color flow mapping to enhance the technique's usefulness.

1. The two commonly used Doppler techniques are continuous wave (CW) and pulsed wave (PW).
   a. The PW technique emits a short burst of ultrasound, and the Doppler echo receiver "listens" for returning information. The PW Doppler can control the site at which the Doppler signals are sampled, but the maximal detectable velocity is limited, making it unusable for quantification of severe obstruction.

TABLE 4.1

NORMAL DOPPLER VELOCITIES IN CHILDREN AND ADULTS: MEAN (RANGES) (M/SEC)

	CHILDREN	ADULTS
Mitral flow	1.0 (0.8–1.3)	0.9 (0.6–1.3)
Tricuspid flow	0.6 (0.5–0.8)	0.6 (0.3–0.7)
Pulmonary artery	0.9 (0.7–1.1)	0.75 (0.6–0.9)
Left ventricle	1.0 (0.7–1.2)	0.9 (0.7–1.1)
Aorta	1.5 (1.2–1.8)	1.35 (1.0–1.7)

From Hatle, L., & Angelsen, B. (1985). *Doppler ultrasound in cardiology* (2nd ed.). Philadelphia: Lea & Febiger.

   b. The CW technique emits a constant ultrasound beam with one crystal, and another crystal continuously receives returning information. The CW Doppler can measure extremely high velocities (e.g., for the estimation of severe stenosis), but it cannot localize the site of the sampling; rather, it picks up the signal anywhere along the Doppler beam.
   c. When these two techniques are used in combination, clinical application expands.
2. Normal Doppler velocities in children and adults are shown in Table 4.1.
   a. Normal Doppler velocity is less than 1 m/sec for the pulmonary valve, but it may be up to 1.8 m/sec for the ascending and descending aortas.
   b. Doppler studies from the AVs. Doppler tracings from the mitral and tricuspid valves provide some indices of ventricular diastolic function. They are obtained from the apical four-chamber view with the Doppler sample volume placed in the valve orifices. There are two flow waves in the AV valves; the E wave (occurring during the early diastolic filling phase) and A wave (occurring during atrial contraction) (Fig. 4.11).
      (1) Normally, the E wave is taller than the A wave, except for the first 3 weeks of life, during which the A wave may be taller than the E wave.
      (2) Normal mitral Doppler indices (for children and young adults) are as follows (mean $\pm$ SD). The average peak E velocity is 0.73 ± 0.09 m/sec, the average peak A velocity is 0.38 ± 0.089 m/sec, and the average E:A velocity ratio is 2.0 ± 0.5.
      (3) With stenosis of the atrioventricular valves, the flow velocities of the E and A waves increase.
3. Measurement of pressure gradients
   a. The simplified Bernoulli equation is used to estimate the pressure gradient across a stenotic lesion, regurgitant lesion, or shunt lesion. One of the following equations may be used.

$$P_1 - P_2 \text{ (mm Hg)} = 4(V2^2 - V1^2)$$
$$P_1 - P_2 \text{ (mm Hg)} = 4(V \text{ max})^2,$$

where ($P_1 - P_2$) is the pressure difference across an obstruction, V_1 is the velocity (m/sec) proximal to the obstruction, and V_2 is the velocity (m/sec) distal to the obstruction in the first equation. When V1 is less than 1 m/sec, it can be ignored, as in the second equation. However, when V_1 is more than 1.5 m/sec, it should be incorporated in the equation to obtain a more accurate estimation of pressure gradients. This is important in the study of the ascending and descending aortas (for possible coarctation) where flow velocities are often more than 1.5 m/sec. Ignoring V_1 may significantly overestimate pressure gradient in patients with AS or coarctation of the aorta.

b. The pressure gradient calculated from the Bernoulli equation is the peak instantaneous pressure gradient, *not* the peak-to-peak pressure gradient measured during cardiac catheterization. The peak instantaneous pressure gradient is generally larger than the peak-to-peak pressure gradient. The difference between the two is more noticeable in patients with mild to moderate obstruction and less apparent in patients with severe obstruction.

4. **Estimation of Intracardiac or Intravascular Pressures.** The Doppler echo allows estimation of pressures in the RV, PA, and LV using the flow velocity of valvular or shunt jets. The following are some examples of such applications.
   a. RV (or PA) systolic pressure (SP) can be estimated from the velocity of the tricuspid regurgitation (TR) jet, if present, by the following equation:

$$\text{RVSP (or PASP)} = 4(V)^2 + \text{RA Pressure},$$

   where V is the TR jet velocity. For example, if the TR velocity is 2.0 m/sec, the instantaneous pressure gradient is $4 \times (2.0)^2 = 4 \times 4.0 = 16$ mm Hg. In most children and adolescents, using an assumed RA pressure of 5 mm Hg, the RV systolic pressure (or PA systolic pressure in the absence of pulmonary stenosis) will come out to be 21 mm Hg.

   b. RV (or PA) systolic pressure can also be estimated from the velocity of the VSD jet by the following equation:

$$\text{RVSP (or PASP)} = \text{Systemic SP (or arm SP)} - 4(V)^2,$$

where V is the VSD jet. For example, if the VSD jet flow velocity is 3 m/sec, the instantaneous pressure drop between the LV and RV is $4 \times 3^2 = 36$ mm Hg. That is, the RV systolic pressure is 36 mm Hg lower than the LV systolic pressure. If the arm systolic blood pressure is

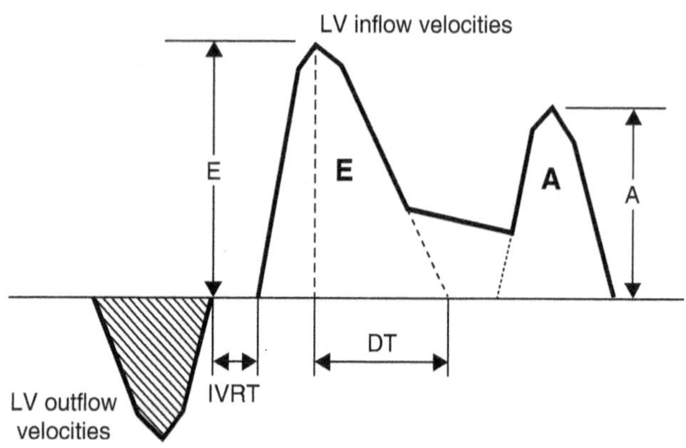

FIG. 4.11

Selected parameters of diastolic function (see text for discussion). *A,* A wave; *DT,* deceleration time; *E,* E wave; *IVRT,* isovolumic relaxation time; *LV,* left ventricle. *(From Park, M. K., & Salamat, M. (2020).* Park's pediatric cardiology for practitioners *(7th ed.). Philadelphia: Mosby.)*

90 mm Hg (which is close to but usually higher than the LV systolic pressure), the RV pressure is estimated to be 90 − 36 = 54 mm Hg. In the absence of PS, the PA systolic pressure will be approximately 54 mm Hg.

5. **Diastolic Function.** As discussed earlier in this chapter, using mitral inflow velocities obtained in the apical four-chamber view, LV diastolic function can be evaluated (Fig. 4.11). Although LV diastolic dysfunction is easy to find, it is usually nonspecific and does not provide independent diagnostic information. Normal values for children and the two well-known patterns of abnormal diastolic function (a decreased relaxation pattern and a "restrictive" pattern) are shown in Fig. 11.2).

II. OTHER ECHOCARDIOGRAPHIC TECHNIQUES

Fetal echo, transesophageal echo, intravascular echo, and tissue Doppler echo are examples of other echo technique. These are briefly summarized.

A.FETAL ECHOCARDIOGRAPHY

Improvement in image resolution has made it possible to visualize fetal CV structure possible, thereby permitting in utero diagnosis of CV anomalies. The optimal timing for performance of a comprehensive transabdominal fetal echo is 18 to 22 weeks of gestation. Images can be more difficult to obtain after 30 weeks of gestation.

Indications for fetal echo are expanding. Increased nuchal translucency present on obstetrical ultrasound at 10 to 13 weeks' gestation has been associated with an increased risk of CHD, even in the absence of chromosomal anomaly. Infants conceived via intracytoplasmic sperm injection and in vitro fertilization have up to a threefold increase in the prevalence of CHDs.

B.TRANSESOPHAGEAL ECHOCARDIOGRAPHY (TEE)

High-quality 2D images can be obtained by way of the esophagus by placing a 2D or multiplane transducer at the end of a flexible endoscope. It may be indicated when satisfactory images of the CV structure are not possible by the usual transthoracic approach, such as those with obesity or chronic obstructive pulmonary disease. The TEE is especially helpful in assessing thrombus in native or prosthetic valves, endocarditis vegetation, thrombi in the left atrium, and aortic dissection. TEE is often used during cardiac surgery to monitor LV function during the surgery as well as to assess cardiac morphology before and after surgical repair. TEE requires general anesthesia or sedation and the presence of an anesthesiologist.

C.INTRAVASCULAR ECHOCARDIOGRAPHY

To provide an intravascular echo, the ultrasonic transducer is placed in a small catheter so that vessels can be imaged by means of the lumen. These devices can evaluate atherosclerotic arteries in adults and coronary artery stenosis or aneurysm in children with Kawasaki's disease.

D.TISSUE DOPPLER ECHOCARDIOGRAPHY

While the conventional Doppler echo assesses the direction and the velocity of blood flow, tissue Doppler echo assesses the velocity of myocardial tissue movement by setting the tissue point at any arbitrary point, such as the annulus of the AV valve. Tissue Doppler echo can be used to study LV systolic or diastolic function.

III. RADIOLOGIC TECHNIQUES

Although the conventional echo study remains the mainstay of noninvasive evaluation of cardiac patients, it has limitations. In addition to being operator dependent, echocardiography may not provide optimal quality of images of CV structures due to postoperative scars, chest wall deformities, overlying lung tissue, large body size in adolescents, and obesity. In particular, extracardiac structures, such as the pulmonary arteries, pulmonary veins, and aortic arch, cannot always be adequately imaged by echo study due to acoustic window limitations. As for the coronary arteries, only the proximal portion can be adequately imaged by echo studies.

BOX 4.1

ADVANTAGES AND DISADVANTAGES OF MRI AND CT

	ADVANTAGES	DISADVANTAGES
MRI	No radiation Excellent in assessment of ventricular function (such as LV and RV volume, mass, and function, including regurgitation fraction) Excellent tissue differentiation Lack of dependence on a rapid bolus of IV contrast	Long scanning time (45–60 min) Need for sedation and anesthesia, requiring close monitoring Metallic artifacts Contraindicated in patients with a pacemaker or ICD
CT	Short total scan time (5–10 min) Fewer requirements of sedation Excellent quality images of extracardiac vasculature (such as pulmonary arteries and veins, aortic arch, coronary arteries, and aortic collaterals) Simultaneous evaluation of lungs and airways High spatial resolution	Radiation exposure Risk of iodinated contrast material Requires breath-hold and low, regular heart rate Lack of information on ventricular function (e.g., RV function, pulmonary regurgitation fraction)

CT, computed tomography; *ICD*, implantable cardioverter defibrillator; *IV*, intravenous; *LV*, left ventricular; *MRI*, magnetic resonance imaging; *RV*, right ventricular.

A. ADVANTAGES AND DISADVANTAGES OF TECHNIQUES

Both magnetic resonance imaging (MRI) and cardiac computed tomography (CT) can provide images of CV structures and other intrathoracic structures that are not usually imaged by echo studies. However, one of the radiologic techniques may be better than the other in its capability and its practicality. Physicians and cardiologists often must decide which noninvasive technique to use to best serve their patients. This section provides some insights into the advantages and disadvantages of MRI and CT (summarized in Box 4.1).

B. CHOICE OF IMAGING MODALITIES ACCORDING TO AGE GROUPS

1. For infants and children younger than 8 years
   a. Echo studies provide accurate diagnosis of even complex CHDs in most cases. Therefore the need for using MRI or CT study arises only rarely.
   b. MRI can be used to answer most of the unanswered questions regarding ventricular size and function and extracardiac vasculature.
   c. When the question is primarily about the extracardiac vasculature, CT can also be used. Its use should be balanced against the risk of ionizing radiation exposure.
2. For adolescents and adults
   a. Although echo remains the primary diagnostic modality, MRI plays an increasing role, especially for the evaluation of the extracardiac

thoracic vasculature, ventricular volume and function, and flow measurement.

b. MRI is usually preferred over CT or cardiac catheterization in this age group because it avoids exposure to ionizing radiation and can provide a wealth of functional information.
c. CT is used in patients with contraindications to MRI, such as those with a cardiac pacemaker or implantable cardioverter defibrillator, and those in whom concomitant evaluation for coronary disease is necessary.

Chapter 5

Other Noninvasive Tools

Besides noninvasive imaging tools, there are other noninvasive investigational tools that are frequently used in the evaluation of cardiac patients. They include exercise stress testing, long-term ECG monitoring, and ambulatory blood pressure (BP) monitoring.

I. EXERCISE STRESS TESTING

Exercise stress testing plays an important role in the evaluation of cardiac symptoms by quantifying the severity of the cardiac abnormality and assessing the effectiveness of management. Although some exercise laboratories have developed bicycle ergometer protocols, the treadmill protocols, such as the Bruce protocol, are well standardized and widely used because most hospitals have treadmills.

A. Monitoring During Exercise Stress Testing

During exercise stress testing, the patient is continually monitored for symptoms such as chest pain or faintness, ischemic changes or arrhythmias on the ECG, oxygen saturation, and responses in heart rate and BP.

1. **Heart rate**. Heart rate is measured from the electrocardiographic (ECG) signal.
   a. The maximal heart rate ranges between 188 and 210 beats/min. The mean maximal heart rates reported are virtually identical for boys and girls: 198 ± 11 for boys and 200 ± 9 for girls.
   b. Heart rate declines abruptly during the first minute of recovery to between 140 and 150 beats/min.
   c. Inadequate increments in heart rate may be seen with sinus node dysfunction, in congenital heart block, and after cardiac surgery.
   d. An extremely high heart rate at low levels of work may indicate physical decondition or marginal circulatory compensation.
2. **Blood pressure**. BP is measured in the arm with the auscultatory method or an oscillometric device. Accuracy of BP measurement, especially systolic BP, is doubtful during exercise.
   a. Systolic pressure increases linearly with progressive exercise. Systolic pressure usually rises to as high as 180 mm Hg with little change in diastolic pressure. Maximal systolic pressure in children rarely exceeds 200 mm Hg. During recovery it returns to baseline in about 10 minutes.
   b. The diastolic pressure ranges between 51 and 76 mm Hg at maximum systolic BP. Diastolic pressure also returns to the resting level by 8 to 10 minutes of recovery.

c. High systolic pressure in the arm, to the level of what is considered hypertensive emergency, raises a concern in both children and adults, but it probably does not reflect the central aortic pressure. The major portion of the rise in arm systolic pressure during treadmill exercise probably reflects peripheral amplification due to vasoconstriction in the nonexercising arms (associated with increased blood flow to vasodilated exercising legs); central aortic pressure would probably be much lower than the systolic pressure in the arm in most cases. Fig. 5.1 is a dramatic illustration of a relationship between the central and peripheral arterial pressures measured directly with arterial cannulas inserted in the ascending aorta and radial artery during upright exercise in young adults. Note that when the radial artery systolic pressure is over 230 mm Hg, the aortic pressure is only 160 mm Hg and there is very little increase in diastolic pressure (Fig. 5.1). This phenomenon is known as peripheral amplification of systolic pressure, discussed in Chapter 1 (see Fig 1.3). Therefore the usefulness of arm BP in assessing CV function during upright exercise is questionable, except in the case of failure to rise.

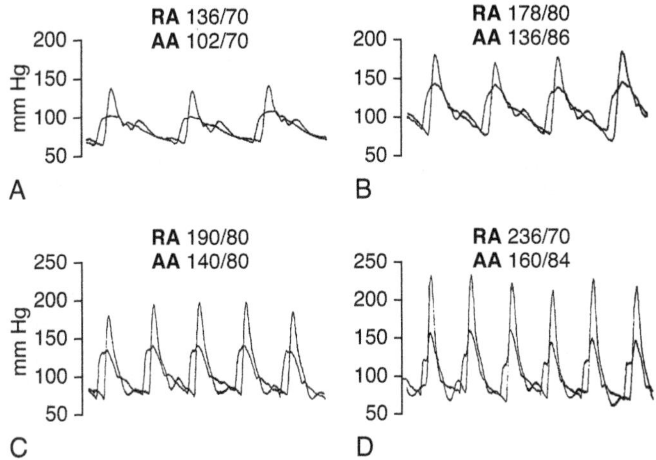

FIG. 5.1

Simultaneously recorded aortic and radial arterial pressure tracings in a young adult during rest (A) and those at 28.2% (B), 47.2% (C), and 70.2% (D) of maximal oxygen uptake during treadmill exercise. *AA*, ascending aorta; *RA*, radial artery. *(From Rowell, L. B., Brengelmann, G. L., Blackmon, J. R., Bruce, R. A., & Murray J. A. (1968). Disparities between aortic and peripheral pulse pressure induced by upright exercise and vasomotor changes in man.* Circulation, 37, *954-964.)*

d. Failure of BP to rise to the expected level may be much more significant than the level of the rise in arm BP. The failure reflects an inadequate increase in cardiac output. This is commonly seen with cardiomyopathy, LVOT obstruction, coronary artery diseases, or the onset of ventricular or atrial arrhythmias.

3. **ECG monitoring**. The major reasons for ECG monitoring are to detect exercise-induced arrhythmias and ischemic changes.
   a. **Exercise**-induced arrhythmias: Arrhythmias that increase in frequency or begin with exercise are usually significant. Type and frequency before and after the exercise and occurrence of new or more advanced arrhythmias should be noted. Occurrence of serious ventricular arrhythmias may be an indication to terminate the test.
   b. **ST**-segment depression is the most common manifestation of exercise-induced myocardial ischemia.
      (1) For children, down-sloping or sustained horizontal depression of the ST segment of 2 mm or greater when measured at 80 msec after the J point is considered abnormal (see Fig. 2.20).
      (2) Most guidelines for adult exercise testing consider ST-segment depression of 1 mm or greater as an abnormal response. If the ST segment is depressed at rest, an additional depression of 1 mm or greater should be present to be significant.
      (3) Specificity of the exercise ECG is poor in the presence of ST-T abnormalities on a resting ECG or with digoxin use.
      (4) When there is an abnormal depolarization (such as BBB, ventricular pacemaker, or WPW preexcitation), interpretation of ST-segment displacement is impossible.
4. **Oximetry**. Normal children maintain oxygen saturation greater than 90% during maximal exercise when monitored by pulse oximetry. Desaturation (<90%) is considered an abnormal response and may reflect pulmonary, cardiac, or circulatory compromise. Children who received lateral tunnel Fontan operations with fenestration may desaturate during exercise due to R-L shunt through the fenestration.

B. Endurance Time

There is a high correlation between the maximum oxygen consumption (Vo_2 max) and endurance time. Thus endurance time is the best predictor of exercise capacity in children. The endurance data reported by Cummings et al. in 1978 have served as the reference for several decades. Two reports from the U.S. (Chatrath et al., 2002; Ahmed et al., 2001) indicate that the endurance time has been reduced significantly since the 1970s. It is concerning that endurance times reported from two other countries (Italy in 1994; Turkey in 1998) are similar to those published by Cummings et al. and are significantly longer than those reported in the two U.S. reports. This may be an indication that U.S. youth are less physically fit than the youth from other countries, which may lead to increased risk of CAD and stroke in the U.S.

TABLE 5.1

PERCENTILES OF ENDURANCE TIME (MIN) BY BRUCE TREADMILL PROTOCOL

	PERCENTILES					
AGE GROUP (YR)	**10**	**25**	**50**	**75**	**90**	**MEAN ± SD**
BOYS						
4-5	6.8	7.0	8.2	10.0	12.7	8.9 ± 2.4
6-7	6.6	7.7	9.6	10.4	13.1	9.6 ± 2.3
8-9	7.0	9.1	9.9	11.1	15.0	10.2 ± 2.5
10-12	8.1	9.2	10.7	12.3	13.2	10.7 ± 2.1
13-15	9.6	10.3	12.0	13.5	15.0	12.0 ± 2.0
16-18	9.6	11.1	12.5	13.5	14.6	12.2 ± 2.2
GIRLS						
4-5	6.8	7.2	7.4	9.1	10.0	8.0 ± 1.1
6-7	6.5	7.3	9.0	9.2	12.4	8.7 ± 2.0
8-9	8.0	9.2	9.8	10.6	10.8	9.8 ± 1.6
10-12	7.3	9.3	10.4	10.8	12.7	10.2 ± 1.9
13-15	6.9	8.1	9.6	10.6	12.4	9.6 ± 2.1
16-18	7.4	8.5	9.5	10.1	12.0	9.5 ± 2.0

From Chatrath, R., Shenoy, R., Serratto, M., & Thoele, D. G. (2002). Physical fitness of urban American children. *Pediatric Cardiology, 23, 608-612.*

5

population. A new set of endurance data from a recent U.S. study is presented in Table 5.1.

C. Indications for Exercise Stress Test

Common indications for exercise testing in children are as follows.

1. To evaluate specific signs or symptoms that are induced or aggravated by exercise, such as chest pain, dizziness, or syncope.
2. To assess or identify abnormal responses to exercise in children with cardiac, pulmonary, or other organ disorders, including the presence of myocardial ischemia and arrhythmias.
3. To assess efficacy of specific medical or surgical treatments.
4. To assess functional capacity for recreational, athletic, and vocational activities.
5. To evaluate prognosis, including both baseline and serial testing measurements.
6. To establish baseline data for institution of cardiac, pulmonary, or musculoskeletal rehabilitation.
7. To evaluate for risk stratification of asymptomatic WPW patients for tachyarrhythmias.

D. Contraindications

1. Absolute contraindications include patients with acute myocardial or pericardial inflammatory diseases or patients with severe obstructive lesions in whom surgical intervention is clearly indicated.
2. Patients with pulmonary hypertension, documented long QT syndrome, uncontrolled hypertension, unstable arrhythmias, or Marfan syndrome and those who have had a heart transplantation are at high risk (and they may be relative contraindications).

E. Termination of Exercise Testing

1. Three general indications to terminate an exercise test are:
   a. When diagnostic findings have been established and further testing would not yield any additional information;
   b. When monitoring equipment fails; and
   c. When signs or symptoms indicate that further testing may compromise the patient's well-being.
2. The following are some indications for termination of exercise testing in the pediatric age group.
   a. Failure of heart rate to increase or a decrease in ventricular rate with increasing workload associated with symptoms (such as extreme fatigue, dizziness)
   b. Progressive fall in systolic pressure with increasing workload
   c. Severe hypertension, >250 mm Hg systolic or 125 mm Hg diastolic, or BP higher than can be measured by the laboratory equipment
   d. Dyspnea that the patient finds intolerable
   e. Symptomatic tachycardia that the patient finds intolerable
   f. Progressive fall in oxygen saturation to <90% or a 10-point drop from resting saturation in a patient who is symptomatic
   g. Presence of ≥3-mm flat or downward sloping ST-segment depression
   h. Increasing ventricular ectopy with increasing workload
   i. Patient requests termination of the study

II. OTHER STRESS TESTING PROTOCOLS

Besides treadmill exercise, there are other types of stress testing, such as the 6-minute walk test, and exercise-induced bronchospasm (EIB) provocation tests.

A. Six-Minute Walk Test

This simple test can be used in individuals with moderate to severe exercise limitation for traditional exercise testing. The patient is instructed to walk as fast as possible (without running) at a steady pace for 6 minutes, to cover as much distance or as many laps possible, around two flagpoles positioned 30 meters apart on a flat ground. The total distance walked is the primary outcome.

The test may be useful in following disease progression and measuring the response to medical interventions, rather than the need to relate the patient's exercise tolerance against a healthy population. Patients using supplemental oxygen should perform the test with oxygen. If monitoring equipment is not available, oxygen saturation and heart rate are monitored before and after the test. At least two practice tests performed on a separate day are advisable.

B. Exercise-Induced Bronchospasm Provocation Test

Exercise in cold or dry air typically induces airway obstruction in asthmatic patients. Bronchial reactivity is measured while a subject exercises for 5 to 8 minutes on a treadmill at an intensity of 80% maximum capacity.

1. Baseline spirometry is obtained before exercise.
2. The exercise protocol used should increase the heart rate to 80% of predicted maximum within 2 minutes; starting with stage 4 of the Bruce protocol may be appropriate. The usual incremental workload used in many exercise tests is not appropriate, because if the intensity of exercise is raised slowly, the patient may develop refractoriness to bronchospasm.
3. Within 6 to 8 minutes of exercise or by the time the heart rate increases to 180 beats/min, symptoms of airway obstruction develop.
4. Spirometry is repeated immediately after exercise and again at minute 5, 10, and 15 of recovery. Most pulmonary function test nadirs occur within 5 to 10 minutes after exercise.
5. Declines of 12% to 15% in forced expiratory volume in 1 second (FEV1) are typically diagnostic.

III. LONG-TERM ECG RECORDING

Long-term ECG recording is the most useful method to document and quantitate the frequency of arrhythmias, correlate the arrhythmia with the patient's symptoms, and evaluate the effect of antiarrhythmic therapy.

A. Indications

Ambulatory ECG monitoring is obtained for the following reasons:

1. To determine whether symptoms such as chest pain, palpitation, or syncope are caused by cardiac arrhythmias
2. To evaluate the adequacy of medical therapy for an arrhythmia
3. To screen high-risk cardiac patients (such as those with hypertrophic cardiomyopathy or those in postoperative status after operations known to predispose to arrhythmias (e.g., Fontan-type operation)
4. To evaluate possible intermittent pacemaker failure in patients who have an implanted pacemaker
5. To determine the effect of sleep on potentially life-threatening arrhythmias

B. Types of Long-Term ECG Recorders

There are several different types of long-term ECG recorders, which detect arrhythmias for varying lengths of time.

1. Holter recording
   a. The Holter monitoring records the heart rhythm continuously for 24 using ECG electrodes attached on the chest. The heart rhythm is recorded on a flash card or wirelessly and then processed at a heart center. Three simultaneous channels are usually recorded to help distinguish artifacts from arrhythmias. The monitor has a built-in timer that is used with the patient's diary to allow subsequent correlation of symptoms and activities with arrhythmias. This type of recording is useful when the child has symptoms almost daily.
   b. The following are suggested formats of interpretation of a Holter recording.
      (1) Describe the basic rhythm and the range of the heart rate.
      (2) For bradycardia, describe its rate, rhythm, and duration (or number of beats) and the presence of escape beats, etc.
      (3) For extreme tachycardia, describe the rate, rhythm, mode of initiation and termination, and its duration.
      (4) Describe any abnormalities in AV conduction.
      (5) Describe any arrhythmias, including their characteristics, duration, and frequency.
      (6) Correlate the arrhythmias with the patient's activities and symptoms.
      (7) If the patient complained of anginal pain, correlate ST-segment changes with activities.
2. Patch ECG recording devices: The advancement in electronic and adhesive technologies has enabled the development of the wearable Patch ECG Monitors (Holter patches) capable of continuously recording ECG signals for 7 to 14 days or an even longer period, which is much longer than the standard Holter monitor can. These monitors attach directly to the skin and record ECG signals without visible electrodes and lead wires. They are waterproof, offer good adhesions to the skin, and can operate as either recorders or wireless streaming devices.
3. Event recorders: Event monitors are devices that are used by patients over a longer period (typically one month). The monitor is used when symptoms suggestive of an arrhythmia occur infrequently. Two general types of cardiac event monitors are available:
   a. Looping memory (presymptom) event monitor. The term "looping" refers to the memory of the monitor to save a preceding or ongoing rhythm in the memory loop. Three to five electrodes are attached on the chest. The monitor is always on but only stores and transmits the patient's rhythm when the patient or caregiver pushes the button or automatically when the monitor detects a heart rate that fulfills preset criteria. The stored ECGs are wirelessly transmitted to the event monitoring center directly.

b. Nonlooping memory (postsymptom) event monitor. It does not have electrodes that are attached to the chest. This device is used to record symptoms that last longer than 45 to 60 seconds. It is a small device that has small metal discs that function as the electrodes. When symptoms occur, the device is pressed against the chest to start the recording. The device records and stores the events in solid-state memory. It can store up to six such events before it is necessary to transmit the information.

4. Implantable loop recorder/insertable cardiac monitor: This device is indicated in patients with very infrequent symptoms, such as once every 6 months. In such patients, magnetic resonance imaging (MRI)-compatible, insertable cardiac monitors, about the size of a 1 3/4-inch paper clip, are implanted beneath the skin in the upper left chest. A reader is activated by the patient and the information is then transmitted via the portal to the health care provider. The device can be "interrogated" through the skin to determine what the heart was doing when the symptoms occurred.

IV. AMBULATORY BLOOD PRESSURE MONITORING

BP is not a static variable; it changes not only from daytime to nighttime but also from minute to minute. In some patients, there is a transient elevation of BP when BP is measured in a health care facility (i.e., "white-coat hypertension"). This could lead to an overdiagnosis of hypertension and to unnecessarily aggressive and costly diagnostic studies and treatment. This test helps identify those with "white coat hypertension." Some researchers advocate the use of ambulatory BP monitoring (ABPM) in all patients with casual BP elevation.

A. Method of Ambulatory BP Monitoring

In ABPM, BP is measured multiple times with a preapplied BP cuff, usually using the oscillometric method for a 24-hour period while children participate in their normal daily activities, during both awake and sleep periods. Typically, BP measurements are programmed to occur every 15 to 20 minutes during awake periods and every 20 to 30 minutes during expected sleep periods. Monitors should be applied to the nondominant arm with appropriate size of BP cuff. Patients' diaries are critical tools and should include the sleep times, nap times, and periods of physical activities. The use of ABPM is usually limited to children 5 to 6 years of age or older. Successful recording has been reported in more than 70% of children younger than 6 years of age. A sufficient number of valid recordings are needed: minimum of 1 reading per hour, including during sleep and at least 40 to 50 readings for a full 24-hour period. Outlier data are first filtered out before making calculations of ABPM. Values that fall outside of the following range should be discarded: systolic BP (SBP), 60 to 220 mm Hg; diastolic BP (DBP), 35 to 120 mm Hg; heart rate, 40 to 180 beats/min; and pulse pressure 40 to 120 mm Hg.

B. Ambulatory BP Standard Calculations

The new 2014 recommendations by the American Heart Association include additional calculations using diastolic BP, which was not included in the 2008 recommendation.

1. The mean systolic and diastolic BP values during the entire 24-hour period, awake, and during sleep periods.
2. BP load, which is defined as the percentage of valid BP measures above the 95th percentile for age, gender, and height.
3. Nocturnal dipping. It is calculated by ([mean awake BP − mean sleep BP ÷ mean awake BP × 100] for both SBP and DBP). Normal nocturnal dipping was generally defined as a ≥ 10% decline in mean SBP and mean DBP from daytime BP levels. Non-dipping was defined as a decline of <10%.

C. Ambulatory PM Standards

The 2014 Update on ABPM (Flynn et al., 2014) has recommended two sets of normative standards for ABPM: one by height and the other by age. Normative data based on age are presented in Appendix B (Table B.8 for boys and Table B.9 for girls).

D. Staging of Ambulatory BP Levels in Children

Table 5.2 provides a suggested schema for staging ABPM by the 2014 Update on ABPM (Flynn et al., 2014).

TABLE 5.2

SUGGESTED REVISED SCHEMA OF AMBULATORY BLOOD PRESSURE LEVELS IN CHILDREN

CLASSIFICATION	OFFICE BP[a]	MEAN AMBULATORY SBP OR DBP[b,c]	SBP OR DBP LOAD[c]
Normal BP	< 90th percentile	< 95th percentile	< 25%
White coat hypertension	≥ 95th percentile	< 95th percentile	< 25%
Pre-hypertension (now called elevated BP)	≥ 90th percentile or > 120/80 mm Hg	< 95th percentile	≥ 25%
Masked hypertension	< 95th percentile	> 95th percentile	≥ 25%
Ambulatory (or sustained) hypertension	> 95th percentile	> 95th percentile	25-50%
Severe ambulatory hypertension (at risk for end-organ damage)	> 95th percentile	> 95th percentile	> 50%

BP, blood pressure; *DBP*, diastolic blood pressure; *SBP*, systolic blood pressure.

[a]Based on National High Blood Pressure Education Program Task Forces normative data

[b]Based on normative ABPM value in Appendix B (Tables B.8 and B.9).

[c]For either the wake or sleep period of the study, or both.

Adapted from Flynn, J. T., Daniels, S. R., Hayman, L. L., Maahs, D. M., Mitsnefes, M., Zachariah J. P., & Urbine, E. M., American Heart Association Atherosclerosis, Hypertension and Obesity in Youth Committee of the Council on Cardiovascular Disease in the Young. (2014). Update: Ambulatory blood pressure monitoring in children and adolescents. A scientific statement from the American Heart Association. *Hypertension, 63, 1116-1135.*

Chapter 6

Invasive Procedures

There are two kinds of invasive procedures that are used in the practice of pediatric cardiology: diagnostic cardiac catheterization (including angiocardiography) and catheter intervention procedures (therapeutic cardiac catheterization).

I. CARDIAC CATHETERIZATION AND ANGIOCARDIOGRAPHY

Cardiac catheterization and angiocardiography are the definitive diagnostic tests for most cardiac patients. They are carried out under sedation or anesthesia.

A. Indications

Accurate diagnosis of most CHDs does not require diagnostic catheterization. With improved capability of noninvasive imaging tools such as echo and color flow Doppler studies and radiologic techniques such as cardiac magnetic resonance imaging and cardiac computed tomography, many cardiac problems are adequately diagnosed and managed without cardiac catheterization studies. Indications for these invasive studies vary from institution to institution and from cardiologist to cardiologist. The following are some circumstances that suggest the need for cardiac catheterization.

1. To perform balloon procedures for angioplasty (with or without stent placement), valvuloplasty, or balloon atrial septostomy in patients with lesions amenable to these procedures
2. To perform pulmonary valve replacement with a tissue valve (Melody valve and Edwards SAPIEN valve) that is sutured to a stent and is deployed percutaneously
3. To determine accurate pressure gradients in combined lesions of AS and AR or PS and PR, or multiple levels of obstruction
4. To assess pulmonary hypertension and its responsiveness to vasodilator therapy
5. To calculate pulmonary vascular resistance as a preoperative study or in the setting of low-flow lesions, such as seen in patients after bidirectional Glenn operation or after complete Fontan operation
6. To determine details of pulmonary vascular supply, the aortopulmonary collateral supply, and the coronary artery anatomy in patients with pulmonary atresia with intact ventricular septum or pulmonary atresia with complex ventricular anatomy
7. To find answers to postoperative problems such as excessive desaturation after a B-T shunt or bidirectional Glenn operation, or when excessive aortopulmonary collateral is suspected

8. To assess post-transplantation vasculopathy and to obtain endomyocardial biopsy for rejection identification in cardiac transplantation patients
9. To assess cardiomyopathy or myocarditis
10. To assess coronary circulation in some cases of Kawasaki disease

B. Sedation

A number of sedatives have been used by different institutions with equal success rates. Smaller doses of sedatives are usually used in cyanotic infants. General anesthesia is usually used, especially when an interventional procedure is planned.

Among the sedatives that have been used are chloral hydrate, diphenhydramine, meperidine (Demerol), promethazine (Phenergan), chlorpromazine (Thorazine), ketamine, and morphine. It should be kept in mind that ketamine has important hemodynamic effects; it increases the SVR and blood pressure.

C. Hemodynamic Values and their Calculations

Pressure and oxygen saturation values for normal children are shown in Fig. 6.1. During cardiac catheterization, cardiac output, cardiac shunt, and vascular resistance are routinely calculated.

1. **Flows (cardiac output)** are calculated by the Fick formula:

$$\text{Pulmonary flow (Qp)} = \frac{VO_2}{C_{PV} - C_{PA}},$$

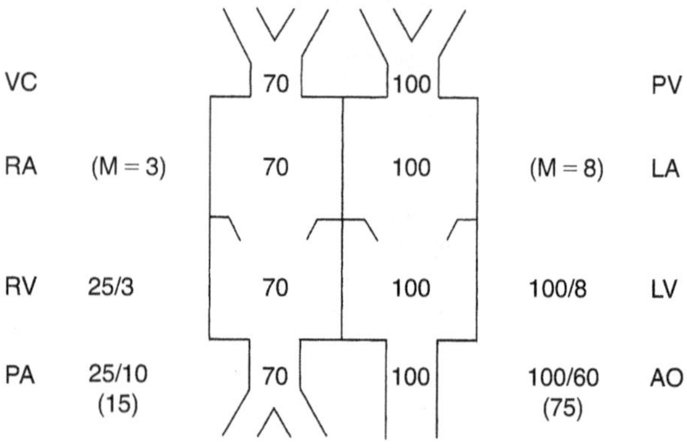

FIG. 6.1

Average values of pressure and oxygen saturation in normal children. *AO*, aorta; *LA*, left atrium; *LV*, left ventricle; *M*, mean pressure; *PA*, pulmonary artery; *PV*, pulmonary vein; *RA*, right atrium; *RV*, right ventricle; *VC*, vena cava.

$$\text{Systemic flow (Qs)} = \frac{VO_2}{C_{AO} - C_{MV}},$$

where flows are in liters per minute, VO_2 is oxygen consumption in milliliters per minute, and C is oxygen content in milliliters per liter at the various positions: the PV, PA, aorta (AO), and mixed systemic venous blood.

Oxygen consumption is either directly measured during the procedure or estimated from a table (see Appendix, Table A.6). Oxygen content (milliliters per 100 mL of blood) is derived by multiplying oxygen capacity by percent saturation. Oxygen capacity (milliliters per 100 mL of blood) is the total content of oxygen that hemoglobin contains when it is 100% saturated (1.36 × hemoglobin in grams per 100 mL). Normal systemic flow (or pulmonary flow in the absence of shunt) is 3.1 ± 0.4 L/min/m^2 (i.e., cardiac index).

2. **The magnitude of the shunt** is calculated as follows:

$$\text{Left-to-right(L-R)shunt} = \text{Qp-Qs}$$

$$\text{Right-to-left(R-L)shunt} = \text{Qs-Qp}$$

In pediatrics, the ratio of pulmonary to systemic flow (Qp/Qs), which does not require an oxygen consumption value, is often used. The ratio provides information on the magnitude of the shunt. Patients with an L-R shunt greater than 2:1 are usually candidates for surgical or percutaneous intervention.

3. **Vascular resistances** are calculated by using formulas derived from Ohm's law ($R = \Delta P/Q$)).

$$\text{PVR} = \frac{\text{Mean PA pressure} - \text{mean LA pressure}}{\text{Qp}}$$

$$\text{SVR} = \frac{\text{Mean PA pressure} - \text{mean LA pressure}}{\text{Qp}}$$

The SVR varies between 15 and 30 units/m^2. The normal PVR is high at birth but reaches near-adult values (1 to 3 units/m^2) after 2 to 4 months. The normal ratio of PVR/SVR ranges from 1:20 to 1:10.

D. Selective Angiocardiography

A radiopaque dye is rapidly injected through a cardiac catheter into a certain site in the cardiovascular system, and angiograms are obtained, often on biplane views. Nonionizing contrast media with low osmolality (e.g., Isovue, Omnipaque) are widely used because of their low incidence of side effects. The dose of angiographic dyes for an angiogram ranges from 1 to 2 mL/kg of body weight, depending on the nature of the defect.

E. Risks

1. The risk of cardiac catheterization and angiocardiography varies with the age and illness of the patient, the type of lesion, and the experience of those doing the procedure. Serious complications can occur, including (rarely) death. About 3% to 5% of patients may have significant nonfatal complications.
2. Complications include serious arrhythmias, heart block, cardiac perforation, hypoxic spells, arterial obstruction, hemorrhage, infection, reactions to the contrast material, intramyocardial injection of the contrast, and renal complications (hematuria, proteinuria, oliguria, and anuria). Hypothermia, acidemia, hypoglycemia, convulsions, hypotension, and respiratory depression are more likely in the newborn infant.

F. Preparation and Monitoring

Adequate preparation of the patient before the procedure and careful monitoring during the procedure can minimize complications and fatality from the invasive studies. Following studies should be considered for children undergoing cardiac catheterization.

1. A 12-lead electrocardiogram (ECG), chest radiographs (both posteroanterior and lateral), two-dimensional echocardiography, urinalysis, and a complete blood count within days or weeks in advance of the study.
2. Baseline coagulation studies and a platelet count for deeply cyanotic children.
3. Blood type and cross-match for infants less than 5 kg of body weight.

The following preparations and monitoring are particularly important in minimizing complications.

1. Avoiding hypothermia when an infant is being studied, by increasing temperature in the cardiac catheterization laboratory, using a warming blanket, and monitoring rectal temperature.
2. Monitoring oxygen saturation transcutaneously, checking arterial blood gases and pH, and correcting acidemia and hypoxemia; correcting hypoglycemia or hypocalcemia before the start of the procedure.
3. Administering oxygen, if indicated, during the procedure.
4. Intubating or readiness for intubating in infants with respiratory difficulties, and having emergency medications (e.g., atropine, epinephrine, bicarbonate) drawn up and ready.
5. Initiating prostaglandin infusion in cyanotic infants who appear to have a ductus-dependent lesion.
6. Angiotensin-converting enzyme inhibitors or angiotensin-receptor blockers should be held 24 hours prior to a planned anesthesia due to increased risk of significant hypotension on induction.
7. Whenever possible, having another physician or an anesthesiologist available to monitor the patient.

II. CATHETER INTERVENTION PROCEDURES

Catheter interventional procedures can save lives of critically ill neonates and may eliminate or delay the need for elective surgical procedures. Blood vessels and heart valves that are too small can be enlarged using balloon catheters and/or implantable stents. Too small an opening in the atrial septum can be enlarged by using balloon or blade catheters. An opening can be created in an intact atrial septum for an L-R or R-L shunt to occur. Abnormal connections within the heart (such as ASD and VSD) can be closed using innovative devices. Abnormal blood vessels (PDA or collaterals) can also be closed using coils or plugging devices. In recent years, percutaneous valve replacement in the aortic or pulmonary position has seen wider use.

A. Atrial Septostomy

In balloon atrial septostomy (Rashkind procedure), an opening is created or enlarged in the atrial septum, using a special balloon-tipped catheter, to improve shunting at the atrial level in patients with serious CHDs (such as TGA, pulmonary atresia, tricuspid atresia, TAPVR, etc.). This procedure is mostly effective in infants younger than 1 month of age.

In infants older than 6 to 8 weeks of age, the atrial septum may be too thick to allow an effective balloon septostomy. In such cases, the atrial septum can be opened using a blade catheter (i.e., Park Blade Septostomy Catheter). The opening can then be torn further with a balloon catheter.

B. Balloon Valvuloplasty

The balloons used in this interventional procedure are made of special plastic polymers and retain their predetermined diameters.

1. **Pulmonary valve stenosis**. Balloon pulmonary valvuloplasty is the treatment of choice for valvular PS in children and, to a large extent, has replaced the surgical pulmonary valvotomy. The procedure is performed antegrade through a femoral vein. Balloon valvuloplasty may be indicated in patients with a maximum instantaneous systolic Doppler gradient as little as 35 mm Hg, when combined with evidence of RVH. A balloon is chosen to be 120% to 130% of the pulmonary valve annulus. When using a double-balloon technique, a combined diameter of 150% to 160% of the pulmonary valve annulus may be used.
2. **Aortic valve stenosis**. This procedure is more difficult and carries a higher complication rate than does pulmonary valvuloplasty, especially for infants. The gradient reduction is less effective than for the pulmonary valve and creating a significant aortic insufficiency is the major risk of the procedure. The procedure is performed retrograde with a catheter introduced into the femoral artery. For a single-balloon technique, the initial balloon is chosen with a diameter about 80% to 90% of the measured aortic annulus. With the double-balloon technique, the combined diameter of the two balloons should be approximately 120% of the aortic annulus.

Indications for balloon valvotomy include peak systolic pressure gradients in excess of 60 mm Hg in asymptomatic children and adolescents. In symptomatic patients (with ischemic or repolarization changes on ECG), a pressure gradient of 50 mm Hg should be used. Newborns or small infants with critical valve obstruction with a dilated LV or poor LV function are also candidates for the procedure, regardless of the measured pressure gradient value. Complications include production or worsening of AR, iliofemoral artery injury and occlusion, ventricular fibrillation, and even death in small infants.

3. **Mitral stenosis**. Balloon dilatation valvuloplasty has been effective for rheumatic mitral stenosis (MS) but less effective for congenital MS.
4. **Stenosis of prosthetic conduits and valves within conduits**. The balloon dilatation procedure may reduce the transconduit gradient across stenotic areas of prosthetic conduits and across valves contained within conduits.

C. Balloon Angioplasty

Balloon catheters similar to those used in balloon valvuloplasties are used for the relief of stenosis of blood vessels. This procedure has been used for coarctation of the AO, PA branch stenosis, and stenosis of the systemic veins. Following the balloon procedure, some blood vessels recoil and do not maintain the dilated caliber of the vessel. Endovascular stents are sometimes used to maintain vessel patency after balloon angioplasty of any vascular structure. After stent placement, the vascular endothelium grows over the struts of the stent over several months, functionally incorporating the stent into the vessel wall. Occasionally, however, the endothelialization may go awry, resulting in a thick neointimal layer causing a functional stenosis.

1. **Recoarctation of the AO**. Balloon angioplasty has become the procedure of choice for patients with postoperative residual obstruction of coarctation of the AP. The procedure's success rate is close to 80%, and late development of an aortic aneurysm rarely occurs. Some centers use a stent to prevent restenosis and to diminish the incidence of late aneurysm formation.
2. **Native (or unoperated) coarctation of the AO**. Balloon angioplasty for native unoperated coarctation is controversial. The rate of recoarctation following the balloon procedure appears higher than that following surgery in infants. The complication rate is 17%, with aortic aneurysm formation (both acute and late) occurring in 6% of the patients. The long-term effects of the procedure on aneurysm formation are unknown. Some centers use cutting balloons or low-profile stents in very sick infants, which may reduce aneurysm formation.
3. **Branch pulmonary artery stenosis**. Surgical treatment of peripheral PA stenosis is often impossible. Hypoplastic and stenotic branch PAs are seen with postoperative TOF, pulmonary atresia, and HLHS. The immediate success rate of the balloon procedure is about 60%, but restenosis occurs in a significant number of patients, and aneurysm

formation occurs in approximately 3% of patients. High-pressure balloons appear to improve the effectiveness. Vessels resistant to high-pressure balloons respond to either cutting balloon angioplasty alone or followed by high-pressure ballooning. Cutting balloons have three or four microsurgical blades with a cutting depth of 0.15 mm, which are activated when the balloons are inflated. Use of an intravascular stent has also improved immediate results and may improve the long-term success rate.

4. **Systemic venous stenosis**. The balloon procedure may be performed for obstructed venous baffles after the Senning operation for TGA.

D. Closure Techniques

Various closure devices have been used for nonsurgical closure of ASD, PDA, and muscular VSD in the cardiac catheterization laboratory.

1. Atrial septal defect.
   a. In the United States, the Amplatzer Septal Occluder (AGA Medical, Golden Valley, MN) is the most commonly used device to close the secundum ASD. The Gore Cardioform Septal Occluder (W. L. Gore and Associates) is less frequently used and appears to be suitable for smaller ASD or PFO up to 17 mm.
   b. The use of the closure device may be indicated to close a secundum ASD measuring 4 mm or more in diameter (but less than 36 mm for the Amplatzer device and less than 17 mm for the Cardioform device), and there must be sufficient rims of atrial septal tissue around the defect. After the device closure, patients take 3 to 5 mg/kg of aspirin daily for 6 months until endothelialization of the device is complete.
   c. Closure rate is excellent with residual shunt present in less than 5% at 1-year follow-up.
2. Ventricular septal defect. Successful closure of a muscular VSD, which is remote from cardiac valves, has been reported, mostly using the Amplatzer VSD device.
3. Patent ductus arteriosus.
   a. Most small PDA closures are now performed using Gianturco vascular occlusion coils. They are small, coiled wires coated with thrombogenic Dacron strands that open like a small "pigtail" when placed in the vessel. Good candidates for the coil occlusion are those children weighing 6 kg and larger with the ductus 4 mm and smaller; however, more recently PDAs in preterm infants with a weight of less than 1000 g have successfully been occluded using percutaneous devices. In 2019, the U.S. Food and Drug Administration approved the Amplatzer Piccolo Occluder for such procedures.
   b. For larger PDAs (but less than 12 mm in diameter), the Amplatzer duct occluder is the most commonly used device in the United States. The devices are implanted antegrade from the femoral vein. There is a $\geq$98% closure rate at 6 months with minimal

complications and no mortality. Very large ducti in small infants are still probably best treated surgically.

4. Occlusion of collaterals and other vessels. This technique closes aortopulmonary collaterals (often seen with TOF), systemic arteriovenous fistulas, pulmonary arteriovenous fistulas, or surgically placed shunts that are no longer needed. When delivered, the coil occludes the vessel by creating a thrombus around the coil. Alternatively, the Amplatzer duct occluder is used. Peripheral embolization of the coil or balloon into the PAs or the AO is a major risk.

E. Percutaenous Valve Placement

Since Bonhoeffer and his colleagues first replaced pulmonary valves by percutaneous techniques in 2000, this technique has gained increasing experience. Candidates for this technique are typically those patients who received surgery for tetralogy of Fallot and late development of severe pulmonary regurgitation. This technique is expected to reduce the need for repeated cardiac surgeries by replacing surgically placed conduits. Most of the reported cases used the Melody transcatheter pulmonary valve (Medtronic, Minneapolis, MN). The Edwards SAPIEN valve (Edwards Lifescience, Irvine, CA) is a newer valve that can be placed in RV outflow tract up to 29 mm in size, compared with the Melody valve with a maximum size of 22 mm.

PART III

CONGENITAL HEART DEFECTS

Congenital heart defects are divided into the following four topics: left-to right shunt lesion, obstructive lesions, cyanotic heart defects, and miscellaneous congenital heart defects.

Chapter 7

Left-to-Right Shunt Lesions

I. ATRIAL SEPTAL DEFECT (OSTIUM SECUNDUM ASD)

A. PREVALENCE

Thirty to 40 percent of all CHDs. Female preponderance (male-to-female ratio of 1:2).

B. PATHOLOGY AND PATHOPHYSIOLOGY

1. Three types of ASDs occur in the atrial septum (Fig. 7.1).
   a. Secundum ASD is in the central portion of the septum and is the most common type (50% to 70% of ASDs).
   b. Primum ASD (or partial ECD) is in the lower part of the septum (30% of ASDs).
   c. Sinus venosus defect is near the entrance of the SVC or IVC to the RA (about 10% of all ASDs). PAPVR is common with a sinus venous defect.
2. An L-R shunt occurs through the defect, with a volume overload to the RA and RV and an increase in pulmonary blood flow.

C. CLINICAL MANIFESTATIONS

1. The patients are usually asymptomatic.
2. A widely split and fixed S2 and a grade 2 to 3/6 systolic ejection murmur at the ULSB are characteristic of moderate-size ASD (Fig. 7.2). With a large L-R shunt, a mid-diastolic rumble (resulting from relative TS) may be audible at the LLSB. The typical auscultatory findings are usually absent in infants and toddlers, even in those with a large defect, because the RV is not compliant enough to result in a large L-R shunt in these patients.
3. The ECG shows RAD (+90 to +180) and mild RVH, RBBB, or IRBBB with an rsR′ pattern in V1.
4. Chest radiographs show cardiomegaly (with RAE and RVE), increased PVM, and a prominent MPA segment when the shunt is moderate or large.
5. Two-dimensional echo shows the position and the size of the defect. Cardiac catheterization is not necessary.
6. Natural history.
   a. Spontaneous closure of the defect occurs in more than 80% of patients with defects of up to 8 mm (diagnosed by echo) before 1{1/2} years of age. An ASD with a diameter >8 mm rarely closes spontaneously. Spontaneous closure is not likely to occur after 4 years of age. The defect may reduce in size in some patients.

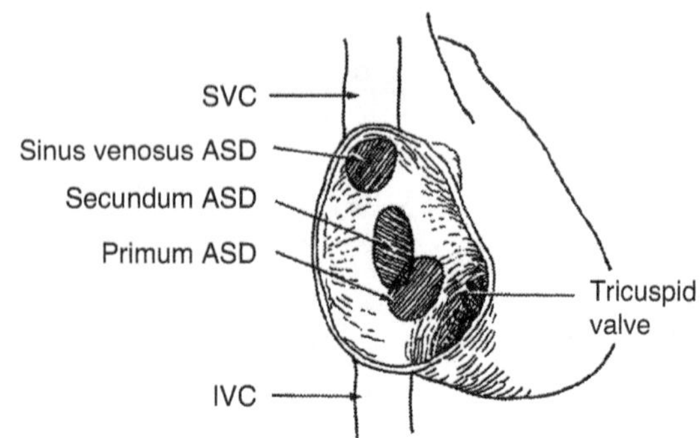

FIG. 7.1

Anatomic types of atrial septal defect (*ASD*) viewed with the right atrial wall removed. *IVC,* inferior vena cava; *SVC,* superior vena cava. *(From Park, M. K., & Salamat, M. (2020).* Park's pediatric cardiology for practitioners *(7th ed.). Philadelphia: Mosby.)*

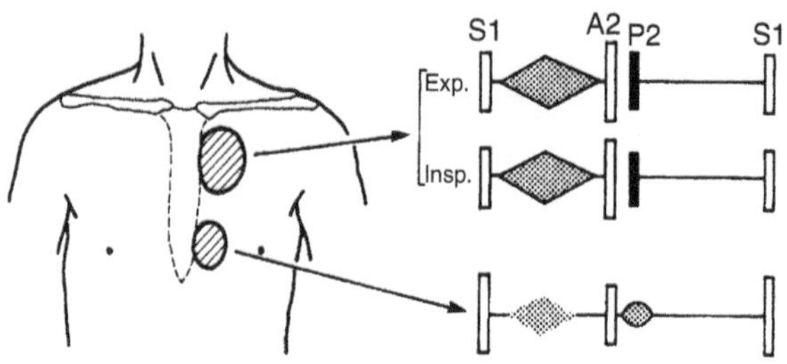

FIG. 7.2

Cardiac findings of ASD. Throughout this book, heart murmurs *with solid borders* are the primary murmurs, and those *without solid borders* are transmitted murmurs or those occurring occasionally. Abnormalities in heart sounds are shown in *black. Exp.*, Expiration; *Insp.*, inspiration. *(From Park, M. K., & Salamat, M. (2020).* Park's pediatric cardiology for practitioners *(7th ed.). Philadelphia: Mosby.)*

b. Spontaneous closure does not occur in primum or sinus venous type.
c. If the defect is large and left untreated, pulmonary hypertension develops in the third and fourth decades of life.
d. Cerebrovascular accident due to paradoxical embolization through an ASD is a rare complication.

D. MANAGEMENT

Medical and Nonsurgical

1. Exercise restriction is not required, unless symptomatic.
2. Nonsurgical closure of the defect using a catheter-delivered closure device has become a preferred method, provided the indications are met. Advantages of nonsurgical closure would include a less-than-24-hour hospital stay, rapid recovery, less pain, and no residual thoracotomy scar.
    a. These devices are applicable only to secundum ASD. The use of the closure device may be indicated for a defect measuring ≥ 5 mm in diameter (but <32 mm for Amplatzer device and <17 mm for Cardioform occluder) with evidence of RA and RV volume overload. In the United States, currently the Amplatzer Septal Occluder (AGA Medical) and Gore CardioForm occluder (W. L. Gore and Associates) are approved for secundum ASD closure.
    b. There must be enough rim of septal tissue around the defect for appropriate placement of the device. The size of the rim around the ASD can be estimated by two-dimensional (2D) echo study as diagrammatically shown in Fig. 7.3. The rim size is estimated in four directions: anterosuperior, anteroinferior, posterosuperior, and posteroinferior.
    c. The ASD devices can be implanted successfully in children younger than 2 years of age, although a weight >15 kg is preferred.
    d. Following the device closure, the patients are placed on aspirin 3-5 mg/kg/day for 6 months.
    e. Closure rates are excellent with small residual shunts seen in less than 5% at 1-year follow-up.

Surgical

For patients with primum ASD and sinus venosus defect, and some patients with secundum ASD for which the device closure is considered inappropriate, surgical closure is indicated when there is a significant L-R shunt with Qp/Qs of 1.5:1 or greater. Surgery is usually delayed until 2 to 4 years of age, unless CHF develops. Open repair with a midsternal incision or minimally invasive cardiac surgical technique (with a smaller skin incision) is used. The surgical mortality rate is less than 1%. High PVR (≥ 10 units/m^2) is a contraindication to surgery.

Follow-Up

1. Periodic follow-up is needed after the ASD closure device implantation for arrhythmia, residual shunt, obstruction of pulmonary and systemic venous returns, interference with the AV valve function, and/or device erosion through the cardiac wall.
2. After surgery, atrial or nodal arrhythmias occur in 7% to 20% of patients. Occasional sick sinus syndrome requires pacemaker therapy.

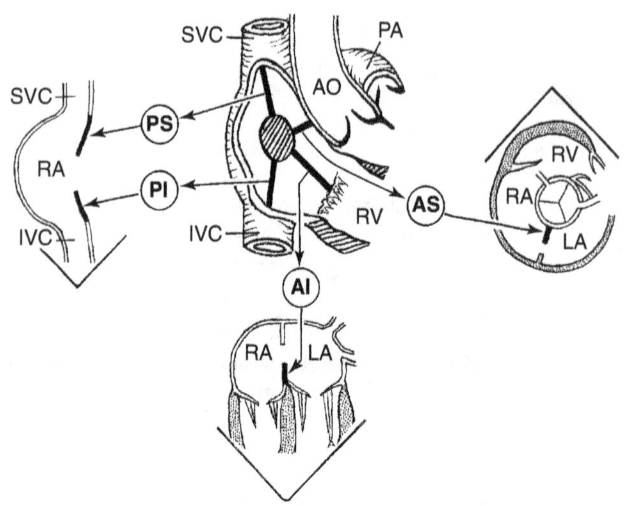

FIG. 7.3

Two-dimensional echo estimates of the atrial septal defect rim size. The posterosuperior (PS) and posteroinferior (PI) rims are estimated in the bi–vena caval view from the subcostal transducer position, the anteroinferior (AI) rim from the apical four-chamber view, and the anterosuperior (AS) (or retro-aortic) rim from the parasternal short-axis view. AO, aorta; IVC, inferior vena cava; LA, left atrium; PA, pulmonary artery; RA, right atrium; RV, right ventricle; SVC, superior vena cava.

II. VENTRICULAR SEPTAL DEFECT

A. PREVALENCE

VSD is the most common form of CHD, accounting for 15% to 20% of all CHDs, not including those occurring as part of cyanotic CHDs.

Pathology and Pathophysiology

1. The ventricular septum consists of a small membranous septum and a larger muscular septum. The muscular septum has three components: the inlet, infundibular, and trabecular (or simply muscular) septa (see Fig. 7.4). A membranous VSD often involves a varying amount of muscular septum adjacent to it (i.e., perimembranous VSD).
2. The frequency of different isolated subtypes of VSD found may be quite different depending on the diagnostic tools used in the study.
   a. By 2D echo, the incidence of muscular VSDs is much higher than perimembranous and other subtypes. Muscular VSDs accounted for

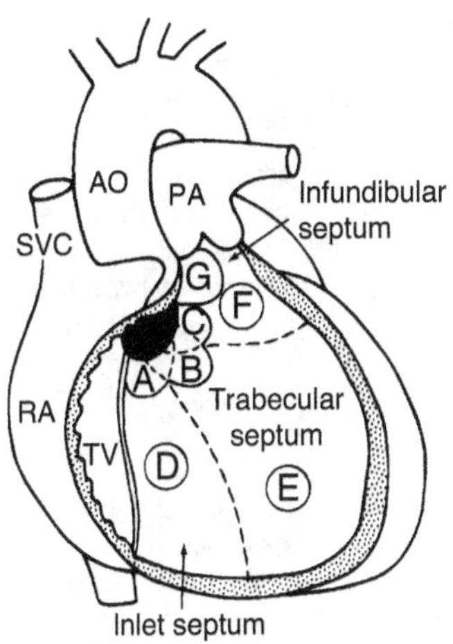

FIG. 7.4
Anatomic locations of various types of ventricular septal defects (VSDs), viewed with the RV free wall removed. The black area is the membranous ventricular septum. (A) Perimembranous inlet ("AV canal-type") VSD. (B) Perimembranous trabecular (typical membranous) VSD. (C) Perimembranous infundibular ("tetralogy-type") VSD. (D) Inlet muscular VSD. (E) Trabecular muscular VSD. (F) Infundibular or outlet muscular VSD. (G) subarterial infundibular (supracristal) VSD. *AO,* aorta; *PA,* pulmonary artery; *RA,* right atrium; *SVC,* superior vena cava; *TV,* tricuspid valve.

59%; perimembranous VSDs, 27%; outlet VSDs, 1%; and inlet VSDs, 1% or combination of these (12%). However, many of the muscular (trabecular) VSDs are small in size, and about 85% to 95% of them close spontaneously.

b. When studied in surgical and autopsy settings, the prevalence of subtypes of VSD is quite different from the abovementioned figures (due in part to small size and spontaneous closure of the muscular VSDs). Perimembranous VSD accounted for 80%; outlet VSD, 5%-7% (29% in the Far Easern countries); inlet VSD, 5%-8% %; and muscular VSD, 5%-20% (McDaniel, 2001).

3. The VSD seen with TOF is a large nonrestrictive perimembranous defect with extension into the subpulmonary region. The inlet VSD is typically seen with endocardial cushion defects.
4. In subarterial infundibular or supracristal VSD, the aortic valve may prolapse through the VSD, with resulting AR and reduction of the VSD shunt. The prolapse and AR may occasionally occur with the perimembranous VSD.

5. In VSDs with small to moderate L-R shunts, volume overload is placed on the LA and LV (but not on the RV). With larger defects the RV is also under volume and pressure overload, in addition to a greater volume overload on the LA and LV. PBF is increased to a varying degree depending on the size of the defect and the pulmonary vascular resistance. With a large VSD, pulmonary hypertension results. With a long-standing large VSD, pulmonary vascular obstructive disease (PVOD) develops, with severe pulmonary hypertension and cyanosis resulting from an R-L shunt. At this stage, surgical correction is nearly impossible.

Clinical Manifestations

1. Patients with small VSDs are asymptomatic, with normal growth and development. With large VSDs, delayed growth and development, repeated pulmonary infections, CHF, and decreased exercise tolerance are relatively common. With PVOD, cyanosis and a decreased level of activity may result.
2. With a small VSD, a grade 2 to 5/6 regurgitant systolic murmur (holosystolic or less than holosystolic) maximally audible at the LLSB is characteristic (Fig. 7.5). A systolic thrill may be present at the LLSB. With a large defect, an apical diastolic rumble is audible, which represents a relative stenosis of the mitral valve due to large pulmonary venous return to the LA (Fig. 7.6). The S2 may split narrowly, and the intensity of the P2 increases if pulmonary hypertension is present (Fig. 7.6).
3. Electrocardiographic (ECG) findings: Small VSD, normal; moderate VSD, LVH, and LAH (±); large VSD, biventricular hypertrophy (BVH) and LAH (±); PVOD, pure RVH.

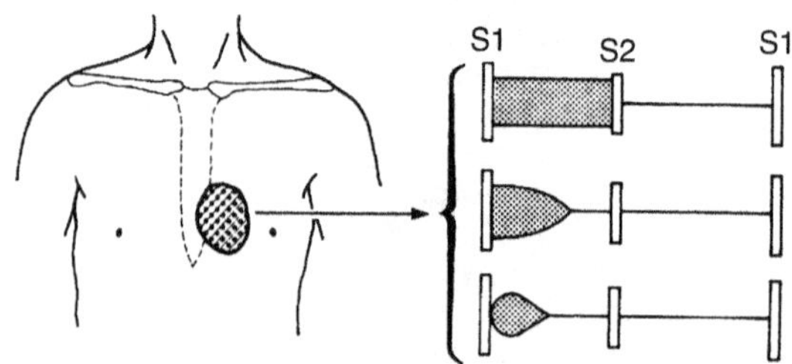

FIG. 7.5

Cardiac findings of a small ventricular septal defect. A regurgitant systolic murmur is best audible at the lower left sternal border (LLSB); it may be holosystolic or less than holosystolic. Occasionally, the heart murmur is in early systole. A systolic thrill may be palpable at the LLSB (*dots*). The S2 splits normally, and the P2 is of normal intensity.

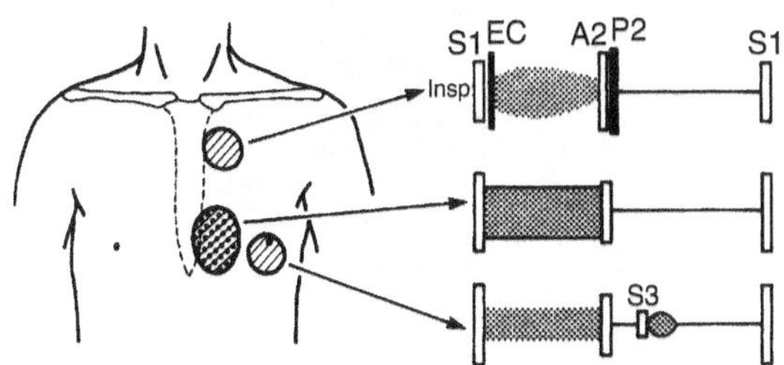

FIG. 7.6
Cardiac findings of a large ventricular separate defect. A classic holosystolic regurgitant murmur is audible at the lower left sternal border. A systolic thrill is also palpable at the same area (*dots*). There is usually a mid-diastolic rumble, resulting from relative mitral stenosis, at the apex. The S2 is narrowly split, and the P2 is accentuated in intensity. Occasionally an ejection click may be audible in the upper left sternal border when associated with pulmonary hypertension. The heart murmurs shown without solid borders are transmitted from other areas and are not characteristic of the defect. Abnormal sounds are shown in *black*.

4. Chest radiographs reveal cardiomegaly of varying degrees with enlargement of the LA, LV, and possibly the RV. PVMs are increased. The degree of cardiomegaly and the increase in PVMs are directly related to the magnitude of the L-R shunt. In PVOD, the heart is no longer enlarged and the MPA and the hilar pulmonary arteries are notably enlarged, but the peripheral lung fields are ischemic.
5. Two-dimensional echo studies provide accurate diagnosis of the position and size of the VSD. LA and LV dimensions provide indirect assessment of the magnitude of the shunt. Fig. 7.7 shows diagrams of 2D echo views of different parts of the ventricular septum, which helps identify different types of VSDs. The Doppler studies of the PA, TR (if present), and the VSD itself are useful in indirect assessment of RV and PA pressures.
6. Natural history.
   a. Spontaneous closure occurs frequently, most often in small muscular VSDs, and more often in the first year of life than thereafter. Large defects tend to become smaller with age.
   b. Inlet and infundibular VSDs do not become smaller or close spontaneously.
   c. CHF develops in infants with a large VSD but usually not until 6 or 8 weeks of age, when the PVR drops below a critical level.
   d. PVOD may begin to develop as early as 6 to 12 months of age in patients with a large VSD or earlier in a patient with trisomy.

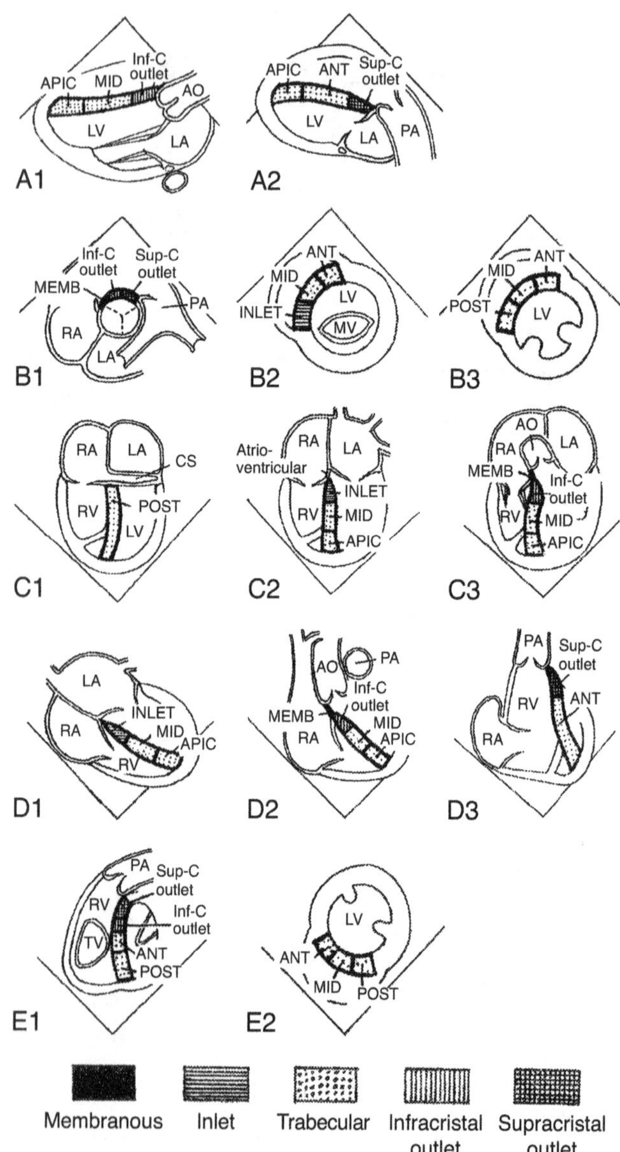
A1
APIC
MID
Inf-C outlet
AO
LV
LA
A2
APIC
ANT
Sup-C outlet
LV
LA
PA
B1
Inf-C outlet
Sup-C outlet
MEMB
PA
RA
LA
B2
ANT
MID
INLET
LV
MV
B3
ANT
MID
POST
LV
C1
RA
LA
CS
RV
POST
LV
C2
Atrio-ventricular
RA
LA
INLET
RV
MID
APIC
C3
AO
RA
LA
MEMB
Inf-C outlet
RV
MID
APIC
D1
LA
INLET
RA
MID
APIC
RV
D2
AO
PA
Inf-C outlet
MEMB
MID
RA
APIC
D3
PA
Sup-C outlet
RV
ANT
RA
E1
PA
Sup-C outlet
RV
Inf-C outlet
TV
ANT
POST
E2
LV
ANT
MID
POST
Membranous
Inlet
Trabecular
Infracristal outlet
Supracristal outlet

B. MANAGEMENT

Medical and Nonsurgical

1. Treatment of CHF with diuretics, afterload reducers, and sometimes digoxin (see Chapter 19).
2. No exercise restriction is required in the absence of pulmonary hypertension.
3. Nonsurgical device closure of selected muscular VSDs is possible when the defect is not too close to cardiac valves and when it is difficult to access surgically. Some centers have used so-called hybrid procedures through left thoracotomy incision and performing "perventricular" device closure without the use of cardiopulmonary bypass to close muscular VSD. Device closure is not popular for the perimembranous VSD because of the potential for postprocedure heart block or development of AR.

Surgical

1. Procedure.
   a. Direct closure of the defect is performed under hypothermic cardiopulmonary bypass, preferably through an atrial approach rather than through a right ventriculotomy.
   b. PA banding is rarely performed unless additional lesions make the complete repair difficult.
2. Indications and timing.
   a. A significant L-R shunt with Qp/Qs of greater than 2:1 is an indication for surgical closure. Surgery is not indicated for a small VSD with Qp/Qs less than 1.5:1.
   b. Timing.
   (1) Infants with CHF and growth retardation unresponsive to medical therapy should be operated on at any age, including early infancy.
   (2) Infants with a large VSD and evidence of increasing PVR should be operated on as soon as possible.
   (3) Infants who respond to medical therapy may be operated on by the age of 12 to 18 months.

◀ **FIG. 7.7**

Selected two-dimensional echo views of the ventricular septum. These schematic drawings are helpful in determining the type of ventricular septal defect. Different shading has been used for easy recognition of different parts of the ventricular septum. Row A, parasternal long-axis views. Row B, parasternal short-axis views. Row C, apical four- and "five-chamber" views. Row D, subcostal long-axis views. Row E, subcostal short-axis views. *ANT,* anterior muscular; *AO,* aorta; *APIC,* apical muscular; *CS,* coronary sinus; *Inf-C outlet,* infracristal outlet muscular; *INLET,* inlet muscular; *LA,* left atrium; *LV,* left ventricle; *MEMB,* membranous; *MID,* mid-muscular; *PA,* pulmonary artery; *POST,* posterior muscular; *RA,* right atrium; *RV,* right ventricle; *Sup-C outlet,* supracristal outlet muscular. *(From Park, M. K., & Salamat, M. (2020).* Park's pediatric cardiology for practitioners *(7th ed.). Philadelphia: Mosby.)*

(4) Asymptomatic children may be operated on between 2 and 4 years of age.

c. Contraindications. PVR/SVR ratio of 0.5 or greater or PVOD with a predominant R-L shunt.

3. Mortality and complications.

Surgical mortality is 0.5%. Up to 3% of patients develop complete heart block, some transient. Residual shunt occurs in less than 5%.

4. Surgical approaches for special situations.
   a. **VSD + large PDA.** If the PDA is large, the ductus alone may be closed in the first 6 to 8 weeks, and the VSD may be closed later. If the VSD is large and nonrestrictive, the VSD should be closed early and the PDA ligated at the time of VSD repair.
   b. **VSD + COA.** Controversies exist. One approach is the repair of COA alone initially and the closure of the VSD later if indicated. Other options include COA repair and PA banding if the VSD appears large or repair of both defects at the same time using one or two incisions.
   c. **VSD + AR** is usually associated with subarterial infundibular (or supracristal) VSD and occasionally with perimembranous VSD. When AR is present, a prompt closure of the VSD is recommended, even if the Qp/Qs is less than 2:1, to abort progression of or to abolish AR. Some centers close the VSD if aortic prolapse is evident even in the absence of AR.

Follow-Up

Postoperatively, an office follow-up should be done every 1 to 2 years. The ECG shows RBBB in 50% to 90% of the patients who had VSD repair through right ventriculotomy and in up to 40% of the patients who had repair through the right atrial approach.

III. PATENT DUCTUS ARTERIOSUS

A. PREVALENCE

Five to 10 percent of all CHDs, excluding those in premature infants.

B. PATHOLOGY AND PATHOPHYSIOLOGY

1. There is a persistent postnatal patency of a normal fetal structure between the PA and the descending aorta.
2. The magnitude of the L-R shunt is determined by the diameter and length of the ductus and the level of PVR. With a long-standing large ductus, pulmonary hypertension and PVOD may develop with an eventual R-L shunt and cyanosis.

C. CLINICAL MANIFESTATIONS

1. The patients are asymptomatic when the ductus is small. When the defect is large, signs of CHF may develop.
2. A grade 1 to 4/6 continuous (machinery) murmur best audible at the ULSB or left infraclavicular area is the hallmark of the condition (Fig. 7.8). An apical diastolic rumble is audible with a large-shunt PDA.

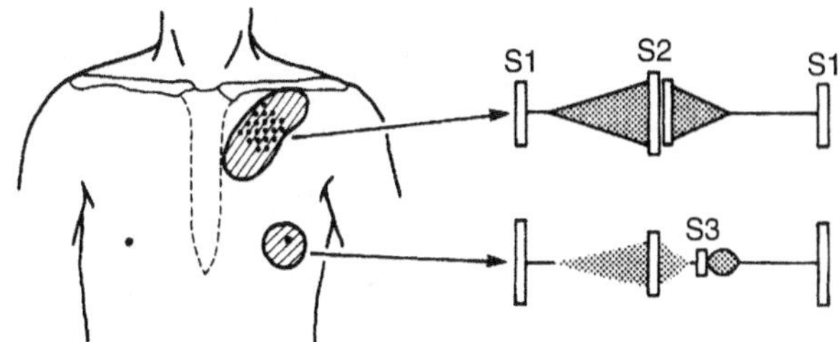

FIG. 7.8
Cardiac findings of patent ductus arteriosus. A continuous murmur, maximally audible at the left upper sternal border or left infraclavicular area, is a typical finding. When the shunt is large, a diastolic rumble is audible at the apex. A systolic thrill may be present in the area shown by *dots*.

Bounding peripheral pulses with wide pulse pressure are present with a large-shunt PDA.

3. ECG findings are similar to those of VSD: normal or LVH in a small to moderate PDA; BVH in a large PDA; RVH if PVOD develops.
4. Chest radiographs are also similar to those of VSD: normal with a small-shunt PDA; with a large-shunt PDA, cardiomegaly (with LA and LV enlargement) and increased PVM are present; with PVOD the heart size is normal, with a marked prominence of the MPA and hilar vessels.
5. The PDA can be directly imaged and its hemodynamic significance determined by 2D echo and color flow Doppler examination. Cardiac catheterization is not indicated in isolated PDA.
6. Natural history: CHF or recurrent pneumonia or both develop if the shunt is large. Spontaneous closure of PDA is rare in term infants if it persists beyond the neonatal period.

D. MANAGEMENT

Medical and Nonsurgical

1. No exercise restriction is required in the absence of pulmonary hypertension.
2. Indomethacin is ineffective in term infants with PDA.
3. Indications for nonsurgical closure of PDA:
   a. Definitely indicated for hemodynamically significant PDA with CHF, failure to thrive, or enlarged LA and LV.
   b. Reasonable to close small PDA when the murmur of PDA is audible.
   c. Controversial for closing so-called silent ductus, which is a small ductus incidentally detected by echo studies but without audible heart murmur.
   d. Contraindicated when PVOD is present.

4. Catheter closure of the ductus may be used. Small ductus <4 mm in diameter are closed by Gianturco stainless coils and larger ones by the Amplatzer PDA device. An optimal candidate for the coil occlusion has the ductus 2.5 mm or less in size, but the use of multiple coils can close a ductus up to 5 mm. The Amplatzer device may be used for PDAs ranging in size from 4 to 12 mm (with 100% closure rate). Complications may include residual leaks, pulmonary artery coil embolization, hemolysis, left PA stenosis, aortic occlusion with the Amplatzer device, and femoral vessel occlusion.

Surgical

Surgical closure is reserved for those patients in whom nonsurgical closure technique is not considered applicable. Ligation and division through left posterolateral thoracotomy without cardiopulmonary bypass is performed. Repair through a smaller incision with video-assisted thoracoscopy is becoming popular. Surgical mortality is near 0%. PVOD is a contraindication to surgery.

E. DIFFERENTIAL DIAGNOSIS

The following conditions require differentiation from PDA because they may present with a heart murmur similar to that of PDA and/or with bounding pulses.

1. Coronary AV fistula (the murmur is audible over the precordium, not at the ULSB).
2. Systemic AV fistula (a wide pulse pressure with bounding pulse, CHF, and a continuous murmur over the fistula [head or liver] are characteristic).
3. Pulmonary AV fistula (a continuous murmur over the back, cyanosis, and clubbing in the absence of cardiomegaly).
4. Venous hum (an innocent condition that disappears when the patient is supine).
5. Murmurs of collaterals in patients with COA or TOF (audible in the intercostal spaces).
6. VSD + AR (maximally audible at the MLSB or LLSB, it is actually a to-and-fro murmur, rather than a continuous murmur).
7. Absence of pulmonary valve (a to-and-fro murmur, or "sawing-wood sound" at the ULSB, large central pulmonary arteries on chest radiographs, RVH on ECG, and cyanosis).
8. Aortopulmonary septal defect (AP window) (bounding peripheral pulses, a murmur resembling that of VSD, and signs of CHF).
9. Peripheral PA stenosis (a continuous murmur may be audible all over the thorax, unilateral or bilateral).
10. Ruptured sinus of Valsalva aneurysm (sudden onset of chest pain and severe heart failure, a continuous murmur or a to-and-fro murmur, and often Marfan features).

IV. PATENT DUCTUS ARTERIOSUS IN PRETERM NEONATES

A. PREVALENCE

Clinical evidence of PDA appears in 45% of infants <1750 g birth weight (with CHF occurring in 15%) and in about 80% of infants <1200 g birth weight (with CHF occurring in 40% to 50%).

B. PATHOLOGY AND PATHOPHYSIOLOGY

1. PDA is a special problem in premature infants with hyaline membrane disease. With improvement in oxygenation, the PVR falls rapidly, but the ductus remains patent because its responsiveness to oxygen is immature in premature newborns. The resulting large L-R shunt makes the lung stiff, and weaning the infant from the ventilator and oxygen therapy becomes difficult.
2. If the ductus is not closed, the infant remains on ventilator therapy, with development of bronchopulmonary dysplasia and pulmonary hypertension with right-sided heart failure.

C. CLINICAL MANIFESTATIONS

1. It is important to predict a significant PDA in a premature neonate, in whom weaning from a ventilator is delayed or fails. Episodes of apnea or bradycardia may be the initial sign of PDA in infants who are not on ventilators.
2. The physical examination reveals bounding peripheral pulses, a hyperactive precordium, and tachycardia with or without gallop rhythm. The classic continuous murmur at the left infraclavicular area or ULSB is diagnostic, but the murmur may be only systolic and is difficult to hear in infants who are on ventilators.
3. The ECG is usually normal but occasionally shows LVH.
4. Chest radiographs show cardiomegaly and increased PVM in larger premature infants who are not intubated. In infants who are intubated and on high ventilator settings, chest radiographs may show the heart to be either of normal size or only mildly enlarged.
5. Two-dimensional echo and color flow Doppler studies (with the sample volume placed at the pulmonary end of the ductus) provide accurate anatomic and functional information, such as ductal shunt patterns (pure L-R, bidirectional, or predominant R-L shunt), pressures in the PA, and magnitude of the ductal shunt or pulmonary perfusion status.

D. MANAGEMENT

For symptomatic infants, either pharmacologic or surgical closure of the ductus is indicated. A small PDA that does not cause symptoms should be followed medically for 6 months because of the possibility of spontaneous closure.

Medical

1. Fluid restriction to 120 mL/kg/day and a diuretic (e.g., chlorothiazide) may be tried for 24 to 48 hours (with a low success rate). Use of furosemide is not recommended, because it is known to stimulate prostaglandin E_2 synthesis and thus dilates the PDA. Digoxin is not used because it has little hemodynamic benefit and a high incidence of digitalis toxicity.
2. Pharmacologic closure of the PDA can be achieved with the following medications.
   a. Intravenous (IV) *indomethacin* (a prostaglandin synthetase inhibitor). Indomethacin inhibits the synthesis and release of prostaglandins, which play a major role in maintaining ductal patency during fetal life. Contraindications to the use of indomethacin include high blood urea nitrogen (>25 ng/dL) or creatinine (>1.8 mg/dL) levels, low platelet count (<80,000/mm^3), bleeding tendency (including intracranial hemorrhage), necrotizing enterocolitis, and hyperbilirubinemia. The following is a dosage regimen. The dose is given every 12 hours a total of 3 doses. For <48 hours old, 0.2 mg/kg is followed by 0.1 mg/kg × 2. For 2-7 days old, 0.2 mg/kg × 3, and for >7 days, 0.2 mg/kg followed by 0.25 mg/kg × 2.
   b. *Ibuprofen,* another inhibitor of prostaglandin synthesis, has also been used in ductal closure in premature infants. Intravenous ibuprofen (10 mg/kg, followed at 24-hour intervals by two doses of 5 mg/kg) starting on the third day of life was equally effective in closing the ductus in preterm newborns as indomethacin. Ibuprofen had a significantly lower incidence of oliguria, and it does not appear to have a deleterious effect on cerebral blood flow.
   c. More recently, *acetaminophen* is being used for PDA closure in preterm infants, with success rates comparable with those of indomethacin or ibuprofen. Acetaminophen is believed to block the peroxidase segment of prostaglandin synthetase, thus inhibiting prostaglandin production. Elevation of transaminase may be a side effect. A current recommended dosing is 15 mg/kg given every 6 hours (oral or IV).
3. Prophylactic use of ibuprofen in small preterm infants does not appear to be useful because, although it reduced the occurrence and the need for surgical ligation of the ductus, it did not reduce the frequency of intraventricular hemorrhage (IVH), mortality, or morbidity.

Surgical

If medical treatment is unsuccessful or if the use of medications is contraindicated, surgical ligation of the ductus is indicated. Many centers now perform PDA ligation in the neonatal intensive care unit at the bedside. The operative mortality is 0% to 3%. The use of minimally invasive video-assisted thoracoscopic surgery (VATS) is popular in the management of PDA in low-birth-weight infants.

Percutaneous

More recently device closures even in neonates with a weight less than 1000 g have successfully been performed with devices such as Amplatzer Piccolo Occluder, which was approved by the FDA in 2019.

V. COMPLETE ENDOCARDIAL CUSHION DEFECT (COMPLETE AV CANAL)

A. PREVALENCE

Five percent of all CHD. Of patients with complete ECD, about 70% are children with Down syndrome.

B. PATHOLOGY AND PATHOPHYSIOLOGY

1. Complete ECD consists of an ostium primum ASD, an inlet VSD, and clefts in the anterior mitral valve leaflet and in the septal leaflet of the tricuspid valve, forming common anterior and posterior cusps of the AV valve (Fig. 7.9C). When the ventricular septum is intact, the defect is termed partial ECD or ostium primum ASD.
2. In complete ECD, a single valve orifice connects the atrial and ventricular chambers, whereas in the partial form, there are separate mitral and tricuspid orifices.
3. In the majority of complete ECDs, the AV valve orifice is equally committed to the RV and LV. In some patients, however, the orifice is committed primarily to one ventricle, with hypoplasia of the other ventricle (i.e., "unbalanced" AV canal with RV or LV dominance).

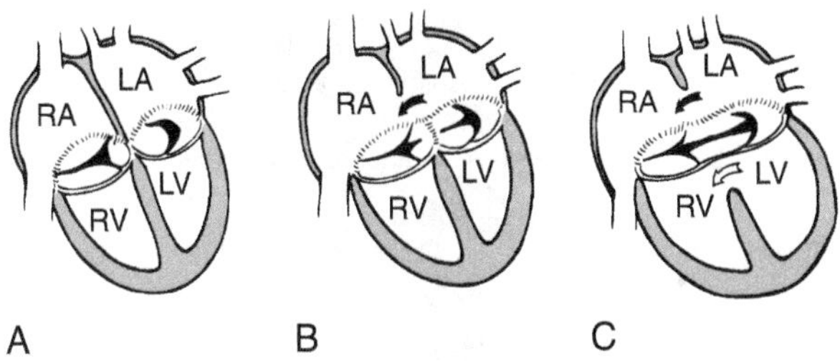

FIG. 7.9

Atrioventricular valve (AV) and cardiac septa in partial and complete endocardial cushion defects (ECDs). (A) Normal AV valve anatomy with no septal defects. (B) Partial ECD with clefts in the mitral and tricuspid valves and an ostium primum ASD (*arrow*). (C) Complete ECD. There is a common AV valve with large anterior and posterior bridging leaflets. An ostium primum ASD (*solid arrow*) and an inlet VSD (*open arrow*) are present. *LA*, left atrium; *LV*, left ventricle; *RA*, right atrium; *RV*, right ventricle.

Hypoplasia of one ventricle may necessitate one ventricular repair (Fontan-type operation).

4. Additional cardiac anomalies may include TOF (called "canal tet," occurring in 6% of patients with ECD), DORV with more than 50% overriding of the aorta (occurring in 6%), and TGA (occurring in 3%). Associated defects are rare in children with Down syndrome.
5. The combination of these defects may result in an interatrial and/or interventricular shunt, AV valve regurgitation, or LV-to-RA shunt. CHF with or without pulmonary hypertension usually develops early in infancy.

C. CLINICAL MANIFESTATIONS

1. Failure to thrive, repeated respiratory infections, and signs of CHF are common during early infancy.
2. Hyperactive precordium with a systolic thrill at the LLSB and a loud S2 are frequent findings. A grade 3 to 4/6 holosystolic regurgitant murmur is audible along the LLSB. The systolic murmur of MR may be audible at the apex. A mid-diastolic rumble at the LLSB or at the apex (from relative stenosis of the tricuspid and/or mitral valve) and gallop rhythm may be present.
3. The ECG finding of a "superior" QRS axis (with the axis between −40 degrees and −150 degrees) is characteristic. RVH or RBBB is present in all, and many have LVH as well. Most patients have a prolonged PR interval (first-degree AV block).
4. Chest radiographs always show cardiomegaly with increased PVMs.
5. Two-dimensional echo and color flow Doppler studies allow imaging of all components of ECD, as well as an assessment of the hemodynamic severity.
6. Natural History. CHF occurs 1 to 2 months after birth, and recurrent pneumonia is commonly seen. Children with Down syndrome and ECD begin to develop PVOD in the latter half of the first year of life. The survivors develop PVOD and die in late childhood or as young adults.

D. MANAGEMENT

Medical

Medical management is recommended initially for small infants with CHF, as surgical mortality is relatively high in this age group.

Surgical

1. PA banding is no longer recommended unless other associated anomalies make complete repair a high-risk procedure.
2. Closure of ASD and VSD and reconstruction of cleft AV valves under cardiopulmonary bypass and/or deep hypothermia are carried out between 2 and 4 months of age. Surgical mortality is about 2.5%. Most

of these infants have CHF that is unresponsive to medical therapy, and some have elevated PVR. Early surgical repair of the defect is especially important for infants with Down syndrome because of their known tendency to develop early PVOD. Complications of the surgery include MR (which is persistent or has been worsened), sinus node dysfunction (with resulting bradyarrhythmias), and complete heart block (occurring in less than 5% of the patients).

3. Patients with unbalanced AV canal (with hypoplasia of right or left ventricle) may be treated by an earlier PA banding and later by a modified Fontan operation.
4. In patients with canal tet who are severely cyanotic, a systemic-to-PA shunt is carried out during infancy and a complete repair done between 2 and 4 years of age.

Follow-Up

For patients with a significant regurgitation of the AV valve or residual ventricular shunts, anticongestive medications (e.g., diuretics, angiotensin-converting enzyme inhibitors, digoxin) may be required. Some restriction of activities may be required if residual hemodynamic abnormalities are present.

VI. PARTIAL ENDOCARDIAL CUSHION DEFECT (OSTIUM PRIMUM ASD)

A. PREVALENCE

One to 2 percent of all CHDs (much lower than secundum ASD).

B. PATHOLOGY AND PATHOPHYSIOLOGY

1. A defect is present in the lower part of the atrium septum near the AV valves, without an interventricular communication (see Fig. 7.9B). The anterior and posterior bridging leaflets are fused by a connecting tongue to form separate right and left AV orifices. Clefts of the mitral and occasionally of the tricuspid valve are present.
2. Less common forms of partial ECD include common atrium (which is a characteristic lesion seen in the Ellis-van Creveld syndrome), VSD of the inlet septum (i.e., AV canal-type VSD), and isolated cleft of the mitral valve.
3. Pathophysiology of ostium primum ASD is similar to that of ostium secundum ASD.

C. CLINICAL MANIFESTATIONS

1. Usually asymptomatic during childhood.
2. Physical findings are identical to those of secundum ASD (see Fig. 7.2), except for a regurgitant systolic murmur of MR, which may be present at the apex.

3. The ECG shows a "superior" QRS axis, as in complete ECD. First-degree AV blocks (50%) and RVH or RBBB (rsR′ pattern in V1) are common.
4. Chest radiographs are identical to those of secundum ASD except for the enlargement of the LA and LV when MR is significant.
5. Two-dimensional echo allows accurate diagnosis of primum ASD.
6. Natural history: CHF may develop in childhood and pulmonary hypertension in adulthood. Spontaneous closure of the defect does not occur. Cardiac arrhythmias (20%) may complicate the defect.

D. MANAGEMENT

Medical

No exercise restriction is required in asymptomatic children. Occasionally, anticongestive measures with diuretic may be indicated.

Surgical

Closure of the primum ASD and reconstruction of the cleft mitral and tricuspid valves are performed electively between 2 and 4 years of age. Surgical mortality is approximately 2.5%.

Follow-Up

Sinus node dysfunction may develop and require pacemaker therapy.

VII. PARTIAL ANOMALOUS PULMONARY VENOUS RETURN

A. PREVALENCE

Less than 1% of all children with CHD.

B. PATHOLOGY AND PATHOPHYSIOLOGY

1. One or more but not all PVs drain into the RA or its venous tributaries, such as the SVC, IVC, coronary sinus, or left innominate vein (Fig. 7.10).
2. The right PVs are involved twice as often as the left PVs. The right PVs may drain into the SVC, often associated with sinus venous ASD (Fig. 7.10A), or drain into the IVC (Fig. 7.10B), in association with an intact atrial septum and bronchopulmonary sequestration.
3. The left PVs either drain into the left innominate vein (Fig. 7.10C) or into the coronary sinus (Fig. 7.10D).
4. The hemodynamic alteration is similar to that seen with ASD. The magnitude of the pulmonary blood flow is determined by the number of anomalous PVs and the presence and size of the ASD.

C. CLINICAL MANIFESTATIONS

1. Children with PAPVR are usually asymptomatic.

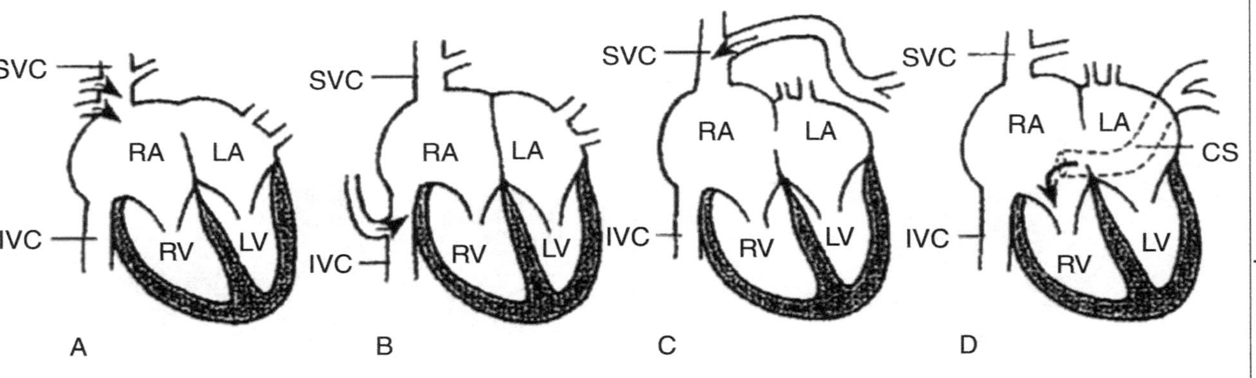

FIG. 7.10
Common types of partial anomalous pulmonary venous drainage. (A) The right pulmonary artery (PA) drains anomalously to the superior vena cava (*SVC*). Sinus venosus atrial septal defect (ASD) is usually present. (B) The right lower PV drains into the inferior vena cava (*IVC*), usually without an associated ASD. (C) The left PVs drain into the left innominate vein. (D) The left PVs drain into the coronary sinus (*CS*). *LA,* left atrium; *LV,* left ventricle: *RA,* right atrium; *RV,* right ventricle.

2. Physical findings are similar to those of ASD (see Fig. 7.2). When associated with ASD, the S2 is split widely and fixed. When the atrial septum is intact, the S2 is normal.
3. The ECG shows RVH or RBBB or is normal.
4. Chest radiographs show RAE, RVE, and increased PVMs.
5. Echo diagnosis of PAPVR is less reliable. Cardiac magnetic resonance imaging can make correct diagnosis of the condition without catheterization.
6. Natural history: If PAPVR is undetected, cyanosis and exertional dyspnea may develop during the third and fourth decades, resulting from pulmonary hypertension and PVOD.

D. MANAGEMENT

Medical

Exercise restriction is not required.

Surgical

1. Surgical correction is carried out when the patient is 2 to 5 years of age. A significant L-R shunt with Qp/Qs greater than 1.5:1 or 2:1 is an indication for surgery. Isolated single lobe anomaly is not ordinarily corrected.
2. Surgical procedures vary according to the site of anomalous drainage.
   a. For the anomalous drainage into the SVC, a tunnel is created between the anomalous vein and the ASD using a Teflon or pericardial patch and the SVC is widened to prevent obstruction of flow.
   b. For the anomalous drainage into the IVC, an intraatrial tunnel drains the venous blood into the LA. When this is associated with the bronchopulmonary sequestration, the involved lobes(s) may be resected (without connecting the anomalous vein to the heart).
   c. To the left innominate vein. The anomalous left pulmonary vein is anastomosed to the base of the amputated left atrial appendage.
   d. When the left PVs drain into the coronary sinus, the sinus is unroofed and the orifice of the coronary sinus is closed.
3. Surgical mortality occurs <1% of the time.

Chapter 8

Obstructive Lesions

I. PULMONARY STENOSIS

A. PREVALENCE

Isolated PS occurs in 4% to 8% of all CHDs.

B. PATHOLOGY AND PATHOPHYSIOLOGY

1. PS may be valvular (90%), subvalvular (infundibular), or supravalvular (i.e., stenosis of the main PA). Stenosis of the PA branches is presented in Chapter 10.
   a. In valvular PS, the pulmonary valve is thickened, with fused or absent commissures and a small orifice. A poststenotic dilatation of the MPA usually develops with valvular PS.
   b. In neonates with critical PS, the RV, tricuspid valve, right ventricular outflow tract (RVOT), and pulmonary artery are commonly underdeveloped.
   c. Dysplastic pulmonary valve (with thickened, irregular, immobile tissue) is frequently seen with Noonan syndrome.
   d. Infundibular PS is usually associated with a large VSD as seen in TOF. The poststenotic dilatation is not seen with subvalvular stenosis.
2. In so-called double-chambered RV, abnormal muscular bands (running between the ventricular septum and the anterior wall) divide the RV cavity into a proximal high-pressure chamber and a distal low-pressure chamber.
3. Pulmonary artery stenosis may occur in the main pulmonary artery, its main branches, or in the small distal pulmonary arteries. This topic is discussed in a separate heading in this chapter.
4. Depending on the severity of PS, a varying degree of RVH develops. The RV is usually normal in size, but in newborns with critical PS, the RV is hypoplastic.

C. CLINICAL MANIFESTATIONS

1. Usually asymptomatic with mild PS. Exertional dyspnea and easy fatigability may be seen in moderately severe cases, and CHF occurs in severe cases. Neonates with critical PS are cyanotic and tachypneic.
2. An ejection click is present at the ULSB with valvular PS (Fig. 8.1). The S2 may split widely, and the P2 may be diminished in intensity. A systolic ejection murmur (grade 2 to 5/6) with or without systolic thrill is best audible at the ULSB and transmits fairly well to the back and

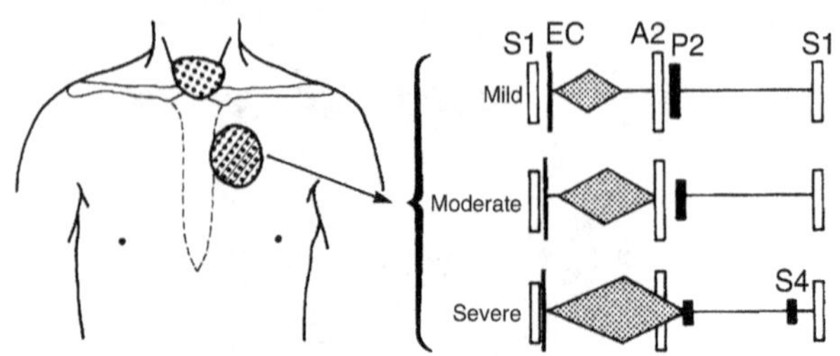

FIG. 8.1

Cardiac findings of pulmonary valve stenosis. Abnormal sounds are shown in *black*. *Dots* represent areas with systolic thrill. *EC*, Ejection click.

axillae. The louder and longer the murmur, the more severe is the stenosis. Neonates with critical PS may have only a faint heart murmur, if any.

3. The electrocardiogram (ECG) is normal in mild PS. RAD and RVH are present in moderate PS. RAH and RVH with "strain" pattern are present in severe PS. Neonates with critical PS may show LVH (due to hypoplastic RV and relatively large LV).
4. Chest radiographs show normal heart size and a prominent MPA segment (i.e., poststenotic dilatation). PVMs are normal but may be decreased in severe PS.
5. Two-dimensional echo and Doppler echo studies:
   a. Thickened pulmonary valve with restricted systolic motion (doming) and a poststenotic dilatation of the MPA are commonly seen.
   b. The severity of PS (by peak Doppler pressure gradient) may be classified as follows:
      (1) Mild: <35 to 40 mm Hg (or RV pressure $<50\%$ of LV pressure).
      (2) Moderate: gradient 40 to 70 mm Hg (or RV pressure 50% to 75% of LV pressure).
      (3) Severe: >70 mm Hg (or RV pressure $\geq 75\%$ of LV pressure).
6. Natural history: The severity of the obstruction is usually not progressive in mild PS, but it tends to progress with age in moderate or severe PS. CHF may develop in patients with severe stenosis. Sudden death is possible in patients with severe stenosis during heavy physical activities.

D. MANAGEMENT

Medical and Nonsurgical

1. For neonates with critical PS and cyanosis, prostaglandin E_1 (PGE_1) infusion should be started to reopen the ductus. Balloon valvuloplasty is

the procedure of choice in critically ill neonates. Immediate reduction in pressure gradient can be achieved in more than 90% of these neonates. Complications of the balloon procedure are more common than in older patients, with a mortality rate of up to 3%. Even dysplastic valves appear to mature after the balloon procedure. About 15% of the patients require reintervention (either repeat valvuloplasty or surgery) at a later time.

2. Balloon valvuloplasty is the procedure of choice for significant pulmonary valve stenosis. Cardiac catheterization is recommended for the balloon procedure in patients with a Doppler pressure gradient near 50 mm Hg. Indications for the balloon procedure may include the following.
   a. Pressure gradient >40 mm Hg with the patient sedated in the catheterization laboratory.
   b. If the catheterization pressure gradient is 30 to 39 mm Hg, the balloon procedure is reasonable.
   c. Symptoms (angina, syncope, or presyncope) attributable to PS with catheter gradient >30 mm Hg.
   d. It is reasonable to try on dysplastic pulmonary valve (with lower success rate of 65%).
3. Complications of the balloon procedure.
   a. PR is common after balloon dilatation (occurring in 10% to 40%). Therefore use of a balloon 120% to 130% of the pulmonary annulus is recommended to reduce the incidence of PR.
   b. Following relief of severe PS (either by balloon or surgery), hypertrophied dynamic infundibulum may cause a persistent pressure gradient, with rare occurrences of fatal outcome ("suicidal right ventricle"); in this case intravenous propranolol could be given during cardiac catheterization. After balloon valvuloplasty oral propranolol may be given to reduce hyperdynamic infundibular obstruction. The reduction of this gradient occurs gradually over weeks
4. Restriction of activity is usually not indicated except for severe PS.

Surgical

1. Surgical valvotomy is occasionally indicated in patients with valvular PS in whom balloon valvuloplasty is unsuccessful.
2. Surgery is indicated in patients with dysplastic pulmonary valves that are resistant to dilatation. Dysplastic valve may need to be completely excised because simple valvotomy may be ineffective.
3. Surgery is also indicated for infundibular stenosis and anomalous RV muscle bundle with significant pressure gradients.
4. If balloon valvuloplasty is unsuccessful, infants with critical PS require surgery on an urgent basis.
5. Stenosis at the main PA requires patch widening of the narrow portion.

Follow-Up

Periodic echo studies are indicated to detect recurrences or worsening of the stenosis.

II. AORTIC STENOSIS

A. PREVALENCE

A group of lesions that produce LV outflow tract obstruction account for 10% of all CHD. Aortic valve stenosis occurs more often in males (male-to-female ratio of 4:1).

B. PATHOLOGY AND PATHOPHYSIOLOGY

1. LVOT obstruction may occur at the valvular, subvalvular, or supravalvular levels (Fig. 8.2).
2. Valvular stenosis may be caused by a bicuspid aortic valve, a unicuspid aortic valve, or stenosis of the tricuspid (or tricommissural) aortic valve (Fig. 8.3).
   a. By far the most common type of aortic valve stenosis is bicuspid aortic valve (BAV), accounting for 75% of AS (Fig. 8.3B). In addition, it is the most common cardiac malformation with prevalence of 0.5% to 2% of the general population, diagnosed by echo studies. Many cases of BAV are nonobstructive during childhood. More than 50% of the patients with BAV have aortic dilatation that is now considered primary aortopathy (rather than the result of hemodynamic abnormality). BAV is believed to be an inheritable disorder (i.e., autosomal dominant disease with incomplete penetrance) with a male-to-female ratio of 3:1.
   b. Much less common is the unicuspid valve with one lateral attachment (Fig. 8.3A).
   c. A valve that has three unseparated cusps with a stenotic central orifice is the least common form (Fig. 8.3C).

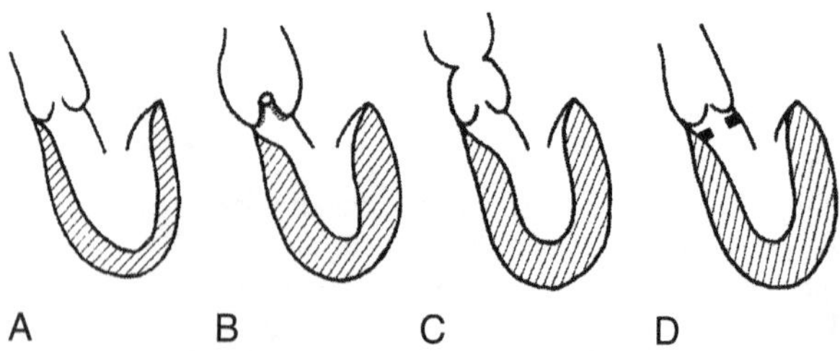

FIG. 8.2

Anatomic types of left ventricular outflow tract obstruction. (A) Normal. (B) Valvular stenosis. (C) Supravalvular stenosis. (D) Discrete subaortic stenosis.

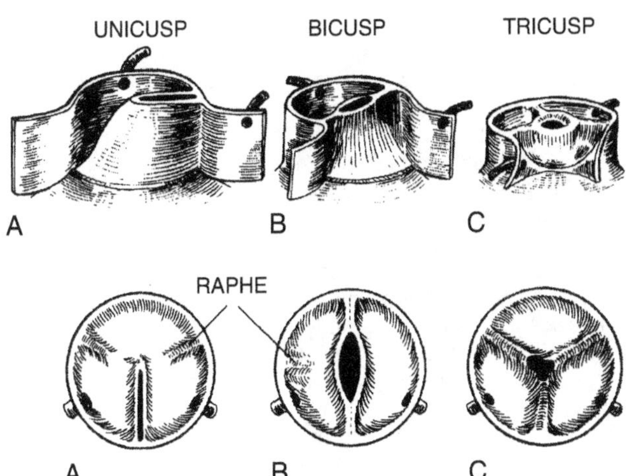

FIG. 8.3

Anatomic types of aortic valve stenosis. The top row shows the side view, and bottom row is the view as seen in surgery during aortotomy. (A) Unicuspid aortic valve. (B) Bicuspid aortic valve. (C) Stenosis of a tricuspid aortic valve. *(From Goor, D. A., & Lillehei, C. W. (1975).* Congenital malformations of the heart. *New York: Grune & Stratton.)*

3. Symptomatic neonates with so-called critical neonatal aortic valve stenosis have primitive, myxomatous valve tissue, with a pinhole opening. The aortic valve ring and ascending aorta, the mitral valve, and the LV cavity are almost always hypoplastic (often requiring Norwood operation followed by Fontan operation).
4. Supravalvular AS occurs at the upper margin of the sinus of Valsalva. This is often associated with Williams syndrome. Patients with supravalvular AS may also have coronary artery ostial stenosis with increased risk of sudden cardiac death.
5. Subvalvular (subaortic) stenosis may be either discrete (simple membrane or fibromuscular ridge) or diffuse tunnel-like fibromuscular narrowing (tunnel stenosis). Discrete subaortic stenosis is more common than the tunnel stenosis and is often associated with other lesions such as VSD, PDA, or COA. Tunnel-like subaortic stenosis is often associated with hypoplasia of the valve ring and the ascending aorta.
6. Natural history: Hypertrophy of the LV may develop if the stenosis is severe. Dilatation of the ascending aorta seen in BAV may progress. AR usually develops with subaortic AS.

C. CLINICAL MANIFESTATIONS

1. Patients with mild to moderate AS and those with BAV are asymptomatic. Exertional chest pain or syncope may occur with severe AS. CHF develops within the first few months of life with critical AS.
2. Blood pressure (BP) is normal in most patients, but a narrow pulse pressure is present in severe AS. Patients with supravalvular AS may have a higher systolic pressure in the right arm than in the left (due to the jet of stenosis directed into the innominate artery, the so-called Coanda effect).
3. A systolic thrill may be present at the URSB, in the suprasternal notch, or over the carotid arteries. An ejection click may be audible with valvular AS. A harsh systolic ejection murmur (grade 2 to 4/6) is best audible at the second right intercostal space or third left intercostal space (Fig. 8.4), with good transmission to the neck and frequently to the apex. A high-pitched, early diastolic decrescendo murmur of AR may be audible in patients with bicuspid aortic valve and those with discrete subvalvular stenosis. In symptomatic infants with critical AS, the heart murmur may be absent or faint, and the peripheral pulses are weak and thready.
4. The ECG is normal in mild cases. LVH with or without a strain pattern is seen in more severe cases.
5. Chest radiographs are usually normal in children, but a dilated ascending aorta may be seen occasionally in valvular AS. A significant cardiomegaly develops with CHF or substantial AR.
6. Echo and Doppler studies are diagnostic.
   a. The parasternal short-axis view of the two-dimensional echocardiography shows the anatomy of the aortic valve: bicuspid, tricuspid, or unicuspid. Normal aortic valves are tricuspid, with three cusps of approximately equal size. In diastole the normal aortic cusp

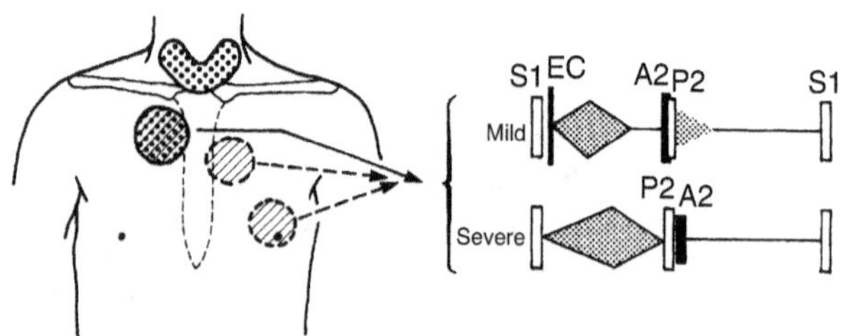

FIG. 8.4

Cardiac findings of aortic valve stenosis. Abnormal sounds are indicated in *black*. Systolic thrill may be present in areas with *dots*. *EC*, Ejection click.

margins form a Y pattern, which opens widely during systole (Fig. 8.5). In systole, a bicuspid aortic valve appears as a noncircular (i.e., football-shaped) orifice (Fig. 8.5). A unicommissural aortic valve, which is seen often in infants with critical AS, is seen as a circular orifice positioned eccentrically within the aortic root and without visible distinct cusps.

b. The Doppler pressure gradient is best obtained in the apical "five-chamber" view. The Doppler pressure gradient (instantaneous gradient) is approximately 20% higher than the peak-to-peak systolic pressure gradient obtained during cardiac catheterization.

c. The severity of the stenosis is defined by a peak velocity across the aortic valve and a mean Doppler gradient across the valve as follows.
   (1) Mild: Peak velocity 2.0–2.9 m/sec (or mean Doppler gradient $\leq$ 20 mm Hg)
   (2) Moderate: Peak velocity 3.0–3.9 m/sec (or mean Doppler gradient between 20 and 39 mm Hg).
   (3) Severe: Peak velocity of $\geq$4.0 m/sec (or mean Doppler gradient of $\geq$40 mm Hg) (or aortic valve area of $\leq$1.0 cm^2 or indexed valve area $\leq$0.6 cm^2/m2).

d. The type of subaortic stenosis is best imaged in the parasternal long-axis view, apical long-axis view, and apical five-chamber view just beneath the aortic valve. One should note whether the stenosis is (a) membrane, (b) fibromuscular ridge, or (c) diffuse tunnel-like fibromuscular narrowing (tunnel stenosis).

e. Supravalvular AS is seen as a narrowing of the ascending aorta in the parasternal long-axis view and apical long-axis view. The suprasternal view best shows diffuse hypoplasia of the ascending aorta.

7. Magnetic resonance imaging (MRI).

   If unclear from echo study, MRI can clarify the level and mechanism of anatomic obstruction. It may be a reliable tool for serial evaluation of aortic dilatation in patients with BAV.

8. Natural history.
   a. Chest pain, syncope, and even sudden death (1%-2% of cases) may occur in children with severe AS.
   b. Heart failure occurs with severe AS during the newborn period or later in adult life.
   c. With BAV, progressive aortic dilatation may occur. Rarely, aortic dilataton may lead to aortic aneurysm.
   d. BAVs are nonobstructive during childhood and become stenotic or significantly regurgitant in adult life due to calcification of the valve. Valve replacement may be required in many adult patients.
   e. Progressive worsening of AR is possible in discrete subaortic stenosis.

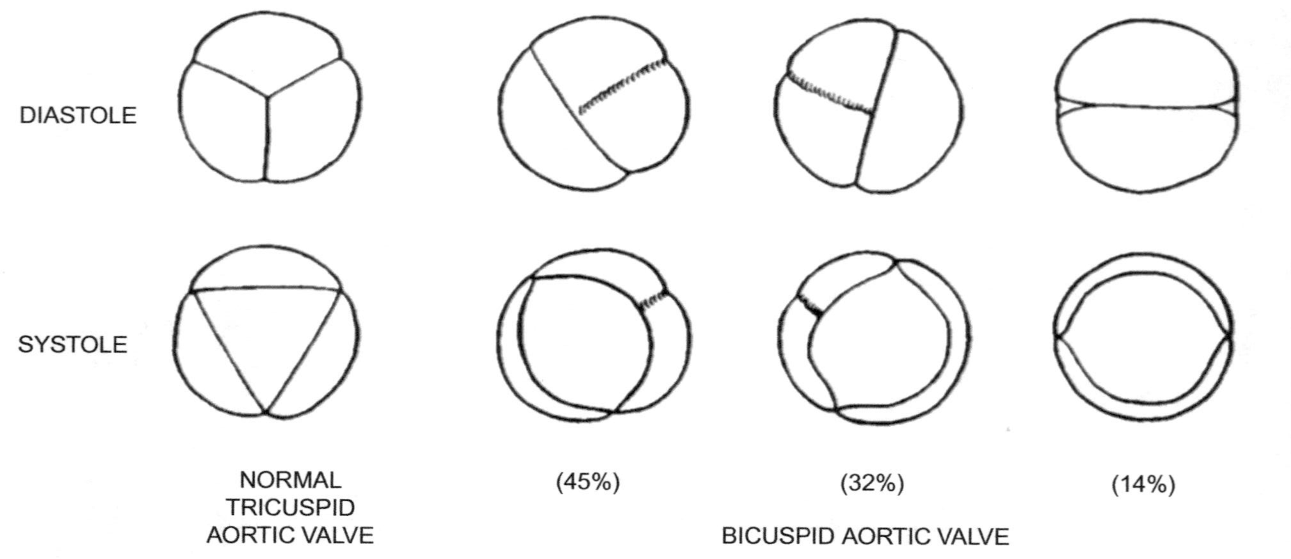

FIG. 8.5

Diagram of parasternal short-axis scan of normal tricuspid (*left column*) and bicuspid aortic valves (*three right columns*) during diastole and systole. The most common pattern of the bicuspid aortic valve demonstrates commissures at the 4- or 5-o'clock and the 9-or 10-o'clock positions, with raphe at the 10 or 2-o'clock position (45%). *(Modified from Brandenburg, R. O., Jr., Tajik, A. J., Edwards, W. D., Reeder, G. S. Shub, C., & Seward, J. B. (1983). Accuracy of 2-dimensional echocardiographic diagnosis of congenitally bicuspid aortic valve: echocardiographic-anatomic correlation in 115 patients.* American Journal of Cardiology, 51*(9), 1469–1473.)*

D. MANAGEMENT

Medical and Nonsurgical

1. In critically ill neonates and infants with CHF, anticongestive measures with fast-acting inotropic agents and diuretics, with or without PGE_1 infusion, are indicated, in preparation for either balloon valvuloplasty or surgery.
2. A serial echo Doppler ultrasound evaluation is needed at 1- to 2-year intervals for patients with mild to moderate stenosis, and more often for severe stenosis.
3. Because of the progressive nature of aortic dilatation in children with BAV, annual echocardiographic measurement of the aortic root and ascending aorta is recommended.
4. Recent American Heart Association recommendations include echocardiographic screening of first-degree relatives of patients with BAV (because approximately 9% of them may have the BAV).
5. Exercise stress testing may be indicated in children with AS who are interested in athletic participation.
6. Activity restrictions. No limitation in activity is required for mild AS. For patients with moderate AS, varying levels of activity restriction are required (see Chapter 25). Patients with severe AS should not participate in any competitive sports.
7. Balloon valvuloplasty.

For moderate to severe valvular AS, percutaneous balloon aortic valvuloplasty has replaced open surgical valvotomy as the treatment of choice.

Indications: The following may be indications for the procedure according to the AHA.

a. Asymptomatic children and young adults, with a (catheter-derived) peak systolic ejection gradient ≥50 mm Hg.
b. Symptomatic patients (with angina, syncope), patients with resting or exercise-induced ECG changes, patients planning to become pregnant, or patients who plan to participate in competitive sports, if they have a gradient ≥40 mm Hg.
c. Infants with valvular AS with depressed LV systolic function, regardless of pressure gradient.
d. Neonates who require maintenance of a patency of ductus arteriosus for adequate systemic perfusion, regardless of pressure gradient.
e. Results of the valvuloplasty: The procedure typically reduces the catheter peak-to-peak systolic gradient to 20 to 35 mm Hg. The optimal ratio of balloon-annulus diameter is 0.8 to 0.9. Larger balloon diameter is associated with a greater risk of developing AR after the procedure. The long-term outcome after a successful valve dilatation is good, but late restenosis and aortic valve regurgitation eventually necessitate reintervention in the majority of patients. The freedom from reintervention for 5 years is 67% for children; it is lower (48%) in newborns.

Surgical

1. For neonates with "critical AS":

   A sick newborn with critical AS who had failed balloon valvuloplasty may have one of the following two.

   a. Closed aortic valvotomy, using calibrated dilators or balloon catheters without cardiopulmonary bypass, may be tried.

   b. In some neonates, Norwood procedure (see Chapter 9) may be necessary due to other associated lesions (i.e., MS, borderline LV size, LVOT obstruction).

2. For valvular AS:

   a. Indications: Failed balloon valvuloplasty or severe AR resulting from the procedure.

   b. Procedures: Either aortic valve commissurotomy, aortic valve replacement (using mechanical or biological valves), or the Ross procedure (see later text) is performed.

      (1) Aortic valve commissurotomy is usually tried if stenosis is the predominant lesion.

      (2) Aortic valve replacement using mechanical or biological valves. The advantage of the mechanical valve is durability, but it has the tendency for thrombus formation with a potential embolization, requiring anticoagulation with warfarin with its attendant risks of bleeding and its known teratogenic effects. Biological valves do not require anticoagulation with warfarin but the deterioration occurs within a decade or two, due to degeneration and calcification. Homografts are preferred for adolescent girls or women in child-bearing age because anticoagulation with warfarin is not required.

      (3) In the ***Ross procedure*** (or pulmonary root autografts), the autologous pulmonary valve replaces the aortic valve, and an aortic or a pulmonary allograft replaces the pulmonary valve (Fig. 8.6). The pulmonary valve autograft has the advantage of longer-term durability; it does not require anticoagulation and there is evidence of the autograft's growth. The patient's own aortic valve may be used for pulmonary position after aortic valvotomy ("double" Ross procedure).

3. For discrete subaortic stenosis:

   a. Indications: Peak gradient >35 mm Hg and at least mild AR are the most commonly accepted indications. Most centers accept the onset of AR as an indication for surgical removal of the membrane.

   b. Procedures: Excision of the membrane is done.

   c. A tendency for recurrence after surgical excision of subaortic membrane has been a concern, with a recurrence rate as high as 25% to 30%. Risk factors for recurrence include (a) younger age (<4 year), (b) high pressure gradient (>50 mm Hg), (c) proximity of the membrane to the aortic valve (<6 mm), and (d) extension of the membrane to the aortic or mitral valves. Some centers delay surgery until after 10 years of age because the recurrence is very

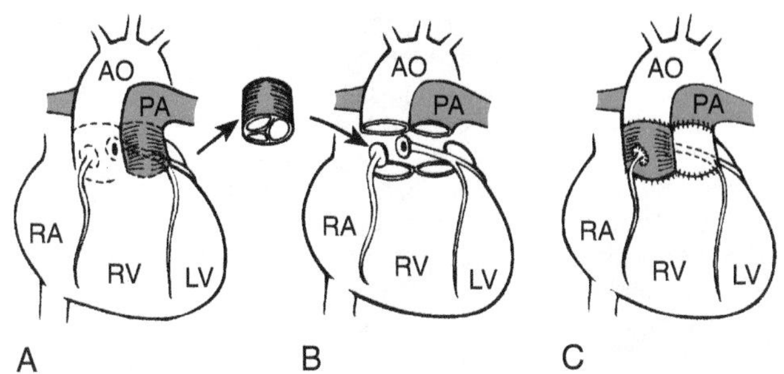

FIG. 8.6
Ross procedure (or pulmonary root autograft). (A) The two horizontal lines on the aorta (*AO*) and pulmonary artery (*PA*) and two broken circles around the coronary artery ostia are lines of proposed incision. The pulmonary valve, with a small rim of right ventricular (*RV*) muscle, and the adjacent PA are removed. (B) The aortic valve and the adjacent aorta have been removed, leaving buttons of aortic tissue around the coronary arteries. (C) The pulmonary autograft is sutured to the aortic annulus and to the distal aorta, and the coronary arteries are sutured to openings made in the PA. The pulmonary valve is replaced with either an aortic or a pulmonary allograft. *LV*, left ventricle; *RA*, right atrium. *(From Park, M. K., & Salamat, M. (2020).* Park's pediatric cardiology for practitioners *(7th ed.). Philadelphia: Mosby.)*

8

rare after this age. More aggressive resection of the membrane and extensive myectomy reduced the recurrence but resulted in a higher complication rate of heart block (14%). Surgical mortality for subaortic membrane is near zero.

d. Patients with the following are considered low risk, and medical follow-up, rather than surgical intervention, is recommended: those with (a) no or trace AR, (b) Doppler gradient ≤30 mm Hg, (c) the membrane not in proximity to the aortic valve (>6 mm), and (d) thin and mobile aortic valve.

4. For tunnel-type subaortic stenosis, a pressure gradient ≥50 mm Hg is an indication for surgery. Valve replacement following aortic root enlargement (Kono procedure) may be performed.
5. For supravalvar AS, peak pressure gradient >50 to 60 mm Hg, severe LVH, or appearance of new AR is an indication for surgery. Widening of the stenotic area using a diamond-shaped fabric patch may be performed.

Follow-Up

1. Annual follow-up is required for all patients who had a balloon or surgical procedure done for the aortic valve because significant AR develops in 10% to 30% of the patients and the discrete subaortic membrane recurs in 25% to 30% after surgical resection.

2. Anticoagulation with warfarin is needed after a prosthetic mechanical valve replacement. The international normalized ratio should be maintained between 2.5 and 3.5 for the first 3 months and between 2.0 and 3.0 beyond that time. Low-dose aspirin (81 mg/day) is also indicated in addition to warfarin.
3. After aortic valve replacement with bioprosthesis, aspirin (81 mg) is indicated (without warfarin).
4. IE prophylaxis is required after placement of prosthetic material or valve when indications arise.
5. Restriction from competitive sports may be necessary for children with moderate residual AS and/or AR.

III. COARCTATION OF THE AORTA

A. PREVALENCE

Four to 8% of all cases of CHD, with a male preponderance (2:1). Thirty percent of patients with Turner syndrome have COA.

B. PATHOLOGY AND PATHOPHYSIOLOGY

1. Narrowing of the upper thoracic aorta is present, most commonly distal to the left subclavian artery.
2. There are two groups of patients with COA: symptomatic infants and asymptomatic children.
   a. In *symptomatic infants* with COA, other cardiac defects (such as aortic hypoplasia, VSD, PDA, and mitral valve anomalies) are often present. These abnormalities may have reduced antegrade flow through the aorta during fetal life and may have caused a poor development of collateral circulation around the COA.
   b. In *asymptomatic children* with COA, associated anomalies are uncommon.
3. COA may occur in association with other CHDs, such as TGA and DORV (e.g., Taussig-Bing abnormality).
4. As many as 85% of patients with COA have a bicuspid aortic valve.
5. Major collateral circulation between the aortic segments proximal and distal to the coarctation consists of (a) the internal mammary artery anteriorly, (b) arteries arising from the subclavian artery by way of the intercostal arteries, and (c) the anterior spinal artery.

The presentation of patients with COA occurs in a bimodal distribution—newborn infants with circulatory symptoms in the first weeks of life and asymptomatic infants and children. Therefore they are presented under a separate heading.

C. CLINICAL MANIFESTATIONS (SYMPTOMATIC INFANTS)

1. Signs of CHF (poor feeding, dyspnea) and renal failure (oliguria, anuria) with general circulatory shock may develop in the first 2 to 6 weeks of life.

2. A loud gallop and week and thready pulses, without heart murmur, are common findings in sick infants. Peripheral pulses may be weak and thready as a result of CHF. A blood pressure differential may become apparent only after improvement of CHF.
3. The ECG usually shows RVH or RBBB, rather than LVH.
4. Chest radiographs show a marked cardiomegaly and signs of pulmonary edema or pulmonary venous congestion.
5. Two-dimensional echo shows the site and extent of the COA and other associated cardiac defects.
   a. In the suprasternal notch view, a thin wedge-shaped "posterior shelf" is imaged distal to the left subclavian artery. Varying degrees of isthmic hypoplasia and hypoplasia of the transverse aortic arch may be present. Poststenotic dilatation of the descending aorta is usually imaged.
   b. Other associated defects such as hypoplastic aorta, bicuspid aortic valve, PDA, VSD, and mitral valve abnormalities can be imaged.
   c. Delayed rate of systolic upstroke and persistent diastolic flow in the abdominal aorta may suggest the diagnosis.
   d. Diagnosis of neonatal COA in the presence of PDA is difficult. The aortic isthmus ≤ 3 mm without PDA or the isthmus ≤ 4 mm in the presence of PDA may be diagnostic of neonatal COA. The ratio of the aortic isthmus to the descending aorta at the diaphragm <0.64 is also a reliable sign of COA in the presence of PDA.
   e. Doppler studies above and below the coarctation site should be obtained in assessing the severity of the coarctation.
6. MRI or computed tomography scanning has become the imaging modality of choice after echo diagnosis of the condition. Cardiac catheterization is performed primarily for interventional treatment.
7. Natural history: Early death from CHF and renal failure is possible.

D. MANAGEMENT (SYMPTOMATIC INFANTS)

Medical and Nonsurgical

1. Intensive anticongestive treatment should be given with fast-acting inotropic agents (catechols), diuretics, and oxygen to stabilize the patient.
2. PGE_1 infusion is indicated to reopen the ductus before any surgical repair or balloon procedure takes place (see Appendix E for the dosage of PGE_1).
3. Balloon angioplasty with or without stent implantation is controversial, but it has emerged as a less invasive alternative to surgery for sick infants. Some centers use cutting balloons or a low-profile stent in very sick infants, which does not require overexpansion of the coarctation segment and thus is less likely to produce aneurysm. When a stent is used, it is usually not expandable to adult size and requires redilatation at a later time.

8

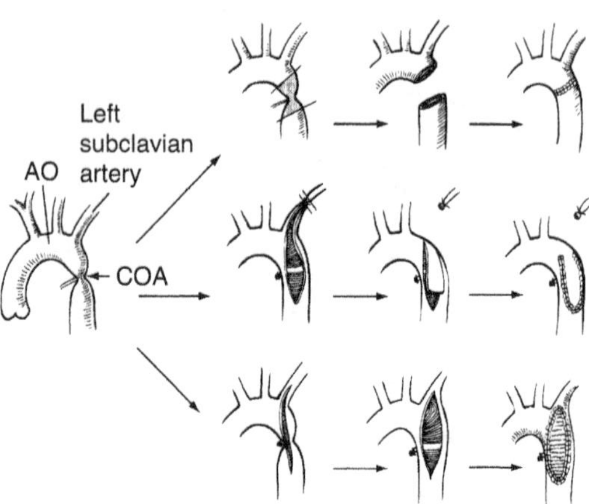

FIG. 8.7

Surgical techniques for repair of coarctation of the aorta. *Top,* End-to-end anastomosis. A segment of coarctation is resected, and the proximal and distal aortas are anastomosed end-to-end. *Middle,* Subclavian flap procedure. The distal subclavian artery is divided, and the flap of the proximal portion of this vessel is used to widen the coarcted segment. *Bottom,* Patch aortoplasty. An elliptic woven Dacron patch is inserted to expand the diameter of the lumen. *(From Park, M. K., & Salamat, M. (2020).* Park's pediatric cardiology for practitioners *(7th ed.). Philadelphia: Mosby.)*

4. Balloon angioplasty is associated with a higher rate of recoarctation (>50%) than surgical repair, and the rate of complications (including femoral artery injury) is high during infancy.

Surgical

1. If CHF develops, the need for surgery or nonsurgical intervention is urgent. Surgical procedure of choice varies from institution to institution.
   a. Simple or extended end-to-end anastomosis is the preferred mode of repair. Rarely, subclavian flap aortoplasty or patch angioplasty is performed (Fig. 8.7).
   b. The mortality rate for isolated COA is less than 1.5%. Postoperative renal failure is the most common cause of death. Residual obstruction and/or recoarctation occur in 6% to 33% of the cases, but the recurrence rate appears lower than that following balloon angioplasty.
2. If it is associated with a VSD, one of the following procedures may be performed.
   a. If the VSD is nonrestrictive, COA and VSD can be repaired in the same operative setting.

b. If the VSD appears restrictive, only coarctation repair is performed. Approximately 40% of restrictive VSD close spontaneously.
c. PA banding is performed if the PA pressure remains high after completing COA surgery. Later the VSD is closed, and the PA band is removed between 6 and 24 months of age.

Follow-Up

1. Reexamination every 6 to 12 months is indicated because recoarctation is possible, especially when surgery is performed in the first year of life.
2. Balloon angioplasty may be performed if a significant recoarctation develops.
3. Surveillance for and treatment of systemic hypertension is needed.

E. CLINICAL MANIFESTATIONS (CHILDREN)

1. These children are usually asymptomatic except for rare complaints of leg pain.
2. The pulse in the leg is absent or weak and delayed. Hypertension in the arm or higher BP readings in the arm than the thigh may be present. An ejection click resulting from the bicuspid aortic valve is frequently audible at the apex and/or base. A systolic ejection murmur, grade 2 to 3/6, is audible at the URSB and MLSB and in the left interscapular area in the back.
3. The ECG usually shows LVH, but it may be normal.
4. Chest radiographs show a normal or slightly enlarged heart. A "3 sign" on overpenetrated films (produced by pre- and poststenotic dilations) may be present. Rib notching may be seen in children after about 5 years of age.
5. Two-dimensional echo studies:
   a. A discrete, shelf-like membrane in the posterolateral aspect of the descending aorta is imaged.
   b. Doppler examination reveals disturbed flow and increased flow velocity distal to the COA.
   c. Continuous wave Doppler flow profile distal to the coarctation is composed of two superimposed signals representing the proximal and distal flows.
   d. The flow velocities proximal and distal to the coarctation site should be used in estimating pressure gradients. This is because the proximal flow velocity is often higher than 1.5 m/sec and it cannot be ignored in the Bernoulli equation.
   e. In severe COA with extensive collaterals, the Doppler-estimated gradient may underestimate the severity of the coarctation.
   f. The bicuspid aortic valve is frequently imaged.

6. MRI with three-dimensional reconstruction, supplemented by gadolinium contrast, has become the imaging modality of choice. Cardiac catheterization is no longer needed for anatomic assessment.
7. Natural history: The bicuspid aortic valve may cause stenosis and/or regurgitation later in life. If a COA is left untreated, LV failure, intracranial hemorrhage, or hypertensive encephalopathy may develop later in life.

F. MANAGEMENT (CHILDREN)

Medical and Nonsurgical

1. Hypertension or hypertensive crisis should be detected and treated. Arm and leg BPs should be checked for increasing pressure differences (possible recurrence). Reduced BP readings in the lower extremities may be due to femoral artery injuries resulting from previous surgeries or interventional procedures.
2. Balloon angioplasty:
   a. Balloon angioplasty without stent placement for native (unoperated) COA is controversial. Some centers use the balloon procedure for the native COA, whereas other centers prefer a surgical approach.
   b. Suggested indications for balloon intervention are as follows:
      (1) Transcatheter systolic gradient across COA of >20 mm Hg and suitable anatomy, irrespective of the patient's age.
      (2) Transcatheter systolic gradient of <20 mm Hg (i) with suitable angiographic anatomy in the presence of extensive collateral vessels, (ii) in patients with univentricular heart, or (iii) in patients with significant LV dysfunction.
      (3) It may be reasonable to consider the procedure for native coarctation as a palliative procedure at any age when there is (i) severe LV dysfunction, (ii) severe mitral regurgitation, or (iii) systemic disease affected by the cardiac condition.
   c. The most common acute complication of the balloon angioplasty is femoral artery injury and thrombosis, especially in small children. There is a possibility of aortic aneurysm formation with serious late complications.
3. Endovascular stent placement: With the advent of new generation stents with higher flexibility, lower profile, and, specifically, the ability to dilate to adult size as well as open cell configuration allowing overlapping of brachiocephalic vessels stent angioplasty, has become the preferred method of intervention for coarctation of aorta even in very young children.
   a. Current AHA recommendations for stent placement in native COA and recoarctation of the aorta are as follows.

(1) For recoarctation, stent placement is indicated in patients who have a transcatheter systolic coarctation gradient >20 mm Hg and are of sufficient size for safe stent placement, which can be expanded to an adult size.
(2) For initial treatment of native COA or recurrent coarctation, it is reasonable to consider stent placement if (a) a transcatheter systolic coarctation gradient of >20 mm Hg, (b) a transcatheter systolic gradient of <20 mm Hg with systolic hypertension caused by the coarctation, or (c) a long segment coarctation with a transcatheter systolic gradient >20 mm Hg is present.
(3) It is reasonable to use stent placement for patients in whom balloon angioplasty has failed in treatment of native or recurrent COA.

b. Advantages of the expandable stent may include the following: (a) it does not require overexpansion of the coarctation segment, thereby reducing the chance of the development of aortic aneurysm; (b) it produces better results with greater reduction of pressure gradient than the balloon procedure alone; and (e) it can be re-expanded to the adult size, avoiding repeat surgical procedures.
c. Successful placement of the stent was reported in 98% of patients with pressure gradient <20 mm Hg. On follow-up, aneurysm was seen in less than 1% of the patients and reintervention was needed in 4%.

Surgical

1. Indications for surgery:
   a. Reduction of aortic diameter by 50% at the level of coarctation (determined by echo or MRI) in the presence of a pressure gradient of more than 20 to 30 mm Hg is considered an absolute indication for surgery.
   b. Significant narrowing of the aorta with a Doppler pressure gradient >20 to 30 mm Hg is considered an indication for surgery in asymptomatic children. (The same degree of pressure gradient by arm and leg BP measurements is a less reliable indication.)
   c. Some recommend surgery if a prominent gradient develops with exercise. This is not reliable; it may be due to peripheral amplification of systolic pressure seen in the arm as discussed in Chapter 5 (see Fig. 5.1).
2. Surgery done before 1 year of age may have lower incidence of hypertension but recurrence rate is high.
3. Resection of the coarctation segment and an end-to-end anastomosis constitute the procedure of choice. Other surgical options are illustrated in Fig. 8.7.

Follow-Up

1. Annual examination is recommended with attention to (a) BP differences in the arm and leg (recoarctation), (b) status of associated abnormalities such as bicuspid aortic valve or mitral valve disease, and (c) possible development of subaortic AS.
2. Possible late complications include aneurysm formation (with likelihood of dissection and rupture), for which MRI or CT angiography is the preferred method (performed every 2 to 5 years).

G. MANAGEMENT ALGORITHM (FOR COA)

Deciding on the optimal treatment for patients with COA can be complicated with different options available, including balloon angioplasty, intravascular stent placement, and surgery. In general, management is dictated by the age at presentation, complexity of the coarctation, native versus recurrent coarctation. The following management algorithm is suggested by Torok, Campbell, Fleming, et al. (2015), although some centers may have different approach.

1. For neonates and infants:
   a. Surgery (preferably extended resection and end-to-end anastomosis) is recommended by most centers. Surgery is more appropriate, especially when the anatomy of the COA is complex, (e.g., transverse arch obstruction) or when repair of associated cardiac defect is required.
   b. It is reasonable to choose balloon angioplasty as a palliative strategy in neonates too sick for major surgical procedure
2. For small children with *native* coarctation:
   a. Most centers prefer surgical repair, especially when the COA is associated with complex anatomy (as described earlier).
   b. Balloon angioplasty is not a good choice because of its long-term risk of aneurysm. Stent placement is also not a good choice because it requires redilatation at a later time and the arteries are too small to accommodate a stent that can be dilated to adult size
3. For small children with *recurrent* coarctation:
   a. Balloon angioplasty without stent is a reasonable approach because the child is too small to receive a stent that can be dilated to adult size.
   b. For those children with complex anatomy (e.g., tortuous segment of recoarctation), surgery should also be considered.
4. For older children, adolescents, and adults:
   a. With a simple, juxtaductal native coarctation, stent placement is a reasonable approach. Stent placement can also be considered for recurrent coarctation. Only stents expandable to an adult size should be used.
   b. Balloon angioplasty (without stent) is not a good choice because it is variably successful and surgical re-intervention may be required.

IV. INTERRUPTED AORTIC ARCH

A. PREVALENCE

About 1% of critically ill infants with CHDs.

B. PATHOLOGY AND PATHOPHYSIOLOGY

1. This extreme form of COA is divided into three types according to the location of the interruption (Fig. 8.8).
   a. In type A, the interruption is distal to the left subclavian artery (occurring in 30% of patients).
   b. In type B, the interruption is between the left carotid and left subclavian arteries (occurs in 43% of cases). DiGeorge syndrome (part of 22q11.2 deletion syndrome) occurs in about 50% of patients with type B interruption.
   c. In type C, the interruption is between the innominate and left carotid arteries (occurs in 17% of cases).
2. PDA and VSD are almost always associated with this defect. A bicuspid aortic valve (60%), mitral valve deformity (10%), persistent truncus arteriosus (10%), or subaortic stenosis (20%) may be present.
3. DiGeorge syndrome occurs in at least 15% of these patients.

C. CLINICAL MANIFESTATIONS

1. Respiratory distress, cyanosis, poor peripheral pulse, or circulatory shock develops in the first few days of life.
2. Cardiac findings are nonspecific.

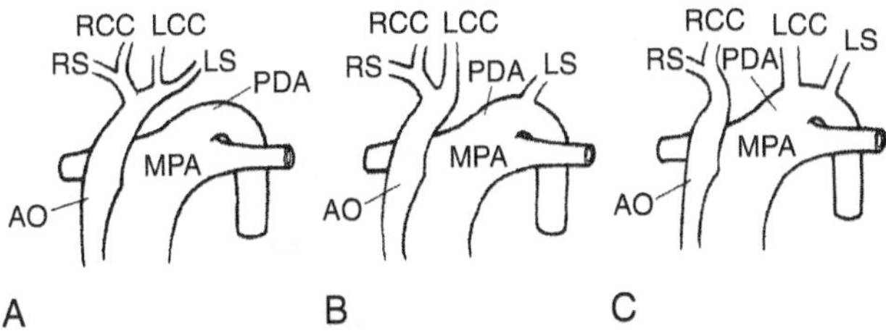

FIG. 8.8

Three types of aortic arch interruption. (A) Type A. (B) Type B. (C) Type C (see text). *AO*, aorta; *LCC*, left common carotid; *LS*, left subclavian; *MPA*, main pulmonary artery; *PDA*, patent ductus arteriosus; *RCC*, right common carotid; *RS*, right subclavian. *(From Park, M. K., & Salamat, M. (2020).* Park's pediatric cardiology for practitioners *(7th ed.). Philadelphia: Mosby.)*

3. Chest radiographs show cardiomegaly, increased PVM, and pulmonary edema. The upper mediastinum may be narrow (due to the absence of thymus [i.e., DiGeorge syndrome]).
4. The ECG may show RVH.
5. Echo studies are useful in the diagnosis of the condition.
6. Cardiac CT or MRI is more frequently used than angiocardiography to clarify the anatomy before surgery.

D. MANAGEMENT

Medical

1. PGE_1 infusion (see Appendix E for dosage), intubation, and oxygen administration.
2. Workup for DiGeorge syndrome (i.e., serum calcium) should be carried out.
3. Citrated blood (that causes hypocalcemia by chelation) should not be transfused. Blood should be irradiated before transfusion in patients with DiGeorge syndrome.

Surgical

1. Surgical repair of the interruption (primary anastomosis, Dacron vascular graft, or venous homograft) and closure of a simple VSD are recommended if possible.
2. If associated with complex defects, repair of the interruption and PA banding are performed, with complete repair at a later time.

V. PULMONARY ARTERY STENOSIS

A. PREVALENCE

PA stenosis accounts for >3% of all CHDs.

B. PATHOLOGY

1. Stenosis of the PA occurs either at the main PA or in the peripheral pulmonary arteries. The most frequent site of stenosis is near the bifurcation as an isolated anomaly.
2. It is associated with other CHDs (such as valvular PS, ASD, VSD, PDA, and TOF).
3. When associated with cyanotic CHDs (such as pulmonary atresia with intact ventricular septum or TOF with pulmonary atresia), the stenosis usually involves multiple branches and multiple sites.
4. It may also be seen in other conditions such as rubella syndrome, Williams syndrome, and Alagille syndrome.
5. Some PA stenosis is secondary to surgical procedures, such as previous B-T shunt.

6. Isolated LPA stenosis may be secondary to coarctation of LPA secondary to connection of the PDA at the base of LPA.

C. CLINICAL MANIFESTATION

1. Mild stenosis of the PAs causes no symptoms. If the stenosis is severe and bilateral, the RV may hypertrophy.
2. An ejection systolic murmur grade 2 to 3/6 is audible at the ULSB, with good transmission to the ipsilateral axilla and back. The S2 is either normal or more obviously split.
3. The ECG is normal with mild stenosis, but it shows RVH with severe stenosis.
4. Chest radiographs usually are normal.
5. Echo and Doppler studies may show stenoses in the main PA or near the bifurcation, but those in smaller branches cannot be imaged by echo.
   a. When unilateral PA stenosis is identified, Doppler evaluation of the severity of the stenosis becomes difficult because of abnormal flow distribution in the lungs (with discrepant blood flow away from the stenotic branch).
   b. Many significant stenoses may not be demonstrable by pressure gradient in a low pulmonary flow situation (such as seen with Glenn shunt and Fontan circulation).
   c. In general, a significant PA stenosis is present when:
      (1) There is a Doppler pressure gradient of >20 to 30 mm Hg,
      (2) RV or main PA pressure is higher than 50% of systemic pressure, or
      (3) Lung perfusion scan shows relative flow discrepancy between two lungs of 35%/65% or worse, rather than the normal right/left perfusion ratio of 55/45%. (Recently the normal right/left perfusion ratio was found to be 52.5/47.5% [± 2.1%].)
6. Lung perfusion scan had been a useful noninvasive method in determining relative pulmonary flow. However, washout effects from additional blood supply to the lung can make flow quantification inaccurate. Currently MRI represents the gold standard for assessing differential blood flow (better than lung perfusion scan).
7. In patients with multiple previous stenting of the pulmonary tree, contrast-enhanced CT imaging is preferred. Angiocardiography is the best invasive tool in the diagnosis of peripheral PA stenosis.

D. MANAGEMENT

1. Mild to moderate PA stenoses usually do not require treatment, but severe ones do.
2. The central (extraparenchymal) type is surgically amenable, but the peripheral (intraparenchymal) type is not correctable by surgery; catheter therapy is often the only option.

3. For peripheral PA stenosis, standard balloon angioplasty, cutting balloons, and the placement of an endovascular stent are available.
   a. Low-pressure balloon angioplasty has a limited success rate (≈50%) and a high (16%) recurrence rate. High-pressure balloon (20 to 25 atm) is more effective.
   b. A balloon-expandable stent may offer better results.
   c. Using a cutting balloon alone or followed by high-pressure ballooning is best suited for small, lobar pulmonary artery branches not amenable to stenting.

Chapter 9

Cyanotic Congenital Heart Defects

A. CYANOSIS

I. PATHOPHYSIOLOGY OF CYANOSIS

Before discussing individual cyanotic CHD, a brief review of pathophysiology of cyanosis is in order.

II. CAUSES OF CYANOSIS

9

Cyanosis is a bluish discoloration of the skin and mucous membranes resulting from an increased concentration of reduced hemoglobin to about 5 g/100 mL in the cutaneous veins. This level of reduced hemoglobin in the cutaneous vein may result from either desaturation of arterial blood (central cyanosis) or increased extraction of oxygen by peripheral tissue in the presence of normal arterial saturation (peripheral cyanosis). Cyanosis is more difficult to detect in children with dark pigmentation.

1. Peripheral cyanosis is due to excessive extraction of oxygen in the venules. Examples of peripheral cyanosis are:
2. Central cyanosis is seen in children with cyanotic CHD, lung disease, or central nervous system (CNS) depression. Rarely cyanosis is caused by methemoglobinema (seen when methemoglobin level is greater than 15% of normal hemoglobin)
   a. Acrocyanosis, a bluish color of the fingers seen in neonates and infants and reflects sluggish blood flow in the fingers.
   b. Circumoral cyanosis refers to a bluish skin color around the mouth, seen in a healthy child with fair skin due to a sluggish capillary blood flow in association with vasoconstriction.

III. INFLUENCE OF HEMOGLOBIN LEVEL ON CYANOSIS

The level of hemoglobin greatly influences the occurrence of cyanosis. Normally, about 2 g/100 mL of reduced hemoglobin is present in the venules so that an additional 3 g/100 mL of reduced hemoglobin in arterial blood is needed to reach 5 g/100 mL of reduced hemoglobin to produce clinical cyanosis.

1. For a normal person with hemoglobin of 15 g/100 mL, 3 g of reduced hemoglobin results from 20% desaturation (because 3 is 20% of 15). Thus cyanosis appears when the oxygen saturation is reduced to about 80%.

2. In a person with polycythemia, cyanosis is recognized at a higher level of oxygen saturation. For example, in a person with hemoglobin of 20 g/100 mL, 3 g of reduced hemoglobin result from only 15% desaturation (or at 85% arterial saturation).
3. In patients with anemia, cyanosis is recognized at a lower level of oxygen saturation. For example, if a patient has a marked anemia (hemoglobin of 6 g/100 mL), 3 g of reduced hemoglobin does not result until the patient's arterial oxygen saturated goes down to 50% desaturation.

IV. CYANOSIS OF CARDIAC VERSUS PULMONARY ORIGIN

Differentiation of cardiac cyanosis from cyanosis caused by pulmonary diseases is crucially important for proper management of cyanotic infants. Traditionally, one tests the response of arterial Po_2 to 100% oxygen inhalation (hyperoxia test). With pulmonary disease, arterial Po_2 usually rises to a level greater than 100 mm Hg. When there is a significant intracardiac R-L shunt, the arterial Po_2 does not exceed 100 mm Hg, and the rise is usually not more than 10 to 30 mm Hg.

V. CONSEQUENCES AND COMPLICATIONS OF CYANOSIS

1. **Polycythemia**. Low arterial oxygen content stimulates bone marrow through erythropoietin release from the kidneys and produces increased number of red blood cells (RBCs). Polycythemia, with a resulting increase in oxygen-carrying capacity, benefits cyanotic children. However, when the hematocrit reaches 65% or higher, a sharp increase in the viscosity of blood occurs, and the polycythemic response becomes disadvantageous.
2. **Clubbing**. Clubbing is caused by soft tissue growth under the nail bed as a consequence of chronic central cyanosis. Clubbing usually does not occur until a child is 6 months or older, and it is seen first and is most pronounced in the thumb. In the early stage, it appears as shininess and redness of the fingertips. When fully developed, the fingers and toes become thick and wide and have convex nail beds. Clubbing may also be seen in patients with liver disease or infective endocarditis and on a hereditary basis without cyanosis.
3. **Central nervous system (CNS) complications**. Very high hematocrit levels place individuals with cyanotic CHD at risk for disorders of the CNS, such as brain abscess and vascular stroke. In the past, cyanotic CHDs accounted for 5% to 10% of all cases of brain abscesses. Vascular stroke caused by embolization arising from thrombus in the cardiac chamber or in the systemic veins may be associated with surgery or cardiac catheterization.
4. **Bleeding disorders**. Disturbances of hemostasis are frequently present in children with severe cyanosis and polycythemia. Most frequently noted are thrombocytopenia and defective platelet aggregation. Other

abnormalities include prolonged prothrombin time and partial thromboplastin time and lower levels of fibrinogen and factors V and VIII. Clinical manifestations may include easy bruising, petechiae of the skin and mucous membranes, epistaxis, and gingival bleeding. RBC withdrawal from polycythemic patients and replacement with an equal volume of plasma tend to correct the hemorrhagic tendency and lower blood viscosity.

5. **Hypoxic spells and squatting**. Although most frequently seen in infants with unrepaired TOF, hypoxic spells may occur in infants with other CHDs (see a later section on TOF for further discussion).

B. CRITICAL CONGENITAL HEART DISEASE (CCHD) SCREENING

I. ROLE OF PULSE OXIMETRY SCREEN IN DETECTION OF HYPOXEMIA

Many neonates with hypoxemia from significant CHDs may not show cyanosis on routine neonatal examination in the first days of life. About one-third of neonates with critical CHD were estimated to be undetected on routine neonatal examination. Pulse oximetry can detect mild degree of arterial hypoxemia without recognizable cyanosis in the newborn.

First developed in 1972 by Takuo Aoyagi and Michio Kishi of Japan, pulse oximetry monitors a person's arterial oxygen saturation noninvasively. The principle of the pulse oximeter is based on the difference in absorption of red light (wavelength of 660 nm) and infrared light (at 940-nm wavelength) by oxygenated hemoglobin and deoxygenaed hemoglobin. Oxygenated hemoglobin absorbs more infrared light and allows more red light to pass through. Deoxygenated hemoglobin absorbs more red light and allows more infrared light to pass through. A pair of small light-emitting diodes (LEDs) in the probe emit red and infrared lights, which go through a translucent part of the body (such as fingertip or earlobe). Red and infrared lights that passed through are detected by a photodiode on the opposite side of the probe. The pulse oximetery detects oxygen saturation of only arterial blood, not the venous or capillary blood. This ability is based on the principle that the amount of red and infrared light absorbed fluctuates with the cardiac cycle as the arterial blood volume increases during systole and decreases during diastole; in contrast, the blood volume in the veins and capillaries remains relatively constant. The processor of pulse oximeters calculates the ratio of the red light detected (transmitted light) to the infrared light detected by the photodiode. This ratio represents the ratio of oxygenated hemoglobin to deoxygenated hemoglobin, and the ratio is then converted to oxygen saturation by the processor.

In 2011, the pulse oximetry screen was made the standard of care in newborn screening and has been endorsed by the American Academy of Pediatrics (AAP), American Heart Association, and American College of Cardiology. The neonatal pulse oximetry screen (POS) can detect cyanotic CHD and other life-threatening noncaardiac neonatal conditions prior to the discharge from the birth hospital. Examples of noncardiac conditions include

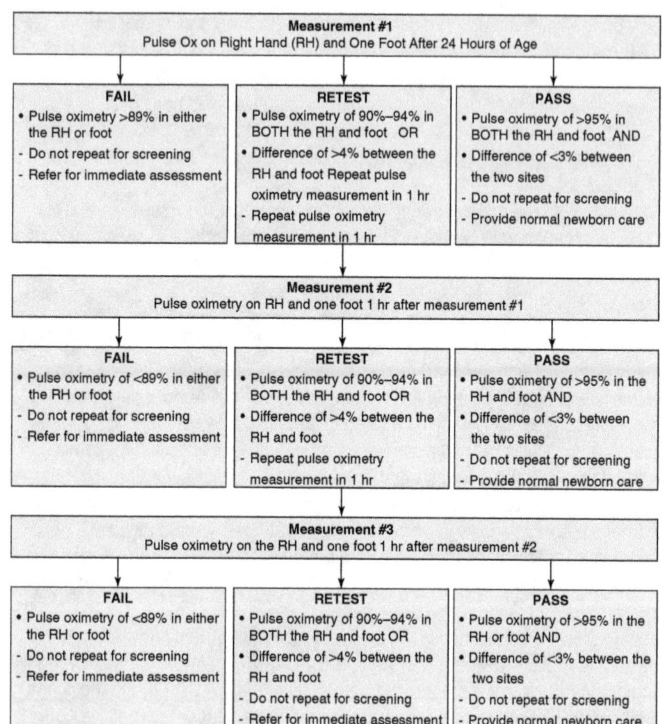

FIG. 9.1

The U.S. Neonatal Pulse Oximetry Screen algorithm. *(From Park, M. K., & Salamat, M. (2020).* Park's pediatric cardiology for practitioners *(7th ed.). Philadelphia: Mosby.)*

hypothermia, infection (including sepsis), lung disease, persistent pulmonary hypertension of the newborn, hemoglobinopathy, and others.

II. NEONATAL PULSE OXIMETRY SCREEN ALGORITHM

The U.S. pulse oximetry (PO) algorithm, which is approved by the AAP, is presented in Fig. 9.1.

1. The screen should be done after 24 hours of life or just prior to early discharge from the hospital. The POS done earlier than 24 hours of age increases false-positive results. Interestingly, however, the false-positive tests detect noncardiac conditions that require prompt attention and treatment.

2. Oxygen saturation should be measured in the right hand (RH) (for preductal arterial saturation) and either foot (for postductal arterial saturation) to detect cyanotic CHDs and ductal-dependent lesions.

Description of the Algorithm

1. **First screening**
   a. Normal neonates should have oxygen (O_2) saturation in the RH and foot higher than 95% and the difference in oxygen saturation between the RH and the foot should be 3% or less (PASS). These infants may be given normal newborn care.
   b. The following are abnormal test results.
      (1) O_2 saturation 89% or less in either the RH or a foot (FAIL). These infants are referred for immediate assessment.
      (2) O_2 saturation between 90% and 94% in the RH and the foot, or difference in the saturation 4% or more between the two sites (RETEST). These infants should be screened again after 1 hour.
2. **Second screening**
   a. Neonates with normal results (PASS) are given routine newborn care.
   b. Neonates with abnormal test results are handled the same way as stated earlier for the first screen. They should be screened again after 1 hour.
3. **Third screening**
   a. Neonates with normal results (PASS) are given routine newborn care.
   b. Neonates with abnormal test results (both RETEST and FAIL categories) are referred for immediate assessment.

What to Do With Infants Who Failed the CCHD Screening

Infants who failed the screen should not be discharged from the hospital without excluding potentially life-threatening conditions; they should undergo evaluation to identify the cause of hypoxemia.

1. An echocardiography and/or cardiology consultation is the next step.
2. However, evaluation of the baby using other means (e.g., chest radiograph, blood work) should not be delayed while awaiting an echocardiogram.
3. If infants with ductal-dependent lesions are found, prostaglandin E_1 (PGE_1) infusion should be initiated to maintain patency of the ductus arteriosus. Cardiology consultation should be requested on an urgent basis. The starting dose of dinoprostone (Prostin) is 0.05 to 0.1 μg/kg/min administered in a continuous intravenous (IV) drip. When the desired effects (increased Po_2, increased systemic blood pressure, improved pH) are achieved, the dose should be reduced step-by-step to 0.01 μg/kg/min. When the initial starting dose has no effect, the dose may be increased up to 0.4 μg/kg/min. Three common side effects of IV infusion of PGE_1 are apnea (12%), fever (14%), and flushing (10%). Less

common side effects include tachycardia or bradycardia, hypotension, and cardiac arrest.

C. CYANOTIC CARDIAC DEFECTS

I. COMPLETE TRANSPOSITION OF THE GREAT ARTERIES

Prevalence

TGA occurs in about 5% to 7% of all CHDs. It is more common in boys (3:1).

Pathology and Pathophysiology

1. The aorta (AO) and the PA are transposed, with the AO arising anteriorly from the RV, and the PA arising posteriorly from the LV. The end result is complete separation of the two circuits, with hypoxemic blood circulating in the body and hyperoxemic blood circulating in the pulmonary circuit (Fig. 9.2) The classic complete TGA is also called D-transposition (D-TGA), denoting D-looping of the cardiac tube during embryogenesis.
2. Defects that permit mixing of the two circulations, such as ASD, VSD, and PDA, are necessary for survival. A VSD is present in 40% of cases. In about 50% of the patients no associated defects are present other than PFO, small ASD, or small PDA.
3. LVOT obstruction (subpulmonary stenosis), either dynamic or fixed obstruction, occurs in about 5% of patients without VSDs. PS occurs in 30% to 35% of patients with VSD.
4. In neonates with poor mixing of the two circulations, progressive hypoxia and acidosis result in early death, requiring an early intervention.

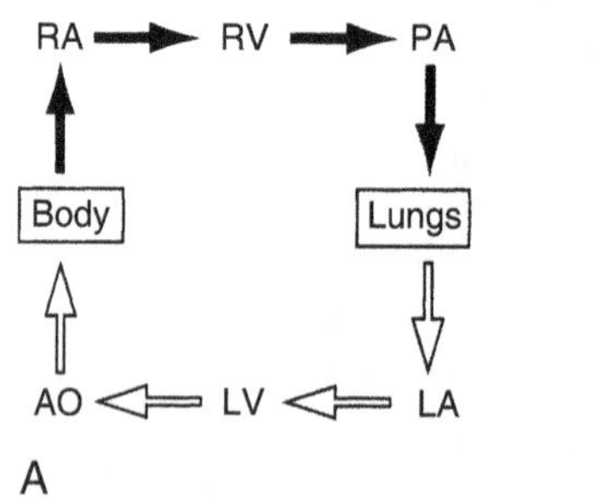

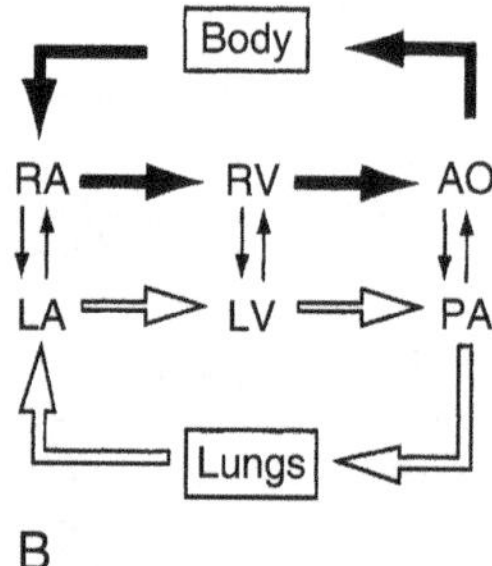

FIG. 9.2

Circulation pathways of normal serial circulation (A) and parallel circulation of TGA (B). *Open arrows* indicate oxygenated blood, and *solid arrows*, desaturated blood. *AO*, aorta; *LA*, left atrium; *LV*, left ventricle; *PA*, pulmonary artery; *RA*, right atrium, *RV*, right ventricle.

Clinical Manifestations

1. Cyanosis and signs of CHF in the newborn period. Severe arterial hypoxemia unresponsive to oxygen inhalation and acidosis are present in neonates with poor mixing (of systemic and pulmonary circulation). Hypoglycemia and hypocalcemia are occasionally present.
2. Moderate to severe cyanosis is present. Auscultatory findings are nonspecific. The S2 is single and loud. No heart murmur is audible in infants with intact ventricular septum. When TGA is associated with VSD or PS, a systolic murmur of these defects may be audible.
3. The electrocardiogram (ECG) shows RAD and RVH. An upright T wave in V1 after 3 days of age may be the only abnormality suggestive of RVH. BVH may be present in infants with large VSDs, PDA, or PS.
4. Chest radiographs show cardiomegaly with increased PVMs. An egg-shaped cardiac silhouette with a narrow superior mediastinum is characteristic.
5. Two-dimensional echo study is diagnostic.
   a. It fails to show a "circle-and-sausage" pattern of the normal great arteries in the parasternal short-axis view. Instead, it shows two circular structures.
   b. Other views show the PA arising from the LV and the aorta arising from the RV.
   c. Associated defects (VSD, LVOT obstruction, PS, ASD, and PDA) can be imaged.
   d. The status of atrial communication, both before and after balloon septostomy, is best evaluated in the subcostal view.
   e. The coronary arteries can be imaged in most patients in the parasternal and apical views.
6. Natural history and prognosis depend on anatomy.
   a. Infants with intact ventricular septum are the sickest group, but they demonstrate the most dramatic improvement following PGE_1 infusion or the Rashkind balloon atrial septostomy.
   b. Infants with VSD or large PDA are the least cyanotic group but are most likely to develop CHF and PVOD (beginning as early as 3 or 4 months of age).
   c. Combination of VSD and PS allows considerably longer survival without surgery, but repair surgery carries a high risk.
   d. Cerebrovascular accident and progressive PVOD, particularly in infants with large VSD or PDA, are rare late complications.

Management

Medical and Nonsurgical

1. Metabolic acidosis, hypoglycemia, and hypocalcemia should be treated if present.
2. PGE_1 infusion is started to raise arterial oxygen saturation by reopening the ductus.

3. Administration of oxygen may help raise systemic arterial oxygen saturation by lowering PVR and increasing PBF, with resulting increase in mixing.
4. A therapeutic balloon atrial septostomy (Rashkind procedure) may be performed. The balloon procedure is needed when (a) there is inadequate atrial mixing through the PFO (evidenced by a high Doppler flow velocity of >1 m/sec) and/or (b) immediate surgical intervention is not ready or planned. Occasionally, blade atrial septostomy may be performed for older infants and those for whom the initial balloon atrial septostomy is not successful.
5. Treatment of CHF may be indicated.

Surgical

Definite treatment is surgical. In the past, prior to the area of arterial switch operation, intracardiac flow pattern was switched at the atrial level (Senning operation) or at the ventricular level (Rastelli operation). At this time, arterial switch operation (Jatene procedure) is clearly the procedure of choice, and intraatrial repair surgeries are very rarely performed only under unusual situations. The indication, timing, and type of surgical treatment vary from institution to institution. For completeness, all of the surgical procedures done in patients with TGA are briefly described with schematic illustrations.

1. Intraatrial repair surgeries (e.g., Senning operation) are no longer performed, except in rare cases, because of undesirable late complications (such as obstruction to the pulmonary or systemic venous return, TR, arrhythmias, and depressed systemic ventricular [i.e., RV] function).
2. Rastelli operation, which redirects the pulmonary and systemic venous blood, is carried out at the ventricular level. It may be carried out in patients with VSD and severe PS. The LV blood is directed to the aorta by creating an intraventricular tunnel between the VSD and the aortic valve. A valved conduit or a homograft is placed between the RV and the PA (Fig. 9.3). This procedure is less popular because of late complications and higher surgical mortality rate. Two alternative procedures are now available: réparation à l'étage ventriculaire (REV) procedure and Nikaidoh procedure (see the following for discussion of these procedures).
3. Arterial switch operation (ASO) is the procedure of choice (Fig. 9.4). This procedure provides anatomic correction with infrequent complications. The proximal portions of the aorta and PA are transected, the coronary arteries are transplanted to the PA, and the proximal great arteries are connected to the distal end of the other great arteries. For this procedure to be successful, the LV pressure should be near systemic levels at the time of surgery, and therefore should be performed before 3 weeks of age. Surgical mortality is down to 2% to 3%. Possible complications

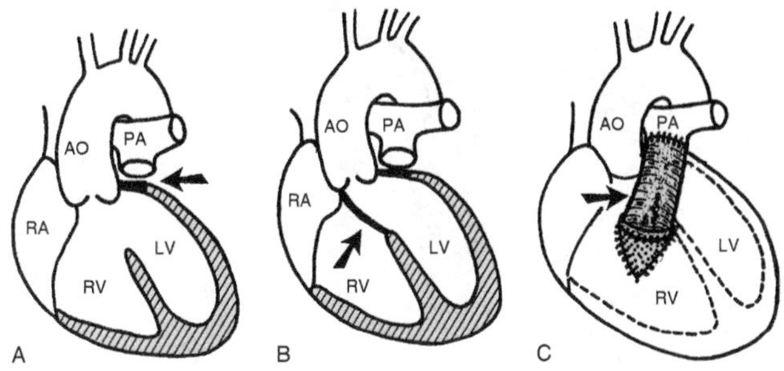

FIG. 9.3

The Rastelli operation. (A) The PA is divided from the LV, and the cardiac end is oversewn (*arrow*). (B) An intracardiac tunnel (*arrow*) is placed between the large VSD and the aorta. (C) The RV is connected to the divided PA by an aortic homograft or a valve-bearing prosthetic conduit. *AO*, aorta; LV, left ventricle*; PA*, pulmonary artery; *RA*, right atrium; *RV*, right ventricle.

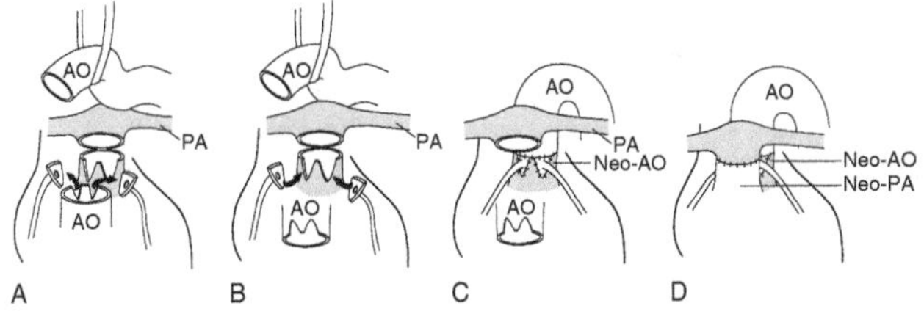

FIG. 9.4

Arterial switch operation. (A) The aorta is transected slightly above the coronary ostia, and the main PA is transected at about the same level. The ascending aorta is lifted, and both coronary arteries are removed from the aorta with triangular buttons. (B) Triangular buttons of similar size are made at the proper position in the PA trunk. (C) The coronary arteries are transplanted to the PA. The ascending aorta is brought behind the PA (Lecompte maneuver) and is connected to the proximal PA to form a neoaorta. (D) The triangular defects in the proximal aorta are repaired, and the proximal aorta is connected to the PA. Note that the neopulmonary artery is in front of the neoaorta. *AO*, aorta; PA, pulmonary artery. *(From Park, M. K., & Salamat, M. (2020).* Park's pediatric cardiology for practitioners *(7th ed.). Philadelphia: Mosby.)*

include coronary artery occlusion, supravalvar PS, supravalvar neoaortic stenosis, and AR.

4. REV procedure may be performed for patients with associated VSD and severe PS (Fig. 9.5). The procedure consists of the following: (1) infundibular resection to enlarge the VSD, (2) intraventricular baffle to

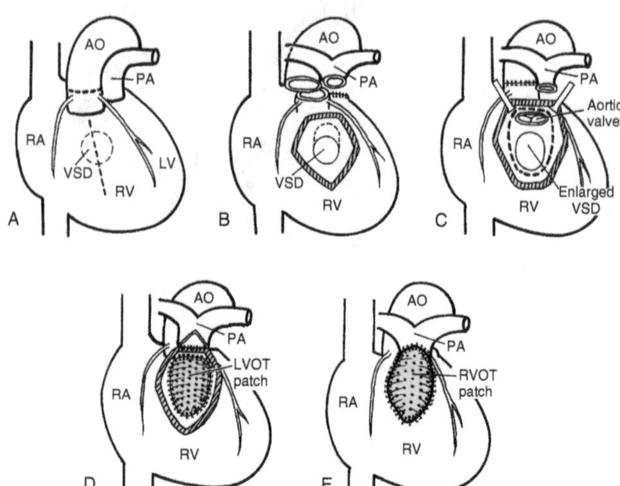

FIG. 9.5

Réparation à l'étage ventriculaire procedure for patients with D-TGA + VSD + severe PS. (A) The *broken lines* indicate the planned aortic and RV incision sites. The *broken circle* indicates a VSD. (B) The aorta and PA have been transected and the RPA is brought anterior to the aorta (Lecompte maneuver). The proximal PA has been oversewn. The VSD is exposed through the right ventriculotomy. *Dotted lines* indicate the portion of the infundibular septum to be excised to enlarge the VSD. (C) The aortic valve is well shown by retractors. The *broken line* indicates the planned site of a patch placement for the LV-AO connection. The transected aorta has been reconnected behind the RPA. (D) The completed LV-to-AO tunnel is shown. The superior portion of the right ventriculotomy is sutured directly to the posterior portion of the main PA. (E) A pericardial or synthetic patch is used to complete the RV-to-PA reconstruction. *AO,* aorta; *LV,* left ventricle; *LVOT,* left ventricular outflow tract; *PA,* pulmonary artery; *RA,* right atrium; RV, right ventricle; *RVOT,* right ventricular outflow tract; *VSD,* ventricular septal defect. *(From Park, M. K., & Salamat, M. (2020).* Park's pediatric cardiology for practitioners *(7th ed.). Philadelphia: Mosby.)*

direct LV output to the aorta, (3) aortic transection in order to perform the Lecompte maneuver (by which the RPA is brought anterior to the ascending aorta), and (4) direct RV-to-PA reconstruction by using an anterior patch (see Fig. 9.5). Lecompte reported surgical mortality of 18%.

5. The Nikaidoh procedure can be performed for patients with associated VSD and severe PS (Fig. 9.6). The repair consists of the following: (1) harvesting the aortic root from the RV (with attached coronary arteries), (2) relieving the LVOT obstruction (by dividing the outlet

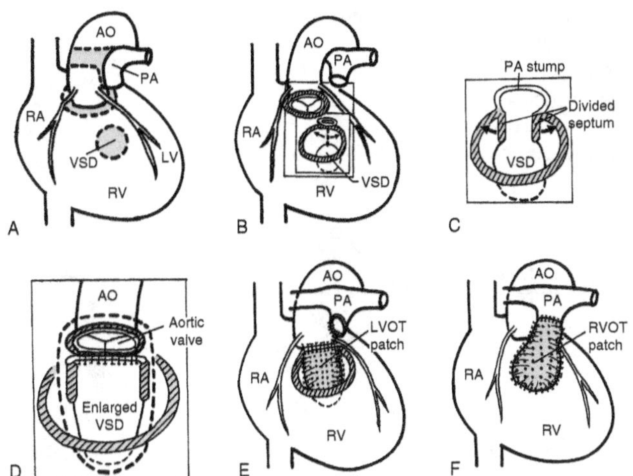

FIG. 9.6

Nikaidoh procedure (for patients with D-TGA, VSD, and severe PS). (A) The *circular broken* line around the aorta is the planned incision site for aortic root mobilization. The smaller *broken circle* indicates a VSD. (B) The aortic root has been mobilized by a circular incision around the aortic root, which leaves an opening in the RV free wall. The main PA is also transected. Through the opening, part of the VSD, ventricular septum, and hypoplastic PA stump are seen. The *dotted vertical line* in the ventricular septum (in the smaller inset in (B)) is the planned incision through the infundibular septum. (C) The incision in the infundibular septum has created a large opening, which includes the PA annulus and stump and the VSD. (D) The posterior portion of the aorta is directly sutured to the PA stump, which results in a large VSD. This completes translocation of the aorta to the original PA position. The thick *oval-shaped broken line* through the front of the transected aortic root is the planned site for placement of the LV outflow tract patch, which will direct the LV flow to the aorta. (E) The completed tunnel is shown (LVOT patch, which directs the LV flow to the aorta). The distal segment of the main PA is fixed to the aorta. Some surgeons use the Lecompte maneuver to bring the RPA in front of the ascending aorta (as shown here). (F) A pericardial patch is oversewn to complete the RV-to-PA connection (RVOT patch). *(From Park, M. K., & Salamat, M. (2020).* Park's pediatric cardiology for practitioners *(7th ed.). Philadelphia: Mosby.)*

septum and excising the pulmonary valve), (3) reconstructing the LVOT (with a patch between the aortic root and the VSD), and (4) reconstructing the RVOT with a pericardial patch or a homograft. In the modified Nikaidoh procedure, one or both coronary arteries are moved to a more favorable position as necessary (not shown) and the Lecompte maneuver is also performed (see Fig. 9.6). The hospital mortality is less than 10%.

The Damus-Kaye-Stansel operation may be performed at 1 to 2 years of age in infants with a large VSD and significant subaortic stenosis. In this procedure, the subaortic stenosis is bypassed by connecting the proximal PA trunk to the ascending aorta. The VSD is closed, and a conduit is placed between the RV and the distal PA (Fig. 9.7). Fig. 9.8 shows a partial listing of surgical approaches used for infants with TGA, including the timing.

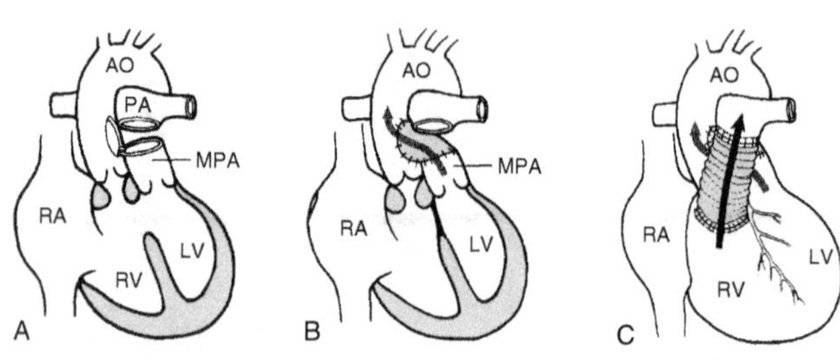

FIG. 9.7
Damus-Kaye-Stansel operation for D-TGA + VSD + subaortic stenosis. (A) The MPA is transected near its bifurcation. An appropriately positioned and sized incision is made in the ascending aorta. (B) The proximal MPA is anastomosed end to side to the ascending aorta, using either a Dacron tube or Gore-Tex. This channel will direct LV blood to the aorta. The aortic valve is either closed or left unclosed. (C) Through a right ventriculotomy the VSD is closed, and a valved conduit is placed between the RV and the distal PA. This channel will carry RV blood to the PA. *AO*, aorta; *LV*, left ventricle; *MPA*, main pulmonary artery; *PA*, pulmonary artery; *RA*, right atrium; *RV*, right ventricle. *(From Park, M. K., & Salamat, M. (2020).* Park's pediatric cardiology for practitioners *(7th ed.). Philadelphia: Mosby.)*

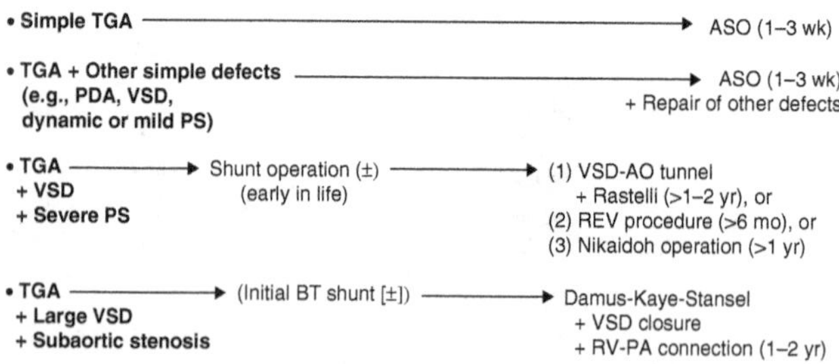

FIG. 9.8
Surgical approaches for TGA. *ASO*, arterial switch operation; *BT*, Blalock-Taussig; PDA, patent ductus arteriosus; PS, pulmonary stenosis; REV, réparation à l'étage ventriculare; *TGA*, transposition of the great arteries; *VSD*, ventricular septal defect. *(From Park, M. K., & Salamat, M. (2020).* Park's pediatric cardiology for practitioners *(7th ed.). Philadelphia: Mosby.)*

Follow-Up

1. Patients who receive an arterial switch operation need to be followed for stenosis of the anastomosis sites in the PA and AO, signs of AR, and possible coronary obstruction (such as myocardial ischemia, LV dysfunction, arrhythmias).
2. Limitation of activity may be indicated if arrhythmias or coronary insufficiency is present.

II. CONGENITALLY CORRECTED TRANSPOSITION OF THE GREAT ARTERIES (L-TGA)

Prevalence

Much less than 1% of all CHDs.

Pathology and Pathophysiology

1. Visceroatrial relationship is normal (the RA on the right of the LA). The RA empties into the anatomic LV through the mitral valve, and the LA empties into the RV through the tricuspid valve. For this to occur, the LV lies to the right of the RV (i.e., ventricular inversion). The great arteries are transposed, with the aorta arising from the RV and the PA arising from the LV. The final result is a functional correction in that oxygenated blood coming into the LA goes out the aorta (Fig. 9.9). This anomaly is

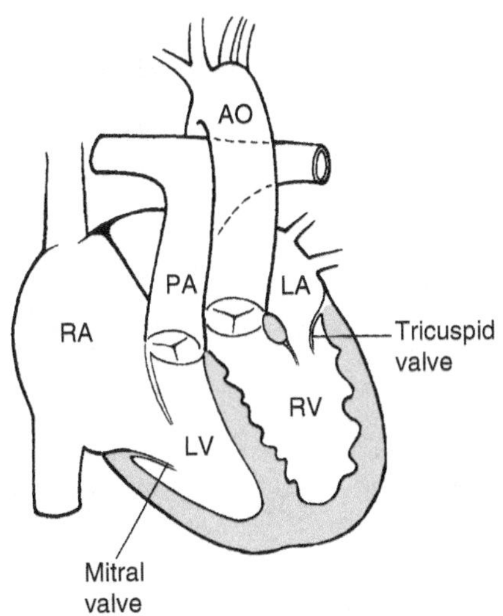

FIG. 9.9

Diagram of congenitally corrected TGA (L-TGA). *AO*, aorta; *LA*, left atrium; *LV*, left ventricle; *PA*, pulmonary artery; *RA*, right atrium; *RV*, right ventricle.

also called L-transposition (L-TGA), indicating *levo* looping of the cardiac tube during embryogenesis.

2. Theoretically, no functional abnormalities exist, but unfortunately most cases are complicated by associated defects. VSD (occurring in 80%) and PS (in 50%) with or without VSD are common, resulting in cyanosis. Regurgitation of the systemic AV valve (tricuspid) occurs in 30% of the patients. Varying degrees of AV block, which are sometimes progressive, and supraventricular tachycardia (SVT) are also frequent.
3. The cardiac apex is in the right chest (dextrocardia) in about 50% of patients.
4. The coronary arteries show a mirror-image distribution. The right-sided coronary artery supplies the anterior descending branch and gives rise to a circumflex; the left-sided coronary artery resembles a right coronary artery.

Clinical Manifestations

1. Patients with associated defects are symptomatic during the first few months of life with cyanosis (VSD + PS) or CHF (large VSD). Patients without associated defects asymptomatic.
2. The S2 is single and loud. A grade 2 to 4/6 harsh holosystolic murmur along the LLSB may indicate a VSD or the systemic AV valve (tricuspid) regurgitation. A grade 2 to 3/6 systolic ejection murmur at the ULSB or URSB may indicate PS.
3. Characteristic ECG findings are the absence of Q waves in V5 and V6 and/or the presence of Q waves in V4R or V1. Varying degrees of AV block (first degree and second degree AV blocks, sometimes progressing to complete heart block) may be present. Atrial and/or ventricular hypertrophy may be present in complicated cases.
4. Chest radiographs may show a characteristic straight left upper cardiac border (formed by the ascending aorta). Cardiomegaly and increased PVMs suggest associated VSD. Dextrocardia is frequent (50%).
5. Two-dimensional echo is diagnostic of the condition and associated defects.
   a. A “double circle” of the semilunar valves is imaged in the parasternal short-axis view. The posterior circle with no demonstrable coronary arteries is the PA. The aorta is usually anterior to and left of the PA.
   b. The LV, which has two well-defined papillary muscles, is seen anteriorly and on the right and is connected to the characteristic “fish mouth” appearance of the mitral valve.
   c. In the apical and subcostal four-chamber views, the LA is seen to connect to the tricuspid valve (which has a more apical attachment to the ventricular septum than the other).
   d. The anterior artery (aorta) arises from the left-sided morphologic RV, and the posterior artery with bifurcation (PA) arises from the right-sided morphologic LV.

   e. The situs solitus of the atria is confirmed.
   f. Associated anomalies such as PS (type and severity), VSD (size and location), and straddling of the AV valve should be checked.
6. Natural history: TR develops in about 30% of patients. Progressive AV conduction disturbances, including complete heart block (up to 30%), may occur.

Management

Medical

1. Treatment of CHF and arrhythmias is indicated, if present.
2. Antiarrhythmic agents are used to treat arrhythmias.

Surgical

1. Palliative procedures: PA banding for uncontrollable CHF due to a large VSD or a B-T shunt for patients with severe PS.
2. Corrective procedures: The presence or absence of TR determines the type of corrective surgery that can be performed, either anatomic repair or classic repair (see Fig. 9.10, surgical summary of L-TGA).

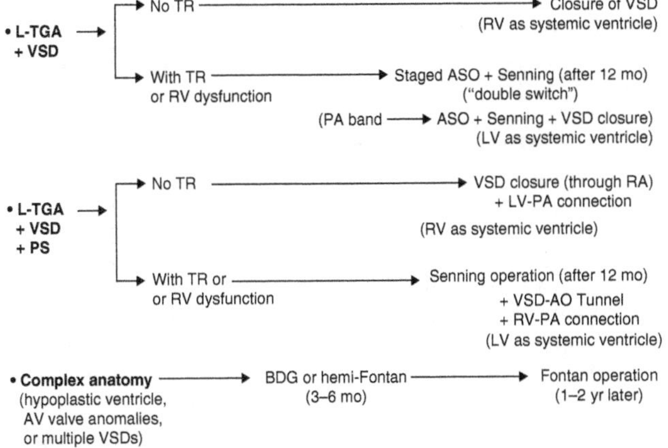

FIG. 9.10

Surgical summary of l-TGA. AO, aorta; ASO, arterial switch operation; OP, operation; PA, pulmonary artery; PS, pulmonary stenosis (= LV outflow tract obstruction); RV, right ventricle; TGA, transposition of the great arteries; TR, tricuspid regurgitation (= left-sided AV valve regurgitation); VSD, ventricular septal defect. *(From Park, M. K., & Salamat, M. (2020).* Park's pediatric cardiology for practitioners *(7th ed.). Philadelphia: Mosby.)*

a. When there is no TR, a classic repair is done, which leaves the anatomic RV as the systemic ventricle.
b. When there is TR or RV dysfunction, attempts are made to make the LV the systemic ventricle (anatomic repair).
c. For complex intracardiac anatomy, a staged Fontan-type operation is performed.

3. Other procedures may be necessary:
   a. Valve replacement for significant TR.
   b. Pacemaker implantation for either spontaneous or postoperative complete heart block.

Follow-Up

1. Follow-up every 6 to 12 months for a possible progression of AV conduction disturbances, arrhythmias, or worsening TR.
2. Routine pacemaker care is needed if a pacemaker is implanted.
3. Varying degrees of activity restriction may be indicated depending on hemodynamic abnormalities or pacemaker status.

III. TETRALOGY OF FALLOT

Prevalence

Five percent to 10% of all CHD.

Pathology and Pathophysiology

1. The original description of TOF included four abnormalities: a large VSD, RVOT obstruction, RVH, and an overriding of the aorta. However, only two abnormalities are important: a VSD large enough to equalize pressures in both ventricles and an RVOT obstruction (Fig. 9.11). The RVH is secondary to the RVOT obstruction and VSD, and the overriding of the aorta varies in degree.
2. The VSD is a perimembranous defect with extension into the infundibular septum and anterior malalignment of the conus. The RVOT may be in the form of infundibular stenosis (50%), pulmonary valve stenosis (10%), or both (30%). The pulmonary annulus and the PA are usually hypoplastic. The pulmonary valve is atretic in 10% of the patients. Abnormal coronary arteries are present in about 5% of the patients, with the most common one being the anterior descending branch arising from the right coronary artery and passing over the RV outflow tract (which prohibits a surgical incision in the region). Right aortic arch is present in 25% of the cases.
3. Because of the nonrestrictive VSD, systolic pressures in the RV and the LV are identical. Depending on the degree of the RVOT obstruction, an L-R, bidirectional, or R-L shunt is present. With a mild PS, an L-R shunt is present ("acyanotic" TOF). With a more severe degree of PS, a predominant R-L shunt occurs (cyanotic TOF). The heart murmur audible in cyanotic TOF originates from the RVOT obstruction, not from the VSD.

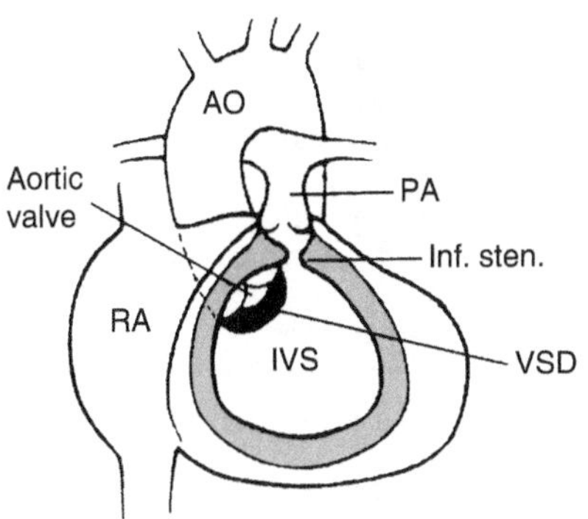

FIG. 9.11
Diagram of TOF. A large subaortic ventricular septal defect (*VSD*) is present through which aortic cusps are visualized. There is a pulmonary stenosis, which is infundibular, valvular, or a combination. The right ventricular muscle is hypertrophied. An infundibular chamber and hypoplastic main pulmonary artery (*PA*) are evident. *AO*, aorta; *Inf. sten.*, infundibular stenosis; *IVS*, interventricular septum; *RA*, right atrium. *(From Park, M. K., & Salamat, M. (2020).* Park's pediatric cardiology for practitioners *(7th ed.). Philadelphia: Mosby.)*

9

Clinical Manifestations

1. Neonates with TOF with pulmonary atresia are deeply cyanotic (see the later separate heading). Most infants with TOF are symptomatic, with cyanosis, clubbing, dyspnea on exertion, squatting, or hypoxic spells. Patients with acyanotic TOF may be asymptomatic.
2. A right ventricular tap and a systolic thrill at the MLSB are usually found. An ejection click of aortic origin, a loud and single S2, and a loud (grade 3 to 5/6) systolic ejection murmur at the middle and upper LSB are present. In the acyanotic form, a long systolic murmur resulting from VSD and infundibular stenosis is audible along the entire LSB, and cyanosis is absent.
3. The ECG shows RAD and RVH. BVH may be seen in the acyanotic form.
4. In cyanotic TOF, chest radiographs show normal heart size, decreased PVMs, and a boot-shaped heart with a concave MPA segment. Right aortic arch is present in 25% of the cases. Chest radiographs of acyanotic TOF are indistinguishable from those of a small to moderate VSD.
5. Two-dimensional echo shows a large subaortic VSD and an overriding of the aorta in the parasternal long-axis view. The anatomy of the RVOT, pulmonary valve, pulmonary annulus, and main PA and its branches is imaged in the parasternal short-axis view. Anomalous coronary artery

distribution can be imaged accurately. The major concern is to rule out any branch of the coronary artery crossing the RV outflow tract. Computed tomography (CT) and magnetic resonance imaging (MRI) angiography may clarify questions on the anomalous coronary arteries. Two-dimensional echo and Doppler studies are the primary method of evaluation before surgery. Cardiac catheterization is reserved only for those patients with specific unanswered questions after the noninvasive studies.

6. Natural history: Children with the acyanotic form of TOF gradually change to the cyanotic form by 1 to 3 years of age. Hypoxic spells may develop in infants (see next section). Brain abscess, cerebrovascular accident, and IE are rare complications. Polycythemia is common, but relative iron deficiency state (hypochromic) with normal hematocrit may be present. Coagulopathies are late complications of a long-standing severe cyanosis.

Hypoxic Spell

Hypoxic spell requires timely recognition and prompt appropriate treatment. The following describes key points of the spell.

1. General description: Hypoxic spell (also called cyanotic spell or "tet" spell) is characterized by (a) a paroxysm of hyperpnea (rapid and deep respiration), (b) irritability and prolonged crying, (c) increasing cyanosis, and (d) decreased intensity of the heart murmur. A severe spell may lead to limpness, convulsion, cerebrovascular accident, or even death. It occurs in young infants, with peak incidence between 2 and 4 months of age.
2. Pathophysiology of hypoxic spell: In TOF, the RV and LV can be viewed as a single pumping chamber, as there are large VSD equalizing pressures in both ventricles (Fig. 9.12). Lowering the SVR or increasing resistance at the RVOT will increase the R-L shunting, and this in turn stimulates the respiratory center to produce hyperpnea. Hyperpnea results in an increase in systemic venous return, which in turn increases the R-L shunt through the VSD, as there is an obstruction at the RVOT. A vicious circle becomes established (Fig. 9.13). Spasm of the RVOT is unlikely cause of the initiation of hypoxic spell; lowering of the SVR probably initiates the spell.
3. Treatment of hypoxic spell: The aim of the treatment is to break the vicious circle of hypoxic spell (as shown in Fig. 9.13). One or more of the following may be used in decreasing order of preference:
   a. Pick up the infant and hold in a knee-chest position.
   b. Morphine sulfate, 0.1 to 0.2 mg/kg subcutaneously or intramuscular, suppresses the respiratory center and abolishes hyperpnea.
   c. Treat acidosis with sodium bicarbonate, 1 mEq/kg IV. This reduces the respiratory center–stimulating effect of acidosis.
   d. Oxygen inhalation has only limited value, because the problem is a reduced PBF, not the ability to oxygenate.

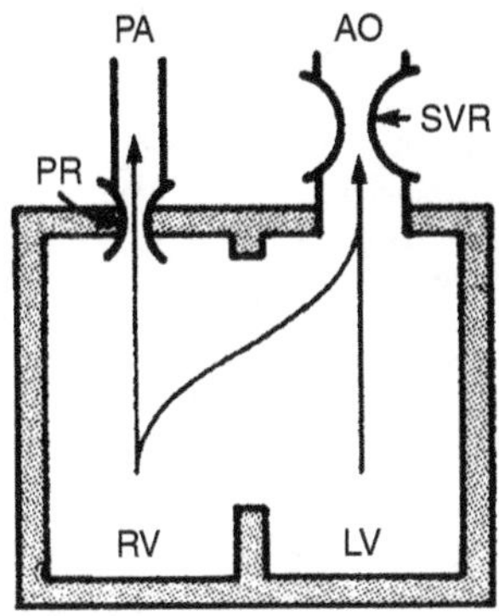

FIG. 9.12
Simplified concept of TOF that demonstrates how a change in the systemic vascular resistance (*SVR*) or right ventricular outflow tract obstruction (pulmonary resistance [*PR*]) affects the direction and the magnitude of the ventricular shunt. *AO*, aorta; *LV*, left ventricle; *PA*, pulmonary artery; *RV*, right ventricle. *(From Park, M. K., & Salamat, M. (2020).* Park's pediatric cardiology for practitioners *(7th ed.). Philadelphia: Mosby.)*

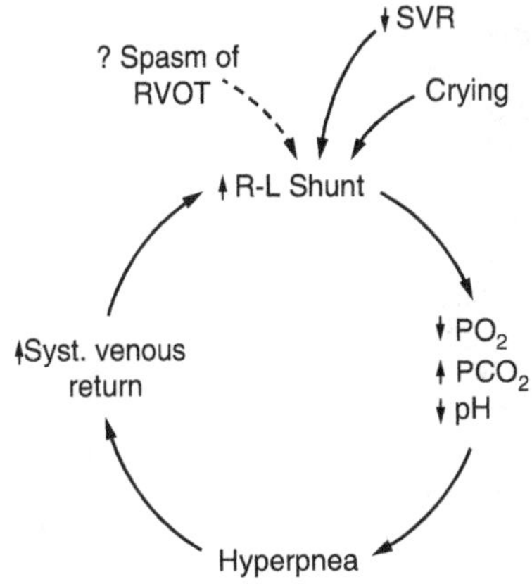

FIG. 9.13
Mechanism of hypoxic spell. *R-L shunt*, right-to-left shunt; *RVOT*, right ventricular outflow tract; *SVR*, systemic vascular resistance. *(From Park, M. K., & Salamat, M. (2020).* Park's pediatric cardiology for practitioners *(7th ed.). Philadelphia: Mosby.)*

e. With these treatments the infant usually becomes less cyanotic and the heart murmur becomes louder, indicating improved PBF.
f. If the spell is not fully under control with the above measures, the following may be tried.
   (1) Ketamine, 1 to 3 mg/kg (average of 2 mg/kg) in a slow IV push, works well (by increasing the SVR and sedating the infant).
   (2) Propranolol, 0.01 to 0.25 mg/kg (average 0.05 mg/kg) in a slow IV push, reduces the heart rate and may reverse the spell.

Management

Medical

1. Hypoxic spells should be recognized and treated appropriately (as described in the preceding section).
2. Oral propranolol, 2 to 4 mg/kg/day, may be used to prevent hypoxic spells while waiting for an optimal time for corrective surgery. The beneficial effect of propranolol may be related to its stabilizing action on peripheral vascular reactivity (and thus prevent sudden fall of the SVR), rather than by prevention of RV outflow tract spasm.
3. Detection and treatment of relative iron deficiency state, if present. Anemic children are particularly prone to cerebrovascular accident.

Surgical

1. Palliative procedures are indicated to increase PBF in infants with severe cyanosis or uncontrollable hypoxic spells on whom the corrective surgery cannot safely be performed, and in children with hypoplastic PA on whom the corrective surgery is technically difficult. Different types of systemic-to-pulmonary (S-P) shunts have been performed (Fig. 9.14).
   a. The B-T shunt (1945) (anastomosis between the subclavian artery and the ipsilateral PA) may be performed in older infants.
   b. Potts operation (1946) (anastomosis between the descending aorta and the left PA) is no longer performed for TOF.
   c. Waterston shunt (1962) (anastomosis between the ascending aorta and the right PA) is no longer performed because of many complications following the operation.
   d. Gore-Tex interposition shunt (modified B-T shunt) between the subclavian artery and the ipsilateral PA is the most popular procedure for any age, especially for infants younger than 3 months of age.
2. Complete repair surgery
   a. Timing:
      (1) Most centers prefer primary elective repair between 3 months and 12 months of age, even if they are asymptomatic, acyanotic (i.e., “pink tet”), or minimally cyanotic.

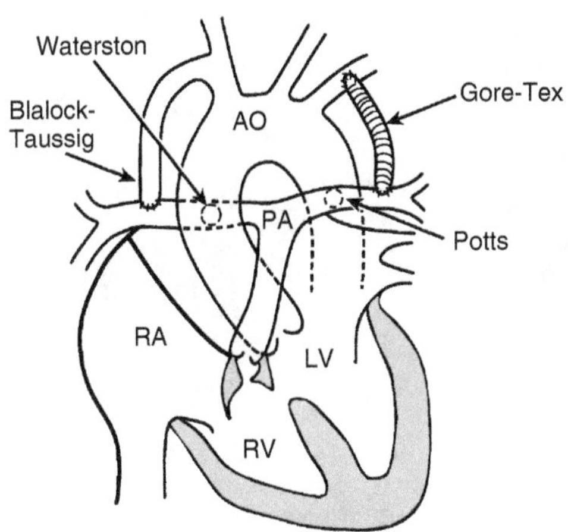

FIG. 9.14
Palliative procedures to increase pulmonary blood flow in patients with cyanosis and decreased PBF. *AO*, aorta; *LV*, left ventricle; *PA*, pulmonary artery; *RA*, right atrium; RV, right ventricle. *(From Park, M. K., & Salamat, M. (2020).* Park's pediatric cardiology for practitioners *(7th ed.). Philadelphia: Mosby.)*

(2) The occurrence of hypoxic spell is generally considered an indication for operation, even in conservative centers.
(3) Mildly cyanotic infants who have had previous shunt surgery may have total repair 1 to 2 years after the shunt operation.
(4) Patients with coronary artery anomalies may have an early surgery at the same time as those without anomalous coronary arteries.

b. Total repair of the defect is carried out under cardiopulmonary bypass. The procedure includes patch closure of the VSD, widening of the RVOT by resection of the infundibular muscle tissue, and pulmonary valvotomy, avoiding placement of a transannular fabric patch (Fig. 9.15). At the present time, surgeons aim to avoid right ventriculotomy and transannular patch whenever possible. However, if the pulmonary annulus and main PA are hypoplastic, transannular patch placement is unavoidable. Some centers advocate placement of a monocusp valve at the time of initial repair, whereas other centers advocate pulmonary valve replacement at a later time if indicated.
c. Surgery for TOF with anomalous anterior descending coronary artery from the right coronary artery (which results in the LAD crossing the RV outflow tract) requires placement of a conduit

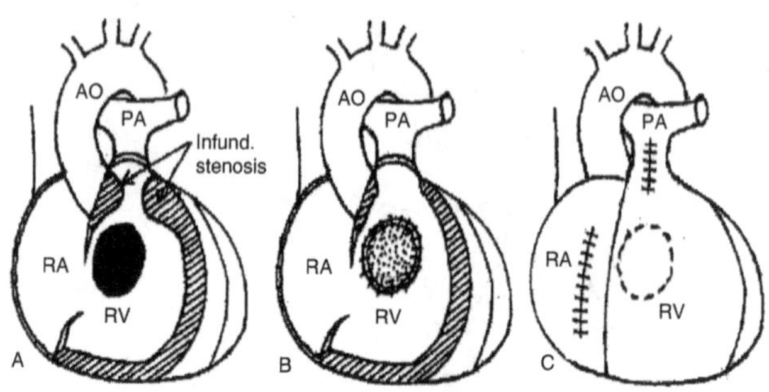

FIG. 9.15

Schematic drawing of surgical correction of tetralogy of Fallot (TOF). (A) Anatomy of TOF showing a large ventricular septal defect (VSD) and infundibular stenosis seen with the anterior walls of the right atrium and right ventricle removed. (B) Patch closure of the VSD is done (through a right atrial incision and through the tricuspid annulus) and the resection of the infundibular stenosis is done (through an incision in the pulmonary artery), avoiding right ventriculotomy. (C) The right atrial incision and the pulmonary artery incision sites are shown. AO, aorta; Infund., infundibular; PA, pulmonary artery; RA, right atrium; RV, right ventricle. *(From Park, M. K., & Salamat, M. (2020).* Park's pediatric cardiology for practitioners *(7th ed.). Philadelphia: Mosby.)*

between the RV and PA. The surgery is usually performed after 1 year of age. A B-T shunt may be necessary initially to palliate the patient. Alternatively, when a small conduit is necessary between the RV and the PA, the native outflow tract should be made as large as possible using transatrial and transpulmonary approach, so that a "double outlet" (the native outlet and the conduit) results from the RV.

Follow-Up

1. Long-term follow-up every 6 to 12 months is recommended, especially for patients with residual VSD shunt, residual RVOT obstruction, residual PA stenosis, arrhythmias, or conduction disturbances.
2. Significant, and usually progressive, pulmonary regurgitation may develop following repair of TOF. Although the PR is well tolerated for a decade or two, it may eventually lead to significant RV enlargement and RV dysfunction. A homograft pulmonary valve may need to be inserted (by either a transcatheter technique or surgery) while the RV function remains reversible. Although the indications for the valve replacement are evolving, the presence of moderate or severe PR (with RV regurgitation fraction 25% or greater), decreased RV function, and/or significant RV dilatation appears to be prerequisite. RV

function and size and regurgitant fraction are best investigated by MRI (or CT).
3. Some patients, particularly those who had Rastelli operation using valved conduit, develop valvular stenosis or regurgitation. Valvular stenosis may improve after balloon dilatation, but PR may worsen. Nonsurgical percutaneous pulmonary valve implantation technique developed by Bonhoeffer et al. has been used successfully.
4. Some children develop late arrhythmias, particularly VT, which may result in sudden death. Arrhythmias are primarily related to persistent RVH as a result of unsatisfactory repair.
5. Pacemaker therapy is indicated for surgically induced complete heart block or sinus node dysfunction.
6. Varying levels of activity limitation may be necessary.
7. For patients who have residual defects or have prosthetic material for repair, IE prophylaxis should be observed throughout life.

IV. TETRALOGY OF FALLOT (TOF) WITH PULMONARY ATRESIA

Prevalence

About 30% of patients with TOF.

Pathology and Pathophysiology

1. In this extreme form of TOF, the intracardiac pathology resembles that of TOF in all respects except for the presence of pulmonary atresia.
2. The PBF is more commonly through a PDA (70%) and less commonly through multiple systemic collaterals (30%), which are called multiple aortopulmonary collateral arteries (or MAPCAs). Both PDA and collateral arteries may coexist as the source of PBF. The ductus is small and long and descends vertically from the transverse arch ("vertical" ductus) and connects to the Pas, which are usually confluent. The subgroup of patients with MAPCAs is associated with nonconfluent PAs, with the right upper lobe and the left lower lobe frequently supplied by systemic collateral arteries. This subgroup is designated as pulmonary atresia and VSD.
3. The central and branch PAs are hypoplastic in most patients but more frequently in patients with MAPCAs than in those with PDA. Incomplete arborization (distribution) of one or both PAs is also more common in patients with nonconfluent PAs than those with confluent PAs.

Clinical Manifestations

1. The patient is cyanotic at birth; the degree of cyanosis depends on whether the ductus is patent and how extensive the systemic collateral arteries are.
2. Usually no heart murmur is audible, but a faint, continuous murmur of PDA may be audible. The S2 is loud and single.

3. The ECG shows RAD and RVH.
4. Chest radiographs show normal heart size, often with a boot-shaped silhouette and a markedly decreased PVM ("black" lung field).
5. Echo studies are diagnostic of the condition, but an angiocardiogram is necessary for complete delineation of the pulmonary artery anatomy and the collaterals. Alternatively, MRI or CT angiography is used for complete anatomic delineation of the aortic collaterals and PA branches.

Management

Medical

1. IV PGE_1 infusion is started to keep the ductus open for cardiac catheterization and in preparation for surgery (see Appendix E for the dosage).
2. Emergency cardiac catheterization or MRI (or CT angiography) is performed to delineate anatomy of the pulmonary arteries and systemic arterial collaterals.

Surgical

1. Primary surgical repair (closure of the VSD, conduit between the RV and the central PA) is possible only when a central PA of adequate size exists and the central PA connects without obstruction to sufficient regions of the lungs (at least equal to one whole lung).
2. Staged repair consists of an initial procedure that increases PBF and induces the growth of the central PA (before 1 or 2 years of age) followed by additional surgical procedure(s) at a later time.
   a. When there is a *confluence* of central PAs, either a B-T shunt or a PA homograft placement can be performed.
      (1) A B-T shunt procedure often results in an iatrogenic stenosis of the PA branch. For a very small confluent central PA, a central end-to-side shunt (Mee procedure) can be performed.
      (2) Initial RVOT reconstruction with a small homograft conduit may need to be replaced with a larger one later. Anastomosis of collateral arteries to the central artery is carried out later. In this case, the VSD may be left open, or closed with a fenestrated patch to maintain an increased PBF (Fig. 9.16, *top row*).
   b. When the central PA is *nonconfluent*, with multiple collaterals supplying different segments of the lungs, a surgical connection between or among the isolated regions of the lungs may be made so they might be perfused from a single source (termed *unifocalization of PBF*) (see Fig. 9.16, *bottom row*). Later, a conduit between the RV and a newly created central PA can be made.
   c. Occlusion of systemic collateral arteries is done by coil embolization preoperatively or at the time of surgery.
3. Fig. 9.17 summarizes surgical approaches for patients with TOF with pulmonary atresia.

Confluent PA and collaterals

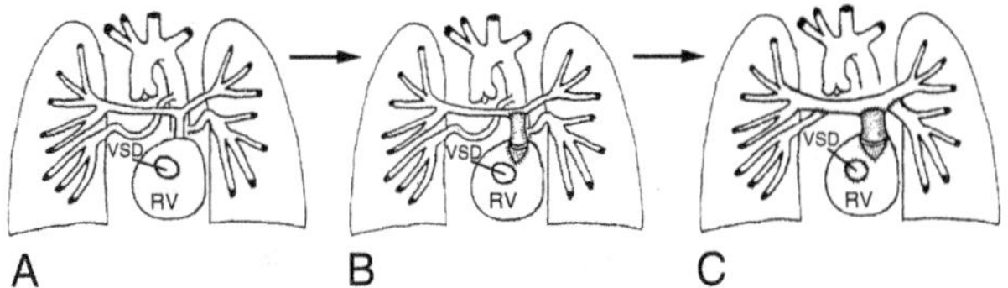

Nonconfluent PA and multiple collaterals

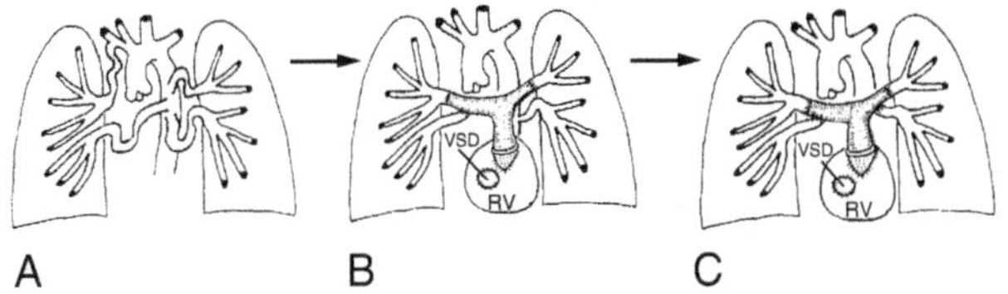

FIG. 9.16
Diagram of staged operation for TOF with pulmonary atresia. Upper row (confluent PA and collaterals). (A) A hypoplastic but confluent central PA and multiple other collateral arteries are shown. (B) A small RV-to-PA connection is made with a pulmonary homograft (shown with shade), with collaterals left alone. (C) The pulmonary artery has grown to a larger size and a larger pulmonary homograft has replaced the earlier small one. Collateral arteries are now anastomosed (unifocalized) to the originally hypoplastic PA branches. VSD may be closed at a later time, usually 1 to 3 years of age. The pulmonary homograft is usually replaced with a larger graft at this time. Bottom row (nonconfluent PA and multiple collaterals): (A) Absent central pulmonary artery and multiple aortic collaterals are shown. B, A small pulmonary homograft (6- to 8-mm internal diameter, shaded) is used to establish RV-to-PA connection with some collaterals connected to it (unifocalized) (performed at 3 to 6 months). Some collaterals are not unifocalized at this time. (C) The homograft conduit has been replaced with a larger one. Remaining collateral arteries are anastomosed to the pulmonary homograft to complete the unifocalization procedure. VSD is closed with or without fenestration, usually at 1 to 3 years. *(From Park, M. K., & Salamat, M. (2020).* Park's pediatric cardiology for practitioners *(7th ed.). Philadelphia: Mosby.)*

Follow-Up

1. Frequent follow-up is needed to assess the palliative surgery, to decide the appropriate time for further operations, and to determine an appropriate time for conduit replacement.
2. IE prophylaxis is indicated for an indefinite period.
3. A certain level of activity restriction is needed for most patients even after surgery.

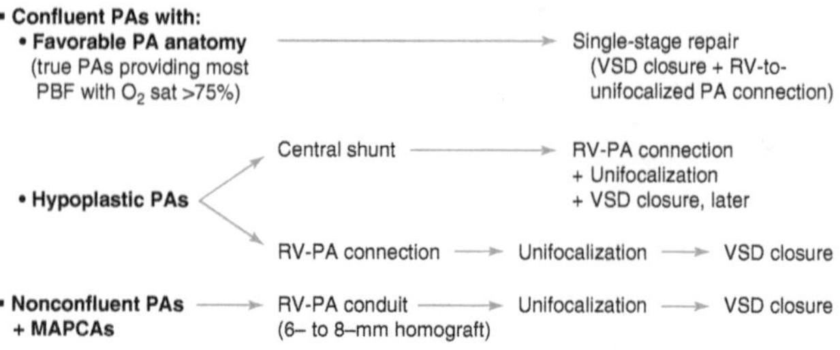

FIG. 9.17

Surgical approaches for TOF with pulmonary atresia (or pulmonary atresia and VSD). *MAPCAs,* multiple aortopulmonary artery collaterals; PA, pulmonary artery; *PBF,* pulmonary blood flow; *RV-PA,* right ventricle-to-pulmonary artery; *VSD,* ventricular septal defect. *(From Park, M. K., & Salamat, M. (2020).* Park's pediatric cardiology for practitioners *(7th ed.). Philadelphia: Mosby.)*

V. TETRALOGY OF FALLOT (TOF) WITH ABSENT PULMONARY VALVE

Prevalence

Approximately 2% to 6% of patients with TOF.

Pathology and Pathophysiology

1. The pulmonary valve leaflets are either absent or rudimentary, and the pulmonary annulus is stenotic, usually in association with TOF.
   A massive aneurysmal dilatation of the PAs develops during fetal life and compresses the lower end of the developing trachea and bronchi. Postnatally, this produces signs of airway obstruction and respiratory difficulties. Pulmonary complications (e.g., atelectasis, pneumonia), rather than the intracardiac defect, are the usual cause of death when managed medically.
2. The ductus arteriosus is frequently absent, with a more severe aneurysmal dilatation of the PAs. A right aortic arch is frequently found (in about 50%)
3. Since the annular stenosis is only moderate, a bidirectional shunt is initially present but it becomes predominantly an L-R shunt beyond the newborn period.

Clinical Manifestations

1. Mild cyanosis may be present in the neonate, but cyanosis disappears and signs of CHF may develop when the PVR falls.
2. A to-and-fro murmur ("sawing-wood sound") at the upper and middle LSB (resulting from PS and PR) is characteristic of the condition. The S2 is loud and single, and RV hyperactivity is palpable.
3. The ECG shows RAD and RVH.

4. Chest radiographs reveal a markedly dilated MPA and hilar PAs. The heart size is either normal or mildly enlarged, and PVMs may be slightly increased. The lung fields may show hyperinflated and/or atelectatic areas.
5. Echo studies reveal a large, subaortic VSD with overriding of the aorta (as seen in TOF), distally displaced pulmonary annulus (with thick ridges instead of fully developed pulmonary valve leaflets), and gigantic aneurysm of the PA and its branches. The RV is markedly dilated, often with paradoxical motion of the ventricular septum. Doppler studies reveal evidence of stenosis and regurgitation at the annulus.
6. Natural history: Most infants with severe pulmonary complications (e.g., atelectasis, pneumonia) die during infancy if treated only medically. The surgical mortality of infants with pulmonary complications is as high as 40%. Therefore surgery should be performed in early infancy before pulmonary complications develop.

Management

Medical

The mortality of medical management is very high. Once the pulmonary symptoms appear, neither surgical nor medical management carries good results.

Surgical

1. Symptomatic neonates should have corrective surgery on an urgent basis. Even asymptomatic infants should have elective primary repair surgery in early infancy. Some use a homograft valve at the pulmonary valve position, and others do not. Some surgeons advocate stenting the airway at the time of surgery.
2. Alternatively, a two-stage operation can be performed. A tight PA banding is performed to eliminate excessive pulsation of the PA along with a B-T shunt, and a complete repair at a later time (at 2 to 4 years of age).

VI. TOTAL ANOMALOUS PULMONARY VENOUS RETURN (TAPVR)

Prevalence

One percent of all CHDs. There is marked male preponderance (4:1) in the infracardiac type.

Pathology and Pathophysiology

1. The PVs drain into the RA or its venous tributaries, rather than directly into the LA. The defects may be divided into the following four types (Fig. 9.18).
   a. Supracardiac (50%): The common PV drains into the SVC via the left SVC (vertical vein) and the left innominate vein.

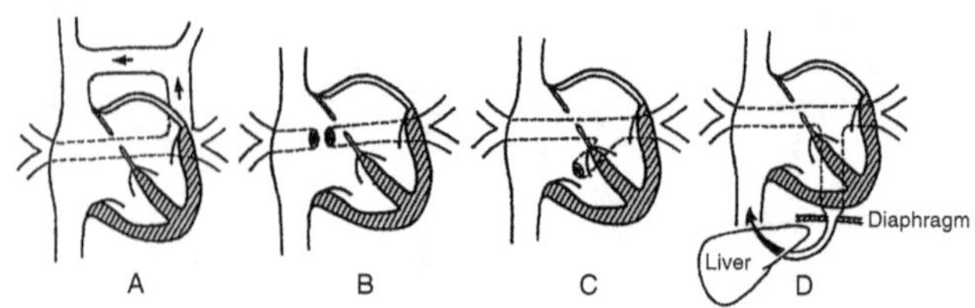

FIG. 9.18

Anatomic classification of TAPVR. (A) Supracardiac. (B) Cardiac, draining into the RA (only two pulmonary veins are shown). (C) Cardiac, draining into the coronary sinus. (D) Infracardiac.

b. Cardiac (20%): The PVs enter the RA separately through four openings (Fig. 9.18B), or the common PV drains into the CS (Fig. 9.18C).
c. Infracardiac (subdiaphragmatic) (20%): The common PV drains to the portal vein, ductus venosus, hepatic vein, or IVC. The common PV penetrates the diaphragm through the esophageal hiatus.
d. Mixed type (10%): A combination of different types.

2. An ASD is necessary for survival. The left side of the heart is relatively small. There is an obstruction of the pulmonary venous return in some patients, especially with the infracardiac type.
3. Pulmonary and systemic venous bloods are completely mixed in the RA. Blood then goes to the LA through an ASD as well as to the RV. Thus oxygen saturations in the systemic and pulmonary circulations are the same, with resulting systemic arterial desaturation.
4. The level of systemic arterial oxygen saturation is proportional to the amount of PBF. When there is no obstruction to PV return (as seen in most of the supracardiac and cardiac types), PV return is large and the systemic arterial blood is only minimally desaturated. When there is obstruction to PV return (as seen in the infracardiac type), PV return is small and the patient is severely cyanotic. Thus clinical manifestations will differ depending on the presence or absence of obstruction to pulmonary venous return.

Clinical Manifestations

Clinical Manifestations Without *Pulmonary Venous (PV) Obstruction*

1. Growth retardation, mild cyanosis, and signs of CHF (tachypnea, tachycardia, and hepatomegaly) are common.
2. Hyperactive RV impulse and characteristic quadruple or quintuple rhythm are present. The S2 is widely split and fixed, and the P2 may be accentuated. A grade 2 to 3/6 systolic ejection murmur is

usually present at the ULSB. A middiastolic rumble is always present at the LLSB (resulting from relative stenosis of the tricuspid valve).
3. The ECG shows RAD, RVH (rsR′ pattern in V1), and occasional RAH.
4. Chest radiographs show moderate to marked cardiomegaly (involving RA and RV) with increased PVMs. A "snowman" sign is seen in older infants with the supracardiac type (usually after 4 months of age).
5. Two-dimensional echo is usually diagnostic. It demonstrates the common PV posterior to the LA without direct communication to the LA. A markedly dilated CS protruding into the LA (seen in TAPVR to the CS) or dilated left innominate vein and SVC (seen in the supracardiac type) may be imaged. An ASD with an R-L shunt and relatively small LA and LV are imaged.
6. Cardiac catheterization is usually not necessary for diagnosis; it is occasionally done to perform atrial septostomy to improve atrial shunt or to identify a complex mixed type of pulmonary venous return. Alternatively, MRI or cardiac CT can be used for diagnosis in cases of complex mixed type; the former is preferable because it does not use ionizing radiation.
7. Natural history: CHF, growth retardation, and repeated pneumonias develop by 6 months of age.

Clinical Manifestations With Pulmonary Venous (PV) Obstruction

1. Marked cyanosis and respiratory distress are present in the neonate.
2. A loud and single S2 and gallop rhythm are present. Heart murmur is usually absent. Pulmonary crackles may be audible.
3. The ECG shows RAD and RVH.
4. The heart size is usually normal on chest radiographs, but the lung fields reveal findings of pulmonary venous congestion or edema.
5. Two-dimensional (2d) echo shows relatively hypoplastic LA and LV. Anomalous PV return below the diaphragm can be directly imaged by 2D echo studies.
6. Cardiac catheterization, MRI, or cardiac CT may be used for complete diagnosis.
7. Natural history: Patients with the infracardiac type rarely survive more than a few weeks without surgery.

Management of Both Groups of Patients

Medical

1. Intensive anticongestive measures are indicated for the nonobstructive type.
2. Oxygen and diuretics are given for pulmonary edema in infants with the obstructive type. Intubation and ventilator therapy with oxygen and positive end-expiratory pressure (PEEP) may be necessary in infants with severe pulmonary edema (due to obstruction to PV return).

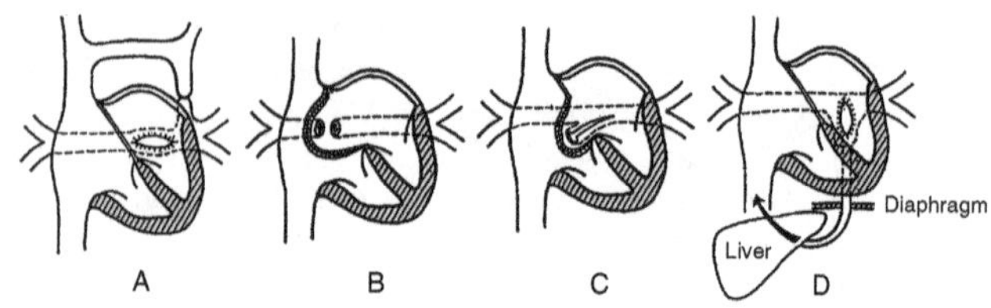

FIG. 9.19
Surgical approaches to various types of total anomalous pulmonary venous return (see text). *(From Park, M. K., & Salamat, M. (2020).* Park's pediatric cardiology for practitioners *(7th ed.). Philadelphia: Mosby.)*

3. In the case of severely restrictive interatrial shunting (restrictive PFO, ASD), balloon atrial septostomy to enlarge the interatrial communication may be beneficial at least temporarily.
4. PGE_1 is not indicated in patients with TAPVR.

Surgical

1. There is no palliative procedure. Corrective surgery is indicated for all patients with this condition. Infants without PV obstruction are operated on as soon as possible after the diagnosis. Infants who do not have PV obstruction but do have heart failure are usually operated on a semi-elective basis.
2. Surgical techniques used for different types of TAPVR are as follows:
   a. **Supracardiac Type**. A large, side-to-side anastomosis is made between the common PV and the LA. The vertical vein is ligated. The ASD is closed with a patch (Fig. 9.19A).
   b. **TAPVR to the Right Atrium**. The atrial septum is excised and a patch is sewn in such a way that the pulmonary venous return is diverted to the LA (Fig. 9.19B).
   c. **TAPVR to the CS**. An incision is made in the anterior wall of the CS ("unroofing") to make a communication between the CS and the LA. A single patch closes the original ASD and the ostium of the CS. This will result in the drainage of CS blood with low oxygen saturation into the LA (Fig. 9.19C).
   d. **Infracardiac Type**. A large vertical anastomosis is made between the common PV and the LA. The common PV is ligated above the diaphragm (Fig. 9.19D).

Follow-Up

Follow-up is needed for possible late development of obstruction to PV return (10%) or atrial arrhythmias, including sinus node dysfunction.

VII. TRICUSPID ATRESIA

Prevalence

One percent to 3% of all CHD in infancy.

Pathology and Pathophysiology

1. The tricuspid valve is absent and the RV and PA are hypoplastic, with decreased PBF. The great arteries are transposed in 30% (mostly D-TGA) and normally related in 70% of the cases. Associated defects such as ASD, VSD, or PDA are necessary for survival.
2. In the most common type (50%), a small VSD and PS (with hypoplasia of the PAs) are present, and the great arteries are normally related. In the second most common type (20%), the great arteries are transposed and the pulmonary valve is normal sized (Fig. 9.20).
3. COA or interrupted aortic arch is a frequently associated anomaly, more commonly seen in cases with TGA.
4. All systemic venous return is shunted from the RA to the LA, with resulting dilatation and hypertrophy of the RA. The LA and LV are large because they handle both systemic and pulmonary venous returns. The level of arterial saturation is positively related to the level of PBF.

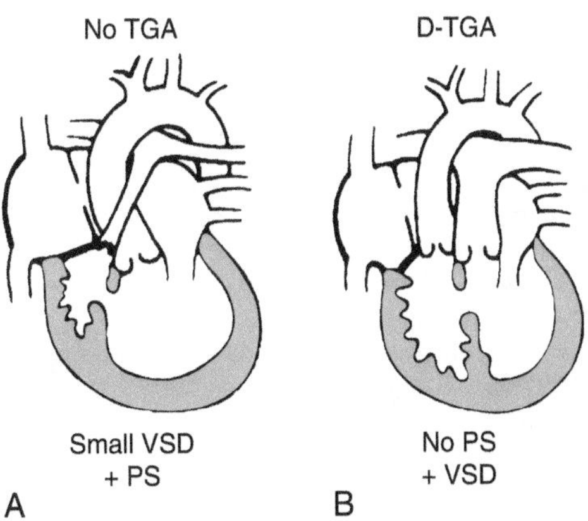

FIG. 9.20

The two most common types of tricuspid atresia. In about 50% of patients, the great arteries are normally related and a small VSD and PS are present (A). When the great arteries are transposed (about 20% of all cases), a VSD is usually present without PS (B). *PS*, pulmonary stenosis; *TGA*, transposition of the great arteries; *VSD*, ventricular septal defect.

Clinical Manifestations

1. Severe cyanosis, tachypnea, and poor feeding are usual.
2. The S2 is single. A grade 2 to 3/6 systolic regurgitant murmur of VSD is usually present at the LLSB. A continuous murmur of PDA is occasionally audible. Hepatomegaly is present when there is an inadequate interatrial communication or CHF.
3. The ECG shows a characteristic "superior" QRS axis (in most patients without TGA and some patients with TGA), RAH or BAH, and LVH.
4. Chest radiographs show normal or slightly increased heart size and decreased PVMs. A boot-shaped heart with a concave MPA segment may be seen. In infants with TGA, PVMs may be increased.
5. Two-dimensional echo shows atretic tricuspid valve, large LV, diminutive RV, and ASD. The presence or absence of TGA, VSD, PDA, and COA is also imaged. The size of the VSD, the presence and severity of PS, and the presence of TGA should all be investigated. Patients with TGA should be examined for possible subaortic stenosis and COA.
6. Cardiac catheterization with atrial septostomy is indicated when atrial communication is inadequate. Cardiac catheterization is generally recommended before a planned surgical intervention other than the B-T shunt or PA banding, to gain information on the PA anatomy, pressure, and vascular resistance and the LV function.
7. Natural history: Few infants survive beyond 6 months of life without surgical palliation. Occasional patients with increased PBF develop pulmonary hypertension and LV failure, which preclude successful Fontan operation.

Management

Medical

1. IV PGE_1 infusion (see Appendix E for dosage) is indicated in cyanotic neonates to maintain the patency of the ductus before planned cardiac catheterization.
2. The balloon atrial septostomy (Rashkind procedure) may be performed to improve the R-L atrial shunt.
3. Rarely, patients in CHF require anticongestive measures.
4. Infants with VSD of adequate size and normal PBF need to be followed closely for decreasing oxygen saturation, which may be caused by reduction in the size of the VSD.

Surgical

The definitive surgery for tricuspid atresia is a Fontan-type operation. One or more palliative procedures are required to produce ideal candidates for Fontan operation. Ideal candidates for a Fontan operation have normal LV function and low PVR.

1. Normal LV function results from prevention of excessive volume overload (by using a relatively small B-T shunt, 3.5 mm for neonates) or pressure loading of the LV (by relieving LV outflow obstruction).

BOX 9.1

FONTAN PATHWAY

Stage I. One of the following procedures is done in preparation for a future Fontan operation.

1. Blalock-Taussig shunt, when PBF is small
2. PA banding, when PBF is excessive
3. Damus-Kaye-Stansel + shunt operation (for TA + TGA + restrictive VSD)

Medical follow-up after stage I. Watch for:

a. Cyanosis (O_2 saturation <75%): cardiac catheterization or MRI to find the cause.
b. Poor weight gain (CHF from too much PBF): tightening of PA band may be necessary.

Stage II (at 3 to 6 months).

1. BDG operation or
2. The hemi-Fontan operation

Medical follow-up after stage II. Watch for the following:

a. A gradual decrease in O_2 saturation (<75%) may be caused by:
   (1) Opening of venous collaterals
   (2) Pulmonary arterio-venous fistula (due to the absence of hepatic inhibitory factor)
   - Perform cardiac catheterization (to find and occlude venous collaterals) or
   - Proceed with Fontan operation
b. Transient hypertension 1 to 2 weeks postoperatively: may use ACE inhibitors
c. Pre-Fontan cardiac catheterization to assess risk factors.

The following are risk factors for the Fontan operation. Presence of ≥2 is a high-risk situation.

(a) Mean PA pressure >18 mm Hg (or PVR >2 U/m^2)
(b) LV end-diastolic pressure >12 mm Hg (or EF <60%)
(c) Atrioventricular valve regurgitation
(d) Distorted PAs secondary to previous shunt operation

Stage III (Fontan operation) at 2 to 5 years of age.

1. Lateral tunnel Fontan (with 4-mm fenestration); device closure of the fenestration 1–2 yr later could be considered, or
2. An extracardiac conduit

ACE, angiotensin-converting enzyme; *BDG*, bidirectional Glenn; *CHF*, congestive heart failure; *EF*, ejection fraction; *LV*, left ventricular; *MRI*, magnetic resonance imaging; *PA*, pulmonary artery; *PBF*, pulmonary blood flow; *PVR*, pulmonary vascular resistance; *TA*, tricuspid atresia; *TGA*, transposition of the great arteries; *VSD*, ventricular septal defect.

2. Low PVR may result from (a) adequate growth of PA branches (b) prevention of distortion of the PA (by avoidance of unnecessary shunt placement, or (c) PA banding in patients with increased PBF.
3. Because the Fontan operation is done for many other complex heart defects, staged approaches to the procedure are discussed in the following section and summarized in Box 9.1 for quick reference.

Staged Approaches to Fontan Operation

Stage I. One of the following three procedures is performed depending on the situation.

1. A B-T shunt (3.5 mm) to the RPA, in patients with decreased PBF.
2. PA banding is rarely necessary for infants with CHF from increased PBF.
3. Damus-Kaye-Stansel and shunt operation for infants with tricuspid atresia + TGA + restrictive VSD. In this procedure, the main PA is transected, and the distal PA is sewn over. The proximal PA is connected end-to-side to the ascending aorta (similar to Fig. 9.7 done for patients with TGA). A B-T shunt is created to supply blood to the lungs.

Medical Follow-Up After Stage I Surgery. The infant should be watched carefully until the time of the stage II palliation with emphasis on the following.

a. Cyanosis (with O_2 saturation <75%): The cause should be investigated by cardiac catheterization or MRI.
b. Poor growth: It may be due to large a PBF and tightening of PA band should be considered.

Stage II. As a stage II operation, either a bidirectional Glenn shunt or rarely the hemi-Fontan operation is performed in preparation for the final Fontan operation.

1. Bidirectional Glenn operation. An end-to-side SVC-to-RPA shunt (also called bidirectional superior cavopulmonary shunt) is performed at 3 to 6 months of age (Fig. 9.21A). Any previous B-T shunt is taken down at the time of the procedure. The azygos vein and the hemiazygos are divided. The IVC blood still bypasses the lungs. Oxygen saturation increases to about 85%. The surgical mortality rate is about 2%.
2. In the hemi-Fontan operation, an anastomosis is made between the superior part of the right atrial appendage and the lower margin of the central portion of the PA. An intraatrial baffle is placed to direct SVC blood to the PAs. The B-T shunt is taken down and the native pulmonary valve is oversewn (Fig. 9.22).

Medical Follow-Up After Stage II Operation should focus on the following. A remarkable improvement in O_2 saturation (approximately 85%) after the surgical procedure may gradually deteriorate. It may be caused by:

a. Development of venous collaterals which decompress the SVC or
b. The development of pulmonary arteriovenous fistula, which may be related to absence of hepatic inhibitory factor. Pulmonary arteriovenous fistula can be investigated by either pulmonary angiography or a bubble contrast echo with injection into branch pulmonary arteries.

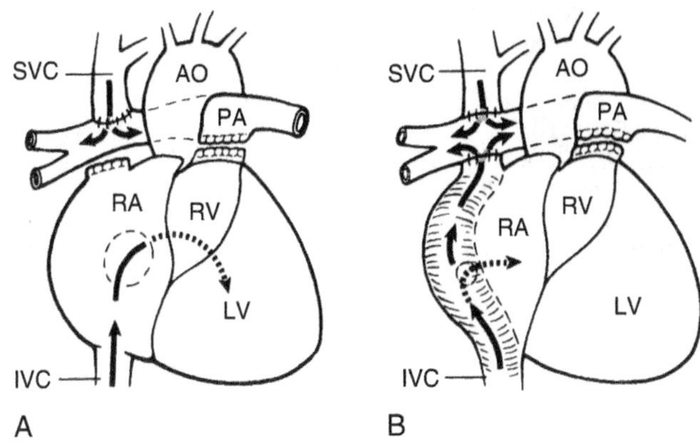

FIG. 9. 21
Bidirectional Glenn operation or SVC-RPA anastomosis (A) and cavocaval baffle-to-PA connection (Fontan operation) with fenestration (B). *AO*, aorta; *IVC*, inferior vena cava; *LV*, left ventricle; *PA*, pulmonary artery; *RA*, right atrium; *RPA*, right pulmonary artery; *RV*, right ventricle; *SVC*, superior vena cava.

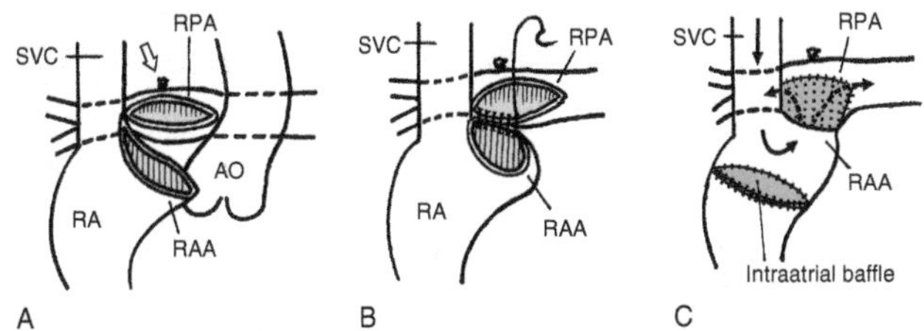

FIG. 9. 22
Hemi-Fontan operation. (A) A B-T shunt is taken down (*arrow*). An incision is made in the superior aspect of the right atrial appendage extending it into the SVC and a horizontal incision is made in the RPA. (B) The lower margin of the RPA incision and the adjacent margin of the incision in the right atrial appendage (*RAA*) and SVC are connected. (C) The connection is completed using a pulmonary allograft. An intraatrial patch is placed to direct SVC blood to the PAs. *(From Park, M. K., & Salamat, M. (2020).* Park's pediatric cardiology for practitioners *(7th ed.). Philadelphia: Mosby.)*

c. If the O_2 saturation drops to 75% or less, it is preferable to proceed with Fontan operation. Alternatively, cardiac catheterization may be performed to find a cause of desaturation (such as systemic veno-venous fistulas, which may be coil occluded).
d. A pre-Fontan cardiac catheterization is performed prior to the planned procedure. The following are risk factors for the Fontan operation:
   (1) A high PVR (>2 U/m^2) or high mean PA pressure (>18 mm Hg);
   (2) Distorted or stenotic PAs secondary to previous shunt operations;
   (3) Poor LV systolic and diastolic functions (LV end-diastolic pressure >12 mm Hg or an ejection fraction $<60\%$); and
   (4) AV valve regurgitation.

The presence of two or more of these risk factors constitutes a high-risk situation.

Stage III. A modified Fontan operation is the definitive procedure for patients with tricuspid atresia. In the Fontan operation, the entire systemic venous return is directed to the pulmonary arteries without an intervening pumping chamber. The Fontan operation is usually completed when the child is 2 to 5 years of age.

1. In patients who had the bidirectional Glenn procedure, an intraatrial tubular pathway (termed *cavocaval baffle* or *lateral tunnel*) is created from the orifice of the IVC to the orifice of the SVC. The cardiac end of the SVC is anastomosed to the undersurface of the RPA to complete the operation (see Fig. 9.21B). Some centers routinely use fenestration in the baffle, and others use it only in high-risk patients. Some centers recommend device closure of the fenestration a year or so after the Fontan procedure. Early survival rates have improved to over 95%.
2. In patients who had the hemi-Fontan operation, the intraatrial patch is excised and a lateral atrial tunnel is constructed, directing flow from the IVC to the previously created amalgamation of the SVC with the RPA (Fig. 9.23).
3. Most centers now perform, as an alternative to a lateral tunnel, an extracardiac conduit may be used to complete the Fontan operation. Extracardiac conduit has a very low operative mortality, a lower incidence of early and late arrhythmias, improved hemodynamics, and fewer postoperative complications. On the other hand, the lack of conduit growth should be considered for the timing of Fontan procedure.
4. Early complications of the Fontan-type operation include the following.
   a. Low cardiac output and/or heart failure.
   b. Persistent pleural effusion occurring more often on the right side.
   c. Supraventricular arrhythmia occurs in the early postoperative period in 15% of patients.
   d. Thrombus formation in the systemic venous pathways.
   e. Although rare, acute liver dysfunction (with alanine aminotransferase >1000 U/L) can occur during the first week after surgery.
   f. The surgical approach for patients with tricuspid atresia is summarized in Fig. 9.24.

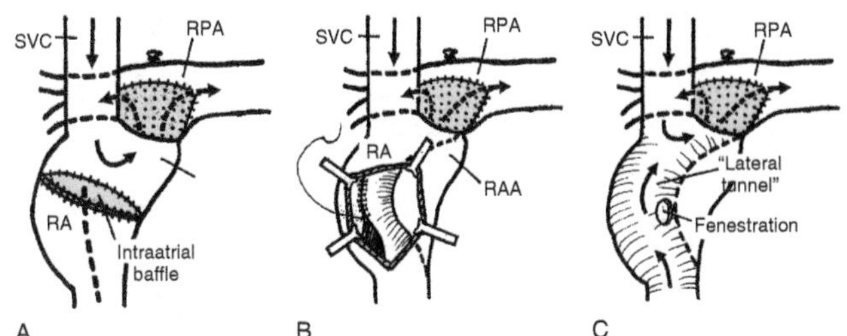

FIG. 9.23
From the hemi-Fontan to Fontan connection. (A) A vertical incision (*heavy broken line*) is made in the anterior RA wall. (B) The intraatrial patch is removed and a lateral tunnel is constructed to direct the IVC blood to the existing conglomerate of RA and RPA. (C) The direction of blood flow from the SVC and IVC is shown. *(From Park, M. K., & Salamat, M. (2020).* Park's pediatric cardiology for practitioners *(7th ed.). Philadelphia: Mosby.)*

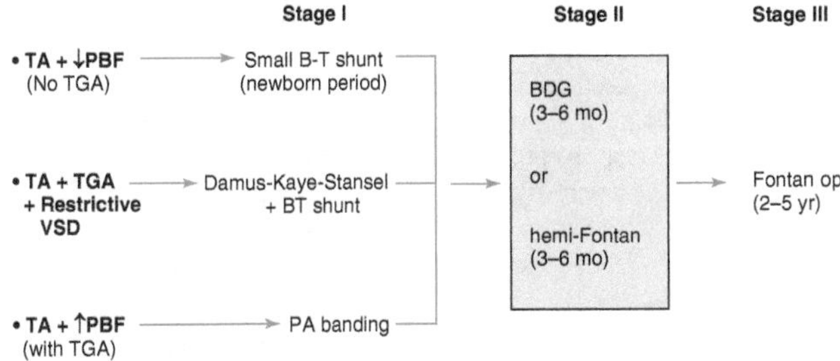

FIG. 9.24
Surgical approaches in tricuspid atresia. *BDG*, bidirectional Glenn; *B-T*, Blalock-Taussig; *op*, operation; *PA*, pulmonary artery; *PBF*, pulmonary blood flow; *TA*, tricuspid atresia; *TGA*, transposition of the great arteries; *VSD*, ventricular septal defect. *(From Park, M. K., & Salamat, M. (2020).* Park's pediatric cardiology for practitioners *(7th ed.). Philadelphia: Mosby.)*

5. Post-Fontan Follow-Up

Regular follow-up is necessary for general management and to detect late complications:

a. Patients should maintain a low-salt diet.
b. Medications:
    i. Some patients need continued digoxin and diuretic therapy.
    ii. An angiotensin-converting enzyme (ACE) inhibitor (such as captopril or enalapril) could be recommended, which is an afterload reducer as well as an antithrombotic agent (by reducing synthesis of plasminogen activator inhibitor-1 [PAI-1]).

iii. Aspirin or even warfarin is used to prevent thrombus formation. Controversy exists as to whether aspirin is adequate for thrombus prophylaxis as compared to warfarin. A recent international report suggests that aspirin (5 mg/kg/day) is as good as properly controlled warfarin therapy.

c. Some centers recommend device closure of the fenestration a year or so after the Fontan procedure. However, about 20% to 40% of fenestrations will close spontaneously in that period of time.
d. Patients should not participate in contact sports while taking warfarin.
e. Antibiotic prophylaxis against IE should be observed when indications arise.
f. Patients should be advised to live at a low elevation, preferably 4000 feet or less. They should avoid vacationing in high altitudes. High altitudes cause pulmonary vasoconstriction and increase PVR. These may lead to Fontan failure, increase Fontan complications (such as protein-losing enteropathy, liver dysfunction), and reduce the rate of long-term survival.

6. Watch for late complications.
   a. Late-onset supraventricular arrhythmia continues to increase with longer follow-up (6% at 1 year and 17% at 5 years).
   b. A progressive decrease in arterial oxygen saturation (which may result from obstruction of the venous pathways, leakage in the intraatrial baffle, or development of pulmonary arteriovenous fistula).
   c. Protein-losing enteropathy can result from increased systemic venous pressure that subsequently causes lymphangiectasis, occurring in 4% of survivors. The prognosis is poor (50% die within 5 years).
   d. As more patients survive into adulthood, Fontan-associated liver disease (FALD) has become more prevalent. This entity requires close follow-ups with periodic laboratory and imaging testing of the liver including (liver enzymes, prothrombin time, bilirubin and ultrasound of liver and spleen).

VIII. PULMONARY ATRESIA

Prevalence

Less than 1% of all CHDs or 2.5% of critically ill infants with CHD.

Pathology and Pathophysiology

1. The pulmonary valve is atretic, and the interventricular septum is intact. An interatrial communication (either ASD or PFO) and PDA are necessary for survival.
2. The RV size is variable and is related to survival.
   a. In the *tripartite type*, all three (inlet, trabecular, and infundibular) portions of the RV are present and the RV is nearly normal in size (Fig. 9.25).

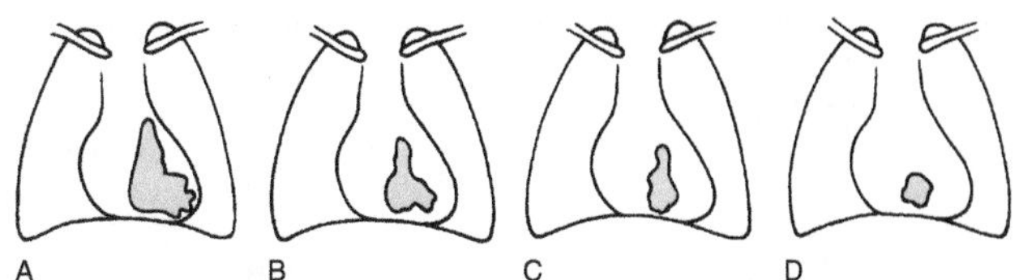

FIG. 9.25

Schematic diagram of right ventriculograms that illustrate three types of pulmonary atresia with intact ventricular septum. ***A***, Normal right ventricle. ***B***, Tripartite type, which shows all three (inlet, trabecular, and infundibular) portions of the RV. ***C***, Bipartite type, in which only the inlet and infundibular portions are present. ***D***, Monopartite type, in which only the inlet portion of the RV is present (almost always associated with coronary sinusoids). *(From Park, M. K., & Salamat, M. (2020).* Park's pediatric cardiology for practitioners *(7th ed.). Philadelphia: Mosby.)*

   b. In the *bipartite type*, the inlet and infundibular portions are present (but the trabecular portion is obliterated).
   c. In the *monopartite type*, only the inlet portion is present. In the monopartite type, the RV is diminutive, and coronary sinusoids are almost always present (Fig. 9.25).
3. Confluent pulmonary arteries are usually present with PBF provided through a PDA. TR is commonly present.
4. This condition is frequently associated with important anomalies of the coronary arteries. The high pressure in the RV is often decompressed through dilated coronary sinusoids into the left or right coronary artery (occurring in 30% to 50% of the patients). Such coronary sinusoids occur only in patients with hypertensive RV but not in patients with TR. Obstruction of the proximal coronary arteries, which is often present, may cause high surgical mortality.
5. RV myocardium shows varying degrees of ischemia, infarction, fibrosis, and endocardial fibroelastosis, with poorly compliant RV, which may contribute to surgical mortality.
6. Pathophysiology is similar to that of tricuspid atresia. The RA hypertrophies and enlarges to shunt systemic venous return to the LA. The LA and LV handle both systemic and pulmonary venous returns and therefore they enlarge. PBF depends on the patency of PDA; closure of PDA after birth results in death.

Clinical Manifestations

1. Severe and progressive cyanosis is present from birth.
2. The S2 is single. Usually no heart murmur is present. A soft, continuous murmur of PDA may be audible at the ULSB.

3. The ECG shows a normal QRS axis (in contrast to the superior QRS axis seen in tricuspid atresia), RAH, and LVH (monopartite type) or occasional RVH (tripartite type).
4. The heart size on chest radiographs may be normal or large (with RA enlargement). The MPA segment is concave, with markedly decreased PVMs.
5. Two-dimensional echo usually demonstrates the atretic pulmonary valve and hypoplasia of the RV cavity and tricuspid valve. The atrial communication and PDA can be imaged and their size estimated.
6. Cardiac catheterization and angiocardiography are required for proper management in most patients with pulmonary atresia. A right ventriculogram demonstrates the size of the RV cavity and the presence or absence of coronary sinusoids, and an ascending aortogram identifies stenosis or interruption of the coronary arteries. Both are important in surgical decision making to rule out RV-dependent coronary circulation to choose between univentricular palliation versus biventricular repair.
7. Natural history: Prognosis is exceedingly poor without neonatal PGE_1 infusion and surgery.

Management

Medical

1. As soon as the diagnosis is suspected, IV PGE_1 infusion is started to maintain ductal patency (see Appendix E for the dosage). For small premature infants, a prolonged course of PGE_1 infusion may be necessary before surgery is undertaken.
2. PDA stenting. In neonates with monopartite RV who are not likely to be candidates for two-ventricular repair (and are likely to require bidirectional Glenn operation or hemi-Fontan in a few months), some centers use PDA stenting instead of the B-T shunt. PDA stenting is likely to last until the time of the bidirectional Glenn or hemi-Fontan procedure.
3. A balloon atrial septostomy may be performed as part of the cardiac catheterization to improve the R-L atrial shunt, but it is recommended only when a two-ventricular repair is considered not possible (due to the presence of RV sinusoids or too small an RV cavity). The balloon atrial septostomy is not performed in patients with the tripartite type. Such patients may become candidates for RVOT patch, in which an elevated RA pressure is important to maximize RV forward output.
4. In patients with membranous atresia, a laser-assisted pulmonary valvotomy with balloon pulmonary valvuloplasty may be a useful alternative to a surgical procedure. (Infundibular atresia is unsuitable for the catheter intervention.)

Surgical

Surgical decision making for this condition depends on the RV size and the presence or absence of RV sinusoids or coronary artery anomalies. The summary of surgical approaches in pulmonary atresia with intact ventricular septum is presented in Fig. 9.26.

1. *Adequate RV size:* In patients with tripartite or bipartite RV, a connection is established between the RV and the MPA (either by transannular patch, closed transpulmonary valvotomy, or laser wire and radiofrequency-assisted valvotomy) in preparation for a possible two-ventricular repair. A B-T shunt is performed at the same time.
   a. If the RV appears to have grown to an adequate size and oxygen saturation is >70% with the B-T shunt temporarily closed during cardiac catheterization, two-ventricular repair with B-T shunt take-down is performed.
   b. If the RV size is considered borderline, *one-and-a-half-ventricular repair* may be performed. In this repair, a bidirectional Glenn operation is combined with an RVOT reconstruction. The bidirectional Glenn anastomosis brings the SVC blood directly to the PA, bypassing the RV,

9

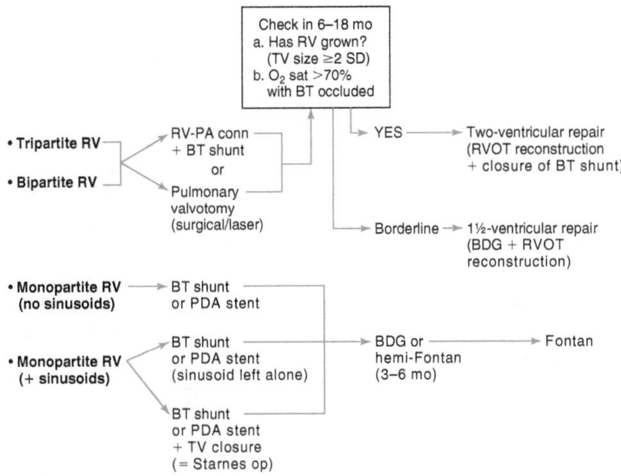

FIG. 9.26

Surgical approach to pulmonary atresia with intact ventricular septum. *BDG,* bidirectional Glenn; *B-T,* Blalock-Taussig; *op,* operation; *RV,* right ventricle; *RVOT,* right ventricular outflow tract; *RV-PA conn.,* right ventricle-to-pulmonary artery connection; *TV,* tricuspid valve.

and the IVC blood goes to the lungs via reconstructed RV outflow tract.

2. In patients with *monopartite RV* with or without coronary sinusoids, a staged Fontan operation is performed (similar to that described for tricuspid atresia). A B-T shunt is performed initially. A PDA stenting may be an alternative to the B-T shunt.
3. For patients with RV sinusoids, the sinusoids may be left alone or the tricuspid valve is closed (Starnes operation). A B-T shunt or PDA stenting is done initially. A bidirectional Glenn or hemi-Fontan operation is done at 3 to 6 months of age, and a Fontan-type operation at 2 to 5 years of age.

Follow-Up

Most patients require close follow-up, because none of the surgical procedures available are curative.

IX. HYPOPLASTIC LEFT HEART SYNDROME (HLHS)

Prevalence

HLHS occurs in 1% of all CHDs.

Pathology and Pathophysiology

1. HLHS includes a group of closely related anomalies characterized by hypoplasia of the LV (in association with atresia or severe stenosis of the aortic and/or mitral valves) and hypoplasia of the ascending aorta and the aortic arch. The LV is small or totally atretic. The atrial septum is intact with a normal patent foramen ovale. A VSD occurs in about 10% of the patients. COA frequently is an associated finding (up to 75%).
2. A high prevalence (up to 29%) of brain abnormalities has been reported, including agenesis of the corpus callosum, holoprosencephaly, microencephaly, and immature cortical mantle.
3. During fetal life the PVR is higher than the SVR, and the dominant RV maintains normal perfusion pressure in the descending aorta through the ductal R-L shunt, even in the presence of the nonfunctioning hypoplastic LV. However, difficulties arise after birth when the ductus closes and the PVR reduces. The end result is a marked decrease in systemic cardiac output and aortic pressure, resulting in circulatory shock and metabolic acidosis. An increase in PBF in the presence of the nonfunctioning LV results in an elevated LA pressure and pulmonary edema.

Clinical Manifestations

1. The neonate is critically ill in the first few hours to days of life, with mild cyanosis, tachycardia, tachypnea, and pulmonary crackles.

2. Poor peripheral pulses and vasoconstricted extremities are characteristic. The S2 is loud and single. Heart murmur is usually absent. Signs of heart failure develop with hepatomegaly and gallop rhythm.
3. The ECG shows RVH. Rarely, an LVH pattern is present (because V5 and V6 electrodes are placed over the dilated RV).
4. Chest radiographs show pulmonary venous congestion or pulmonary edema. The heart is only mildly enlarged.
5. Severe metabolic acidosis (caused by markedly decreased cardiac output) in the presence of slightly decreased arterial Po_2 and a normal PCO_2 are characteristic of the condition.
6. Echo findings are diagnostic and usually obviate cardiac catheterization. Severe hypoplasia of the aorta and aortic annulus and the absent or distorted mitral valve are usually imaged. The LV cavity is diminutive. The LV endocardium may show diffuse endocardial thickening, suggestive of damaged myocardium secondary to continuously elevated LV wall tension. The RV cavity is markedly dilated, and the tricuspid valve is large. A partially constricted PDA may be imaged.
7. Natural history: Pulmonary edema, CHF, progressive hypoxemia, and acidosis result in death without surgery, usually in the first month of life.

9

Management

Medical

1. IV infusion of PGE_1 (alprostadil, Prostin VR Pediatric) should be started as soon as the diagnosis is verified by echocardiogram to reopen the ductus arteriosus (see Appendix E for the dosage).
2. Intubation is not necessary routinely unless patient has a respiratory indication (i.e. apnea). It is preferred to maintain a fraction of inspired oxygen (Fio_2) of 21% to avoid pulmonary overcirculation.
3. Metabolic acidosis should be corrected.
4. Balloon atrial septostomy may help decompress the LA in the case of severely restrictive intraatrial shunting.
5. A neurologic evaluation, including imaging of the head, should be obtained because of a high prevalence of neurodevelopmental abnormalities seen in this condition. MRI of the head appears to be more sensitive than the head ultrasound scan and the latter shows frequent false-positive results.

Surgical

Three options are available in the management of these infants: (1) the Norwood operation (followed by a Fontan-type operation), (2) a hybrid operation (followed by a Fontan-type operation), and (3) cardiac

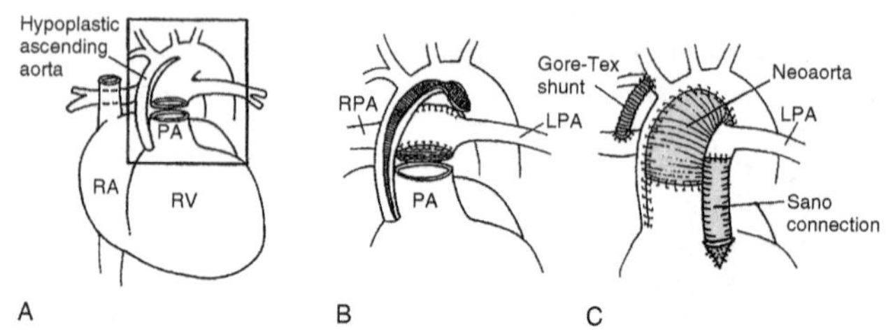

FIG. 9.27

Schematic diagram of Norwood procedure. (A) The heart with aortic atresia and hypoplasia of the ascending aorta and aortic arch is shown. The MPA is transected. (B) The distal PA is closed with a patch. An incision is made in the ascending aorta that extends around the aortic arch to the level of the ductus. The ductus is ligated. (C) A modified right Blalock-Taussig (BT) shunt is created between the right subclavian artery and the RPA as the sole source of pulmonary blood flow. (The Sano central shunt may be used instead of a B-T shunt.) Using an aortic (or pulmonary arterial) allograft (*shaded area*), the PA is anastomosed to the ascending aorta and the aortic arch to create a large arterial trunk. The procedure to widen the atrial communication is not shown. *LPA*, left pulmonary artery; *PA*, pulmonary artery; *RA*, right atrium; *RPA*, right pulmonary artery; *RV*, right ventricle.

transplantation. Only the first two options are presented because they are more popular than transplantation. A rare subgroup of patients with normal-sized LV (due to a large VSD) can have a two-ventricular repair rather than a Fontan operation.

1. The Norwood Approach.
   a. The first-stage (Norwood) operation is performed in the neonatal period and followed later by the Fontan-type operation. The operation consists of the following procedures (Fig. 9.27):
      (1) The main PA is divided, the distal stump is closed, and the ductus arteriosus is ligated and divided.
      (2) A neo-aorta is created by using an allograft that connects the proximal PA and the hypoplastic ascending aorta and aortic arch.
      (3) Pulmonary blood flow is established by either a right-sided B-T shunt or by using a homograft conduit between the RV and PA bifurcation (Sano connection). The Sano central shunt may promote symmetrical growth of the pulmonary arteries and provides a higher aortic diastolic pressure and thus a better coronary artery perfusion than the B-T shunt.)
      (4) Excision of the atrial septum.
   b. The surgical mortality rate is relatively high (7% to 19%). Post-Norwood, nonacute medical management may include the use

of medications (small-dose diuretic, digoxin (±), captopril, and aspirin) and nutritional support.

c. Second-stage operation for HLHS is either the bidirectional Glenn procedure or the hemi-Fontan procedure. These procedures are performed at 3 to 6 months of age (see the section on tricuspid atresia for a description of the procedures).
d. A modified Fontan operation is performed at 2 to 5 years of age (see section on tricuspid atresia for a description of the procedures and see Figs. 9.21 through 9.23). Five important hemodynamic and anatomic features considered essential to a successful Fontan operation for patients with HLHS include (1) unrestrictive interatrial communication, (2) competence of the tricuspid valve, (3) unobstructed PA-to-descending aorta anastomosis, (4) undistorted PAs and low pulmonary vascular resistance, and (5) preservation of RV function.
e. The operative mortality of the Fontan procedure is less than 3%. The overall survival rate after the Fontan operation is better than 95% at follow-up of 50 months.

2. The hybrid approach
   a. Introduced by Galantowicz et al. in 2008, this procedure is now used by some centers as an alternative to Norwood (stage I).
      (1) Performed in the first week of life, the hybrid approach consists of (1) bilateral PA banding (using a 1- to 2-mm ring from 3.5-mm Gore-Tex graft) to provide adequate PBF but without causing pulmonary hypertension and (2) insertion of a PDA stent in the same setting to ensure adequate systemic and coronary perfusion (Fig. 9.28). It can palliate the infant without the use of CBP and delays bidirectional Glenn or hemi-Fontan operation until 3 to 6 months of age.
      (2) As a separate procedure, reliable atrial shunt is established by atrial septostomy.
   b. Comprehensive stage 2 surgery (performed at 3 to 6 months of age) combines the Norwood operation and bidirectional Glenn operation. It includes (1) removal of PDA stent and PA bands, (2) repair of aortic arch and the pulmonary arteries, (3) reimplantation of the diminutive ascending aorta into the pulmonary root, (4) atrial septostomy, and (5) bidirectional Glenn operation. Surgical mortality rate is 8%.
   c. A Fontan-type operation is performed at age 2 to 5 years (as described under "Tricuspid Atresia").
   d. Fig. 9.29 summarizes surgical approaches for HLHS.

Follow-Up

Postoperative follow-up plans are similar to those described for tricuspid atresia.

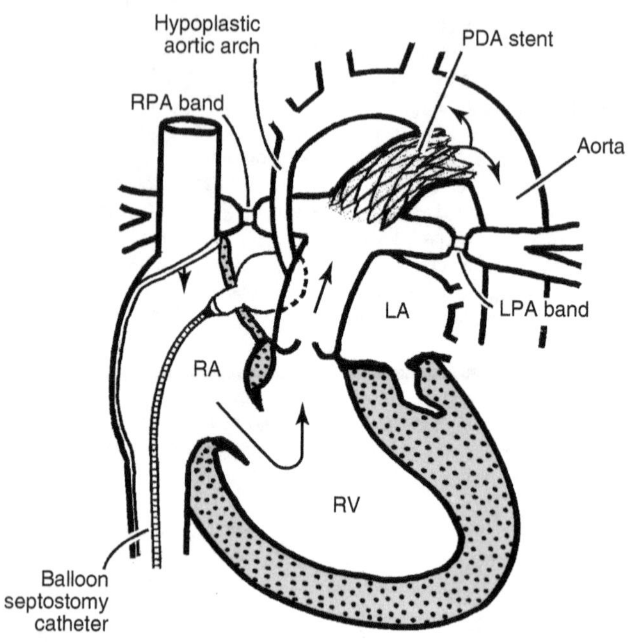

FIG. 9.28

Hybrid stage I intervention for HLHS. Surgical bands around the right and left pulmonary arteries limit blood flow to the lungs, and a stent in the ductus arteriosus holds it open and maintains adequate blood flow to the body. A balloon atrial septostomy allows unobstructed return of pulmonary venous blood to the right side of the heart. *LA*, left atrium; *LPA*, left pulmonary artery; *RA*, right atrium; *RV*, right ventricle; *RPA*, right pulmonary artery.

X. EBSTEIN ANOMALY

Prevalence

Less than 1% of all CHDs.

Pathology and Pathophysiology

1. The septal and posterior leaflets of the tricuspid valve are displaced into the RV cavity, so that a portion of the RV is incorporated into the RA (atrialized RV), resulting in functional hypoplasia of the RV and TR (Fig. 9.30).
2. Tricuspid valve regurgitation is usually present. The RA is massively dilated and hypertrophied. The RV free wall is often thin. Myocardial

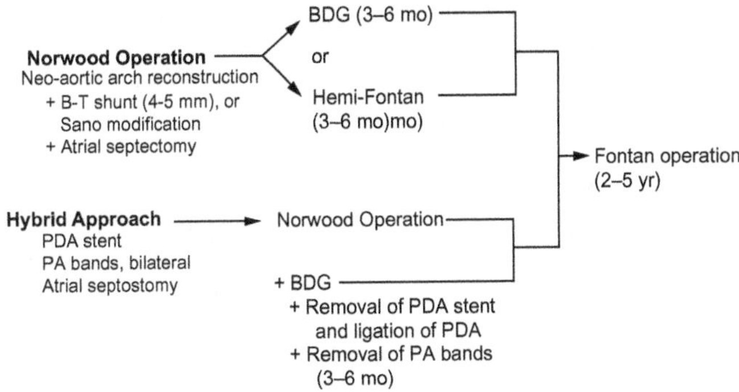

FIG. 9.29

Surgical approaches to hypoplastic left heart syndrome. *BDG*, bidirectional Glenn; *B-T*, Blalock-Taussig. *(From Park, M. K., & Salamat, M. (2020).* Park's pediatric cardiology for practitioners *(7th ed.). Philadelphia: Mosby.)*

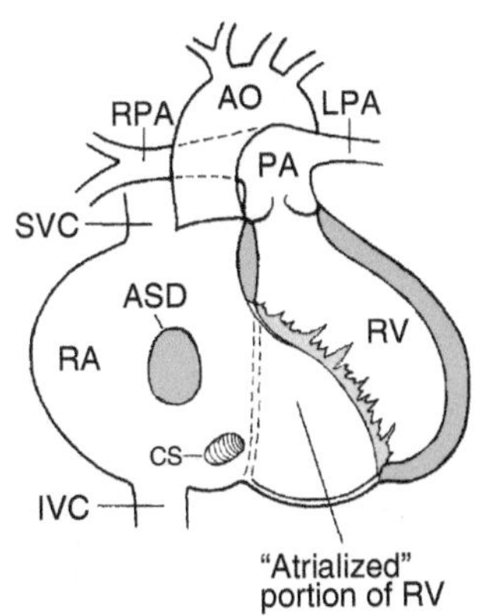

FIG. 9.30

Ebstein anomaly of the tricuspid valve. There is a downward displacement of the tricuspid valve into the RV. Part of the RV is incorporated into the RA (atrialized portion of the RV). Regurgitation of the tricuspid valve results in an enlargement of the RA. An ASD is usually present. *AO*, aorta; *ASD*, atrial septal defect; *CS*, coronary sinus; *IVC*, inferior vena cava; *LPA*, left pulmonary artery; *PA*, pulmonary artery; *RA*, right atrium; *RPA*, right pulmonary artery; *RV*, right ventricle; *SVC*, superior vena cava.

fibrosis is present in the RV and LV free walls (which may cause ventricular dysfunction).

3. An interatrial communication is present, with resulting R-L atrial shunt (and varying degree of cyanosis).
4. WPW preexcitation is frequently associated with the anomaly and predisposes to attacks of SVT.

Clinical Manifestations

1. In severe cases, cyanosis and CHF develop in the first few days of life, with some subsequent improvement. In milder cases, dyspnea, fatigue, and cyanosis on exertion may be present in childhood.
2. The S2 is widely split. Characteristic triple or quadruple rhythm, consisting of split S1, split S2, S3, and S4, is present. A soft regurgitant systolic murmur of TR is usually audible at the LLSB.
3. Characteristic ECG findings are RBBB and RAH. WPW preexcitation, SVT, and first-degree AV block are occasionally present.
4. Chest radiographs may show extreme cardiomegaly, involving principally the RA, and decreased PVMs.
5. Two-dimensional echo shows the apical displacement of the septal leaflet of the tricuspid valve. In the apical four-chamber view, the septal leaflet of the tricuspid valve normally inserts on the ventricular septum slightly more apicalward than the insertion of the mitral valve. In patients with Ebstein anomaly, this normal displacement is exaggerated. A diagnosis of Ebstein anomaly is made when the displacement is more than 8 mm/m^2 of body surface area. The tricuspid valve is elongated and dysplastic with resulting TR and occasionally causes RV outflow tract obstruction. A small RV cavity, a large RA, and an ASD (with R-L shunt) are also imaged.
6. Cardiac catheterization is rarely necessary in patients with Ebstein anomaly. In current era, echocardiography and MRI provide superior images.
7. Natural history: Some 18% of symptomatic newborns die in the neonatal period; 30% of patients die before the age of 10 years, usually from CHF. Cyanosis of neonates tends to improve as the PVR falls. Patients with less severe forms of the defect may be asymptomatic or only mildly symptomatic. Attacks of SVT are common. Other possible complications include CHF, LV dysfunction with fibrosis, and cerebrovascular accident.

Management

Medical

1. In severely cyanotic neonates, intensive treatment with mechanical ventilation, IV PGE_1 infusion, inotropic agents, and correction of metabolic acidosis may be necessary.

2. Infants and children with mild Ebstein anomaly require only regular observation. If CHF develops, anticongestive measures, including diuretics, are indicated.
3. Acute episodes of SVT may be treated most effectively with adenosine. β-Blockers are the most appropriate agents for prevention of SVT of undetermined mechanism. For those patients with recurrent SVT due to AV reentrant mechanism, radiofrequency catheter ablation techniques may be indicated.
4. Varying degrees of activity restriction may be necessary.

Surgical

1. Palliative procedures are performed for critically ill neonates.
   a. B-T shunt (with enlargement of ASD), especially in the presence of RVOT obstruction. A Fontan-type operation is performed later.
   b. If the LV is "pancaked" by large RV or RA, the Starnes operation (pericardial closure of the tricuspid valve), plication of large atrialized RV, enlargement of ASD, and a B-T shunt using a 4-mm tube may be performed. A Fontan-type operation is performed later.
   c. Classic Glenn anastomosis (anastomosis of the SVC to the right PA) or its modification may be considered in severely cyanotic infants.
2. Two-ventricular repair (tricuspid valve repair or replacement) is indicated in children with good RV size and function.
   a. Tricuspid valve repair surgeries (Danielson or Carpentier procedure) are preferable to valve replacement. The Danielson technique plicates the atrialized portion of the RV, narrows the tricuspid orifice in a selective manner, and results in a monoleaflet tricuspid valve. The ASD is closed at the time of surgery. The mortality rate of the Danielson procedure is about 5%, which is lower than that for valve replacement. The Carpentier technique is similar to the Danielson technique, but the valvular repair is done in a direction that is at right angles to that used by Danielson. The surgical mortality rate is 15%.
   b. Tricuspid valve replacement (with allograft or heterograft valve) and closure of the ASD is a less desirable surgical approach but may be necessary for 20% to 30% of patients with Ebstein anomaly who are not candidates for reconstructive surgery. The surgical mortality rate ranges from 5% to 20%.
3. One-ventricular repair: For patients with inadequate size of the RV, the Fontan-type operation is usually performed in stages.
4. Other procedures: For patients with WPW syndrome and recurrent SVT, surgical interruption of the accessory pathway is recommended at the time of surgery.
5. Surgical approaches for Ebstein anomaly are summarized in Fig. 9.31.

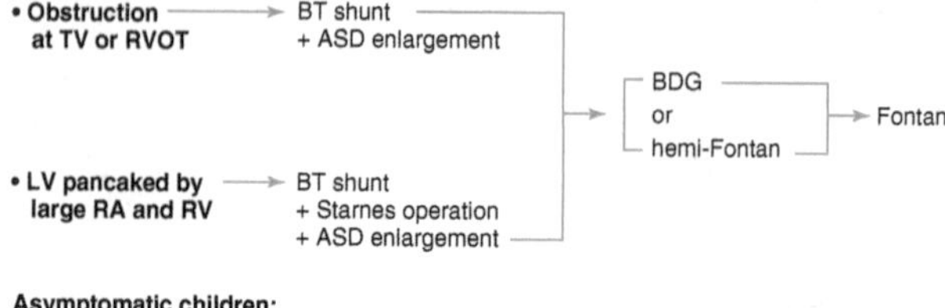

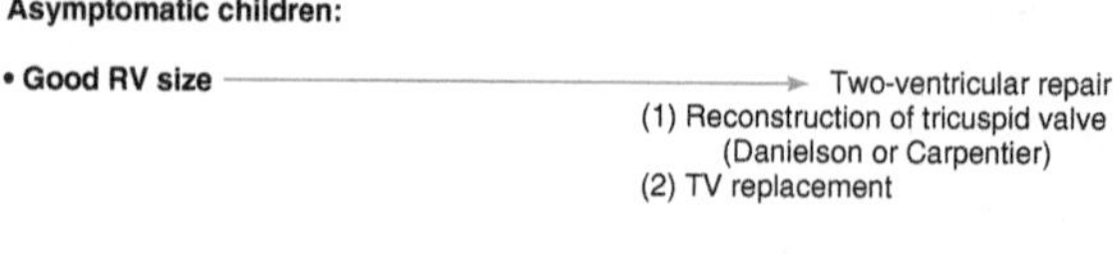

FIG. 9.31

Surgical approaches for Ebstein anomaly of the tricuspid valve. *ASD*, atrial septal defect; *BDG*, bidirectional Glenn; *B-T*, Blalock-Taussig; *LV*, left ventricle; *RA*, right atrium; *RV*, right ventricle; *RVOT*, right ventricular outflow tract; *TV*, tricuspid valve. *(From Park, M. K., & Salamat, M. (2020).* Park's pediatric cardiology for practitioners *(7th ed.). Philadelphia: Mosby.)*

Follow-Up

1. Frequent follow-up is necessary because of the persistence of arrhythmias after surgery, which occurs in 10% to 20% of patients, and because of possible problems associated with tricuspid valve surgery that require reoperation.
2. Some patients may need to be prohibited from participating in competitive or strenuous sports.

XI. PERSISTENT TRUNCUS ARTERIOSUS

Prevalence

Less than 1% of all CHDs.

Pathology and Pathophysiology

1. Only a single arterial trunk (with a truncal valve) leaves the heart and gives rise to the pulmonary, systemic, and coronary circulations. A large VSD is always present. A right aortic arch is present in 30% of patients.
2. Collette and Edwards' classification divides this anomaly into four types (Fig. 9.32): type I (affects 60%); type II (20%); type III (10%); and type IV (10%). Type IV is not a true persistent truncus arteriosus; it is a severe form of TOF with pulmonary atresia with aortic collaterals supplying the lungs. Van Praagh classification divides the defects into

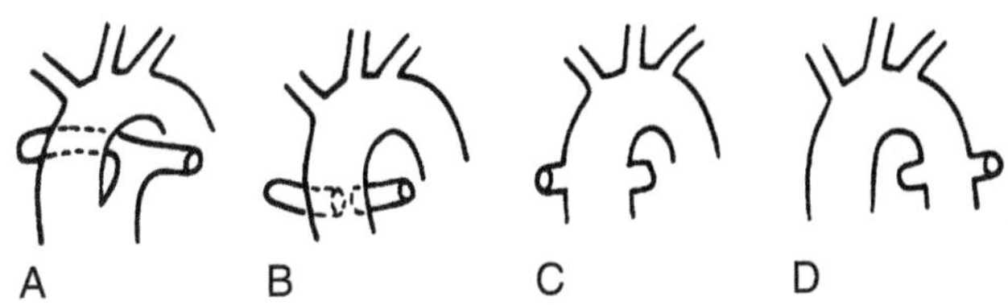

FIG. 9.32
Anatomic types of persistent truncus arteriosus determined by the branching pattern s of the pulmonary arteries (Collette and Edwards classification). (A) Type I. (B) Type II. (C) Type III. (D) Type IV, or pseudotruncus arteriosus.

the following four types. Type A1 is the same as type I by Collette and Edwards. Type A2 corresponds to types II and III. Type A3 reflects the absence of the origin of one of the pulmonary arteries from the proximal trunk. Type A4 is truncus arteriosus with interrupted aortic arch.

3. The pulmonary blood flow is usually increased in type I, nearly normal in types II and III, and decreased in type IV. With decreased PBF, cyanosis is notable. With increased PBF, cyanosis is minimal, but CHF may develop.
4. Coronary artery abnormalities (stenotic coronary ostia, abnormal branching and course) are common, contributing to a high surgical mortality.
5. Interrupted aortic arch is seen in 13% of cases (type A4 of van Praagh classification). A right aortic arch is present in 30% of patients.
6. DiGeorge syndrome with hypocalcemia is present in about 30% of patients.

Clinical Manifestations

1. Cyanosis may be noted immediately after birth. Signs of CHF may develop within several weeks.
2. A systolic click is frequently audible at the apex and ULSB. The S2 is single. A grade 2 to 4/6 systolic ejection murmur may be audible from truncal stenosis or PA branch stenosis. A high-pitched diastolic decrescendo murmur of truncal valve regurgitation is occasionally present. An apical diastolic rumble may be audible when PBF is large. Wide pulse pressure and bounding arterial pulses may be present.
3. The ECG shows BVH (70% of patients); RVH or LVH is less common.
4. Chest radiographs usually show cardiomegaly (biventricular and LA enlargement) and increased PVMs. A right aortic arch is seen in 30% of patients.
5. Two-dimensional echo demonstrates a large VSD directly under the truncal valve (similar to TOF). The pulmonary valve cannot be imaged (because it is absent). A large single great artery (truncus arteriosus)

arises from the heart. The type of persistent truncus arteriosus and the size of the PAs can be determined. An artery branching posteriorly from the truncus is the PA.

6. CT or MRI may be necessary to evaluate arch anatomy and/or PA anatomy. Preoperative cardiac catheterization is now rarely necessary in the neonate.
7. Natural history: Without surgery, most infants die of CHF within 6 to 12 months. Clinical improvement occurs if the infant develops PVOD. Truncal valve regurgitation, if present, worsens with time.

Management

Medical

1. Vigorous anticongestive measures with diuretics and ACE inhibitors are required.
2. Pay attention to the following when DiGeorge syndrome (22q11.2 deletion) is suspected or confirmed:
   a. Serum calcium (Ca) and magnesium (Mg) levels should be obtained (because supplementation of Ca and Mg may be needed).
   b. Only irradiated blood product should be used (to prevent transfusion-acquired acute graft-versus-host disease [GVHD], which destroys lymphocytes).
   c. Immunization with live vaccine should be avoided.
3. Prophylaxis against IE should be observed when indications arise.

Surgical

1. PA banding may be occasionally indicated in small infants with large PBF and CHF, but the mortality is high and the result not satisfactory. Therefore primary repair of the defect is recommended by many centers.
2. Various modifications of the Rastelli procedure are performed, ideally in the first week of life. The VSD is closed so that the LV ejects into the truncus. For type I, an aortic homograft 9 to 11 mm is placed between the RV and the PA. For types II and III, a circumferential band of the truncus, which contains both PA orifices, is removed. This cuff is tailored and then connected to the distal end of the RV-to-PA homograft. Aortic continuity is restored with a tubular Dacron graft.
3. A regurgitant truncal valve is preferably repaired, rather than replaced.

Follow-Up

1. Follow-up every 4 to 12 months is required to detect late complications or problems.
   a. Truncal valve insufficiency may develop or progress.

b. A small conduit needs to be replaced with a larger one, usually by 2 to 3 years of age.
c. Calcification of the valve in the conduit may occur within 1 to 5 years.
d. Ventricular arrhythmias may develop because of right ventriculotomy.

2. Balloon dilatation and stent implantation in the RV-to-PA conduit can prolong conduit longevity and delay the need to surgically replace the conduit.
3. For valvular regurgitation following balloon dilatation of the conduit valve, nonsurgical percutaneous pulmonary valve implantation technique (Bonhoeffer et al., 2000) may be used.
4. IE prophylaxis should be observed throughout the lifetime.

XII. SINGLE VENTRICLE

Prevalence

Single ventricle occurs in <1% of all CHDs.

9

Pathology and Pathophysiology

1. Both AV valves empty into a common main ventricular chamber (double-inlet ventricle). A rudimentary infundibular chamber communicates with the main chamber through the bulboventricular foramen (BVF). One great artery arises from the main chamber, and the other usually arises from the rudimentary chamber. If the main chamber has anatomic characteristics of the LV (80%), it is called double-inlet LV. If the main chamber has anatomic characteristics of the RV, it is called double-inlet RV. Rarely, both atria empty via a common AV valve into the main chamber (common-inlet ventricle).
2. Either D- or L-TGA is present in 85% of patients, and pulmonary stenosis or atresia is present in 50% of patients. COA and interrupted aortic arch are also common.
3. The most common form of single ventricle is double-inlet LV with L-TGA in which the aorta arises from the rudimentary chamber (Fig. 9.33). This type occurs in 70% to 75% of single ventricle.
4. The BVF frequently becomes obstructive, with resulting increase in PBF and decreasing systemic blood flow. This has important hemodynamic and surgical implications (see "Surgical Management").
5. There is a complete mixing of systemic and pulmonary venous blood in the ventricle, and therefore the oxygen saturation in the aorta and PA are identical. The systemic oxygen saturation is proportional to the amount of PBF. With decreased PBF (seen in patients with associated PS), marked cyanosis results. In patients without PS, PBF is large and the patient is minimally cyanotic and may develop CHF.

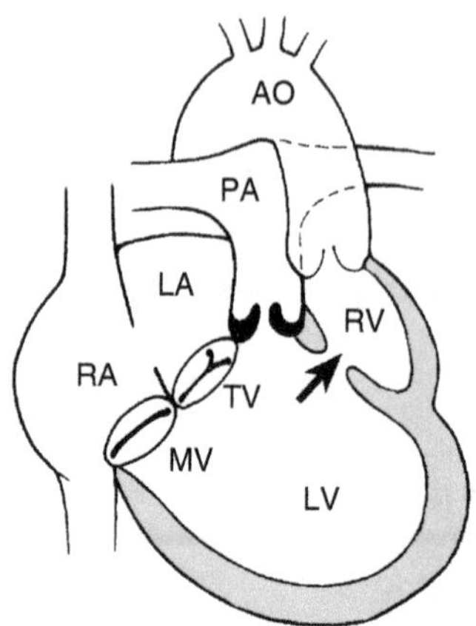

FIG. 9.33
The most common form of single ventricle. The single ventricle is anatomic LV. The great arteries have L-transposition. Stenosis of the pulmonary valve is present in about 50% of patients (shown as thick valves). The bulboventricular foramen (*thick arrow*) connects the main and the rudimentary ventricles. This type accounts for 70% to 75% of cases of single ventricle. *AO*, aorta; *LA*, left atrium; *LV*, left ventricle; *MV*, mitral valve; *PA*, pulmonary artery; *RA*, right atrium; *RV*, right ventricle; *TV*, tricuspid valve.

Clinical Manifestations

1. Cyanosis of a varying degree is present from birth. Symptoms and signs of CHF, failure to thrive, and bouts of pneumonia are commonly reported.
2. Physical findings depend on the magnitude of PBF. With increased PBF, physical findings resemble those of TGA with large VSD. With decreased PBF, physical findings resemble those of TOF.
3. ECG findings may include the following:
   a. An unusual ventricular hypertrophy pattern with similar QRS complexes across most or all precordial leads (RS, rS, or QR pattern) appears.
   b. Abnormalities in the Q wave take one of the following forms: (1) Q waves in the RPLs, (2) no Q waves in any precordial leads, or (3) Q waves in both the RPLs and LPLs.
   c. First- or second-degree AV block or arrhythmias may be present.
4. When PBF is increased, chest radiographs show cardiomegaly and increased PVMs. When PBF is normal or decreased, the heart size is normal and the PVMs are normal or decreased.

5. The diagnostic sign of single ventricle by 2D echo study is the presence of a single ventricular chamber into which two AV valves open. The following anatomic and functional information is important from a surgical point of view.
   a. Morphology of the single ventricle (e.g., double-inlet LV, double-inlet RV).
   b. Is D-TGA or L-TGA present?
   c. Location of the rudimentary outflow chamber, which is usually left and anterior.
   d. Is the BVF adequate or stenotic? The foramen is considered stenotic if the Doppler flow velocity is more than 1.5 m/sec or if the area of the foramen is <2 cm^2/m^2. A foramen that is nearly as large as the aortic annulus is considered ideal.
   e. Presence of PS or AS and the size of the pulmonary arteries.
   f. Anatomy of the AV valves (stenosis, regurgitation, or straddling).
   g. The size of the ASD.
   h. Is PDA, COA, or interrupted aortic arch present?
6. Natural history: Presence or absence of PS, the size of the BVF, and the presence of AV valve regurgitation affect clinical course. Complete heart block may develop (12%). CHF or arrhythmia can cause death.

Management

Medical

1. Neonates with severe PS and those with COA or interrupted aortic arch require IV PGE_1 infusion and other supportive measures before surgery.
2. Anticongestive measures with diuretics are indicated if CHF develops.

Surgical

Patients with single ventricle eventually require one-ventricular repair (i.e., Fontan operation) through a staged approach. The purpose of the first-stage operation is to make them acceptable candidates for the bidirectional Glenn or hemi-Fontan procedure. Summary of the surgical approach is shown in Fig. 9.34.

1. Initial palliative procedures: The type of initial surgery is influenced by the presence or absence of PS and the size of BVF.
   a. No PS + unobstructed BVF (with large PBF and CHF): PA banding is done with a high mortality rate (25% or higher). The banding is done only when the BVF is normal or unobstructed. Obstruction of BVF can develop following the PA banding.
   b. No PS + obstructed BVF: Damus-Kaye-Stansel operation (transection of the MPA, anastomosis of the proximal PA to the aorta) and bidirectional Glenn operation or a B-T shunt.

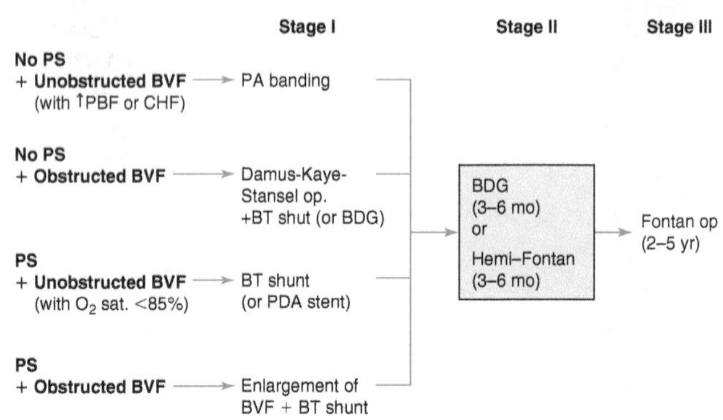

FIG. 9.34

Surgical approach for single ventricle. *BDG*, bidirectional Glenn; *B-T*, Blalock-Taussig; *BVF*, bulboventricular foramen; *CHF*, congestive heart failure; NB, newborn; *PBF*, pulmonary blood flow; *PS*, pulmonary stenosis; *RPA*, right pulmonary artery. *(From Park, M. K., & Salamat, M. (2020).* Park's pediatric cardiology for practitioners *(7th ed.). Philadelphia: Mosby.)*

   c. PS + unobstructed BVF: A B-T shunt or PDA stenting.
   d. PS + obstructed BVF: A B-T shunt and enlargement of the BVF.
2. Second-stage palliative procedures: Either the bidirectional Glenn operation or hemi-Fontan operation (see Figs. 9.21 and 9.22) is carried out between the ages of 3 and 6 months.
3. The Fontan-type operation is performed at 2 to 5 years of age (see "Tricuspid Atresia" for a detailed discussion of the Fontan procedure).

Follow-Up

Close follow-up is necessary for early and late complications, as discussed in "Tricuspid Atresia."

XIII. DOUBLE-OUTLET RIGHT VENTRICLE (DORV)

Prevalence

Less than 1% of all CHDs.

Pathology and Pathophysiology

1. Both the aorta and the PA arise side-by-side from the RV. The only outlet from the LV is a large VSD. The aortic and pulmonary valves are at the same level. Subaortic and subpulmonary coni separate the aortic and pulmonary valves from the tricuspid

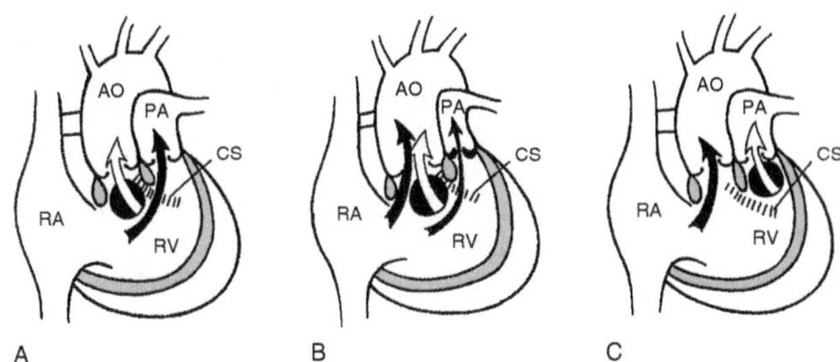

FIG. 9.35

Three representative types of DORV, viewed with the RV free wall removed. (A) Subaortic VSD. (B) Subpulmonary VSD (Taussig-Bing anomaly). (C) Subaortic VSD with PS. Doubly committed and remote VSDs are not shown. *AO*, aorta; *CS*, crista supraventricularis; *PA*, pulmonary artery; *RA*, right atrium; *RV*, right ventricle.

and mitral valves, respectively. DORV may be subdivided according to the position of the VSD and further by the presence of PS (Fig. 9.35).

   a. Subaortic VSD (occurring in 50% to 70% of the patients) (Fig. 9.35A)
   b. Subpulmonary VSD with malposed great arteries (Taussig-Bing anomaly) (Fig. 9.35B).
   c. Subaortic VSD + PS (50% of patients with subaortic VSD) (Fig. 9.35C).
   d. Doubly committed VSD.
   e. Remote VSD.

2. Pathophysiology of DORV is also determined primarily by the position of the VSD and the presence or absence of PS.
   a. With subaortic VSD (Fig. 9.35A), oxygenated blood (open arrow) from the LV is directed to the AO, and desaturated systemic venous blood (*solid arrow*) is directed to the PA, producing mild or no cyanosis. Clinical pictures resemble those of a large VSD with pulmonary hypertension and CHF.
   b. With subpulmonary VSD (Fig. 9.35B), oxygenated blood from the LV is directed to the PA, and desaturated blood from the systemic vein is directed to the aorta, producing severe cyanosis. Thus clinical pictures resemble those of TGA with CHF.
   c. In the presence of PS (Fallot type), clinical pictures resemble those of TOF (Fig. 9.35C).
   d. With the VSD close to both semilunar valves (doubly committed VSD) or remotely located from these valves (remote VSD), mild cyanosis is present and the PBF is increased.

Clinical Manifestations

1. Subaortic VSD without PS: Physical findings resemble those of a large VSD with pulmonary hypertension and CHF. The ECG often resembles that of ECD (superior QRS axis, LAH, RVH, or BVH and occasional first-degree AV block). Chest radiographs show cardiomegaly with increased PVMs and a prominent MPA segment.
2. Subpulmonary VSD (Taussig-Bing malformation): Physical findings resemble those of TGA with severe cyanosis in newborn infants. Signs of CHF supervene later. The ECG shows RAD, RAH, and RVH. LVH may be seen during infancy. First-degree AV block is frequently present. Chest radiographs show cardiomegaly with increased PVMs.
3. Fallot-type DORV with PS: Physical findings are similar to those seen in cyanotic TOF. The ECG shows RAD, RAH, and RVH or RBBB. Chest radiographs show normal heart size (with upturned apex) and decreased PVMs.
4. Echo findings (for all types):
   a. Diagnostic 2D echo signs include (1) both great arteries arising from the RV and running a parallel course in their origin, (2) absence of the LVOT and demonstration of a VSD as the only outlet from the LV, and (3) the mitral-semilunar discontinuity (or absence of normal aortic-mitral continuity).
   b. The size and position of the VSD should be determined in relation to the great arteries.
   c. Associated anomalies such as valvular and/or subvalvular PS and other L-R shunt lesions (e.g., ASD, PDA) should be looked for.

Management

Medical

Medical treatment of CHF if present.

Surgical

1. Palliative procedures
   a. For infants with remote or multiple VSDs (with large PBF and CHF), a PA banding is occasionally performed. For subaortic, subpulmonary, or doubly committed VSD, primary repair is a better choice.
   b. For infants with subpulmonary VSD, enlarging the ASD by the balloon or blade atrial septectomy is important for decompression of the LA and better mixing of pulmonary and systemic venous blood.
   c. For infants with subaortic VSD and PS and decreased PBF (Fallot type), a B-T shunt may be indicated.
2. Corrective surgeries
   a. Subaortic VSD and doubly committed VSD: Creation of an intraventricular tunnel between the VSD and the subaortic outflow

tract in the neonatal period or at least in early infancy. The surgical mortality rate is <5%.

b. Subpulmonary VSD (Taussig-Bing malformation): There are two possible surgical approaches. The surgery should be carried out by 3 to 4 months of age because of the rapid development of PVOD in this subtype.
   (1) The procedure of choice is the creation of an intraventricular tunnel between the VSD and the PA (resulting in TGA), which is then corrected by the arterial switch operation.
   (2) Creation of VSD-to-PA tunnel, followed by Damus-Kaye-Stansel operation and RV-to-PA conduit, is another possibility.
c. Fallot type: There are three surgical options: (1) an intraventricular VSD-to-aorta tunnel plus RV-to-PA homograft valved conduit at 6 months to 2 years of age, (2) REV procedure (see Fig. 9.5), or (3) Nikaidoh procedure (see Fig. 9.6).
d. Remote VSD: When possible, an intraventricular tunnel procedure (between remote VSD and the aorta) is preferred (performed at age 2 to 3 years). PA banding is usually needed in infancy to control CHF. Some patients with remote or multiple VSD may require Fontan operation.

3. Summary of surgical approach is shown in Fig. 9.36.

Follow-Up

Long-term follow-up at 6- to 12-month intervals is necessary to detect late complications (such as the need to reoperate and ventricular arrhythmias).

XIV. HETEROTAXIA (ATRIAL ISOMERISM, SPLENIC SYNDROMES)

There is a failure of differentiation into right-sided and left-sided organs in heterotaxia (splenic syndrome or atrial isomerism), with resulting congenital malformations of multiple organ systems, including complex malformation of the CV system.

1. Asplenia syndrome (Ivemark syndrome, right atrial isomerism) is associated with absence of the spleen (a left-sided organ) and a tendency for bilateral right-sidedness.
2. In polysplenia syndrome (left atrial isomerism), multiple splenic tissues are present, with a tendency for bilateral left-sidedness.
3. Paired organs, such as the lungs, commonly show pronounced isomerism; unpaired organs, such as the stomach, seem to be located in a random fashion.
4. Complex cardiac malformations are almost always present, especially with asplenia syndrome. In general, asplenia syndrome has more severe abnormalities of the cardiovascular system.
5. It is important to know which type of isomerism one has from the point of prophylaxis against bacterial infection. Patients with asplenia

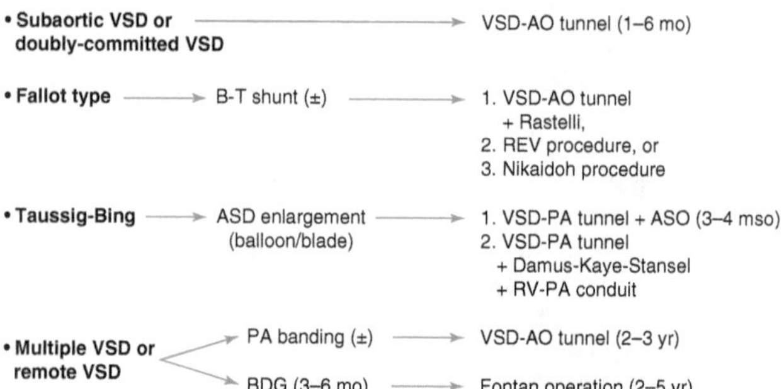

FIG. 9.36

Surgical approach for DORV. *AO*, aorta; *ASD*, atrial septal defect; *ASO*, arterial switch operation; *B-T*, Blalock-Taussig; *PA*, pulmonary artery; *REV*, réparation à l'étage ventriculaire; *RV*, right ventricle; *RV-PA*, RV-to-pulmonary artery; *VSD*, ventricular septal defect; *VSD-AO*, VSD-to-aorta; *VSD-PA*, VSD-to-pulmonary artery. *(From Park, M. K., & Salamat, M. (2020).* Park's pediatric cardiology for practitioners *(7th ed.). Philadelphia: Mosby.)*

syndrome are prone to fulminating sepsis and should be given daily antibiotic prophylaxis and vaccinated against pneumococcus, *Haemophilus influenzae* type b, and meningococcus.

6. Table 9.1 compares CV abnormalities seen in asplenia and polysplenia syndromes. The abnormalities that help differentiate the two are shown with asterisks; the IVC appears to have the most significant differential power (see following text).

1. Asplenia syndrome

Prevalence

One percent of newborns with symptomatic CHD, seen more often in males than in females.

Pathology and Pathophysiology

The spleen, a left-sided organ, is absent in asplenia syndrome. A striking tendency for bilateral right-sidedness characterizes malformations of the major organ systems.

1. Noncardiovascular malformations include bilateral, three-lobed lungs (i.e., two right lungs) with bilateral eparterial bronchi; various gastrointestinal malformations (occurring in 20% of cases); a

TABLE 9.1

CARDIOVASCULAR MALFORMATIONS IN ASPLENIA AND POLYSPLENIA SYNDROMES

STRUCTURE	ASPLENIA SYNDROME	POLYSPLENIA SYNDROME
Systemic veins	Normal IVC in all but may be left-sided (35%)	[a]Absent hepatic segment of IVC with azygos continuation, right or left (85%)
Pulmonary veins	[a]TAPVR with extracardiac connection (75%), often with PV obstruction	Normal PV return (50%) Right PVs to right-sided atrium; left PVs to left-sided atrium (50%)
Atrium and atrial septum	Bilateral right atria (bilateral sinus node) Primum ASD (100%) + secundum ASD (66%)	Bilateral left atria (no sinus node) Single atrium, primum ASD (60%), or secundum ASD (25%)
AV valve	[a]Single AV valve (90%)	Normal AV valve (50%); single AV valve (15%)
Ventricles	Single ventricle (50%); two ventricles (50%)	Two ventricles almost always present; VSD (65%); DORV (20%)
Great arteries	[a]Transposition (70%) (D-TGA, L-TGA) [a]Stenosis (40%) or atresia (40%) of pulmonary valve	Normal great arteries (85%); transposition (15%) Normal pulmonary valve (60%); pulmonary stenosis or atresia (40%)
ECG	Normal P axis, or in the +90° to +180° quadrant	[a]Superior P axis (70%)

[a]Important differentiating points.

symmetrical midline liver; and malrotation of the intestines are all present. The stomach may be located on either the right or the left.

2. Complex cardiac malformations are always present. CV malformations involve all parts of the heart, the systemic and pulmonary veins, and the great arteries. Two sinoatrial nodes are present (due to the presence of two right atria). Table 9.1 summarizes and compares these malformations with those of polysplenia syndrome.
3. The following are CV anomalies that help distinguish asplenia syndrome from polysplenia syndrome.
    a. A normal IVC is present in asplenia syndrome. In polysplenia syndrome, the hepatic portion of the IVC is usually absent (with azygous continuation draining into the SVC).
    b. TGA with PS or pulmonary atresia occurs in about 80% of asplenia syndrome cases, but TGA is present in only 15% of patients with polysplenia syndrome.
    c. Single ventricle and common AV valve occur with greater frequency in asplenia syndrome. In polysplenia syndrome, two ventricles are usually present.

   d. TAPVR to extracardiac structures occurs in more than 75% of cases of asplenia syndrome, but PV return is normal in 50% of patients with polysplenia syndrome.
4. Due to stenosis or atresia of the pulmonary valve, PBF is reduced and severe cyanosis results in patients with asplenia syndrome.

Clinical Manifestations

1. History of severe cyanosis shortly after birth.
2. Heart murmurs of PS and VSD are frequently audible. A midline liver is palpable.
3. The ECG may show a superior QRS axis (as a result of ECD). The P axis is either normal (0 to + 90 degrees) or alternating between the lower left and lower right quadrants (due to the presence of two sinus nodes). RVH, LVH, or BVH is present.
4. Chest radiographs show normal or slightly increased heart size with decreased PBF. The heart is in the right chest, left chest, or midline (mesocardia). A midline liver is a striking feature. Tracheobronchial symmetry with bilateral, eparterial bronchi is usually identified.
5. Imaging and other investigations:
   a. When the systematic approach is used, 2D echo and color flow Doppler studies can detect most, but not all, of the CV anomalies listed in Table 9.1. The anatomy of the IVC and great arteries, and the presence of PS (or pulmonary atresia) are important in differentiating the two syndromes.
   b. Cardiac MRI or CT is usually indicated to diagnose anomalies of pulmonary and systemic venous returns, which cannot always be imaged accurately by echo studies. Diagnosis of the obstructive type of TAPVR should be made before performing a B-T shunt surgery (because the missed diagnosis leads to pulmonary edema).
   c. Howell-Jolly and Heinz bodies seen on the peripheral smear suggest asplenia syndrome. However, these bodies may also be found in some normal newborns and in septic infants.
   d. A radioactive splenic scan may be useful in older infants but is of limited value in extremely ill neonates.
6. Without palliative surgical procedures, more than 95% of patients with asplenia syndrome die within the first year of life. Fulminating sepsis is one cause of death.

Management

Medical

1. In severely cyanotic newborns, prostaglandin E1 infusion is given to reopen the ductus. Cardiac MRI, CT scan, or pulmonary angiogram should be obtained while the ductus is open by PGE1 infusion to rule

out or confirm obstructive anomalous PV return (which is quite common in asplenia syndrome).

2. The risk of fulminating infection, especially by Streptococcus pneumoniae, is high. Daily antibiotic prophylaxis using oral penicillin V or amoxicillin should be given. Erythromycin can be used for children who are allergic to penicillin. The antibiotic prophylaxis can be discontinues at 5 years of age (but other experts continue it throughout childhood and into adulthood).
3. Asplenic patients are required to receive immunizations to prevent septicemia. The most common pathogen causing septicemia in children with asplenia is S. pneumoniae. Less common causes include H. influenzae type b, Neisseria meningitidis, and others. A series of pneumococcal conjugate and polysaccharide vaccines, H. influenza (Hib) immunization, and meningococcal conjugate vaccine should be administered to all children with asplenia (Refer to Red Book for complete information regarding the immunizations by the American Academy of Pediatrics).

Surgical

1. For severely cyanotic patients, a systemic-to-PA shunt is usually necessary during the newborn period or infancy.
2. Patients with the obstructive type of TAPVR may develop pulmonary edema following the shunt surgery. In these infants, a successful connection can be made between the pulmonary venous confluence and the RA without cardiopulmonary bypass.
3. A staged Fontan-type operation can be performed later as outlined under "Tricuspid Atresia" (but with the surgical mortality as high as 65% because of the AV valve regurgitation).

2. Polysplenia syndrome

Prevalence

Less than 1% of all CHD. It occurs usually in females (70%).

Pathology and Pathophysiology

Multiple splenic tissues are present. A tendency for bilateral left-sidedness characterizes this syndrome.

1. Noncardiovascular malformations include bilateral, bilobed lungs (i.e., two left lungs), bilateral, hyparterial bronchi, symmetrical (midline) liver (25%), occasional absence of the gallbladder, and some degree of intestinal malrotation (80%).

2. Cardiovascular malformations are similar to those seen in asplenia syndrome but have a lower frequency of pulmonary valve stenosis or atresia. Occasionally, a normal heart or minimal malformation of the heart is present (approximately 13%).
3. Important features of polysplenia syndrome that distinguish it from asplenia syndrome include the following:
   a. Interrupted IVC: Absence of the hepatic segment of the IVC with azygos or hemiazygos continuation is seen in 85% of patients. This abnormality is rarely present in asplenia syndrome.
   b. Two ventricles are usually present. On the contrary, single ventricle with a common AV valve is common in asplenia syndrome.
   c. TGA, PS or pulmonary atresia, and TAPVR occur less often than they do in asplenia syndrome.
   d. The ECG shows a superiorly oriented P axis, resulting from absence of the sinus node.
   e. Polysplenia syndrome occurs more often in females (70%).
4. Because PS or pulmonary atresia occurs less frequently, cyanosis is not intense, if it is present at all. Rather, CHF often develops because of increased PBF.

Clinical Manifestations

1. History of CHF is more common than that of cyanosis.
2. Heart murmur of VSD may be audible. A symmetrical liver is usually palpable.
3. The ECG shows ectopic atrial rhythm with a superiorly oriented P axis (−30 to −90 degrees) because there is no sinus node (in the two left atria). A superior QRS axis is present as a result of the presence of ECD. RVH or LVH is common. Complete heart block occurs in about 10% of patients.
4. Chest radiography: Mild to moderate cardiomegaly with increased pulmonary vascular markings, midline liver, and bilateral, hyparterial bronchi may be present.
5. Imaging studies:
   a. Two-dimensional and Doppler echo studies reveal all or most of the CV malformations listed in Table 9.1 and help to differentiate this syndrome from asplenia syndrome.
   b. Cardiac MRI or CT is often indicated when polysplenia syndrome is suspected because many patients have complex anomalies of pulmonary and systemic venous returns.
   c. The radioactive splenic scan may show multiple splenic tissues.
6. Natural history: The first-year mortality rate is 60% (in comparison with >95% in asplenia syndrome). The heart rate remains lower than normal (due to the absence of sinus node). Excessive junctional bradycardia or cardiac arrhythmias (usually supraventricular) may develop requiring medications.

Management

Medical

1. CHF should be treated, if present.
2. Although multiple splenic tissues may be present, they may be dysfunctional (functional asplenia). Their functionality needs to be confirmed by scintigraphy. In the case of functional asplenia, antibiotic prophylaxis is the same as with asplenia syndrome.

Surgical

1. PA banding should be performed if intractable CHF develops with large PBF.
2. Total correction of the defect is possible in some children. If total correction is not possible, at least a Fontan-type operation can be performed.
3. Occasionally, pacemaker therapy is required for children with excessive junctional bradycardia and CHF.

XV. PERSISTENT PULMONARY HYPERTENSION OF THE NEWBORN (PPHN)

Prevalence

PPHN (or persistence of the fetal circulation) occurs in approximately 1 in 1500 live births.

Pathology and Pathophysiology

1. This neonatal condition is characterized by persistence of pulmonary hypertension, which in turn causes a varying degree of cyanosis from an R-L shunt through the PDA or PFO. No other underlying CHD is present.
2. Various causes have been identified, but they can be divided into three groups by the anatomy of the pulmonary vascular bed as shown in Box 9.2. In general, pulmonary hypertension caused by the first group is relatively easy to reverse, and that caused by the second group is more difficult to reverse than that caused by the first group. Pulmonary hypertension caused by the third group is the most difficult or impossible to reverse.
3. Varying degrees of myocardial dysfunction often occur in association with PPHN, manifested by a decrease in the LV fractional shortening or TR, which are caused by myocardial ischemia and are aggravated by hypoglycemia and hypocalcemia.

Clinical Manifestations

1. Full-term or postterm neonates are often affected. Symptoms begin 6 to 12 hours after birth, with cyanosis and respiratory difficulties (with retraction and grunting). A history of meconium staining or birth asphyxia is often present. A history of maternal ingestion of

BOX 9.2

CAUSES OF PERSISTENT PULMONARY HYPERTENSION OF THE NEWBORN

I. Pulmonary vasoconstriction in the presence of a normally developed pulmonary vascular bed may be caused by or seen in the following:
   - Alveolar hypoxia (meconium aspiration syndrome, hyaline membrane disease, hypoventilation caused by central nervous system anomalies)
   - Birth asphyxia
   - Left ventricular dysfunction or circulatory shock
   - Infections (such as group B hemolytic streptococcal infection)
   - Hyperviscosity syndrome (polycythemia)
   - Hypoglycemia and hypocalcemia

II. Increased pulmonary vascular smooth muscle development (hypertrophy) may be caused by the following:
   - Chronic intrauterine asphyxia
   - Maternal use of prostaglandin synthesis inhibitors (aspirin, indomethacin) resulting in early ductal closure

III. Decreased cross-sectional area of pulmonary vascular bed may be seen in association with the following:
   - Congenital diaphragmatic hernia
   - Primary pulmonary hypoplasia

nonsteroidal antiinflammatory drugs (in the third trimester) may be present.

2. A prominent RV impulse and a single and loud S2 are usually found. Occasional gallop rhythm (from myocardial dysfunction) and a soft regurgitant systolic murmur of TR may be audible. Systemic hypotension may be present with severe myocardial dysfunction.
3. Arterial desaturation is found in blood samples obtained from an umbilical artery catheter. Arterial Po_2 is lower in the umbilical artery line than in the preductal arteries (the right radial, brachial, or temporal artery) by 5 to 10 mm Hg, because of an R-L ductal shunt. In severe cases, differential cyanosis may appear (with a pink upper body and a cyanotic lower body). If there is a prominent R-L intracardiac shunt (through PFO or ASD), the preductal and postductal arteries may not show a large Po_2 difference.
4. The ECG usually is normal for age but occasional RVH is present. T-wave abnormalities suggestive of myocardial dysfunction may be seen.
5. Chest radiographs reveal a varying degree of cardiomegaly with or without hyperinflation or atelectasis. The PVM may appear normal, increased, or decreased.
6. Echo and Doppler studies show no evidence of cyanotic CHD. The only structural abnormality is the presence of a large PDA with an R-L or bidirectional shunt. The atrial septum bulges toward the left due to a

higher pressure in the RA, with or without an ASD or PFO. Pulmonary veins are normal (TAPVR can mimic PPHN). The LV dimension may be increased, and the fractional shortening or ejection fraction may be decreased.

Management

The goals of therapy are to (1) lower the PVR and PA pressure through the administration of oxygen, the induction of respiratory alkalosis, and the use of pulmonary vasodilators, (2) correct myocardial dysfunction, and (3) stabilize the patient and treat associated conditions. Only principles of management are presented in the following text.

1. General supportive therapy includes monitoring oxygen saturation; detecting and treating acidosis, hypoglycemia, hypocalcemia, hypomagnesemia, and polycythemia; and maintaining body temperature between 98° and 99°F (36.6° and 37.2°C).
2. To increase arterial Po_2 levels, 100% oxygen is administered, initially without intubation. Intubation plus continuous-positive airway pressure at 2 to 10 cm of water may be effective. If still ineffective, mechanical ventilation is used to produce respiratory alkalosis. Fio_2 is adjusted to maintain preductal oxygen saturation of 90% to 95%. Ventilator settings are initially set to achieve Po_2 of 50 to 70 mm Hg and Pco_2 of 40 to 50 mm Hg. The patient is sedated (i.e, morphine, fentanyl) or even paralyzed with pancuronium (Pavulon).
3. Inhalation nitric oxide (iNO) is a potent and selective pulmonary vasodilator. The usual dose is 20 ppm. Most newborn infants require iNO for fewer than 5 days. The use of iNO in PPHN has decreased the need for extracorporeal membrane oxygenation (ECMO) by approximately 40%.
4. A high-frequency oscillatory ventilator is effective in patients with severe PPHN. Through the use of this device; about 40% of patients who would be candidates for ECMO can avoid this procedure.
5. For myocardial dysfunction, dopamine is used with tolazoline to improve cardiac output. Correction of acidosis, hypocalcemia, and hypoglycemia helps improve myocardial function. Diuretics may be included in the regimen. For chronic myocardial dysfunction, ACE inhibitors, or digoxin may be added at a later stage.
6. ECMO has been shown to be effective in the management of selected patients with severe PPHN. However, this treatment may require ligation of a carotid artery and the jugular vein, and cerebrovascular accidents have been reported.

Prognosis

1. Prognosis generally is good for neonates with mild PPHN who respond quickly to therapy. Most of these neonates recover without permanent lung damage or neurologic impairment.

2. For those requiring a maximal ventilator setting for a prolonged time, the chance of survival is smaller, and many survivors develop bronchopulmonary dysplasia and other complications.
3. Patients with developmental decreases in cross-sectional areas of the pulmonary vascular bed usually do not respond to therapy, and their prognosis is poor.
4. Neurodevelopmental abnormalities may manifest.

Chapter 10

Miscellaneous Congenital Heart Diseases

I. ANOMALOUS ORIGIN OF THE LEFT CORONARY ARTERY (BLAND-WHITE-GARLAND SYNDROME, ALCAPA SYNDROME)

A. PATHOLOGY AND PATHOPHYSIOLOGY

The left coronary artery (LCA) arises abnormally from the main PA. Postnatal decrease in the PA pressure results in ineffective perfusion of the LCA, producing ischemia and infarction of the LV that is normally perfused by the LCA.

B. CLINICAL MANIFESTATIONS

1. The newborn patient is usually asymptomatic until the PA pressure falls to a critical level. Symptoms appear at 2 to 3 months of age and consist of recurring episodes of distress (anginal pain) with signs of CHF. Heart murmur usually is absent.
2. Chest radiographs show cardiomegaly. The ECG shows anterolateral myocardial infarction pattern consisting of abnormally deep and wide Q waves, inverted T waves, and ST-segment shift in leads I, aVL, and most precordial leads (V2 through V6).
3. Two-dimensional echo with color flow mapping is diagnostic and has replaced cardiac catheterization. The absence of normal LCA arising from the aorta raises the possibility of the condition. Instead, the LCA is seen to connect to the main PA. Color Doppler examination may show retrograde flow into the main PA from the LCA. The right coronary artery may be enlarged. The left ventricle may enlarge with reduced LV systolic function. Increased echogenicity of papillary muscles and adjacent endocardium suggests fibrosis and fibroelastosis.
4. Computed tomography (CT) scans show high-resolution definition of coronary artery anatomy.
5. Cardiac troponin I level may be increased.

C. MANAGEMENT

Medical treatment alone carries a very high mortality (80% to 100%). All patients with this diagnosis need surgery.

1. Palliative surgery (simple ligation of the anomalous LCA close to its origin from the PA) may be performed in very sick infants to prevent steal into the PA. This should be followed later by an elective bypass procedure.

2. Most centers prefer definitive surgery unless the patient is critically ill, but the optimal operation remains controversial. One of the following two-coronary system surgeries may be performed.
   a. Intrapulmonary tunnel operation (Takeuchi repair). Initially a 5- to 6-mm AP window is created between the ascending aorta and the MPA at the level of the takeoff of the LCA. In the posterior wall of the MPA, a tunnel is created that connects the opening of the AP window and the orifice of the anomalous LCA. The mortality rate is near 0%, but a rate as high as over 20% has been reported. Late complications of the procedure include supravalvar PA stenosis by the tunnel (75%), baffle leak (52%) causing coronary-PA fistula, and AR.
   b. LCA implantation. In this procedure, the anomalous coronary artery is excised from the PA along with a button of PA wall, and the artery is reimplanted into the anterior aspect of the ascending aorta. The early surgical mortality rate is 15% to 20%.
   c. Tashiro repair. A narrow cuff of the main PA, including the orifice of the LCA, is transected. The upper and lower edges of the cuff are closed to form a new left main coronary artery, which is anastomosed to the aorta. The divided main PA is anastomosed end-to-end.
   d. Subclavian-to-LCA anastomosis. In this technique, the end of the left subclavian artery is turned down and anastomosed end-to-side to the anomalous LCA.

II. AORTOPULMONARY SEPTAL DEFECT

A. PATHOLOGY AND PATHOPHYSIOLOGY

In aortopulmonary septal defect (also known as aortopulmonary [AP] window), a large defect is present between the ascending aorta and the main PA. This condition results from failure of the spiral septum to completely divide the embryonic truncus arteriosus. Unlike persistent truncus arteriosus, two separate semilunar valves are present in this condition.

B. CLINICAL MANIFESTATIONS

1. Clinical manifestations are similar to those of persistent truncus arteriosus and are more severe than those of PDA. CHF and pulmonary hypertension appear in early infancy. Peripheral pulses are bounding, but the heart murmur is usually of the systolic ejection type (rather than continuous murmur) at the base.
2. The natural history of this defect is similar to that of a large untreated PDA, with development of pulmonary vascular obstructive disease in surviving patients.

C. MANAGEMENT

Prompt surgical closure of the defect under CPB is indicated. The surgical mortality rate is very low.

III. ARTERIOVENOUS FISTULA, CORONARY

A. PATHOLOGY AND PATHOPHYSIOLOGY

Coronary artery fistulas occur in one of two patterns:

1. True coronary arteriovenous fistula. It represents a branching tributary from a coronary artery coursing along a normal anatomic distribution, with blood emptying into the coronary sinus. This type occurs in only 7% of patients.
2. Coronary artery fistula. In most patients the fistula is the result of an abnormal coronary artery system with aberrant termination. In most cases the fistula terminates in the right side of the heart and the PA (40% in the RV, 25% in the RA, and 20% in the PA).

B. CLINICAL MANIFESTATIONS

1. The patient is usually asymptomatic. A continuous murmur similar to the murmur of PDA is audible over the precordium.
2. The ECG is usually normal, but it may show T-wave inversion, RVH, or LVH if the fistula is large. Myocardial infarction pattern can occur. Chest radiographs usually show normal heart size.
3. Echo studies usually suggest the site and type of the fistula. Presence of a massively dilated proximal portion of one coronary artery suggests a coronary artery fistula or an arteriovenous fistula. One can follow the course of the dilated coronary artery to its site of entry.
4. Often selective coronary artery angiography is necessary for accurate diagnosis before intended intervention.

C. MANAGEMENT

1. A tiny coronary artery fistula to the main PA (coronary artery-to-PA fistula) that is detected incidentally by an echo study should be left alone. Spontaneous closure may occur in some small fistulae, but some of them may progress and require intervention.
2. Small fistulous connections in the asymptomatic patient may be monitored.
3. For moderate or large coronary artery fistula, transcatheter occlusion is reasonable using coils or other occluding devices.
4. Elective surgery is indicated if not amenable to catheter occlusion. Using CPB, the fistula is ligated as proximally as possible without jeopardizing flow in the normal arteries and also ligated near its entrance to the cardiac chamber. The surgical mortality rate is zero to 5%.

IV. ARTERIOVENOUS FISTULA, PULMONARY

A. PATHOLOGY AND PATHOPHYSIOLOGY

1. There is direct communication between the PAs and pulmonary veins (PVs), bypassing the pulmonary capillary circulation. It may take the

form of either multiple tiny angiomas (telangiectasis) or a large PA-to-PV communication.

2. About 60% of patients with pulmonary AV fistulas have Osler-Weber-Rendu syndrome. Rarely, chronic liver disease or a previous bidirectional Glenn operation may cause the fistula.

B. CLINICAL MANIFESTATIONS

1. Cyanosis and clubbing are present, with a varying degree of arterial desaturation ranging from 50% to 85%. Polycythemia is usually present. A faint systolic or continuous murmur may be audible over the affected area. The peripheral pulses are not bounding.
2. Chest radiographs show normal heart size (unlike systemic AV fistula). One or more rounded opacities of variable size may be present in the lung fields. The electrocardiogram (ECG) is usually normal.
3. The diagnosis can be made through contrast two-dimensional (2D) echo. In this technique, 4 to 10 mL of saline that has been agitated is injected into a peripheral vein while monitoring the appearance of bubbles in the left atrium.
4. CT typically shows one or more enlarged arteries feeding a serpiginous or lobulated mass, and one or more draining veins. Pulmonary angiography remains the gold standard to determine the position and structure of the fistula prior to intervention.
5. Stroke, brain abscess, and rupture of the fistula with hemoptysis or hemothorax are possible complications.

C. MANAGEMENT

1. Transcatheter occlusion is recommended for all symptomatic patients and for asymptomatic patients with discrete lesions with feeding arteries ≥3 mm in diameter.
2. Diffuse microscopic pulmonary AV malformations are not amenable to transcatheter occlusion. Surgical resection of the lesions, with preservation of as much healthy lung tissue as possible, may be attempted in symptomatic children, but the progressive nature of the disorder calls for a conservative approach.

V. ARTERIOVENOUS FISTULA, SYSTEMIC

A. PATHOLOGY AND PATHOPHYSIOLOGY

1. Systemic AV fistulas may be limited to small cavernous hemangiomas or may be extensive. In large AV fistulas, there is direct communication (either a vascular channel or angiomas) between the artery and a vein without the interposition of the capillary bed.
2. The two most common sites of large systemic AV fistulas are the brain and liver.
   a. In the brain, it is usually a large type occurring in newborns in association with a vein of Galan malformation.

b. In the liver, hemangioendotheliomas (densely vascular benign tumors) are more common than fistulous arteriovenous malformation.

3. In the large type, cardiomegaly, tachycardia, and even CHF may result because of decreased peripheral vascular resistance and increased stroke volume.

B. CLINICAL MANIFESTATIONS

1. A systolic or continuous murmur is audible over the affected organ. The peripheral pulses may be bounding. A gallop rhythm may be present with CHF.
2. Chest radiographs show cardiomegaly and increased PVMs. The ECG may show hypertrophy of either or both ventricles.

C. MANAGEMENT

1. In patients with large cerebral AV fistulas (and CHF), surgical ligation of the affected artery to the brain is rarely possible without infarcting the brain. Many of these infants die in the neonatal period.
2. In hepatic fistulas, surgical treatment is often impossible because they are widespread throughout the liver. However, hemangioendotheliomas often disappear completely.
   a. Large liver hemangiomas have been treated with corticosteroids, aminocaproic acid, local radiation, or partial embolization, but the beneficial effects of these management options are not fully established.
   b. Catheter embolization is becoming the treatment of choice for many symptomatic patients with hepatic AV fistula.

VI. COR TRIATRIATUM

In this rare cardiac anomaly, the LA is divided into two compartments by a fibromuscular septum with a small opening, producing obstruction of pulmonary venous (PV) return. Embryologically, the upper compartment is a dilated common PV and the lower compartment is the true LA. Hemodynamic abnormalities of this condition are similar to those of MS in that both conditions produce pulmonary venous and arterial hypertensions.

1. Important physical findings include dyspnea, basal pulmonary crackles, a loud P2, and a nonspecific systolic murmur. The ECG shows RVH, and occasional RAH. Chest radiographs show evidence of pulmonary venous congestion or pulmonary edema, prominent MPA segment, and right-sided heart enlargement. Two-dimensional echo is diagnostic. It demonstrates a linear structure within the LA cavity. Degree of obstruction and pulmonary hypertension can be easily estimated by echo study.

2. This is a curable form of pulmonary hypertension. Surgical correction is always indicated. Pulmonary hypertension regresses rapidly in survivors if the correction is made early.

VII. DEXTROCARDIA AND MESOCARDIA

The terms *dextrocardia* (heart in the right side of the chest) and *mesocardia* (heart in midline of the thorax) express the position of the heart as a whole but do not specify the segmental relationship of the heart. A normally formed heart can be in the right chest because of extracardiac abnormalities. On the other hand, a heart in the right chest may be a sign of a serious cyanotic heart defect. The segmental approach is used to examine the significance of abnormal position of the heart.

A. THE SEGMENTAL APPROACH

The heart and the great arteries can be viewed as three separate segments: the atria, the ventricles, and the great arteries. These three segments can vary from their normal positions either independently or together, resulting in many possible sets of abnormalities. Accurate mapping can be accomplished by echo and angiocardiography, but chest radiographs and ECG are helpful also.

1. Localization of the atria.
   a. Chest radiographs
      (1) Right-sided liver shadow and left-sided stomach bubble indicate situs solitus of the atria. Left-sided liver shadow and right-sided stomach bubble indicate situs inversus of the atria.
      (2) A midline (symmetrical) liver shadow on chest radiograph suggests heterotaxia.
   b. The ECG: The sinoatrial (SA) node is always located in the RA. Therefore the P axis of the ECG can be used to locate the atria.
      (1) When the P axis is in the 0 to +90 degrees quadrant, situs solitus of the atria is present.
      (2) When the P axis is in the +90 to +180 degrees quadrant, situs inversus of the atria is present.
   c. Two-dimensional echo identifies the IVC and/or pulmonary veins. The atrial chamber that is connected to the IVC is the RA. The morphology of the atrial appendages further helps differentiate the atria, with the right atrial appendage being broad and triangular and left atrial appendage being narrow and fingerlike. Cardiac magnetic resonance imaging (MRI), angiocardiography, and surgical inspection aid further in the diagnosis of atrial situs.
2. **Localization of the ventricles**. Ventricular localization can be accomplished by the ECG and 2D echo.
   a. ECG: The depolarization of the ventricular septum normally takes place from the embryonic LV to the RV, producing Q waves in the precordial leads that lie over the anatomic LV.
      (1) If Q waves are present in V5 and V6 but not in V1, D-Loop of the ventricle (as in normal persons) is likely.

(2) If Q waves are present in V4R, V1, and V2 but not in V5 and V6, L-loop of the ventricles is likely (ventricular inversion, as seen in L-TGA).

b. Two-dimensional echo: The tricuspid valve leaflet inserts on the interventricular septum more toward the apex than does the mitral septal leaflet.

(1) The ventricle that is attached to the tricuspid valve is the RV.

(2) The ventricle that has two papillary muscles is the LV.

(3) Furthermore, the trabeculations in the RV are more coarse, and the LV endocardial surface is more smooth.

3. **Localization of the great arteries**. Echo studies can locate the great arteries accurately, but the ECG is not helpful in finding them.

B. COMMON TYPES OF DISPLACEMENT

The four most common types of dextrocardia are (1) classic mirror-image dextrocardia, (2) normal heart displaced to the right side of the chest, (3) congenitally corrected TGA, and (4) mal-differentiated ventricle such as seen with asplenia or polysplenia syndrome (Fig. 10.1). All these abnormalities may result in mesocardia. Echo study can make accurate diagnosis of the segmental relationship in dextrocardia or mesocardia. However, chest radiographs and ECGs can be used to deduce the nature of segmental abnormalities, as described earlier.

1. Classic mirror-image dextrocardia (Fig. 10.1A) shows left-sided liver shadow on chest radiographs. The ECG shows the P axis between +90 and +180 degrees and the Q waves in V5R and V6R.
2. Normally formed heart shifted toward the right side of the chest (dextroversion) (Fig. 10.1B) shows the liver shadow on the right on chest radiographs, the P axis between 0 and +90 degrees, and the Q waves in V5 and V6 on the ECG.
3. Congenitally corrected L-TGA (Fig. 10.1C) shows situs solitus of abdominal viscera on chest radiographs. The ECG shows the P axis in the normal quadrant (0 to +90 degrees) and the Q waves on the right precordial leads (V3R, V1, or V2) but no Q waves on V5 and V6.
4. Undifferentiated cardiac chambers (Fig. 10.1D) are often associated with heterotaxia (with complicated cardiovascular defects) and may show midline liver on chest radiographs. The ECG may show the P axis shifting between the 0 to +90 degree quadrant and +90 to +180 degree quadrant in asplenia syndrome (with two sinus nodes). In polysplenia syndrome, the P axis may be superiorly directed (due to ectopic atrial pacemaker). Abnormal Q waves may be seen in the precordial leads.

VIII. HEMITRUNCUS ARTERIOSUS

In hemitruncus arteriosus, one of the PAs, usually the right PA, arises from the ascending aorta, rather than the main PA. Hemodynamically, one lung receives blood directly from the aorta (as in PDA) with resulting volume and/or

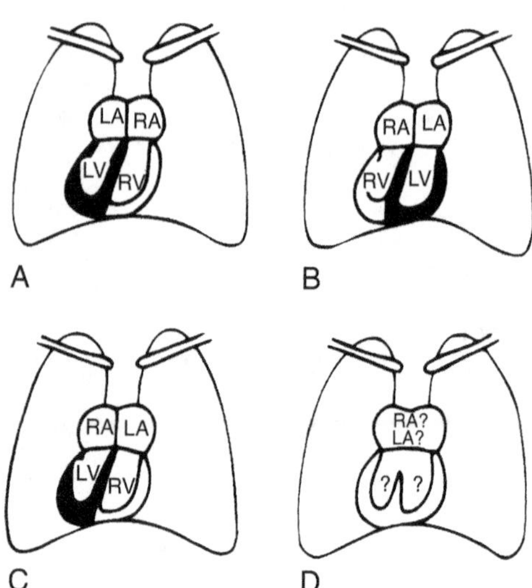

FIG. 10.1

Examples of common conditions when the apex of the heart is in the right side of the chest. (A) Classic mirror-image dextrocardia. (B) Normally formed heart displaced to the right side of the chest. (C) Congenitally corrected transposition of the great arteries. (D) Mal-differentiated ventricle such as seen with asplenia or polysplenia syndrome. *(From Park, M. K., & Guntheroth, W. G. (2006).* How to read pediatric ECGs *(4th ed.). Philadelphia: Mosby.)*

pressure overload, and the other lung receives the entire RV output, resulting in volume overload of that lung. Therefore pulmonary hypertension of both lungs develops. Associated defects such as PDA, VSD, and TOF are occasionally present.

CHF develops early in infancy, with respiratory distress and poor weight gain. A continuous murmur and bounding pulses may be present. The ECG shows BVH, and chest radiographs show cardiomegaly and increased pulmonary vascular markings.

Early surgical correction (anastomosis of the anomalous PA to the main PA) is indicated.

IX. MITRAL STENOSIS, CONGENITAL

A. PATHOLOGY AND PATHOPHYSIOLOGY

1. Isolated congenital MS is very rare. The mitral obstruction usually occurs at more than one level; it may be at the valve leaflets (fusion of the leaflets), the valve ring itself (hypoplastic valve ring), the papillary muscle (single papillary muscle or "parachute mitral valve"), the

chordae (thickened and fused chordae), or the supravalvar region (supravalvar mitral ring). The mitral commissures are poorly developed.
2. Parachute mitral valve is a condition in which all chordae insert to a single papillary muscle causing obstruction to the entry of blood to the LV.
3. Congenital MS is often part of "Shone complex," which consists of all or some of the following abnormalities: supravalvar mitral ring, MS (of various types as described earlier), subvalvular and/or valvular AS, aortic arch hypoplasia, and COA.

B. CLINICAL MANIFESTATIONS

1. With severe MS, tachypnea and dyspnea, pulmonary venous congestion and/or edema, and right heart failure may develop.
2. With milder stenosis, clinical findings are similar to those described for acquired form (i.e., rheumatic MS) (see Chapter 13).

C. MANAGEMENT

1. Mild to moderate MS can be managed with the usual anticongestive measures or β-blockers.
2. For infants and children with severe MS, balloon procedure or surgical intervention may be indicated.
   a. Balloon dilatation of the valve may be attempted but is usually unsuccessful in congenital stenosis.
   b. Surgery may be indicated for failed balloon dilatation or severe MR resulting from the balloon procedure.
   c. Surgically, a supravalvar ring can be removed and thickened and fused chordae can be split apart, but commissurotomy is usually not possible. Occasionally, mitral valve replacement may be necessary. A conduit from the LA to the LV is an unusual option.
3. Recurrent atrial fibrillation, thromboembolic phenomenon, and hemoptysis are indications for intervention.

X. PULMONARY VEIN STENOSIS

This very rare anomaly can be either congenital (or "primary") or acquired.

A. PRIMARY PULMONARY VEIN STENOSIS

1. Pathology

1. Although it can involve a single PV, most often multiple veins are involved and the severity can be progressive leading to partial or total obstruction of flow. The number and severity of the stenosis of the PVs involved determine timing and severity of symptoms.
2. More than 50% of patients with PV stenosis have associated cardiac defects (such as Ebstein anomaly or common AV canal).

3. Pathophysiology is similar to that of MS, leading to pulmonary edema and pulmonary arterial hypertension.
4. Pulmonary vein stenosis may develop in the first few months of life in an extremely premature infant despite unobstructed pulmonary veins at birth.

2. *Clinical Manifestations*

1. Infants with the disease present early with respiratory symptoms (tachypnea and recurrent pneumonias).
2. Chest radiographs may show localized or diffuse pulmonary edema depending on the number of PVs involved.
3. Two-dimensional echo studies of the PVs often reveal signs of PV stenosis. Turbulent pulmonary venous flow on color Doppler should raise the suspicion of PV stenosis. Monophasic flow or flow velocities >1.7 m/sec indicate functionally significant stenosis. Normally, early diastolic flow velocity is <1 m/sec, and presystolic flow velocity is much less than that.
4. Diagnosis is established by multidetector CT angiography. Angiography provides the most selective detailed views of the PVs. Radionuclide imaging may demonstrate reduced flow to the affected portion of the lung that receives blood through affected PV(s).
5. Prognosis is exceedingly poor in patients with involvement of most or all of the PVs. Patients with only one or two PVs involved have much more benign courses.

3. *Management*

Surgical as well as catheter intervention have a uniformly bad long-term outcome with recurrence within 1 to 6 months. Surgery can widen the narrowed veins and interventional procedures can stretch the vessels, but the result is usually a short-term solution since the stenosis typically recurs within a month to 6 weeks. Lung transplantation can be an option in selected patients.

B. ACQUIRED PULMONARY VEIN STENOSIS

1. *Causes*

1. After surgery for TAPVR in children (occurring in about 10% of patients).
2. In adults, the most common cause of PV stenosis is radiofrequency ablation procedures done for treatment of atrial fibrillation. Neoplasm growth, sarcoidosis, or fibrosing mediastinitis are rare causes.

2. *Management*

Balloon angioplasty of the involved vessels usually leads to a reasonably good initial result but restenosis occurs in >50% of patients within 1 year. Use of cutting balloon angioplasty and stents may be more successful.

XI. SYSTEMIC VENOUS ANOMALIES

There are wide ranges of abnormalities of the systemic venous system, some of which have little physiologic importance. Others have surgical significance or produce cyanosis. Two well-known anomalies of systemic veins are (1) persistent left SVC and (2) infrahepatic interruption of the IVC with azygos continuation.

A. ANOMALIES OF THE SUPERIOR VENA CAVA

1. Persistent left SVC draining into the RA.
   a. The left SVC is connected to the coronary sinus as part of the bilateral SVC (Fig. 10.2A). Rarely, the right SVC is absent and the blood from the right upper part of the body drains through the right innominate vein (RIV) to the left SVC (Fig. 10.2B).
   b. Isolated persistent left SVC does not produce symptoms or signs. Cardiac examination is entirely normal. Chest radiographs may show the shadow of the left SVC along the left upper border of the mediastinum. There is a high prevalence of leftward P axis (+15 degrees or less, including "coronary sinus rhythm") on the ECG. Imaging of an enlarged coronary sinus by 2D echo is often the first clue to the diagnosis of persistent left SVC.
   c. Treatment for isolated persistent left SVC is not necessary.
2. Persistent left SVC draining into the LA (Fig. 10.2C).
   a. Persistent left SVC rarely drains into the LA in the absence of the coronary sinus, producing cyanosis (in 8% of abnormal SVC cases).

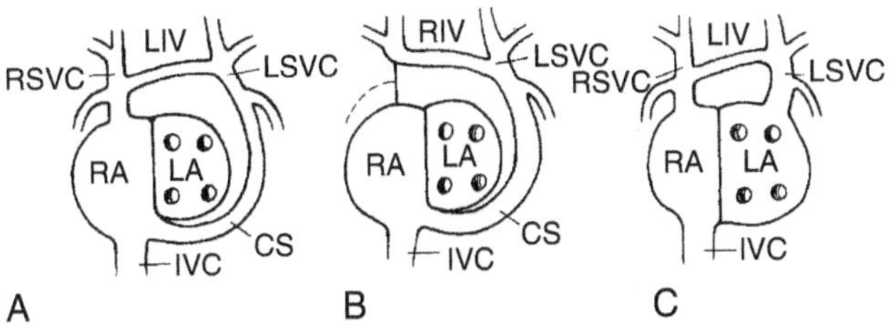

FIG. 10.2

Schematic diagram of persistent left superior vena cava *(LSVC)*. (A) LSVC drains via coronary sinus *(CS)* into the RA. The left innominate vein *(LIV)* and the right superior vena cava *(RSVC)* are adequate. (B) Uncommonly, the RSVC may be atretic. The CS is large because it receives blood from both the right and left upper parts of the body. (C) The CS is absent and LSVC drains directly into the LA. The atrial septum is intact. *IVC*, inferior vena cava; *LA*, left atrium; *RA*, right atrium; *RIV*, right innominate vein.

10

Associated cardiac anomalies, usually of the complex cyanotic type, are almost invariably present.

b. Surgical correction is necessary.

B. ANOMALIES OF THE INFERIOR VENA CAVA

1. Interrupted IVC with azygos continuation.
   a. Instead of receiving the hepatic veins and entering the RA, the IVC drains via an enlarged azygos system into the right SVC and eventually to the RA (Fig. 10.3A). The hepatic veins connect directly to the RA. Bilateral SVC is also common. This type has been reported in about 3% of children with CHDs
   b. Azygos continuation of the IVC is often associated with complex cyanotic CHDs, including polysplenia syndrome. No case has been reported in association with asplenia syndrome.
   c. This condition is readily diagnosed by echo studies as well as by MRI.
   d. Although this anomaly dose not result in clinical manifestations, it creates difficulties in manipulating catheters during cardiac catheterization and can render surgical correction of an underlying cardiac defect more difficult.
   e. There is no need for surgical correction of this venous anomaly per se.
2. **IVC connecting to the LA**. This is an extremely rare condition in which the IVC receives the hepatic veins, curves toward the LA, and makes a

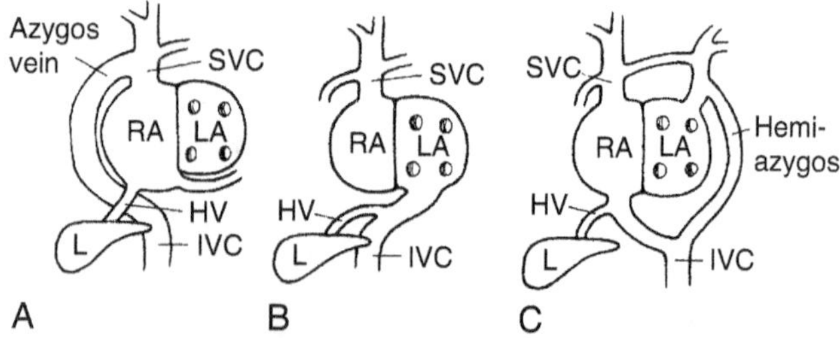

FIG. 10.3

Schematic diagram of selected abnormalities of the IVC. (A) Interrupted IVC with azygos continuation, the most common abnormality of the IVC. The hepatic vein *(HV)* connects directly to the RA. (B) Right IVC draining into the LA. Absence of the lower right IVC. The IVC drains into the left superior vena cava and LA and to the RA through the hepatic portion of the IVC. *IVC*, inferior vena cava; *L*, liver; *LA*, left atrium; *RA*, right atrium; *SVC*, superior vena cava.

	Anatomy	Ba-Esophag.	Chest Film	Symptoms	Treatment
Double Aortic Arch	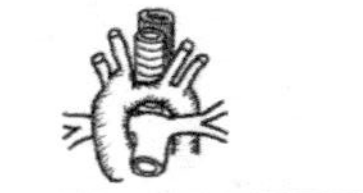	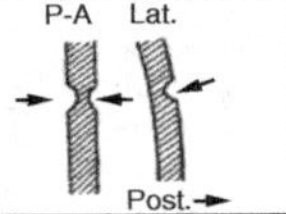 P-A Lat. Post.	Anterior compression of trachea	Respiratory difficulties in early infancy Swallowing dysfunction	Surgical division of the smaller arch
Right Aortic Arch with Left Lig. Arteriosum	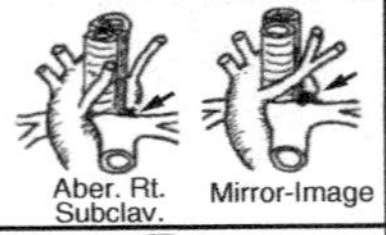 Aber. Rt. Subclav. Mirror-Image	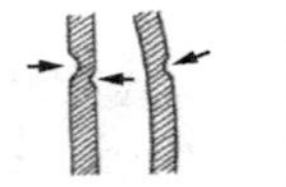	Right aortic arch	Mild respiratory difficulties late in infancy Swallowing dysfunction	Surgical division of left lig. arteriosum
Anomalous Innominate Artery	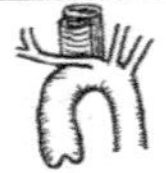	Normal	Anterior compression of trachea	Stridor and/or cough in infancy	Conservative management Surgical suturing of the artery to the sternum (±)
Aberrant Right Subclavian Artery	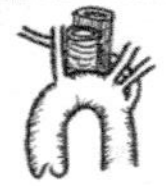	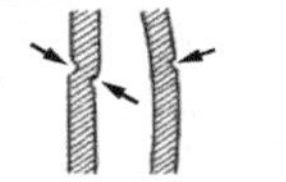		Occasional swallowing dysfunction	Usually no treatment is necessary
"Vascular Sling"	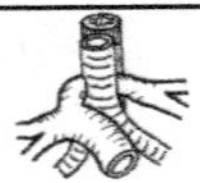	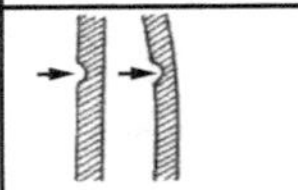	Right-sided emphysema/ atelectasis Posterior compression of trachea	Wheezing and cyanotic episodes since birth	Surgical division of the anomalous LPA (from the RPA) and anastomosis to the MPA

FIG. 10.4

Summary and clinical features of vascular ring. *Aber. Rt. Subclav.*, aberrant right subclavian; *Ba-Esophag.*, barium esophagogram; *Lat.*, lateral view; lig., ligamentum; *LPA*, left pulmonary artery; *MPA*, main pulmonary artery; *P-A*, posteroanterior view; *Post.*, posterior; *RPA*, right pulmonary artery.

direct connection with the LA (Fig. 10.3B), producing cyanosis. Surgical correction is indicated.

3. **Absent right IVC**. Dominant left LVC, in the absence of right IVC, drains into the LA through the left-sided hemiazygos system and persistent left SVC, producing cyanosis (Fig. 10.3C).

XII. VASCULAR RING

A. PREVALENCE

Vascular ring reportedly constitutes less than 1% of all congenital cardiovascular anomalies, but this is probably an underestimation.

B. PATHOLOGY

1. Vascular ring refers to a group of anomalies of the aortic arch and pulmonary artery that cause respiratory symptoms or feeding problems.
2. The vascular ring may be divided into two groups: complete (or true) and incomplete.
   a. In complete vascular ring, the abnormal vascular structures form a complete circle around the trachea and esophagus. They include (1) double aortic arch and (2) right aortic arch with left ligamentum arteriosum.
   b. Incomplete vascular ring comprises vascular anomalies that do not form a complete circle around the trachea and esophagus but do compress these structures. These include (1) anomalous innominate artery, (2) aberrant right subclavian artery, and (3) anomalous left PA ("vascular sling").
3. Pathology of five major vascular rings is presented in the following sections.
   a. **Double aortic arch** is the most common vascular ring (40%) (Fig. 10.4). The right and left aortic arches completely encircle and compress the trachea and esophagus, producing respiratory distress and feeding problems in early infancy. Both aortic arches give off two branches, each giving off the common carotid and the subclavian arteries. The right aortic arch is usually larger than the left arch. This condition is usually an isolated anomaly but is occasionally associated with CHDs such as TGA, VSD, persistent truncus arteriosus, TOF, and COA.
   b. **Right aortic arch with left ligamentum arteriosum**. Depending on the morphology of arch branching, different types may occur.
      (1) In the most frequent form (65%), the right arch first gives off the left carotid artery, then the right carotid artery, followed by the right subclavian artery, and lastly the left subclavian artery (left figure of the anatomy in Fig. 10.4). The ring is completed by a left-sided ligamentum arteriosum connecting the subclavian artery to the left PA. The aberrant left subclavian artery often arises from a retroesophageal diverticulum (called diverticulum of Kommerell). About 10% of this form is associated with an intracardiac defect.

(2) In the second type (occurring in about 35%), the left innominate artery originates from the right arch in mirror image fashion as the first branch, followed by the right carotid and right subclavian arteries. A left-sided ductus (or ligament) connects the descending aorta and the proximal left PA (right figure of the anatomy in Fig. 10.4). More than 90% of patients with this anomaly have associated CHDs, notably TOF and persistent truncus arteriosus.

c. In **anomalous innominate artery** the artery takes off too far to the left from the arch and compresses the trachea, producing mild respiratory symptoms (see Fig. 10.4). This anomaly is commonly associated with other CHDs such as VSD.

d. In **aberrant right subclavian artery** the artery arises independently from the descending aorta and courses behind the esophagus, producing mild feeding problems (see Fig. 10.4). It is the most common arch anomaly (occurring in 0.5% of the general population) without producing symptoms. It is often an isolated anomaly but may be associated with TOF with left arch, COA, or interrupted aortic arch. Its incidence is very high (38%) in Down syndrome with CHD.

e. **Anomalous left PA ("vascular sling")** is a rare anomaly in which the left PA arises from the right PA (see Fig. 10.4). To reach the left lung, the anomalous artery courses over the proximal portion of the right main-stem bronchus, behind the trachea, and in front of the esophagus to the hilum of the left lung. Therefore both respiratory symptoms and feeding problems (such as coughing, wheezing, stridor, and episodes of choking, cyanosis, or apnea) may occur. This anomaly is often associated with other CHDs, such as PDA, VSD, ASD, AV canal, or single ventricle.

C. CLINICAL MANIFESTATIONS

1. Respiratory distress and feeding problems of varying severity appear at varying ages.
2. Physical examination reveals varying degrees of rhonchi. Cardiac examination is normal.
3. The ECGs are normal.
4. Chest radiographs may reveal compression of the air-filled trachea, aspiration pneumonia, or atelectasis. Barium esophagogram is usually diagnostic (see Fig. 10.4) except in anomalous innominate artery.
5. Echo is very helpful but limited for complete diagnosis of the vascular ring and associated intracardiac defects.

D. DIAGNOSIS

1. **Barium esophagogram** is usually diagnostic of most vascular ring (see barium esophagograms in Fig. 10.4).

   a. In double aortic arch, two large indentations are present in both sides (with the right one usually larger) in the posteroanterior (P-A) view, and a posterior indentation is seen on the lateral view.
   b. In right aortic arch with left ligamentum arteriosum, a large right-sided indentation and a much smaller left-sided indentation are present. A posterior indentation, either small or large, also is present on the lateral view.
   c. In anomalous left innominate artery, barium esophagogram is normal.
   d. In aberrant right subclavian artery, a small oblique indentation extending toward the right shoulder on the P-A view and a small posterior indentation on the lateral view are present.
   e. In vascular sling, an anterior indentation of the esophagus seen in the lateral view at the level of the carina is characteristic. This is the only vascular ring that produces an anterior esophageal indentation. A right-sided indentation usually is seen on the P-A view. The right lung is either hyperlucent or atelectatic with pneumonic infiltrations.
2. CT and MRI are often used in the final diagnosis of the anomaly. They are very useful because they reveal not only the position of vascular structures but also of the tracheobronchial and esophageal structures and their relationships to the vascular structures. MRI has been proposed as an excellent substitute for angiography.
3. Occasionally, angiography is indicated to confirm the diagnosis

E. MANAGEMENT

1. Medical

1. Asymptomatic patients need no surgical treatment.
2. For infants with mild symptoms, careful feeding with soft foods and aggressive treatment of pulmonary infections are indicated.

2. Surgical

1. **Indications and timing.** Respiratory distress and a history of recurrent pneumonia and apneic spells are indications for surgical intervention.
2. Surgical procedures.
   a. Double aortic arch. Division of the smaller of the two arches is performed. Knowing which arch is the dominant arch is very important, because thoracotomy is typically performed on the side of the smaller arch. The surgical mortality rate is <5%.
   b. Right aortic arch and left ligamentum arteriosum. Ligation and division of the ligamentum is performed through a left thoracotomy. If a Kommerell diverticulum is found, the diverticulum is resected and the left subclavian artery is transferred to the LCA. The mortality rate is <5%.

c. Anomalous innominate artery. Through right anterolateral thoracotomy, the innominate artery is suspended to the posterior sternum.
d. Aberrant right subclavian artery. The procedure consists of division of the aberrant artery and translocation to the right common carotid artery. It is performed only in symptomatic patients with dysphagia.
e. Anomalous left PA. Surgical division and reimplantation of the left PA to the main PA is performed, usually through a median sternotomy and with the use of CPB.

3. **Complications.** In infants who have had surgery for severe symptoms, airway obstruction may persist for weeks or months after surgery. Careful respiratory management is required in the postoperative period.

PART IV

ACQUIRED HEART DISEASES

In this part, cardiomyopathies, infective endocarditis, myocarditis, pericarditis, Kawasaki disease, acute rheumatic fever, valvular heart disease, cardiac tumors, and cardiac problems that may be associated with selected systemic diseases are presented.

Chapter 11

Primary Myocardial Diseases (Cardiomyopathy)

Primary myocardial disease affects the heart muscle itself and is not associated with congenital, valvular, or coronary heart disease or systemic disorders. Cardiomyopathy has been classified into three types based on anatomic and functional features: (1) hypertrophic, (2) dilated (or congestive), and (3) restrictive (Fig. 11.1). In 1995, two other categories were added: arrhythmogenic cardiomyopathy and left ventricular noncompaction. Different subtypes of cardiomyopathy are functionally different from one another, and the demands of therapy are also different.

I. HYPERTROPHIC CARDIOMYOPATHY

In about 50% of cases, HCM appears to be genetically transmitted as an autosomal dominant trait, and in the remainder, it occurs sporadically. HCM usually is seen in adolescents and young adults, with equal gender distribution. It is the most common cause of sudden cardiac death in teens and young adults, especially among athletes.

A. PATHOLOGY AND PATHOPHYSIOLOGY

1. A massive ventricular hypertrophy is present. Although asymmetric septal hypertrophy (ASH), formerly known as IHSS, is the most common type, a concentric hypertrophy with symmetric thickening of the LV sometimes occurs. Occasionally an intracavitary obstruction may develop during systole, partly because of systolic anterior motion (SAM) of the mitral valve against the hypertrophied septum, called hypertrophic obstructive cardiomyopathy (HOCM). In some patients, midcavity obstruction is caused by anomalous insertion of anterolateral papillary muscle into the anterior mitral leaflet, rather than SAM.
2. So-called apical hypertrophic cardiomyopathy is a variant of HCM in which hypertrophy is confined to the left ventricular apex, without intracavitary obstruction (and with giant negative T waves on the electrocardiogram [ECG]). This subtype is present in about 25% of patients with HCM in Japan and less than 10% in other parts of the world.
3. The myocardium itself has an enhanced contractile state, but diastolic ventricular filling is impaired because of abnormal stiffness of the LV. This may lead to LA enlargement and pulmonary venous congestion, producing congestive symptoms (exertional dyspnea, orthopnea, paroxysmal nocturnal dyspnea).

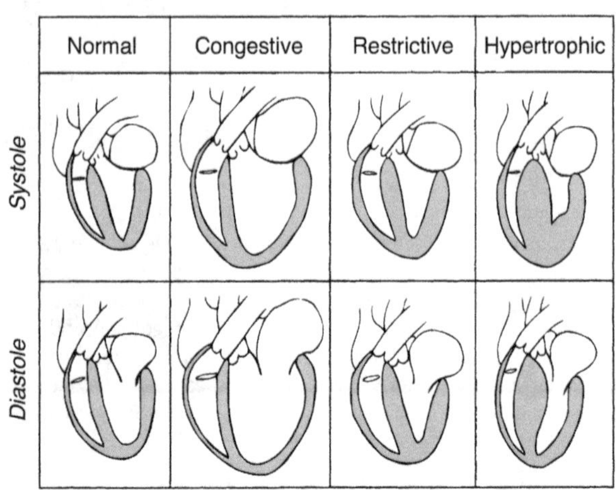

FIG. 11.1
Diagram of left anterior oblique view of heart in different types of cardiomyopathy at end-systole and end-diastole. *Congestive* corresponds to *dilated* cardiomyopathy as used in the text. *((From Goldman, M. R., & Boucher, C. A. (1980). Values of radionuclide imaging techniques in assessing cardiomyopathy.* American Journal of Cardiology, *46(7), 1232–1236).)*

4. About 80% of LV stroke volume occurs in the early part of systole when little or no obstruction exists, resulting in a sharp upstroke of arterial pulse.
5. A unique aspect of HOCM is the variability of the degree of obstruction from moment to moment.
   a. The obstruction to LV output worsens when LV volume is reduced (as seen with positive inotropic agents, reduced blood volume, lowering of SVR).
   b. The obstruction lessens when the LV systolic volume increases (negative inotropic agents, leg raising, blood transfusion, increasing SVR).
6. Ten percent to 20% of infants of diabetic mothers develop a transient form of HCM with or without LVOT obstruction. Children with Noonan syndrome commonly have HOCM (see Table 1.1).

B. CLINICAL MANIFESTATIONS

1. Easy fatigability, dyspnea, palpitation, anginal chest pain, or syncope may be the presenting complaint. Some 30% to 60% of cases are seen in adolescents and young adults with positive family history.

2. A sharp upstroke of the arterial pulse is characteristic. A late systolic ejection murmur may be audible at the MLSB and LLSB or at the apex. A holosystolic murmur (of MR) is occasionally present. The intensity and even the presence of the heart murmur vary from examination to examination in patients with HOCM.
3. The ECG may show LVH, ST-T changes, abnormally deep Q waves with diminished or absent R waves in the left precordial leads (LPLs), and arrhythmias. Occasionally "giant" negative T waves are seen in the LPLs in patients with apical hypertrophic cardiomyopathy. Occasionally, cardiac arrhythmia or first-degree AV block is seen.
4. Chest radiographs may show mild LV enlargement with globular heart.
5. Echo studies may demonstrate the following.
   a. LV hypertrophy can be seen as concentric hypertrophy, localized segmental hypertrophy, ASH, or localized to the apex. ASH is present when the septal thickness is 1.4 times or greater than the posterior LV wall thickness.
   b. In obstructive type, SAM of the mitral valve may be demonstrated. Doppler peak gradient in the LVOT of ≥30 mm Hg indicates an obstructive type.
   c. In adults, LV diastolic wall thickness ≥15 mm (or on occasion, 13 or 14 mm), usually with LV dimension <45 mm, is accepted as HCM. For children, *z* score of ≥2 relative to body surface area (BSA) is compatible with the diagnosis.
   d. Highly trained athletes may show LV hypertrophy, but the LV wall thickness ≥13 mm is very uncommon. In addition, it is always associated with an enlarged LV cavity (with LV diastolic dimension >54 mm, with ranges of 55 to 63 mm). Therefore trained adult athletes with LV wall thickness >16 mm and a nondilated LV cavity are likely to have HCM.
   e. The Doppler examination of the mitral inflow demonstrates signs of diastolic dysfunction with a decreased E velocity, an increased A velocity, and a decreased E:A ratio (usually <0.8) (Fig. 11.2). These abnormalities are, however, nonspecific for HCM; they are also seen with dilated cardiomyopathy.
6. Natural history.
   a. Obstruction may be absent, stable, or progressive (especially in genetically predisposed individuals).
   b. Sudden and unexpected death may occur during sports or vigorous exercise, due to ventricular fibrillation.
   c. Atrial fibrillation may cause stroke or heart failure.

C. MANAGEMENT

1. The goals of management are to (a) reduce LVOT obstruction (by reducing LV contractility and by increasing LV volume), (b) increase ventricular compliance, and (c) prevent sudden death (by preventing or

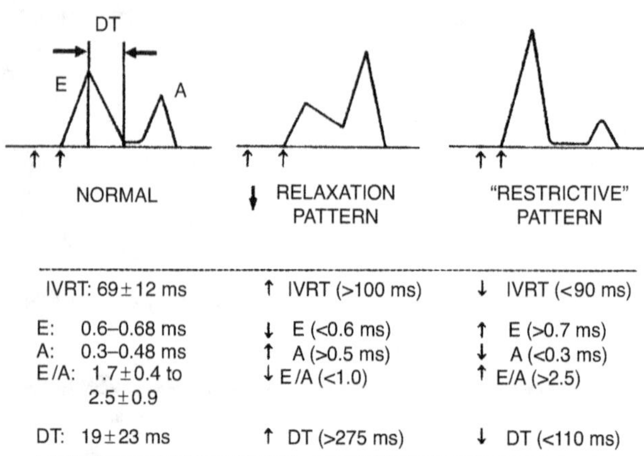

FIG. 11.2

Examples of diastolic dysfunction seen in different types of cardiomyopathy. *A*, A wave (the velocity of a second wave that coincides with atrial contraction); *DT*, deceleration time (time from the peak of the E wave to the point where the decelerating diastolic velocity reaches the baseline); *E*, E wave (the velocity of an early peak that coincides with the early ventricular filling); E:A, ratio of E wave to A wave velocity; *IVRT*, isovolumic relaxation time (measured from the cessation of ventricular outflow to the onset of the E wave; between the two *small arrows*). *(From Park, M. K., & Salamat, M. (2020).* Park's pediatric cardiology for practitioners *(7th ed.). Philadelphia: Mosby.)*

treating ventricular arrhythmias). However, most therapeutic modalities used do not significantly reduce mortality rate.

2. General care.
   a. Patients with HCM should avoid strenuous exercise or competitive sports, regardless of age, gender, symptoms, LVOT obstruction, or treatment.
   b. Genetic testing for HCM sequencing and deletion/duplication panels are available from blood, oral rinse, or buccal (cheek) swabs.
   c. First-degree relatives and other family members should be screened.
3. A β-adrenergic blocker (such as propranolol, atenolol, or metoprolol) or a calcium channel blocker (principally verapamil) is the drug of choice in the obstructive subgroup. These drugs reduce the degree of obstruction, decrease the incidence of anginal pain, and have antiarrhythmic actions.
   a. A combination therapy with atenolol and verapamil may be considered in those patients with excessive LV hypertrophy and severe LVOT obstruction.

b. In small children, propranolol is the drug of choice due to liquid formulation and a low side effect profile. The dosage is 2 to 4 mg/kg/day given in three divided doses, with the heart rate goal of 80 to 100 beats/min.
c. In older children, metoprolol is typically used.
d. In infants of diabetic mothers, β-adrenergic blockers are used when the LVOT obstruction is present. In most of these infants, LV hypertrophy spontaneously resolves within the first 6 to 12 months of life.

4. Prophylactic therapy with either β-adrenergic blockers or verapamil is controversial in patients without LVOT obstruction. Some favor prophylactic use of these drugs even in the absence of LVOT obstruction; others limit prophylactic drug therapy to young patients with a family history of premature sudden death and those with particularly marked LVH.
5. The following drugs are contraindicated: digitalis, other inotropic agents, and vasodilators tend to increase LVOT obstruction; diuretics may reduce LV volume and increase LVOT obstruction (but may be used in small doses to improve respiratory symptoms).
6. For drug-refractory patients with obstruction, Morrow's myotomy-myectomy or percutaneous alcohol ablation may be considered.
   a. In Morrow's procedure, hypertrophied LV septum is resected through a transaortic approach to reduce the obstruction.
   b. In alcohol ablation, absolute alcohol is injected into a target septal perforator branch of the left anterior descending coronary artery to produce "controlled" myocardial infarction.
7. Implantable cardioverter defibrillator (ICD) has been proved to be effective in preventing sudden death. The following are risk factors for sudden death in HCM and may be indications for an ICD.
   a. Prior cardiac arrest (ventricular fibrillation)
   b. Spontaneous sustained ventricular tachycardia (defined as three or more beats at ≥120 beats/min on Holter ECG)
   c. Family history of premature sudden death
   d. Unexplained syncope, particularly in young patients
   e. LV thickness ≥30 mm, particularly in adolescents and young adults
   f. Nonsustained VT
   g. Abnormal exercise blood pressure (BP) (attenuated response or hypotension)
8. Cardiac arrhythmias.
   a. Ventricular arrhythmias are treated with propranolol, amiodarone, and other antiarrhythmic agents, guided by serial ambulatory ECG monitoring.
   b. Atrial fibrillation (AF) occurs more often in patients with LA enlargement. For new-onset AF, electrical cardioversion followed by anticoagulation with warfarin (superior to aspirin) is recommended. Amiodarone is generally considered as the most effective agent for preventing recurrence of AF.
9. Infants of diabetic mothers

In most cases, the LV hypertrophy spontaneously resolves within the first 6 to 12 months of life. β-Adrenergic blockers, such as propranolol, may help the LVOT obstruction, but treatment usually is not necessary. Digitalis and other inotropic agents are contraindicated because they may worsen the obstruction.

II. DILATED (CONGESTIVE) CARDIOMYOPATHY

Dilated cardiomyopathy (DCM) is the most common form of cardiomyopathy in children.

A. CAUSES

1. The cause of the condition is idiopathic in about 50% of the cases. Twenty percent to 35% of patients with idiopathic cardiomyopathy have been shown to have inherited familial DCM. Among the familial types, an autosomal dominant inheritance pattern is most frequent (occurring in 30% to 50%); X-linked, autosomal recessive; and mitochondrial inheritance patterns are less common.
2. Among the known causes of DCM are myocarditis (46%) and neuromuscular diseases (≈25%), followed by familial cardiomyopathy, active myocarditis, and others. The most frequently recognized familial form is Duchenne muscular dystrophy. Some cases of idiopathic dilated cardiomyopathy may be the result of subclinical myocarditis.
3. Some patients with idiopathic DCM may have tachycardia-induced cardiomyopathy, which is related to chronic tachycardia (usually atrial or supraventricular tachycardia).
4. Other rare causes of DCM include infectious causes other than viral infection (bacterial, fungal, protozoan, rickettsial), endocrine-metabolic disorders (hyperthyroidism and hypothyroidism, excessive catecholamines, diabetes, hypocalcemia, hypophosphatemia, glycogen storage disease, mucopolysaccharidoses), and nutritional disorders (kwashiorkor, beriberi, carnitine deficiency).
5. Cardiotoxic agents such as doxorubicin and systemic diseases (such as connective tissue diseases) can also cause dilated cardiomyopathy.

B. PATHOLOGY AND PATHOPHYSIOLOGY

1. In DCM, a weakening of systolic contraction is associated with dilatation of all four cardiac chambers. Dilatation of the atria is in proportion to ventricular dilatation.
2. Intracavitary thrombus formation is common in the apical portion of the ventricular cavities and in atrial appendages, and it may give rise to pulmonary and systemic embolization.
3. Histologic examinations from endomyocardial biopsies show varying degrees of myocyte hypertrophy and fibrosis. Inflammatory cells are usually absent, but a varying incidence of inflammatory myocarditis has been reported.

C. CLINICAL MANIFESTATIONS

1. Fatigue, weakness, and symptoms of left heart failure (e.g., dyspnea on exertion, orthopnea) may be present.
2. On physical examination, signs of CHF (e.g., tachycardia, pulmonary crackles, weak pulses, distended neck veins, hepatomegaly) may be present. A prominent S3 with or without gallop rhythm is present. A soft systolic murmur of MR or TR may be audible.
3. The ECG commonly shows sinus tachycardia, LVH, and ST-T changes.
4. Chest radiographs show generalized cardiomegaly, often with signs of pulmonary venous congestion.
5. Echo studies are diagnostic and may include unexpected findings in an asymptomatic patient.
   a. The LV and RV are markedly dilated with poor contractility. The LA may be enlarged.
   b. Fractional shortening (FS) and ejection fraction (EF) are reduced.
   c. Intracavitary thrombus and pericardial effusion may be present.
   d. The mitral inflow Doppler tracing demonstrates a reduced E velocity and a decreased E:A ratio: nonspecific signs (see Fig. 11.2).
6. Laboratory tests: The following lab tests may help identify the causes of DCM.
   a. Urine for organic and amino acids, 3-methylglutaconic acid (i.e., Barth syndrome)
   b. Blood studies for complete blood count, comprehensive metabolic panel, lactate, calcium, magnesium, carnitine/acylcarnitine, thyroid function, creatine kinase and its MB fraction (CK-MB), troponin, brain natriuretic peptide (BNP) or its N-terminal fragment (NT-proBNP)
   c. Genetic testing for DCM sequencing and deletion/duplication panels are available from blood, oral rinse or buccal (cheek) swabs.
7. Although echo study is diagnostic, cardiac catheterization can be helpful (1) to exclude anomalous coronary artery, (2) to predict etiology and prognosis by obtaining endomyocardial biopsy, and (3) to evaluate for possible cardiac transplantation including measurement of pulmonary vascular resistance.
8. **Natural history.** Progressive deterioration is the rule rather than the exception for many patients. Cardiac arrhythmias, systemic or pulmonary embolization, and CHF are common causes of death. Review of literature in children has suggested approximately one-third of patients die, one-third recover completely, and one-third improve with some residual cardiac dysfunction.

D. MANAGEMENT

When no identifiable and treatable cause of DCM is found, therapy is supportive and consists of (a) anticongestive regimens, (b) control of significant arrhythmias, and (c) minimizing the risk of thromboembolic complications.

1. **Anticongestive treatment.** Angiotensin-converting enzyme (ACE) inhibitors, β-adrenergic blockers, or combination of both are used. Diuretics and digoxin may also be added.
   a. ACE inhibitors (captopril, enalapril) are the first line of drug to use, along with pulsed use of diuretics. ACE inhibitors reduce congestive symptoms by moving the Frank-Starling curve to the left and upward with resulting reduction in cardiac afterload and increase in stroke volume (see Fig 19.1).
   b. The beneficial effects of carvedilol, a β-adrenergic blocking agent, have been reported in adult patients as well as children with DCM. The use of β-adrenergic blocking agents is somewhat unorthodox, given poor contractility of the ventricle. Studies suggest that activation of the sympathetic nervous system may have deleterious cardiac effects (rather than being an important compensatory mechanism, as traditionally thought). β-Adrenergic blockers may exert beneficial effects by a negative chronotropic effect with reduced oxygen demand, reduction in catecholamine toxicity, inhibition of sympathetically mediated vasoconstriction, or reduction of potentially lethal ventricular arrhythmias.
   c. Diuretics (furosemide) and digoxin are also frequently added to the treatment. Aldosterone antagonists (spironolactone) have also been shown to be beneficial with a decrease in the risk of death.
2. Antiplatelet agents (aspirin) should be initiated. The propensity for thrombus formation in these patients may prompt use of anticoagulation with warfarin. If thrombi are detected, they should be treated aggressively with heparin initially and later switched to long-term warfarin therapy.
3. Control of significant arrhythmias.
   a. Amiodarone is effective and relatively safe in children.
   b. For symptomatic bradycardia, a cardiac pacemaker may be necessary.
   c. An implantable ICD may be considered for high-risk patients. Children who are considered to have risk factors for sudden death in DCM include (a) LV end-diastolic dimension *z* score >2.6, (b) age at diagnosis <14 years, and (c) an LV posterior wall thickness–to–end-diastolic dimension ratio of <0.14.
4. If carnitine deficiency is considered as the cause for the cardiomyopathy, carnitine supplementation should be started.
5. Beneficial effects of growth hormone (for 3 to 6 months) were reported in adults as well as children with DCM. Administration of recombinant human growth hormone (0.025-0.04 mg/kg/day for 6 months) may improve LVEF, increase LV wall thickness, reduce the chamber size, and improve cardiac output.
6. Many of these children may become candidates for cardiac transplantation.

III. DOXORUBICIN CARDIOMYOPATHY

A. ETIOLOGY AND PATHOLOGY

1. Doxorubicin cardiomyopathy, a form of dilated cardiomyopathy, is one of the common causes of chronic CHF in children. Its prevalence is nonlinearly dose related, occurring in 2% to 5% of patients who have received a cumulative dose of 400 to 500 mg/m^2 and up to 50% of patients who have received more than 1000 mg/m^2 of doxorubicin (Adriamycin).
2. Risk factors for developing doxorubicin cardiomyopathy include the following.
   a. Patients who received cumulative dose of anthracyclines >360 mg/m^2 are 40 times more likely to die than those who received <240 mg/m^2.
   b. Age younger than 4 years.
   c. Concomitant cardiac irradiation.
   d. A dosing regimen with larger and less frequent doses has been raised as a risk factor but not proved.
3. Dilated LV, decreased contractility, and elevated LV filling pressure are present.

B. CLINICAL MANIFESTATIONS

1. Patients have a history of receiving doxorubicin, with the onset of symptoms 2 to 4 months, and rarely years, after completion of therapy.
2. Patients are usually asymptomatic until signs of CHF develop. Tachypnea and exertional dyspnea are the usual presenting complaints. Signs of CHF may be present on physical examination.
3. Chest radiographs show cardiomegaly with or without pulmonary congestion or pleural effusion.
4. The ECG frequently shows sinus tachycardia with occasional ST-T changes. During doxorubicin therapy, a prolonged QTc interval occurs in 40% of patients immediately after a single dose.
5. Echocardiographic abnormalities of DCM occur within a year after doxorubicin treatment and may include the following.
   a. The LV size is slightly increased and the LV wall thickness slightly decreased.
   b. LV contractility (either EF or fractional shortening) is decreased. Cardiotoxicity is defined as an LVEF decline of ≥5% to <55% with heart failure symptoms or an asymptomatic decrease of LVEF ≥10% to <55%
   c. During doxorubicin therapy, echo may show reduced EF or fractional shortening (but stopping therapy based on these changes may not be justified).
6. Symptomatic patients have a high mortality rate. The 2-year survival rate is about 20%, and almost all patients die by 9 years after the onset of the illness.

C. MANAGEMENT

1. Attempts to reduce anthracycline cardiotoxicity have been directed toward (a) anthracycline dose limitation; (b) method of drug administration; (c) developing less cardiotoxic analogs; (d) concurrently administering cardioprotective agents to attenuate the cardiotoxic effects of anthracycline to the heart; and (e) secondary prevention strategies of early detection of cardiotoxicity and early initiation of therapy.
   a. Limiting the total cumulative dose to 400 to 500 mg/m^2 reduces the incidence of CHF to 5%, but this dose may not be effective in treating some malignancies.
   b. Continuous infusion therapy may reduce cardiac injury by avoiding peak levels, but a recent study reports no cardioprotection of continuous infusion.
   c. Liposomal doxorubicin (which contains doxorubicin wrapped up in a fatty covering called liposome) preserves anticancer properties of the drug but reduces cardiotoxicity.
   d. Concurrent administration of the cardioprotective agents such as dexrazoxane (an iron chelator), carvedilol (a β-receptor antagonist with antioxidant property), and coenzyme Q10 have shown some protective effects, without attenuating the antimalignancy effect of the drug. Among these, dexrazoxane appears to be most cardioprotective.
   e. Early detection of cardiotoxicity by echo study (LVEF < 55%) and early initiation of drug therapy with enalapril + carvedilol appear to make LV systolic function recovery more likely.
2. When anthracycline cardiomyopathy is diagnosed, management is the same as discussed earlier for dilated cardiomyopathy in general. Currently, the following medications are used.
   a. Afterload-reducing agents (ACE inhibitors [e.g., enalapril]), diuretics, and digoxin are useful.
   b. β-Blockers have been shown to be beneficial in some children with chemotherapy-induced cardiomyopathy, similar to what has been reported in adults. Carvedilol, a nonselective β-blocker, also has vasodilator effect and antioxidant activity.
3. Cardiac transplantation may be an option for selected patients.

IV. RESTRICTIVE CARDIOMYOPATHY

A. PREVALENCE AND CAUSES

1. Restrictive cardiomyopathy is an extremely rare form of cardiomyopathy, accounting for 5% of cardiomyopathy cases in children.
2. It may be idiopathic, or it may be associated with a systemic infiltrative disease (such as scleroderma, amyloidosis, and sarcoidosis) or an inborn error of metabolism (mucopolysaccharidosis). Malignancies or radiation therapy may result in restrictive cardiomyopathy.

B. PATHOLOGY AND PATHOPHYSIOLOGY

1. This condition is characterized by markedly dilated atria and normal or decreased volume of both ventricles. Ventricular diastolic filling is impaired, resulting from excessively stiff ventricular walls. Systolic function of the ventricle is normal (or near normal). Therefore this condition resembles constrictive pericarditis in clinical presentation and hemodynamic abnormalities.
2. There are areas of myocardial fibrosis and hypertrophy of myocytes, or the myocardium may be infiltrated by various materials, as seen in such conditions as amyloidosis, sarcoidosis, hemochromatosis, glycogen deposit, Fabry disease (with deposition of glycosphingolipids), or neoplastic infiltration
3. Development of pulmonary hypertension due to diastolic dysfunction is a significant problem in children as is in adults.

C. CLINICAL MANIFESTATIONS

1. History of exercise intolerance, weakness and dyspnea, or chest pain may be present.
2. Jugular venous distention, hepatomegaly, a loud S2 (P2), gallop rhythm, and a systolic murmur of MR or TR may be present.
3. Chest radiographs show cardiomegaly, pulmonary congestion, and pleural effusion.
4. The ECG usually shows RAH and/or LAH. It may show atrial fibrillation and paroxysms of SVT.
5. Echo studies reveal the following:
   a. Marked biatrial enlargement with normal dimension of the LV and RV, almost diagnostic signs.
   b. Normal LV systolic function (EF) until the late stages of the disease.
   c. Abnormal diastolic function (with increased E velocity and increased E:A ratio, and shortened deceleration time (see Fig. 11.2).
   d. Possible atrial thrombus.
6. Differentiation of restrictive cardiomyopathy from *constrictive pericarditis* is important because the latter can be treated successfully with pericardiotomy.
   a. In constrictive pericarditis, echo shows a thickened pericardium and Doppler studies show a marked respiratory variation in the filling phase, although both conditions show similar Doppler findings of diastolic dysfunction.
   b. Cardiac catheterization shows similar hemodynamic data in both conditions, although pulmonary hypertension is worse in restrictive cardiomyopathy.
   c. Endomyocardial biopsy reveals myocyte hypertrophy and interstitial fibrosis; it may also reveal a specific cause.
   d. Rarely, surgical exploration may be needed.

D. MANAGEMENT

Treatment is directed at alleviating symptoms. In general, medical therapy does not improve survival. The prognosis is poor.

1. Diuretics are beneficial by relieving congestive symptoms, but they should be used judiciously because they can reduce end-diastolic pressure, making symptoms worse.
2. Calcium channel blockers may be used to increase diastolic compliance.
3. Digoxin is not indicated, because systolic function is unimpaired.
4. ACE inhibitors should not be used because they may reduce systemic BP without increasing cardiac output.
5. Anticoagulants (warfarin) and antiplatelet drugs (aspirin and dipyridamole) may help prevent thrombosis.
6. Permanent pacemaker is indicated for complete heart block.
7. Cardiac transplantation may be an option before pulmonary hypertension develops.

V. ARRHYTHMOGENIC CARDIOMYOPATHY

This cardiomyopathy is also known as arrhythmogenic RV dysplasia, arrhythmogenic RV cardiomyopathy, RV dysplasia, or RV cardiomyopathy.

A. PREVALENCE AND PATHOLOGY

1. This rare anomaly of unknown etiology is more prevalent in northern Italy.
2. The myocardium of the RV is partially or totally replaced by fibrous or adipose tissue. The RV wall may rarely assume a paper-thin appearance because of the total absence of myocardial tissue, but in others, RV wall thickness is normal or near normal. The LV is also often affected.
3. Histologic sections show a variable reduction in myofibrils and inflammation associated with interstitial infiltration by histiocytes and lymphocytes.

B. CLINICAL MANIFESTATIONS

1. The onset is in infancy, childhood, or adulthood (but usually before age 20 years), with history of palpitation, syncopal episodes, or both. It accounts for about 5% of sudden cardiac death.
2. Presenting manifestations may be arrhythmias (VT, SVT) or signs of CHF.
3. The ECG is helpful in suspecting the diagnosis.
   a. Tall P waves in lead II (RAH) and decreased RV forces may be present.
   b. Inverted T waves in the right precordial leads (V1-V4) may be significant (although this pattern is normally seen in young children).
   c. The ECG may show PVCs or ventricular tachycardia with LBBB morphology.
   d. An incomplete RBBB pattern may be present (in >30% of the cases).

4. Chest radiographs usually show cardiomegaly.
5. Echo studies show selective RV enlargement, extreme thinning of the RV free wall, often with systolic bulging, the hallmark of the condition.
6. Cardiac MRI and RV angiogram show similar findings as echo studies.
7. Cardiac catheterization may show an elevated right atrial "a" wave. An RV angiogram usually shows RV systolic dysfunction. The hallmark of the disease is systolic bulging of the RV free wall. Endomyocardial biopsy of the RV septum shows classic pathologic changes in more than 90% of the patients but with a high false-negative rate.
8. A substantial portion of patients die before 5 years of age from CHF and intractable ventricular tachycardia.

C. MANAGEMENT

1. Various antiarrhythmic agents are often unsuccessful in abolishing ventricular arrhythmias.
2. Surgical intervention (ventricular incision or complete electrical disarticulation of the RV free wall) may be tried if antiarrhythmic therapy is unsuccessful.
3. ICD may be indicated in selected patients.

VI. NONCOMPACTION CARDIOMYOPATHY

A. CAUSE

This condition results from an intrauterine arrest of normal compaction of the loose interwoven meshwork of the ventricular myocardium (which normally occurs during the first month of fetal life). Several gene mutations in patients with noncompaction cardiomyopathy have been reported; thus the genetic testing of the relatives of an index case is recommended. Familial occurrence has been reported in up to 25% with a less severe form of the disease.

B. CLINICAL MANIFESTATIONS

1. Most patients with this disorder are asymptomatic. Occasionally, they may present with signs and symptoms of heart failure during infancy.
2. Cardiac examination may be entirely normal. Signs of LV dysfunction may be present or eventually develop. Associated dysmorphic facial features may be seen in 14%. Nearly 30% of the patients have neurologic disorders, including seizures, hypotonia, myopathy, or mental/motor retardation.
3. The ECG may show giant QRS complexes, sometimes with WPW preexcitation.
4. Chest radiographs are usually normal.
5. Echo findings:
   a. Characteristic echo findings are segmental thickening of the LV wall consisting of two layers with a thin, compacted epicardial layer and an extremely thickened noncompacted endocardial layer with prominent trabeculations and deep recesses. Apical and

midventricular segments of both the inferior and lateral walls are most commonly affected.

b. LV systolic dysfunction is seen in 35% to 90% of pediatric patients. LV diastolic dysfunction is often present.

6. **Natural history.** Heart failure usually worsens despite optimal treatment. Arrhythmias and thromboembolic events are mostly seen in adults, but they may also be seen in children.

C. TREATMENT

1. Anticongestive measures with digoxin, diuretic, and afterload-reducing agents are usually used. The use of carvedilol, a β-blocker, should be considered in patients with LV dysfunction; it has been shown to improve LV dysfunction.
2. All patients should be on an antiplatelet dose of aspirin. If thrombosis is detected, anticoagulation with warfarin should be started.
3. Appropriate antiarrhythmic therapy is indicated. Implantation of ICD may be considered for life-threatening ventricular arrhythmias.
4. Patients with dysmorphic features or neurologic manifestations may need detailed metabolic screening (e.g., fatty acid oxidation disorder or mitochondrial disease).
5. Heart transplantation is a possible option for selected patients.

Chapter 12

Cardiovascular Infections and Related Conditions

I. INFECTIVE ENDOCARDITIS (SUBACUTE BACTERIAL ENDOCARDITIS)

A. PREVALENCE

Subacute bacterial endocarditis (SBE) affects 0.5:1000 to 1:1000 hospital patients, excluding those with postoperative endocarditis.

B. PATHOLOGY AND PATHOGENESIS

1. Two factors are important in the pathogenesis of IE: (a) structural abnormalities of the heart or great arteries with a significant pressure gradient or turbulence, with resulting endothelial damage and platelet-fibrin thrombus formation; and (b) bacteremia, even if transient, with adherence of the organisms and eventual invasion of the underlying tissue.
2. Those with a prosthetic heart valve or prosthetic material in the heart are at particularly high risk for IE because these promote deposition of sterile thrombus.
3. Almost all patients who develop IE have a history of congenital or acquired heart disease. Drug addicts may develop endocarditis in the absence of known cardiac anomalies.
4. Dental procedures or chewing with diseased teeth or gums may be the most frequent cause of bacteremia.

C. MICROBIOLOGY

1. In the past, *Streptococcus viridans*, enterococci, and *Staphylococcus aureus* were responsible for over 90% of cases of IE. In recent years, this frequency has decreased to 50% to 60%, with a concomitant increase in cases caused by fungus and HACEK organisms (*Haemophilus, Actinobacillus, Cardiobacterium, Eikenella*, and *Kingella*). HACEK organisms are particularly common in neonates and immunocompromised children.
2. α-Hemolytic streptococci (*S. viridans*) are the most common cause of IE following dental procedures or in those patients with carious teeth or periodontal disease.
3. Staphylococci (*S. aureus* and coagulase-negative staphylococci) account for more cases than *S. viridans* in developed countries, usually health care–associated infections, such as postoperative endocarditis,

indwelling vascular catheters, prosthetic material, prosthetic valve, among newborn infants, and intravenous drug abusers.

4. Enterococci are the organisms most often found after genitourinary or gastrointestinal surgery or instrumentation.
5. Fungal endocarditis (which has a poor prognosis) may occur in sick neonates, in patients receiving long-term antibiotic or steroid therapy, or after open heart surgery.
6. **Culture-negative endocarditis.** Diagnosis of this condition is made when a patient has clinical and/or echocardiographic evidence of endocarditis but persistently negative blood cultures. This occurs in about 5% to 7% of endocarditis in the United States. The most common cause of the condition is current or recent antibiotic therapy. It can be caused by a fastidious organism that grows poorly in vitro and rarely by fungus. At times, the diagnosis can be made only by removal of vegetation (during surgery).

D. CLINICAL MANIFESTATIONS

1. Most patients are known to have an underlying heart disease. A history of toothache, recent dental procedure, or tonsillectomy is occasionally present. A history of recent cardiovascular procedures or surgeries may be present. The onset is usually insidious with prolonged low-grade fever of 38°C but fever may fluctuate up to 39.5°C.
2. Heart murmur is almost always present and splenomegaly is common (70%).
3. Skin manifestations (50%) may be present in the following forms:
   a. Petechiae on the skin, mucous membranes, or conjunctivae are frequent.
   b. Osler nodes (tender, pea-sized red nodes at the ends of the fingers or toes) are rare in children.
   c. Janeway lesions (small, painless, hemorrhagic areas on the palms or soles) are rare.
   d. Splinter hemorrhages (linear hemorrhagic streaks beneath the nails) also are rare.
4. Embolic or immunologic phenomena in other organs are present in about 50% of cases.
   a. Pulmonary emboli or hematuria and renal failure may occur.
   b. Seizures and hemiparesis (20%) may occur.
   c. Roth spots (oval, retinal hemorrhages with pale centers located near the optic disc) occur in <5% of patients.
5. Laboratory studies.
   a. Positive blood cultures are obtained in more than 90% of patients in the absence of previous antimicrobial therapy.
   b. Anemia and leukocytosis with a shift to the left are common.
   c. The sedimentation rate is increased unless there is polycythemia.
   d. Microscopic hematuria is found in 30% of patients.

6. **Echocardiography.** Although standard transthoracic echo (TTE) is sufficient in most cases, transesophageal echo (TEE) may be needed in obese or very muscular adolescents.
   a. The following echo findings are included as major criteria in the modified Duke criteria: (1) oscillating intracardiac mass on valve or supporting structures, in the path of regurgitation jets or on implanted material; (2) abscesses; (3) new partial dehiscence of prosthetic valve; and (4) new valvular regurgitation.
   b. The absence of vegetations on echo does not in itself rule out IE. False-negative diagnosis is possible if vegetations are small or have already embolized.
   c. Conversely, a false-positive diagnosis is possible. An echogenic mass may represent a sterile thrombus, sterile prosthetic material, normal anatomic variation, an abnormal uninfected valve (previous scarring, severe myxomatous changes), or improper gain of the echo machine. Echo evidence of vegetation may persist for months or years after bacteriologic cure.
   d. Certain echo features suggest a high-risk case or a need for surgery: (1) large vegetations (greatest risk when the vegetation is >10 mm), (2) severe valvular regurgitation, (3) abscess cavities, (4) pseudoaneurysm, (5) valvular perforation or dehiscence, or (6) decompensated heart failure.

E. DIAGNOSIS

The diagnosis of infective endocarditis is challenging. The modified Duke criteria are used in the diagnosis. There are three categories of diagnostic possibilities using the modified Duke criteria: definite, possible, and rejected (Box 12.1). Box 12.2 shows definitions of major and minor clinical criteria. It is imperative for readers to carefully read and understand the statements in these boxes (Boxes 12.1 and Box 12.2).

1. A diagnosis of "***definite***" IE is made when (a) pathologic evidence ***and*** (b) fulfillment of certain clinical criteria (listed in Box 12.1) are present.
2. The category of ***"possible"*** IE is made when (a) one major criterion and one minor criterion ***or*** (b) three minor criteria are present.
3. The category of "***rejected***" IE is made when one of the four statements in Box 12.1 is present.

F. MANAGEMENT

1. Blood cultures are indicated for all patients with fever of unexplained origin and a pathologic heart murmur, a history of heart disease, or previous endocarditis.
   a. Usually three blood cultures are drawn over 24 hours, unless the patient is very ill. In 90% of cases, the causative agent is recovered from the first two cultures.

BOX 12.1

DEFINITION OF INFECTIVE ENDOCARDITIS ACCORDING TO THE MODIFIED DUKE CRITERIA

DEFINITE IE

A. Pathologic criteria
   1. Microorganisms demonstrated by culture or histologic examination of a vegetation, a vegetation that has embolized, or an intracardiac abscess specimen; or
   2. Pathologic lesions; vegetation or intracardiac abscess confirmed by histologic examination showing active endocarditis

B. Clinical criteria
   1. Two major criteria; or
   2. One major criterion and three minor criteria; or
   3. Five minor criteria

POSSIBLE IE

1. One major criterion and one minor criterion; or
2. Three minor criteria

REJECTED

1. Firm alternative diagnosis explaining evidence of IE; or
2. Resolution of IE syndrome with antibiotic therapy for <4 days; or
3. No pathological evidence of IE at surgery or autopsy, with antibiotic therapy for <4 days; or
4. Does not meet criteria for possible IE as above

IE, infective endocarditis.

From Baddour, L. M., Wilson, W. R., Bayer, A. S., et al. (2005). Infective endocarditis: diagnosis, antimicrobial therapy, and management of complications: a statement for healthcare professionals from the Committee on Rheumatic Fever, Endocarditis, and Kawasaki Disease, Council on Cardiovascular Disease in the Young, and the Councils on Clinical Cardiolgoy, Stroke, and Cardiovascular Surgery and Anesthesia, American Heart Association. *Circulation, 111*(23):e394-e433.

   b. If there is no growth by the second day of incubation, two more cultures may be obtained. There is no value in obtaining more than five blood cultures over 2 days unless the patient received prior antibiotic therapy.
   c. Aerobic incubation alone suffices because it is rare for IE to be due to anaerobic bacteria.

2. Initial empirical therapy is started with the following antibiotics while awaiting the results of blood cultures. Consultation from a local infectious disease specialist is strongly recommended.
   a. The usual initial regimen is an antistaphylococcal semisynthetic penicillin (nafcillin, oxacillin, or methicillin) and an aminoglycoside (gentamicin). This combination covers against *S. viridans, S. aureus,* and gram-negative organisms.

BOX 12.2

DEFINITION OF MAJOR AND MINOR CLINICAL CRITERIA FOR THE DIAGNOSIS OF INFECTIVE ENDOCARDITIS

MAJOR CRITERIA

A. Blood culture positive for IE
   1. Typical microorganisms consistent with IE from two separate blood cultures: *Viridans* streptococci, *Streptococcus bovis*, HACEK group, *Staphylococcus aureus*; or community-acquired enterococci in the absence of a primary focus; or
   2. Microorganisms consistent with IE from persistently positive blood cultures defined as follows: at least two positive cultures of blood samples drawn >12 hours apart; or all of three or a majority of ≥4 separate cultures of blood (with first and last sample drawn at least 1 hour apart)
   3. Single positive blood culture for *Coxiella burnetii* or anti–phase I IgG antibody titer >1:800

B. Evidence of endocardial involvement

Echocardiogram positive for IE (TEE recommended for patients with prosthetic valves, rated at least "possible IE" by clinical criteria, or complicated IE [paravalvular abscess]; TTE as first test in other patients) defined as follows:
   1. Oscillating intracardiac mass on valve or supporting structures, in the path of regurgitant jets, or on implanted material in the absence of an alternative anatomic explanation; or
   2. Abscess; or
   3. New partial dehiscence of prosthetic valve; or
   4. New valvular regurgitation (worsening or changing or preexisting murmur not sufficient)

MINOR CRITERIA

1. Predisposition, predisposing heart condition, or injection drug users
2. Fever, temperature >38°C
3. Vascular phenomena: major arterial emboli, septic pulmonary infarcts, mycotic aneurysm, intracranial hemorrhage, conjunctival hemorrhages, and Janeway lesions
4. Immunologic phenomena: glomerulonephritis, Osler nodes, Roth spots, and rheumatoid factor
5. Microbiologic evidence: positive blood culture but does not meet a major criterion as noted above[a] or serologic evidence of active infection with organism consistent with IE

[a]Excludes single positive cultures for coagulase-negative staphylococci and organisms that do not cause endocarditis.

HACEK, *Haemophilus*, *Actinobacillus*, *Cardiobacterium*, *Eikenella*, and *Kingella*; *IE*, infective endocarditis; *IgG*, immunoglobulin G; *TEE*, transesophageal echo; *TTE*, transthoracic echo.

From Baddour, L. M., Wilson, W. R., Bayer, A. S., et al. (2005). Infective endocarditis: diagnosis, antimicrobial therapy, and management of complications: a statement for healthcare professionals from the Committee on Rheumatic Fever, Endocarditis, and Kawasaki Disease, Council on Cardiovascular Disease in the Young, and the Councils on Clinical Cardiology, Stroke, and Cardiovascular Surgery and Anesthesia, American Heart Association. *Circulation, 111*(23), e394-e433.

b. If a methicillin-resistant *S. aureus* is suspected, vancomycin should be substituted for the semisynthetic penicillin.
c. Vancomycin can be used in place of penicillin or a semisynthetic penicillin in penicillin-allergic patients.

3. The final selection of antibiotics for native valve IE depends on the organism isolated and the results of an antibiotic sensitivity test.
   a. Streptococcal infective endocarditis
      (1) For highly sensitive *S. viridans*, IV penicillin (or ceftriaxone given once daily) for 4 weeks is sufficient. Alternatively, penicillin, ampicillin, or ceftriaxone combined with gentamicin for 2 weeks may be used.
      (2) For penicillin-resistant streptococci, 4 weeks of penicillin, ampicillin, or ceftriaxone combined with gentamicin for the first 2 weeks is recommended.
   b. Staphylococcal endocarditis
      (1) For methicillin-susceptible staphylococci IE, one of the semisynthetic β-lactamase–resistant penicillins (nafcillin, oxacillin, or methicillin) for a minimum of 6 weeks (with or without gentamicin for the first 3 to 5 days) is used.
      (2) For patients with methicillin-resistant IE, vancomycin for 6 weeks (with or without gentamicin for the first 3 to 5 days) is used.
   c. *Enterococcus*-caused endocarditis usually requires a combination of IV penicillin or ampicillin together with gentamicin for 4 to 6 weeks. If patients are allergic to penicillin, vancomycin combined with gentamicin for 6 weeks is required.
   d. For HACEK organisms, ceftriaxone or another third-generation cephalosporin alone or ampicillin plus gentamicin for 4 weeks is recommended. IE caused by other gram-negative bacteria (such as *Escherichia coli*, *Pseudomonas aeruginosa*, or *Serratia marcescens*) is treated with piperacillin or ceftazidime together with gentamicin for a minimum of 6 weeks.
   e. Fungal endocarditis is very difficult to treat. Amphotericin B, with or without flucytosine, is most often used, but surgical replacement of the infected valve (native or prosthetic) is usually required.
   f. In culture-negative endocarditis, treatment is directed against staphylococci, streptococci, and the HACEK organisms using ceftriaxone and gentamicin. When staphylococcal IE is suspected, nafcillin should be added to the above therapy.
4. Patients with prosthetic valve endocarditis should be treated for 6 weeks based on the organism isolated and the results of the sensitivity test. Operative intervention may be necessary before the antibiotic therapy is completed if the clinical situation warrants (such as progressive CHF, significant malfunction of prosthetic valves, persistently positive blood cultures after 2 weeks' therapy). Bacteriologic relapse after an appropriate course of therapy also calls for operative intervention.

G. PROGNOSIS

The overall recovery rate is 80% to 85%; it is 90% or better for *S. viridans* and enterococci, and about 50% for *Staphylococcus* organisms. Fungal endocarditis is associated with a very poor outcome.

H. PREVENTION

Until 2007, antibiotic prophylaxis for IE was routinely recommended before dental procedures for almost all CHDs (with exception of ASD), rheumatic and other valvular diseases, hypertrophic cardiomyopathy, and all other conditions included in the current recommendation. In 2007, the American Heart Association (AHA) made a major change in the antibiotic prophylaxis against IE.

1. The following are the updated recommendations for antibiotic prophylaxis.
   a. Antibiotic prophylaxis is recommended only for cardiac conditions listed in Box 12.3, which was updated in 2017.
   b. Procedures for which antibiotic prophylaxis is recommended and those not recommended are listed in Box 12.4.
   c. Antibiotic choices and dosages for dental procedures are shown in Table 12.1.
2. Special situations.
   a. For patients receiving rheumatic fever prophylaxis, use other antibiotics, such as clindamycin, azithromycin, or clarithromycin, rather than using a higher dose of the same antibiotic.
   b. When the patient is already receiving a course of an antibiotic for other reasons (such as tonsillitis), delay a dental procedure, if possible, until at least 10 days after completion of the antibiotic therapy.
3. For patients who undergo cardiac surgery, the following applies:
   a. A careful preoperative dental evaluation is recommended so that required dental treatment may be completed before cardiac surgery.
   b. Prophylaxis at the time of surgery should be directed primarily against staphylococci and should be of short duration.

12

BOX 12.3

2017 AHA/ACC UPDATED RECOMMENDATION ON CARDIAC CONDITIONS FOR WHICH PROPHYLAXIS WITH DENTAL PROCEDURES IS RECOMMENDED

Prophylaxis against IE is reasonable before dental procedures that involve manipulation of gingival tissue, manipulation of the peripheral region of teeth, or perforation of the oral mucosa in patients with the following:

1. Prosthetic cardiac valves, including transcatheter-implanted prostheses and homografts.
2. Prosthetic material used for cardiac valve repair, such as annuloplasty rings and chords.
3. Previous IE.
4. Unrepaired cyanotic congenital heart disease or repaired congenital heart disease, with residual shunts or valvular regurgitation at the site of or adjacent to the site of a prosthetic patch or prosthetic device.
5. Cardiac transplant with valve regurgitation due to a structurally abnormal valve.[a]

[a]The risk of IE is highest in the first 6 months after transplantation because of endothelial disruption, high-intensity immunosuppressive therapy, frequent central venous catheter access, and frequent endomyocardial biopsies.

IE, infective endocarditis.

Adapted from Nishimura RA, Otto CM, Bonow RO, et al: 217 AHA/ACC focused update of the 2014 AHA/ACC guidelines for the management of patients with valvular heart disease: a report of the American College of Cardiology/American Heart Association Task Force on Clinical Practice Guidelines, *Circulation* 2017;135(25): e1159-e1195.

BOX 12.4

PROCEDURES FOR WHICH ENDOCARDITIS PROPHYLAXIS IS RECOMMENDED

1. Dental procedures

   All dental procedures that involve manipulation of gingival tissue of the periapical region of teeth or perforation of the oral mucosa. Antibiotic choices and dosages for dental procedures are shown in Table 12.1.
2. Respiratory tract procedures
   a. Prophylaxis is recommended for the procedures that involve incision or biopsy of the respiratory mucosa, such as tonsillectomy and adenoidectomy.
   b. Prophylaxis is not recommended for bronchoscopy (unless it involves incision of the mucosa, such as for abscess or empyema).
3. GI and GU procedures
   a. No prophylaxis for diagnostic esophagogastroduodenoscopy or colonoscopy.
   b. Prophylaxis is reasonable in patients with infected GI or GU tract (with amoxicillin or ampicillin to cover against enterococci).
4. Skin, skin structure, or musculoskeletal tissue.
   a. Prophylaxis is recommended for surgical procedures that involve infected skin, skin structure, or musculoskeletal tissue (with antibiotics against *Staphylococcus* and β-hemolytic *Streptococcus*, such as antistaphylococcal penicillin or a cephalosporin).
   b. Vancomycin or clindamycin is administered if unable to tolerate β-lactam or if infection is caused by methicillin-resistant *Staphylococcus*.

GI, gastrointestinal; *GU*, genitourinary.

TABLE 12.1

PROPHYLACTIC REGIMENS FOR DENTAL PROCEDURES

		SINGLE DOSE 30-60 MIN BEFORE PROCEDURE	
SITUATION	**AGENT**	**CHILDREN**	**ADULTS**
Oral	Amoxicillin	50 mg/kg	2 g
Unable to take oral medications	Ampicillin, or cefazolin or ceftriaxone	50 mg/kg (IM, IV) 50 mg/kg (IM, IV)	2 g (IM, IV) 1 g (IM, IV)
Allergic to penicillin or ampicillin—oral	Cephalexin[a,b] or clindamycin, or azithromycin or clarithromycin	50 mg/kg 20 mg/kg 15 mg/kg 15 mg/kg	2 g 600 mg 500 mg 500 mg
Allergic to penicillin or ampicillin and unable to take oral medication	Cefazolin, or ceftriaxone	50 mg/kg (IM, IV)	1 g (IM, IV)
	Clindamycin	20 mg/kg (IM, IV)	600 mg (IM, IV)

IM, intramuscular; *IV*, intravenous

[a]Or other first- or second-generation oral cephalosporin in equivalent adult or pediatric dosage.

[b]Cephalosporins should not be used in an individual with a history of anaphylaxis, angioedema, or urticaria with penicillin or ampicillin.

c. Prophylaxis should be initiated immediately before the operative procedure, repeated during prolonged procedures to maintain serum concentrations intraoperatively, and continued for no more than 48 hours postoperatively.

II. MYOCARDITIS

A. PREVALENCE

Myocarditis severe enough to be recognized clinically is rare, but the prevalence of mild and subclinical cases is probably much higher.

B. ETIOLOGY

1. Infections: Viruses (such as adenovirus, coxsackieviruses, echoviruses, and many others) are the most common cause of myocarditis in North America. In South America, Chagas disease (caused by *Trypanosoma cruzi*, a protozoan) is far more common. Rarely, bacteria, rickettsia, fungi, protozoa, and parasites are the causative agents.
2. Immune-mediated diseases: ARF, Kawasaki disease.
3. Autoimmune disorders: sarcoidosis, systemic lupus erythematosus.
4. Toxic myocarditis (drug ingestion, diphtheria exotoxin, and anoxic agents).

C. PATHOLOGY

1. The principal mechanism of cardiac involvement in viral myocarditis is believed to be a cell-mediated immunologic reaction, not merely myocardial damage from viral replication. Isolation of virus from the myocardium is unusual at autopsy.
2. Microscopic examination reveals patchy infiltrations by plasma cells, mononuclear leukocytes, and some eosinophils during the acute phase and giant cell infiltration in the later stages.

D. CLINICAL MANIFESTATIONS

1. History of an upper respiratory tract infection may be present in older children. The onset of illness may be sudden in neonates and small infants, causing anorexia, vomiting, lethargy, and occasionally circulatory shock. In older children, a gradual onset of CHF and arrhythmia are commonly seen.
2. A soft, systolic ejection murmur and irregular rhythm caused by supraventricular or ventricular ectopic beats may be audible. Hepatomegaly (evidence of viral hepatitis) may be present.
3. The ECG may show any one or a combination of the following: low QRS voltages, ST-T changes, prolongation of the QT interval, and arrhythmias, especially premature contractions.

4. Cardiomegaly on chest radiograph is the most important clinical sign of myocarditis.
5. Echo studies reveal cardiac chamber enlargement and impaired LV systolic function. Occasionally, LV thrombi are found.
6. **Laboratory studies.** Cardiac troponin (I and T) levels and myocardial enzymes (creatine kinase [CK], MB isoenzyme of CK [CK-MB]) may be elevated. Troponin levels may be more sensitive than the cardiac enzymes. The normal value of cardiac troponin I in children is 2.0 ng/mL or less. B-type natriuretic peptide (BNP) and N-terminal-pro-BNP levels are elevated at the time of the diagnosis and they aid for management and evaluation of treatment progress.
7. Cardiac magnetic resonance imaging (MRI) has become the diagnostic tool of choice in diagnosis of acute or chronic phase of myocarditis. Cardiac MRI has mostly replaced radionuclide scanning in identifying inflammatory and necrotic changes characteristic of myocarditis. In additional, it aids the evaluation of cardiac function, pericardial effusion, and/or edema. Myocarditis can be confirmed by an endomyocardial biopsy.
8. **Natural history.** The mortality rate is as high as 75% in symptomatic neonates with acute viral myocarditis. In children, the majority of patients, especially those with mild inflammation, recover completely. Some patients develop subacute or chronic myocarditis with persistent cardiomegaly with or without signs of CHF and ECG evidence of LVH or BVH. Clinically, these patients are indistinguishable from those with dilated cardiomyopathy. Myocarditis may be a precursor to some cases of idiopathic dilated cardiomyopathy. Some patients develop refractory heart failure and may become candidates for heart transplantation.

E. MANAGEMENT

1. Virus identification by viral cultures from the blood, stool, or throat washing should be attempted, and comparison of acute and convalescent sera may be made for serologic titer rise.
2. Oxygen and bed rest are recommended. Use of a "cardiac chair" or "infant seat" relieves respiratory distress.
3. Bed rest and limitation in activities are recommended during the acute phase.
4. Anticongestive medications are used for symptomatic patient with heart failure.
   a. Rapid-acting diuretics (furosemide or ethacrynic acid) and angiotensin-converting enzyme (ACE) inhibitors (captopril) or angiotensin receptor blockers are beneficial in the acute phase
   b. Rapid-acting inotropic agents (such as dobutamine, dopamine, or inodilator, milrinone) are useful in critically ill children; however, they have the potential for arrhythmia.

c. Use of digoxin is not recommended, because some patients with myocarditis are found to be exquisitely sensitive to the drug.
d. β-Blockers are not recommended in the acute phase but may be required as long-term maintenance drug.
e. Nonsteroidal antiinflammatory agents are not recommended during acute and subacute phase.
f. The role of corticosteroids is unclear at this time, except in the treatment of severe rheumatic carditis.

5. Some centers have reported beneficial effects of intravenous immunoglobulin (IVIG) (2 g/kg, over 24 hours) (with better survival and better LV function by echo) as seen with Kawasaki disease; however, the routine use of IVIG remains controversial and is not recommended broadly.
6. Arrhythmias should be treated aggressively and may require the use of IV amiodarone. In patients with significant AV conduction disturbance, permanent pacemaker may be necessary

III. PERICARDITIS

A. ETIOLOGY

1. Viral infection is probably the most common cause of pericarditis, particularly in infancy. Viral causes include coxsackie virus, herpesvirus, mumps virus, and human immunodeficiency virus (HIV), among others.
2. Bacterial infection (purulent pericarditis) is rare. Commonly encountered are *S. aureus, Streptococcus pneumoniae, Haemophilus influenzae, Neisseria meningitidis*, and streptococci.
3. ARF is a common cause of pericarditis in older children in certain parts of the world.
4. Tuberculosis (an occasional cause of constrictive pericarditis with insidious onset).
5. Heart surgery (postpericardiotomy syndrome).
6. Collagen disease such as rheumatoid arthritis.
7. A complication of oncologic disease or its therapy, including radiation.
8. Uremia (uremic pericarditis).

B. PATHOLOGY AND PATHOPHYSIOLOGY

1. Pericardial effusion may be serofibrinous, hemorrhagic, or purulent. Effusion may be completely reabsorbed or may result in pericardial thickening or chronic constriction (constrictive pericarditis). Findings of myocarditis are also present in about one-third of the patients.
2. Symptoms and signs of pericardial effusion are determined by two factors: speed of fluid accumulation and competence of the myocardium. A rapid accumulation of a large amount of pericardial fluid produces more serious circulatory embarrassment. A slow accumulation of a large amount of fluid may be well tolerated by

stretching of the pericardium, if the myocardium is intact. A rapid accumulation of even a small amount of fluid in the presence of myocarditis can produce circulatory embarrassment.

3. When the pericardial effusion builds up, resulting in compression of the heart, it is called cardiac tamponade. Onset may be rapid or gradual. With the development of pericardial tamponade, several compensatory mechanisms are called on: systemic and pulmonary venous constriction (to improve diastolic filling), an increase in the SVR (to raise falling blood pressure), and tachycardia (to improve cardiac output).

C. CLINICAL MANIFESTATIONS

1. Precordial or substernal pain (sharp, dull, aching, or stabbing) with occasional radiation to the shoulder and neck may be a presenting complaint. The pain may be relieved by leaning forward and made worse by supine position or deep inspiration.
2. Pericardial friction rub is the pathognomonic physical sign. The heart is hypodynamic, and heart murmur is usually absent. In children with purulent pericarditis, septic fever (101° to 105°F [38° to 41° C), tachycardia, chest pain, and dyspnea are almost always present. Signs of cardiac tamponade may be present (distant heart sounds, tachycardia, pulsus paradoxus, hepatomegaly, neck vein distention, and occasional hypotension with peripheral vasoconstriction).
3. The ECG may show a low-voltage QRS complex, ST-segment shift, and T-wave inversion.
4. Chest radiographs may show a varying degree of cardiomegaly. Water bottle–shaped heart and increased pulmonary venous markings are seen with large effusion.
5. Echo is the most useful tool in establishing the diagnosis of pericardial effusion. It appears as an echo-free space between the epicardium (visceral pericardium) and the parietal pericardium.
    a. Small pericardial effusion first appears posteriorly in the dependent portion of the pericardial sac. A small amount of fluid, which appears only in systole, is normal. With larger effusion, the fluid also appears anteriorly. With very large effusions, the swinging motion of the heart may be imaged.
    b. The following are helpful 2D echo findings of cardiac tamponade.
        (1) Tamponade usually occurs with circumferential effusion.
        (2) Collapse of the RA in late diastole (Fig. 12.1) is seen in subcostal views (because the pressure in the pericardial sac exceeds the pressure within the RA at end-diastole when the atrium has emptied).
        (3) Diastolic collapse or indentation of the RV free wall, especially the outflow tract, best seen in parasternal long axis view.

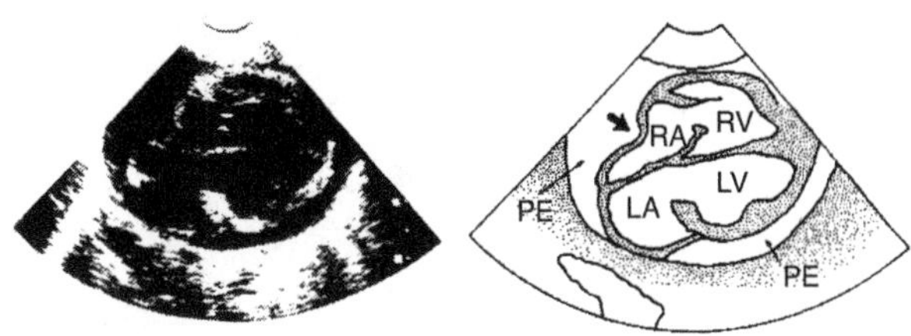

FIG. 12.1

Subcostal four-chamber view demonstrating pericardial effusion (*PE*) and collapse of the right atrial wall (*arrow*), a sign of cardiac tamponade.

D. MANAGEMENT

1. Pericardiocentesis or surgical drainage to identify the cause of the pericarditis is mandatory, especially when purulent or tuberculous pericarditis is suspected. A drainage catheter may be left in place with intermittent low-pressure drainage.
2. Pericardial fluid studies include blood cell counts and differential, glucose, and protein concentrations; histologic examination of cells; Gram and acid-fast stains; and viral, bacterial, and fungal cultures.
3. For cardiac tamponade, urgent decompression by surgical drainage or pericardiocentesis should be carried out. While preparing for the procedure, fluid push with crystalloids and colloids should be given to increase central venous pressure and thereby improve cardiac filling, which can provide temporary emergency stabilization. Medications that decrease systemic pressure such as vasodilators and diuretics should be avoided.
4. Urgent surgical drainage of the pericardium is indicated when purulent pericarditis is suspected. This must be followed by IV antibiotic therapy for 4 to 6 weeks.
5. There is no specific treatment for viral pericarditis.
6. Salicylates are given for precordial pain in patients with nonbacterial or rheumatic pericarditis.
7. Corticosteroid therapy may be indicated in children with severe rheumatic carditis or postpericardiotomy syndrome.

IV. CONSTRICTIVE PERICARDITIS

A. CAUSES AND PATHOLOGY

1. Although rare in children, constrictive pericarditis may be associated with an earlier viral pericarditis, tuberculous pericarditis, incomplete

drainage of purulent pericarditis, hemopericardium, mediastinal irradiation, neoplastic infiltration, or connective tissue disorders.
2. In this condition, a fibrotic, thickened, and adherent pericardium restricts diastolic filling of the heart.

B. CLINICAL MANIFESTATIONS

1. Distended jugular veins, hepatomegaly with ascites, and systemic edema may be present. Auscultation of the heart may reveal diastolic pericardial knock, which resembles the opening snap, along the left sternal border in the absence of heart murmur.
2. Chest radiographs may show calcification of the pericardium, enlargement of the superior SVC and LA, and pleural effusion.
3. The ECG may show low QRS voltages, T-wave inversion or flattening, and LAH. Atrial fibrillation occasionally is seen.
4. Echo findings.
    a. Two-dimensional echo shows (1) a thickened pericardium, (2) dilated IVC and hepatic vein, and (3) paradoxical septal motion and abrupt displacement of the interventricular septum during early diastolic filling ("septal bounce") (not specific for this condition).
    b. M-mode echo may reveal two parallel lines representing the thickened visceral and parietal pericardia or multiple dense echoes.
    c. Doppler examination of the mitral inflow reveals findings of diastolic dysfunction (see Fig. 11.2) and a marked respiratory variation in diastolic inflow tracings.
5. Cardiac catheterization may document the presence of constrictive physiology.
    a. The RA and LA pressures, ventricular end-diastolic pressures, and PA wedge pressure are all elevated and usually equalized.
    b. Ventricular pressure waveforms demonstrate the characteristic "square root sign" (in which there is an early rapid fall in diastolic pressure followed by a rapid rise to an elevated diastolic plateau).

C. TREATMENT

The treatment for constrictive pericarditis is complete resection of the pericardium; symptomatic improvement occurs in 75% of patients.

V. KAWASAKI DISEASE

A. ETIOLOGY AND EPIDEMIOLOGY

1. The cause of Kawasaki disease (KD) is not known. It may be related to abnormalities of the immune system initiated by an infectious insult. Children of all racial and ethnic groups are affected, although it is more common in Asians and Pacific islanders.
2. It peaks in winter and spring in the United States. It occurs primarily in young children; 80% of the patients are younger than age 4 years, 50%

are younger than age 2 years, and cases in children older than 8 years and younger than 3 months are rarely reported.

B. PATHOLOGY

1. During the first 10 days after the onset of fever, a multisystem vasculitis develops, which has the greatest predilection for the coronary arteries. Other arteries such as iliac, femoral, axillary, and renal arteries are less frequently involved.
2. Coronary artery (CA) aneurysm may develop in 15% to 20% of patients.
3. There is also pancarditis, involving the AV conduction system (which can produce AV block), myocardium (myocardial dysfunction, CHF), pericardium (pericardial effusion), and endocardium (with AV valve involvement).
4. Late changes (after 40 days) consist of healing and fibrosis in the CAs, with thrombus formation and stenosis in the postaneurysmal segment and myocardial fibrosis from old myocardial infarction.
5. The elevated platelet count seen in this condition contributes to coronary thrombosis.
6. Fate of aneurysms. Mildly dilated arteries may be able to return to normal. Large saccular aneurysms have lost their intima, media, and elastica, which cannot be regenerated. Fusiform aneurysms with partially preserved media can thrombose or develop progressive stenosis. Large or giant CA aneurysms >8 mm do not resolve, regress, or remodel. They rarely rupture and always contain thrombi that can become occlusive.

C. CLINICAL MANIFESTATIONS

The clinical course of the disease may be divided into three phases: acute, subacute, and convalescent.

1. Acute phase (first 10 days)
   a. Six signs that comprise the principal clinical features of KD are present during the acute phase (see Box 12.5).
      (1) Abrupt onset of fever, usually >39°C (102°F) and often >40°C (104°F); fever persists for a mean of 11 days without treatment.
      (2) Bilateral conjunctivitis without exudate, which resolves rapidly.
      (3) Changes in the lips and oral cavity: erythema, dryness, fissuring, and bleeding of the lips, "strawberry tongue," and diffuse erythema of the oropharynx.
      (4) Changes in extremities: erythema of the palms and soles, firm edema, and sometimes painful induration.
      (5) Diffuse maculopapular eruption involving the trunk, extremities, and perineal region; desquamation usually occurs by days 5 to 7.
      (6) Unilateral cervical lymphadenopathy, usually >1.5 cm, in approximately 50% of patients.

BOX 12.5

DIAGNOSIS OF CLASSIC KAWASAKI DISEASE

- Fever persisting at least 5 days
- Presence of at least four of the following principal features:
  1. Erythema and cracking of lips, strawberry tongue, and/or erythema of oral and pharyngeal mucosa
  2. Bilateral bulbar conjunctival injection without exudates.
  3. Rash: maculopapular, diffuse erythroderma, or erythema multiform–like
  4. Erythema and edema of the hands and feet in acute phase and/or periungual desquamation in subacute phase
  5. Cervical lymphadenopathy (>1.5 cm in diameter), usually unilateral.
- Exclusion of other diseases with similar findings (see Differential Diagnosis).

Adapted from McCrindle, B. W., Rowley, A. H., Newburger, J. W., et al. (2017). Diagnosis, treatment, and long-term management of Kawasaki disease: a scientific statement for Health Professionals from the American Heart Association. *Circulation, 135*(17), e927-e999.

b. Abnormal CV findings may include some or all of the following: tachycardia, gallop rhythm, and/or other signs of heart failure, MR murmur, cardiomegaly on chest radiographs. The ECG may show arrhythmias, prolonged PR interval (occurring in up to 60%), nonspecific ST-T change, or abnormal Q waves (wide and deep) suggestive of myocardial infarction. Chest radiographs may show cardiomegaly if myocarditis or significant CA abnormality or valvular regurgitation is present.

c. Echocardiography
   (1) CA aneurysm rarely occurs before day 10 of illness; it appears at the end of the first week through the second week of illness. However, other suggestive signs including dilatation of proximal CA segments may appear.
   (2) Aneurysms of the CA are classified as saccular (nearly equal axial and lateral diameters), fusiform (symmetric dilatation with gradual proximal and distal tapering), and ectatic (dilated without segmental aneurysm). "Giant" aneurysm is present when the diameter of the aneurysm is ≥8 mm.
   (3) During the acute phase (before CA aneurysm appears), other echo findings suggestive of cardiac involvement may appear: perivascular brightness and ectasia (dilatation), LV enlargement with decreased LV systolic function, mild MR, and pericardial effusion.
   (4) During the acute phase, detection of dilated proximal CA segments is important in the diagnosis of the disease. All major proximal CA segments (left main CA [LMCA], left anterior descending [LAD], and right CA [RCA]) should be measured and compared with normal values (see Table D.6, Appendix D). A coronary dimension that is greater than +3 standard deviations (SDs) in one of the three segments (left main CA

[LMCA], left anterior descending [LAD], and right CA [RCA]) or one that is greater than +2.5 SD in two proximal segments is considered abnormal.

d. Involvement of other organ systems is also frequent during the acute phase.
   (1) Arthritis or arthralgia of multiple joints (30%)
   (2) Sterile pyuria (60%)
   (3) Abdominal pain with diarrhea (20%), liver dysfunction (40%), hydrops of the gallbladder (10%, demonstrable by abdominal ultrasound) with jaundice
   (4) Irritability, lethargy or semicoma, and aseptic meningitis (25%)
   (5) Desquamating rash in groin
e. Laboratory studies. Even though laboratory results are nonspecific, they provide support for a diagnosis of KD in patients with nonclassic but suggestive clinical features.
   (1) Acute-phase reactant levels (C-reactive protein levels [CRP], erythrocyte sedimentation rate [ESR]) are always elevated, which is uncommon with viral illnesses. The CPR is more useful as a marker of inflammation than the ESR in KS; IVIG infusion therapy can cause an elevated ESR (but not CRP).
   (2) Marked leukocytosis with a shift to the left and anemia are common during acute phase. (Leukopenia and lymphocyte predominance suggest a viral illness.)
   (3) Thrombocytosis (usually >450,000/mm^3) is a characteristic feature of KD but does not occurs until after day 7 of the illness, sometimes reaching 600,000 to >1 million/mm^3 during the subacute phase. Low platelet count suggests viral illness.
   (4) Elevated liver enzymes (transaminases) (>2 times the upper limit of normal) in 40% of patients; hypoalbuminemia, and mild hyperbilirubinemia may be present in 10%.
   (5) Decreased albumin <3 g/dL may occur.
   (6) Pyuria (due to urethritis) is seen in up to 80% of children with KD.
   (7) Elevated serum cardiac troponin I may occur, which suggests myocardial damage.

2. Subacute phase (11 to 25 days after onset)

   The following clinical findings are seen during the subacute phase.
   a. Desquamation of the tips of the fingers and toes takes place (within 2 to 3 weeks of illness).
   b. Rash, fever, and lymphadenopathy disappear.
   c. Significant cardiovascular changes, including coronary aneurysm (seen in approximately 20%), pericardial effusion, CHF, and myocardial infarction, can occur in this phase.
   d. Thrombocytosis also occurs during this period (peaking at 2 weeks or more after the onset of the illness).

3. Convalescent phase

   This phase lasts until the elevated ESR and platelet count return to normal. Deep transverse grooves (Beau lines) may appear across the fingernails and toenails.

D. NATURAL HISTORY

1. It is a self-limited disease for most patients.
2. However, CA aneurysm occurs in 15% to 25% of patients and is responsible for myocardial infarction (fewer than 5%) and mortality (1% to 5%). If the CA remains normal throughout the first month after onset, subsequent development of a coronary lesion is extremely unusual. However, it may be wise to repeat the echo study at 8 weeks after the onset of the illness to comfortably rule out CA involvement.
3. CA aneurysm has a tendency to regress within a year in about 50% of patients, but these arteries do not dilate normally in response to exercise or coronary vasodilators.
4. In some patients, stenosis, tortuosity, and thrombosis of the coronary arteries result.

E. DIAGNOSIS

1. The diagnosis of KD is based on clinical findings. Box 12.5 lists the principal clinical features that establish the diagnosis.
   a. Fever for ≥5 days and at least four of the five principal criteria establish the diagnosis of KD (see Box 12.5). Lymphadenopathy is present only in 50% of cases.
   b. When CA abnormality is detected, fever for ≥5 days and fewer than four criteria can be diagnosed as having KD. Indeed, a substantial fraction of children with KD with CA anomalies never meet the diagnostic criteria. However, CA aneurysm rarely occurs before day 10 of the disease. During this period, perivascular brightness or ectasia (dilatation) of the CA, decreased LV systolic function, mild MR, or pericardial effusion may be present instead.
2. Incomplete (preferable to "atypical") KD with two or three principal features creates a management problem (due to serious consequences of not giving IVIG). Incomplete KD is more common in young infants than older children. Therefore, physicians should not wait for full manifestation of the disease and should consider other laboratory findings and abnormal echo findings in deciding whether or not to initiate treatment. Fig. 12.2 is an algorithm proposed by the AHA (McCrindle, 2017).
   a. Acute-phase reactants (with abnormal values): CRP (≥3.0 mg/dL) and ESR (≥40 mm/hr) are very helpful. In the presence of abnormal CRP or ESR, the presence of three or more abnormal laboratory findings (listed in following text) or positive echocardiogram satisfied

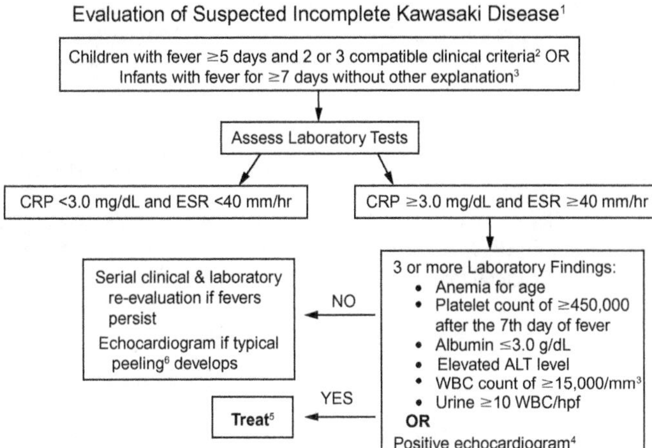

FIG. 12.2

Algorithm for evaluation of suspected incomplete Kawasaki disease. Notes: (1) The algorithm is not evidence based; it represents the informed opinion of the expert committee. (2) Clinical findings of Kawasaki disease are listed in Box 12.5. Characteristics suggesting that another diagnosis should be considered include exudative conjunctivitis, exudative pharyngitis, ulcerative intraoral lesions, bullous or vesicular rash, generalized adenopathy, or splenomegaly. (3) Infants ≤6 months of age are the most likely to develop prolonged fever without other clinical criteria or Kawasaki disease; these infants are at particularly high risk of developing coronary artery (CA) abnormalities. (4) Echocardiography is considered positive for purposes of this algorithm if any of three conditions are met: (a) *z* score of left anterior descending CA or right CA ≥2.5; (b) CA aneurysm is observed; or (c) ≥3 other suggestive features exist, including decreased left ventricular function, mitral regurgitation, pericardial effusion, or *z* score in left anterior descending CA or right CA of 2 to 2.5. (5) If the echocardiogram findings are positive, treatment should be given within 10 days of fever onset or after the 10th day of fever in the presence of clinical and laboratory signs CRP or ESR of ongoing inflammation. (6) Typical peeling begins under the nail beds of fingers and toes. *ALT*, alanine aminotransferase; *CPR*, C-reactive protein; *ESR*, erythrocyte sedimentation rate; *WBC*, white blood cell. *(Adapted from McCrindle, B. W., Rowley, A. H., Newburger, J. W., et al. (2017). Diagnosis, treatment, and long-term management of Kawasaki disease: a scientific statement for Health Professionals from the American Heart Association.* Circulation, 135*(17), e927-e999.)*

the diagnosis of incomplete KD. Even if there are less than three abnormal lab tests, abnormal echo findings qualifies for treatment.

b. Other supplemental laboratory tests (with their abnormal values) are as follows: (a) anemia for age, (b) platelets ≥450,000/mm^3 after 7 days, (c) serum albumin (≤3.0 g/dL), (d) elevated alanine aminotranferase (> 50 or 60 U/L), (e) white blood cell count (≥15,000/mm^3), and (f) urine white cell (≥10 cells/high-power field).

F. DIFFERENTIAL DIAGNOSIS

a. Measles and group A β-hemolytic streptococcal infection most closely mimic KD.
b. Others include viral infections (e.g., measles, adenovirus, enterovirus, Epstein-Barr virus), scarlet fever, staphylococcal scalded skin syndrome, toxic shock syndrome, bacterial cervical lymphadenopathy, drug hypersensitivity reaction, Stevens-Johnson syndrome, juvenile rheumatoid arthritis, and Rocky Mountain spotted fever.

G. MANAGEMENT

Two goals of therapy are (a) reduction of inflammation within the CA (by high-dose IVIG) and (b) prevention of thrombosis by inhibition of platelet aggregation (by aspirin).

1. A high dose of IVIG (2 g/kg) is given as a single infusion (given slowly in a 10- to 12-hour infusion). It should be given ideally by 7 days of illness but at least within the first 10 days of illness. Following IVIG infusion, two-thirds of patients become afebrile by 24 hours after completion of infusion; 90% are afebrile by 48 hours.
2. Aspirin (ASA) in high dose (80 to 100 mg/kg/day, administered every 6 hours) is given for its antiinflammatory and antipyretic effects. In most centers, after fever has resolved for 48 to 72 hours, the aspirin dose is lowered to 3 to 5 kg/day given in single dose. The low-dose aspirin is continued for 6 to 8 weeks when no evidence of coronary changes exists. For children with coronary abnormalities, aspirin may be continued indefinitely.

   In Japan and Western Europe, the antiplatelet dose (3 to 5 mg/kg/day) of aspirin is given from the onset, because the high-dose aspirin does not have antiplatelet effect, does not appear to reduce coronary aneurysm, and may result in increased frequency of hepatotoxicity, gastrointestinal irritation and bleeding, and Reye syndrome.
3. Other antiinflammatory agents, such as corticosteroids, abciximab, and infliximab, have been reported to have varying levels of beneficial effects on the CA aneurysm. Because the data on IVIG efficacy are so clear, these antiinflammatory drugs are not considered reasonable monotherapy. Some of them may be used in select patients with special problems (as discussed in the following text).
4. **IVIG-resistant patients** (defined as those patients who develop recrudescent or persistent fever at least 36 hours after the end of their IVIG infusion, occurring in 10% to 20% of KD patients). The following are the 2017 AHA recommendations (McCrindle, 2017).

a. A second dose of IVIG (2 g/kg) may be given to patients with persistent or recrudescent fever at least 36 hours after the end of the first IVIG infusion.
b. The following medications may be tried as an *alternative* to a second infusion of IVIG.
   (1) High-dose pulse steroids (usually methylprednisolone 20 to 30 mg/kg intravenously for 3 days, with or without a subsequent course of oral prednisone).
   (2) Infliximab (5 mg/kg).
c. A longer (e.g., 2 to 3 weeks) tapering course of prednisolone or prednisone, *together with* IVIG 2 g/kg and ASA.
d. The following may be tried on patients who have failed after a second IVIG infusion plus other regimens: (1) cyclosporine; (2) immunomodulatory monoclonal antibody therapy (except tumor necrosis factor-α blockers).

5. Prevention of thrombosis during the acute illness (McCrindle, 2017).
   a. Low-dose ASA (3 to 5 mg/kg/day) should be administered to patients without evidence of CA changes until 4 to 6 weeks after onset of illness.
   b. For patients with rapidly expanding CA aneurysms, systemic anticoagulation with low-molecular-weight heparin (LMWH) or warfarin (international normalized ratio target 2.0 to 3.0) in addition to low-dose ASA is reasonable.
   c. For patients with large or giant aneurysms (≥8 mm) or *z* score ≥ 10 and a recent history of CA thrombosis, triple therapy with ASA, a second antiplatelet agent (e.g., dipyridamole [Persantine] or clopidogrel [Plavix]), and anticoagulation with warfarin or LMWH may be considered.
6. Treatment of CA thrombosis.
   a. CA thrombosis with actual or impending occlusion of the arterial lumen should be treated with thrombolytic therapy or in patients of sufficient size, by mechanical restoration of CA blood flow at cardiac catheterization.
   b. Thrombolytic agents should be administered together with low-dose ASA and low-dose heparin, with careful monitoring for bleeding.

H. NATURAL HISTORY

Kawasaki's disease is a self-limited disease for most patients. Cardiovascular involvement is the most serious complication.

1. Coronary aneurysm develops in 15% to 25% of untreated patients and is responsible for myocardial infarction (<5%) and mortality (1% to 5%). Significantly higher temperature (101.3°F [38.5°C] on days 9 to 12) and longer duration of fever (> 14 days) appear to be risk factors for coronary aneurysm.
2. Angiographic resolution of aneurysm 1 to 2 years after the illness occurs in 50% to 67% of the patients, but these arteries do not dilate in response to exercise or coronary vasodilators.

3. More than 70% of myocardial infarctions occur in the first year after onset of the disease. Giant aneurysm (>8 mm) is associated with a greater morbidity and mortality (because of thrombotic occlusion or stenotic obstruction and subsequent myocardial infarction).
4. If the coronary arteries remain normal throughout the first month after the onset, subsequent development of a new coronary lesion is extremely unusual.

I. LONG-TERM FOLLOW-UP

Serial cardiology follow-up is important for evaluation of the cardiac status. The recommendations of the AHA Rheumatic Fever, Endocarditis, and Kawasaki Disease Committee (Newburger et al., 2004) are summarized in Table 12.2.

1. For children with no or transient coronary abnormalities, aspirin is discontinued after 6 to 8 weeks. No follow-up diagnostic tests are indicated.
2. If there is coronary aneurysm, low-dose ASA is continued indefinitely. With large aneurysm, a combination of aspirin and warfarin is indicated.
3. Varying levels of activity restriction are indicated in patients who have CA aneurysm.
4. **Echocardiography.** If significant abnormalities of the coronary vessels, LV dysfunction, or valvular regurgitation are found, the echo should be repeated at 6- to 12-month intervals. In the absence of CA abnormalities in the first 6 to 8 weeks, follow-up echoes are not indicated.
5. Exercise stress testing or myocardial perfusion evaluation is indicated in children with CA aneurysms at 1- to 2-year intervals.
6. Occasionally, coronary angiography may be indicated in infants with large aneurysms or stenosis, in patients with symptoms suggestive of ischemia, in patients with positive exercise tests or thallium studies, and/or those with evidence of myocardial infarction.
7. Rarely for patients with evidence of reversible ischemia from CA stenosis (demonstrable on stress imaging tests), percutaneous intervention, such as balloon angioplasty, rotational atherectomy, stenting, or a combination of these procedures may be indicated. On rare occasions, CA bypass surgery may be indicated. The internal mammary artery graft may be used for bypass surgery.

VI. ACUTE RHEUMATIC FEVER

A. PREVALENCE

Acute rheumatic fever (ARF) is a relatively uncommon disease in the United States and developed countries. However, in the past few decades, new outbreaks have occurred and new sporadic cases are being reported in the United States. The disease usually affects children 6 to 15 years of age (with a park incidence at 8 years of age).

TABLE 12.2

FOLLOW-UP RECOMMENDATIONS ACCORDING TO THE DEGREE OF CORONARY ARTERY INVOLVEMENT

RISK LEVEL	PHARMACOLOGIC THERAPY	PHYSICAL ACTIVITY	FOLLOW-UP AND DIAGNOSTIC TESTING	INVASIVE TESTING
I No CA changes at any stage of illness	None beyond first 6-8 weeks (Aspirin for first 6-8 weeks only)	No restrictions beyond first 6-8 weeks	Cardiovascular risk assessment, counseling at 5-year intervals	None recommended
II Transient CA ectasia disappears within first 6-8 weeks	None beyond first 6-8 weeks (Aspirin for first 6-8 weeks only)	No restrictions beyond initial 6-8 weeks	Cardiovascular risk assessment and counseling at 3- to 5-year intervals	None recommended
III One small to medium CA aneurysm/major CA	Low-dose aspirin (3-5 mg/kg/day), at least until aneurysm regression documented	For patients <11 years old, no restrictions beyond initial 6—8 weeks For patients 11-20 years old, physical activity guided by stress test or myocardial perfusion scan every 2 years Contact or high-impact sports discouraged for patients taking antiplatelet agents	Annual cardiology follow-up with echocardiogram and ECG Cardiovascular risk assessment and counseling Stress test with myocardial perfusion scan every 2 years in patients >10 years old	Angiography if noninvasive test suggests ischemia

TABLE 12.2 *(continued)*

FOLLOW-UP RECOMMENDATIONS ACCORDING TO THE DEGREE OF CORONARY ARTERY INVOLVEMENT

RISK LEVEL	PHARMACOLOGIC THERAPY	PHYSICAL ACTIVITY	FOLLOW-UP AND DIAGNOSTIC TESTING	INVASIVE TESTING
IV One or more large or giant CA aneurysms, or multiple or complex aneurysms in same CA without obstruction	Long-term aspirin (3-5 mg/kg/day) and warfarin (target: INR 2.0-2.5) or low-molecular heparin (target: antifactor Xa level 0.5-1.0 U/ml) should be combined in giant aneurysm	Contact or high-impact sports should be avoided because of risk of bleeding Other physical activity recommendations guided by annual stress test or myocardial perfusion evaluation	Cardiology follow-up with echocardiogram and ECG every 6 months Annual stress test with myocardial perfusion evaluation For females of child-bearing age, reproductive counseling is recommended	First angiography at 6-12 months or sooner if clinically indicated Repeat angiography if noninvasive test, clinical, or laboratory findings suggest ischemia Elective repeat angiography under some circumstances (atypical anginal pain, inability to do stress testing, etc.)
V CA obstruction	Long-term low-dose aspirin (3-5 mg/kg/day) Warfarin or low-molecular- weight heparin if giant aneurysm persists Consider use of β-blocker to reduce myocardial oxygen consumption	Contact or high-impact sports should be avoided because of risk of bleeding Other physical activity recommendations guided by stress test or myocardial perfusion scan	Cardiology follow-up with echocardiogram and ECG every 6 months Annual stress test or myocardial perfusion scan For females of child-bearing age, reproductive counseling is recommended	Angiography recommended to address therapeutic options of bypass grafting or catheter intervention

CA, coronary artery; *ECG*, electrocardiogram; *INR*, international normalized ratio.

Modified from Newburger, J. W., Takahashi, M., Gerber, M. A., et al. (2004). Diagnosis, treatment, and long-term management of Kawasaki disease: a statement for health professionals from the Committee on Rheumatic Fever, Endocarditis, and Kawasaki Disease, Council on Cardiovascular Disease in the Young, American Heart Association. *Pediatrics, 114*(6), 1708-1733.

B. ETIOLOGY AND PATHOLOGY

1. ARF is believed to be an immunologic response that occurs as a delayed sequela of group A streptococcal (GAS) infection of the pharynx, but not of the skin.
2. The inflammatory lesion is found in many parts of the body, most notably in the heart, brain, joints, and skin. Although rheumatic carditis was considered to be pancarditis, valvulitis is much more important than myocardial and pericardial involvements.
3. The mitral valve is most frequently involved and most severely affected. Mitral regurgitation occurs in about 95% of the patients and aortic regurgitation in 20% to 25% of the patients.

C. CLINICAL MANIFESTATIONS

1. History of streptococcal pharyngitis 1 to 5 weeks (average 3 weeks) before the onset of symptoms may be elicited. The latent period may be as long as 2 to 6 months (average 4 months) in cases of isolated chorea.
2. Clinical manifestations of ARF may be grouped into (a) five major criteria, (b) four minor criteria, and (c) supporting evidence of preceding streptococcal infection (Box 12.6). Among the five major manifestations, carditis (50% to 79%) and arthritis (35% to 66%) are more common

BOX 12.6

REVISED JONES CRITERIA (2015)[a]

Major Criteria	Minor Criteria
• Carditis (clinical and/or subclinical)	• Polyarthralgia
• Arthritis (polyarthritis only)	• Fever ≥38.5°C
• Chorea	• ESR ≥60 mm/hr and/or CRP ≥3.0 mg/dL
• Erythema marginatum	• Prolonged PR interval for age
• Subcutaneous nodules	

Evidence of Prior Group A Streptococcal Infection (any one of the following)

- Increased or rising ASO titer (or anti-DNASE B)
- Positive throat culture for group A β-hemolytic streptococci
- Positive rapid group A streptococcal carbohydrate antigen

Diagnosis

Initial ARF:	2 Major criteria, or 1 Major criterion + 2 Minor criteria
Recurrent ARF:	2 Major criteria, or 1 Major criterion + 2 Minor criteria, or 3 Minor criteria + Evidence of preceding GAS infection

[a]For low-risk population only. Note that for moderate- or high-risk population areas, a lighter requirement for the diagnosis of ARF exists.

ARF, acute rheumatic fever; *ASO*, antistreptolysin O; *CRP*, C-reactive protein; *ESR*, *GAS*, group A streptococcal.
Modified from Gewitz, M. H., Baltimore, R. S., Tani, L. Y., et al. (2015). Revision of the Jones criteria for the diagnosis of acute rheumatic fever in the era of Doppler echocardiography: a scientific statement from the American Heart Association. *Circulation, 131*(2), 1806-1818.

than the others. These are followed by chorea (10% to 30%), subcutaneous nodules (0% to 10%), and lastly erythema marginatum (<6%).

3. Major manifestations
   a. Carditis is in the most common manifestation of ARF (50% to 79%)
      (1) Tachycardia (out of proportion to the degree of fever) is common. A heart murmur of MR and/or AR is almost always present. Clinical presentation may be quite variable from the asymptomatic patients with characteristic heart murmur to the critically ill patients presenting in heart failure (occurring in 15% to 25%).
      (2) Echo examination can determine the presence and severity of MR and AR more objectively than auscultation can. Inclusion of echo/Doppler findings can enhance correct diagnosis of acute rheumatic carditis, including those with *subclinical carditis* (see later text for further discussion). Other abnormal echo findings may include pericardial effusion, increased LV dimension, or impaired LV function.
      (3) Concept of subclinical carditis. In the past, clinical evidence of carditis was based solely on the presence of heart murmur of MR and/or AR on auscultation. With increasing availability of echo/Doppler studies, more cases of cardiac involvement are being accurately detected than previously. *Subclinical carditis* refers to the circumstance in which auscultatory findings of MR and/or AR are not recorded, but echo/Doppler studies reveal evidence of mitral and/or aortic valvulitis (Box 12.7). The prevalence of subclinical carditis may reach as high as 50%. Therefore echo/Doppler studies should be performed in all cases of confirmed and suspected cases of ARF. Echo/Doppler studies should be performed strictly fulfilling the findings noted in Box 12.7 to assess whether carditis is present in the absence of auscultatory findings. Findings not consistent with carditis should exclude the diagnosis of rheumatic carditis.
   b. Arthritis involving large joints (knees, ankles, elbows, wrists) is the second most common manifestation (35% to 66%). Often more than one joint, either simultaneously or in succession, is involved, with the characteristic migratory nature of the arthritis. Swelling, heat, redness, severe pain, tenderness, and limitation of motion are common. The arthritis responds dramatically to antiinflammatory salicylate therapy; if patients treated with salicylates do not improve within 48 hours, the diagnosis of ARF probably is incorrect. Arthritis subsides in a few days to weeks even without treatment and does not cause permanent damage.
   c. Subcutaneous nodules (0% to 10%) are hard, painless, nonpruritic, freely movable swellings, 0.5 to 2 cm in diameter. They are usually found symmetrically, singly, or in clusters on the extensor surfaces of

BOX 12.7

ECHOCARDIOGRAPHY AND DOPPLER FINDINGS IN RHEUMATIC VALVULITIS

MORPHOLOGIC FINDINGS	DOPPLER FINDINGS

• Acute mitral valve changes
  • Annular dilation
  • Chordal elongation
  • Chordal rupture resulting in flail leaflet with severe mitral regurgitation
  • Anterior (or less commonly posterior) leaflet tip prolapse
  • Beading/nodularity of the leaflet tips
• Chronic mitral valve changes: not seen in acute carditis
  • Leaflet thickening
  • Chordal thickening and fusion
  • Restricted leaflet motion
  • Calcification
• Aortic valve changes in either acute or chronic carditis
  • Irregular or focal leaflet thickening
  • Coaptation defect
  • Restricted leaflet motion
  • Leaflet prolapse
	• Pathologic mitral regurgitation (all 4 criteria met)
	  • Seen in at least 2 views
	  • Jet length ≥2 cm in at least 1 view
	  • Peak velocity >3 m/sec
	  • Pansystolic jet in at least 1 envelope
	• Pathologic aortic regurgitation (all 4 criteria met)
	  • Seen in at least 2 views
	  • Jet length ≥1 cm in at least 1 view
	  • Peak velocity >3 m/sec
	  • Pandiastolic jet in at least 1 envelope

Modified from Gewitz, M. H., Baltimore, R. S., Tani, L. Y., et al. (2015). Revision of the Jones criteria for the diagnosis of acute rheumatic fever in the era of Doppler echocardiography: a scientific statement from the American Heart Association. *Circulation, 131*(2), 1806-1818.

both large and small joints, over the scalp, or along the spine. They are not transient, lasting for weeks, and have a significant association with carditis. They are also found in conditions other than rheumatic fever (such as rheumatoid arthritis and systemic lupus erythematosus).

d. Erythema marginatum (<6%), with the characteristic nonpruritic serpiginous or annular erythematous rashes, is most prominent on the trunk and the inner proximal portions of the extremities. The rashes are evanescent, disappearing on exposure to cold and reappearing after a hot shower or when the patient is covered with a warm blanket.
e. Sydenham chorea, or St. Vitus dance (10% to 30%), is found more often in prepubertal (8 to 12 years) girls than in boys. It is a neuropsychiatric disorder consisting of both neurologic disorders (choreic movement and hypotonia) and psychiatric components (such as emotional lability, hyperactivity, separation anxiety, obsessions, and compulsions). It begins initially with emotional lability and personality changes, soon (in 1 to 4 weeks) replaced by

the characteristic spontaneous, purposeless movement of chorea, which is followed by motor weakness. The choreic movements last for an average of 7 months (and up to 17 months) before slowly waning in severity. It is often an isolated manifestation; the patient may have no fever, and ESR and antistreptolysin O (ASO) titers may be normal. Recently, elevated titers of "antineuronal antibodies" recognizing basal ganglion tissues have been found in over 90% of patients, suggesting that chorea may be related to dysfunction of basal ganglia and cortical neuronal components.

4. Four minor manifestations include fever, arthralgia, elevated acute-phase reactants (elevated ESR and CRP), and prolonged PR interval (see Box 12.6).
   a. Polyarthralgia refers to multiple joint pain without the objective changes of arthritis.
   b. Fever (usually with a temperature of at least 101.3°F [38.5°C]) is present early in the course of untreated rheumatic fever.
   c. Elevated acute-phase reactants (elevated CRP levels and elevated ESR) are objective evidence of an inflammatory process.
   d. A prolonged PR interval on the ECG is neither specific for ARF nor an indication of active carditis.
5. Evidence of antecedent group A streptococcal infection.
   Laboratory evidence of antecedent group A streptococcal infection is needed for the diagnosis. Exception to this includes chorea, which usually has a long latent period, and insidious onset of the illness. Any one of the following can serve as evidence of preceding infection according to a recent AHA statement.
   a. Increased or rising ASO titer or other streptococcal antibodies (anti-DNASE B).
   b. Positive throat culture for group A β-hemolytic streptococcus.
   c. A positive rapid group A Streptococcus carbohydrate antigen test in a child whose clinical presentation suggests a high pretest probability of streptococcal pharyngitis.

D. DIAGNOSIS

ARF is diagnosed by the use of revised Jones criteria (updated in 2015; see Box 12.6). The criteria are three groups of important clinical and laboratory findings: (1) five major criteria, (2) four minor criteria, and (3) supporting evidence of preceding GAS infection.

1. A diagnosis of ARF is highly probable when either two major criteria or one major and two minor criteria, plus evidence of antecedent streptococcal infection, are present.
2. For recurrent ARF (in individuals with previous history of ARF or those with RHD), a less rigid criteria is used because they are at high risk for recurrent attacks if reinfected with GAS. In addition to the same criteria as mentioned earlier, only three minor criteria in the presence of evidence of preceding GAS infection suffice.

3. Exceptions to the Jones criteria include the following two specific situations:
   a. Chorea may occur as the only manifestation of ARF.
   b. Indolent carditis may be the only manifestation in patients who come to medical attention months after the onset of rheumatic fever.
4. The following tips help in applying the Jones criteria:
   a. Two major criteria are always stronger than one major plus two minor criteria.
   b. Polyarthralgia or a prolonged PR interval cannot be used as a minor criterion when using arthritis and carditis, respectively, as major criterion.

E. CLINICAL COURSE

1. Only carditis can cause permanent cardiac damage. Signs of mild carditis disappear rapidly in weeks, but those of severe carditis may last for 2 to 6 months.
2. Arthritis subsides within a few days to several weeks, even without treatment, and does not cause permanent damage.
3. Chorea gradually subsides in 6 to 7 months or longer and usually does not cause permanent neurologic sequelae.

F. MANAGEMENT

1. When ARF is suggested by history and physical examination, one should obtain the following laboratory studies: complete blood count, acute-phase reactants (ESR and CRP), throat culture, ASO titer (and a second antibody titer, particularly with chorea), chest radiography films, and ECG. Cardiology consultation is indicated to clarify whether there is cardiac involvement; two-dimensional echo and Doppler studies are usually performed at that time.
2. Benzathine penicillin G, 0.6 to 1.2 million units intramuscularly, is given to eradicate streptococci. This serves as the first dose of penicillin prophylaxis as well (see later discussion). In patients allergic to penicillin, erythromycin, 40 mg/ kg per day in 2 to 4 doses for 10 days, may be substituted for penicillin.
3. Antiinflammatory or suppressive therapy with salicylates or steroids must not be started until a definite diagnosis is made. Early suppressive therapy may interfere with a definite diagnosis of ARF by suppressing full development of joint manifestations and suppressing acute-phase reactants.
4. Therapy with antiinflammatory agents should be started as soon as ARF has been diagnosed.
   a. For mild to moderate carditis, ASA alone is recommended in a dose of 90 to 100 mg/kg per day in 4 to 6 divided doses. An adequate blood level of salicylates is 20 to 25 mg/100 mL. This dose is

continued for 4 to 8 weeks, depending on the clinical response. After improvement, the therapy is withdrawn gradually over 4 to 6 weeks while monitoring acute-phase reactants.

b. For severe carditis, prednisone (2 mg/kg per day in 4 divided doses) for 2 to 6 weeks is indicated. The dose of prednisone should be tapered and ASA started during the final week of prednisone to prevent rebound.

c. For arthritis, ASA therapy is continued for 2 weeks and gradually withdrawn over the following 2 to 3 weeks.

5. When the diagnosis of ARF is confirmed, one must educate the patient and parents about the need to prevent subsequent streptococcal infection through continuous antibiotic prophylaxis.
6. Bed rest of varying duration is recommended. The duration depends on the type and severity of the manifestations and may range from a week (for isolated arthritis) to several weeks for severe carditis. Bed rest is followed by a period of indoor ambulation of varying duration before the child is allowed to return to school. The ESR is a helpful guide to the rheumatic activity and therefore to the duration of restriction of activities. Full activity is allowed when the ESR has returned to normal, except in children with significant cardiac involvement. Table 12.3 is a general guide to the period of bed rest and indoor ambulation.
7. CHF may be treated with complete bed rest, prednisone for severe carditis of recent onset, furosemide (1 mg/kg every 6 to 12 hours, if indicated) and an afterload reducing agent.
8. Management of Sydenham chorea:
   a. Reduce physical and emotional stress and use protective measures as indicated to prevent physical injuries.
   b. Give benzathine penicillin G, 1.2 million units, initially for eradication of streptococcus and also every 28 days for prevention of recurrence, just as in patients with other rheumatic manifestations. Without the prophylaxis, about 25% of patients with isolated chorea (without

TABLE 12.3

GENERAL GUIDELINES FOR BED REST AND INDOOR AMBULATION

	ARTHRITIS ALONE	MILD CARDITIS[a]	MODERATE CARDITIS[b]	SEVERE CARDITIS[c]
Bed rest	1-2 wk	3-4 wk	4-6 wk	As long as congestive heart failure is present
Indoor ambulation	1-2 wk	3-4 wk	4-6 wk	2-3 mo

[a]Questionable cardiomegaly.

[b]Definite but mild cardiomegaly.

[c]Marked cardiomegaly or heart failure.

carditis) develop rheumatic valvular heart disease in 20-year follow-up.

c. Antiinflammatory agents are not needed in patients with isolated chorea.
d. For severe cases, any of the following drugs may be used: phenobarbital, haloperidol, valproic acid, chlorpromazine (Thorazine), diazepam (Valium), or steroids.
e. Results of plasma exchange (to remove antineuronal antibodies) and IVIG therapy (to inactivate the effects of the antineuronal antibodies) are promising in decreasing the severity of chorea and they were better than prednisone (Garvey et al., 2005).

G. PROGNOSIS

The presence or absence of permanent cardiac damage determines the prognosis. The development of residual heart disease is influenced by the following three factors.

1. The more severe the cardiac involvement at the time the patient is first seen, the greater the incidence of residual heart disease.
2. The severity of valvular involvement increases with each recurrence.
3. Regression of heart disease. Evidence of cardiac involvement at the first attack may disappear in 10% to 25% of patients 10 years after the initial attack. Valvular disease resolves more frequently when prophylaxis is followed.

H. PREVENTION

1. Primary Prevention (Subhead to Prevention)

Primary prevention of rheumatic fever is possible in some patients by appropriate antibiotic treatment of streptococcal pharyngitis. However, it is not possible to treat all patients because about 30% of the patients develop subclinical pharyngitis and not all symptomatic patients seek medical care.

2. Secondary Prevention (subhead)

An individual with a previous attack of rheumatic fever is at high risk of a recurrent attack of rheumatic fever. Prevention of recurrent rheumatic fever requires continuous antimicrobial prophylaxis.

1. Patients with documented histories of rheumatic fever, including those with isolated chorea and those without evidence of rheumatic heart disease, must receive prophylaxis.
2. Ideally, patients should receive prophylaxis indefinitely. The duration of prophylaxis varies with the presence and severity of cardiac involvement (see Table 12.4).
3. Choice of antibiotics.

TABLE 12.4

RECOMMENDED DURATION OF SECONDARY RHEUMATIC FEVER PROPHYLAXIS

CATEGORY	DURATION AFTER LAST ATTACK
Rheumatic fever with carditis and residual heart disease (persistent valvular disease[a])	10 years or until 40 years of age (whichever is longer)
Rheumatic fever with carditis but no residual heart disease (no valvular disease[a])	10 years of until 21 years of age (whichever is longer)
Rheumatic fever without carditis disease)	5 years or until 21 years of age (whichever is longer)

[a]Clinical or echocardiographic evidence.

From Gerber, M. A., Baltimore, R. S., Eaton, C. B., et al. (2009). Prevention of rheumatic fever and diagnosis and treatment of acute streptococcal pharyngitis: a scientific statement from the American Heart Association Rheumatic Fever, Endocarditis, and Kawasaki Disease Committee of the Council on Cardiovascular Disease in the Young, the Interdisciplinary Council on Functional Genomics and Translational Biology, and the Interdisciplinary Council on Quality of Care and Outcome Research. *Circulation 119*(11), 1541-1551.

a. Benzathine penicillin G, 600,000 units given intramuscularly every 28 days (not once a month) for children <27 kg (60 lb) and 1.2 million units for children >60 lb is the drug of choice.
b. Alternatively, penicillin V (250 mg twice a day, oral); or sulfadiazine (oral), 0.5 g once daily for children <27 kg (60 lb); 1.0 g once a day for children >60 lb.
c. For individuals allergic to penicillin and sulfadiazine, macrolide or azalide may be given.

Chapter 13

Valvular Heart Disease

Valvular heart disease is either congenital or acquired. Many congenital valvular abnormalities are associated with other major defects. A relatively isolated form of valvular heart disease is rheumatic in origin, which still occurs in some parts of the world. Among rheumatic heart disease, mitral valve involvement occurs in about three-fourths and aortic valve involvement in about one-fourth of cases. Rheumatic involvement of the tricuspid and pulmonary valves almost never occurs. Although the cause of mitral valve prolapse (MVP) is not entirely clear, it is discussed in this chapter.

I MITRAL STENOSIS

A. PREVALENCE

MS of rheumatic origin is rare in children (because it requires 5 to 10 years from the initial attack to develop the condition), but it is the most common valvular involvement in adult rheumatic patients in areas where rheumatic fever is still prevalent. Congenital MS occurs in 0.2 to 0.6% of CHDs, usually as part of other defects.

B. PATHOLOGY AND PATHOPHYSIOLOGY

1. Congenital MS encompasses different types of obstructions occurring at different levels near the mitral valve position. The stenosis may be due to obstruction at the valve level (fusion of the leaflets), at the papillary muscle level (single papillary muscle seen with parachute mitral valve), at the chordae (thickened and fused chordae seen in single papillary muscle), or at the supravalvar region (supravalvar mitral ring), and it may be due to the hypoplasia of the valve ring itself (as seen with HLHS). Some of these anomalies are associated with other CHD.
2. In rheumatic MS, thickening of the leaflets and fusion of the commissures dominate the pathologic findings. Calcification with immobility of the valve results over time.
3. Regardless of the etiology, a significant MS results in the enlargement of the LA, pulmonary venous hypertension, and pulmonary artery hypertension with resulting enlargement and hypertrophy of the right side of the heart.
4. In patients with severe MS, pulmonary congestion and edema, fibrosis of the alveolar walls, hypertrophy of the pulmonary arterioles, and loss of lung compliance result.

C. CLINICAL MANIFESTATIONS

1. In infants with severe MS, symptoms develop early with shortness of breath and failure to thrive. Children with mild MS are asymptomatic.

With significant MS, dyspnea with or without exertion is the most common symptom in older children. Orthopnea, nocturnal dyspnea, or palpitation is present in more severe cases.

2. Neck veins are distended if right-sided heart failure supervenes. A loud S1 at the apex and a narrowly split S2 with accentuated P2 are audible if pulmonary hypertension is present (Fig. 13.1). In older children, an opening snap (a short snapping sound accompanying the opening of the mitral valve) and a low-frequency mitral diastolic rumble may be present at the apex. A crescendo presystolic murmur may be audible at the apex. Occasionally, a high-frequency diastolic murmur of PR (Graham Steell murmur) is present at the ULSB in patients with pulmonary hypertension.
3. The electrocardiogram (ECG) may show RAD, LAH, and RVH (caused by pulmonary hypertension). AF is rare in children.
4. Chest radiographs show enlargement of the LA and RV. The main PA segment is usually prominent. Lung fields show pulmonary venous congestion, interstitial edema shown as Kerley B lines (dense, short, horizontal lines most commonly seen in the costophrenic angles), and redistribution of pulmonary blood flow with increased pulmonary vascularity to the upper lobes.
5. Echo studies provide accurate diagnosis and severity of MS.
    a. Dilated LA, RV, and RA and prominent main PA are imaged.
    b. A mean Doppler gradient of <4 to 5 mm Hg results from mild stenosis, 6 to 12 mm Hg from moderate stenosis, and >13 mm Hg from severe stenosis.
    c. RV systolic pressure can be estimated from the TR jet velocity.

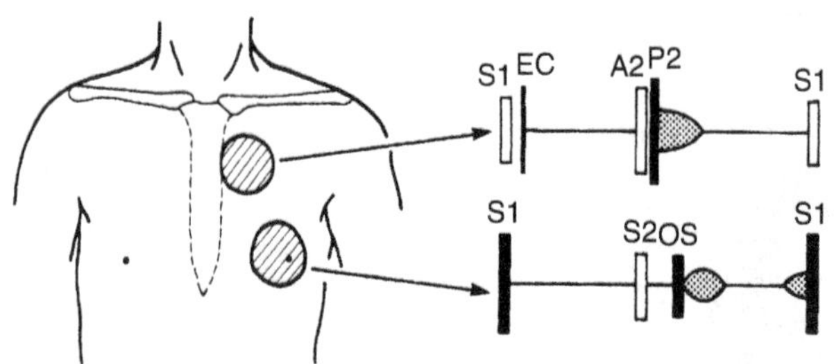

FIG. 13.1

Cardiac findings of MS. Abnormal sounds are shown in black and include a loud S1, an ejection click (*EC*), a loud S2, and an opening snap (*OS*). Also note the mid-diastolic rumble and presystolic murmur. The murmur of pulmonary insufficiency indicates long-standing pulmonary hypertension.

C. NATURAL HISTORY

1. Infants with significant MS with failure to thrive require either balloon or surgical intervention.
2. Most children with mild MS are asymptomatic but become symptomatic with exertion.
3. For rheumatic MS, recurrence of rheumatic fever worsens the stenosis.
4. Atrial flutter or fibrillation and thromboembolism (related to the chronic atrial arrhythmias) are rare in children.
5. Hemoptysis can develop from the rupture of small vessels in the bronchi as a result of long-standing pulmonary venous hypertension.

D. MANAGEMENT

Different management plans apply to congenital MS and rheumatic MS.

E. FOR CONGENITAL MITRAL STENOSIS

1. Patients with mild or moderate stenosis usually do not warrant surgery or catheter intervention.
   a. Diuretic therapy and/or varying degrees of restriction of activity may be indicated.
   b. If atrial fibrillation (AF) develops, medical treatment with propranolol, verapamil, or digoxin may be used. Cardioversion may be indicated for patients with chronic AF. Quinidine may prevent recurrence.
   c. Recurrent AF, thromboembolic phenomenon, and hemoptysis may be indications for surgery in children.
2. Patients with severe MS require relief of obstruction. Options of intervention include balloon mitral valvuloplasty, surgical valvuloplasty, or surgical valve replacement. Surgical management is challenging due to the limited life span of prosthesis, need for replacement due to growth, and need for chronic anticoagulation. Therefore in some infants with severe pathology, a Norwood or hybrid approach (as used for HLHS) early in life may be an option.

F. FOR RHEUMATIC MITRAL STENOSIS

1. For patients with rheumatic MS, secondary prevention of rheumatic fever with penicillin or sulfonamide is indicated (see Chapter 12).
2. 2014 American Heart Association/American College of Cardiology (AHA/ACC) guidelines recommend the following (Nishimura et al., 2014).
   a. Anticoagulation with warfarin or heparin is indicated in patients with (1) MS and AF or (2) MS and a prior embolic event, or (3) MS and a left atrial thrombus.
   b. Percutaneous mitral balloon commissurotomy is recommended for symptomatic patients with severe MS (defined as mitral valve area $\leq 1.5\ cm^2$, stage D) and favorable valve morphology in the absence of left atrial thrombus or moderate-to-severe MR.

c. Mitral valve surgery (repair, commissurotomy, or valve replacement) is indicated in severely symptomatic patients with severe MS (as defined earlier) who are not at high risk for surgery and who are not candidates for or who have failed previous percutaneous mitral balloon commissurotomy.

3. **Mitral valve replacement surgery**. A prosthetic valve insertion carries a surgical mortality of 0 to 19%. All mechanical valves require anticoagulation with warfarin. Reoperation may become necessary due to valve deterioration or malfunction.

G. POSTINTERVENTION FOLLOW-UP

1. Regular checkups every 6 to 12 months with echo and Doppler studies should be done for possible dysfunction of the repaired or replaced valve.
2. After replacement with a *mechanical valve*, warfarin is indicated to achieve an international normalized ratio (INR) of 2.5 to 3.5. Low-dose aspirin is also indicated.
3. After replacement with a *bioprosthesis*, if there are risk factors (e.g., AF, a prior embolic event, and a left atrial thrombus), warfarin is also indicated. When there are no risk factors, aspirin alone is indicated at 75 to 100 mg per day.

II MITRAL REGURGITATION

A. PREVALENCE

MR is more common than MS. Congenital MR is most often associated with AV canal defect. MR of rheumatic origin is rare but it is the most common valvular involvement in children with rheumatic heart disease.

B. PATHOLOGY

1. Congenital MR associated with AV canal defects occurs through the cleft in the mitral valve (with eccentric regurgitation). Rheumatic MR results from the shortening of the mitral leaflet by fibrosis (with central regurgitation).
2. With increasing severity of MR, dilatation of the LA and LV results and the mitral valve ring may become dilated. Pulmonary hypertension may eventually develop but is less common than with MS.

C. CLINICAL MANIFESTATIONS

1. Patients are usually asymptomatic with mild MR. With increasing severity of MR, a history of fatigue and palpitation may be present.
2. The S2 may split widely as a result of shortening of the LV ejection and early closure of the aortic valve. A loud S3 is common. The hallmark of MR is a grade 2 to 4/6 regurgitant systolic murmur at the apex, with good transmission to the left axilla (best demonstrated in the left decubitus position). A short, low-frequency diastolic rumble may be present at the apex (Fig. 13.2).

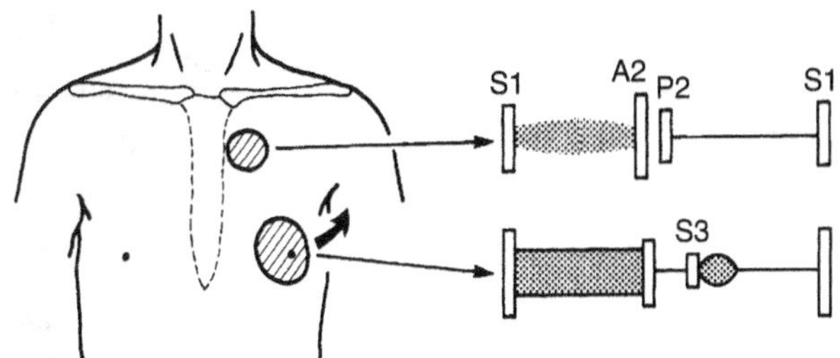

FIG. 13.2
Cardiac findings of MR. The *arrow* near the apex indicates the direction of radiation of the murmur toward the left axilla.

3. The ECG is normal in mild cases. With moderate to severe MR, LVH (or LV dominance) with or without LAH may be present. AF is rare in children but frequent in adults.
4. Chest radiographs may show LA and LV enlargement. Pulmonary venous congestion may develop if CHF supervenes.
5. Two-dimensional echo shows dilated LA and LV; the degree of the dilatation is related to the severity of MR. Color flow mapping of the regurgitant jet into the LA and Doppler studies can assess the severity of the regurgitation. The MR is central with rheumatic MR (and eccentric with congenital cleft mitral valve).
6. Natural history. Patients are relatively stable for a long time with MR. LV failure and consequent pulmonary hypertension may develop in adult life.

D. MANAGEMENT

1. Medical

1. Prophylaxis against recurrence of rheumatic fever is important.
2. Activity need not be restricted in mild cases.
3. Afterload-reducing agents (such as angiotensin-converting enzyme [ACE] inhibitors) are useful in maintaining the forward cardiac output.
4. Anticongestive therapy is provided if CHF develops.
5. If AF develops (rare in children), propranolol, verapamil, or digoxin is indicated to slow the ventricular rate.

1. Surgical

a. Indications

1. It is generally advised to delay surgery in infants and small children until the onset of severe symptoms, such as intractable CHF or progressive cardiomegaly with symptoms.

2. Mitral valve surgery is recommended for symptomatic patients with severe MR and LV ejection fraction (LVEF) greater than 30%.
3. Mitral valve surgery is recommended for asymptomatic patients with severe AR and LV systolic dysfunction (LVEF 30% to 60% and/or LV end-systolic dimension ≥40 mm).

2. Procedures and Mortality

1. Surgical repair (such as cleft repair, annuloplasty, chordal shortening, etc.) is preferable to valve replacement whenever possible. Valve repair has a lower mortality rate (<1%), and anticoagulation is not necessary.
2. Valve replacement is rarely necessary for unrepairable regurgitation. Frequently used low-profile prostheses are the Bjork-Shiley tilting disk and the St. Jude pyrolitic carbon valve. Valve replacement has a higher mortality rate (2% to 7%) than the repair surgery and anticoagulation therapy must be continued.

3. Postoperative Follow-Up

1. Valve function (of either the repaired natural valve or the replacement valve) should be checked by echo and Doppler studies every 6 to 12 months.
2. After replacement with a mechanical valve, even with no risk factors (such as AF, previous thromboembolism, LV dysfunction, and hypercoagulable state), warfarin is indicated (INR of 2.5 to 3.5) along with a low-dose aspirin.
3. After replacement with a bioprosthesis with no risk factors, aspirin alone is indicated at the dose of 75 to 100 mg per day. When there are risk factors, warfarin is also indicated.

III AORTIC REGURGITATION

A. PREVALENCE

AR is more often congenital than rheumatic in origin. AR of rheumatic origin is almost always associated with mitral valve disease

B. PATHOLOGY

1. Congenital causes of AR include bicuspid aortic valve, those associated with VSD (either subpulmonary or membranous), secondary to subaortic stenosis, and those associated with dilated aortic root (Marfan syndrome or Ehlers-Danlos syndrome).
2. Acquired type of AR is seen in rheumatic heart disease or following aortic balloon valvuloplasty.

C. CLINICAL MANIFESTATIONS

1. Patients with mild AR are asymptomatic. Exercise tolerance is reduced with more severe AR.

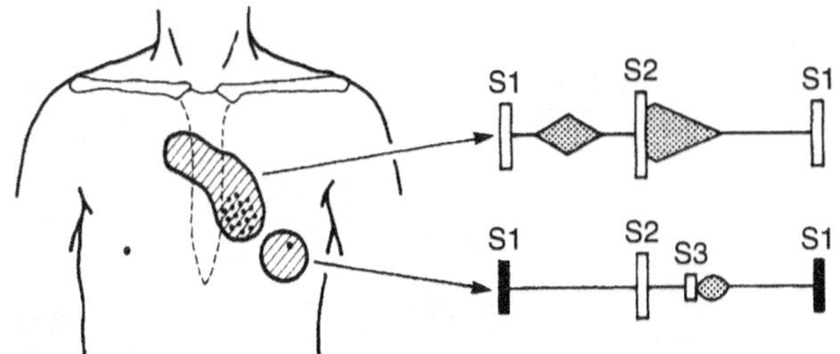

FIG. 13.3
Cardiac findings of AR. The S1 is abnormally soft (*black bar*). The predominant murmur is a high-pitched, diastolic decrescendo murmur at the third left intercostal space.

2. With moderate or severe AR, hyperdynamic precordium is present. A wide pulse pressure and a bounding water-hammer pulse may be present with severe AR. The S2 may be normal or single. A high-pitched diastolic decrescendo murmur, best audible at the third or fourth left intercostal space, is the auscultatory hallmark (Fig. 13.3). This murmur is more easily audible with the patient sitting and leaning forward. The longer the murmur, the more severe is the regurgitation. A mid-diastolic mitral rumble (Austin Flint murmur) may be present at the apex when the AR is severe.
3. The ECG is normal in mild cases. In severe cases, LVH usually is present with or without LAH.
4. Chest radiographs show cardiomegaly of varying degrees involving the LV.
5. Echo studies demonstrate an increased LV dimension. The LV diastolic dimension is proportional to the severity of AR. Color flow and Doppler examination can estimate the severity of AR. LV systolic dysfunction develops at a later stage in severe AR.
6. Natural history. Patients with mild to moderate AR remain asymptomatic for a long time, but once symptoms begin to develop, many patients deteriorate rapidly. Anginal pain, CHF, and multiple PVCs are unfavorable signs occurring with severe AR.

D. MANAGEMENT

1. Medical

1. Varying degrees of activity restriction are indicated in more severe cases.
2. When used on a long-term basis, the ACE inhibitors have been shown to reduce (or even reverse) the dilatation and hypertrophy of the LV in children with AR but without CHF.

3. If CHF develops, digoxin, diuretics, and ACE inhibitors may be temporarily beneficial, but the benefits are rarely maintained.
4. In patients with rheumatic AR, antibiotic prophylaxis (with penicillin or sulfonamide) to prevent the recurrence of rheumatic fever is indicated.

2. Surgical

a. Indications

Ideally, surgery should be performed before irreversible dilatation of the LV develops, but there is no reliable method of detecting that point. The following are recommendations of ACC/AHA 2014 guidelines for adults with chronic AR (Nishimura et al., 2014). Similar indications may apply for adolescents and younger children.

1. Aortic valve replacement (AVR) is indicated for symptomatic patient with severe AR regardless of LV systolic function.
2. AVR is indicated for asymptomatic patients with chronic severe AR and LV systolic dysfunction (LVEF $<50\%$)
3. AVR is reasonable for asymptomatic patients with severe AR with normal LV systolic function (LVEF $\geq 50\%$) but with severe LV dilatation (LV end-systolic dimension >50 mm or indexed LV end-systolic dimension $>25mm/m^2$).

3. Procedure and Mortality

Aortic valve repair is favored over valve replacement whenever possible. Valve replacement does not incorporate growth potential, except for the Ross procedure. The mortality rate for valve repair is near zero and that for valve replacement is about 2% to 5%.

1. Valve repair may include repair of simple tears or valvuloplasty for prolapsed cusps, etc. with the mortality rate of near zero.
2. Valve replacement surgery. The antibiotic-sterilized aortic homograft has been widely used and appears to be the device of choice. The porcine heterograft has the risk of accelerated degeneration, and the mechanical prostheses require anticoagulation therapy.
3. A pulmonary root autograft (Ross procedure) may be an attractive alternative to the conventional valve replacement surgery (see Fig. 8.6) in selected adolescents and young adults. In this procedure, the patient's own pulmonary valve is used to replace the diseased aortic valve. The surgical mortality rate is near zero. This procedure does not require anticoagulant therapy, the autograft may last longer than a porcine bioprosthesis, and there is a growth potential for the autograft pulmonary valve.

4. Follow-Up

1. Regular follow-up is required every 6 to 12 months with echo and Doppler studies after intervention.
2. Anticoagulation is needed after a prosthetic mechanical valve replacement (with INR 2.5 to 3.5 for the first 3 months and 2.0 to 3.0

beyond that time). Low-dose aspirin (81 mg/day for adolescents) is also indicated in addition to warfarin.

3. After aortic valve replacement with bioprosthesis and no risk factors, low-dose aspirin (81 mg) is indicated, but warfarin is not indicated. When there are risk factors (such as AF, previous thromboembolism, LV dysfunction, and hypercoagulable state), warfarin is indicated to achieve an INR of 2.0 to 3.0.
4. Following Ross procedure, anticoagulation is not indicated.

IV MITRAL VALVE PROLAPSE

A. PREVALENCE

The reported incidence of MVP of 2% to 5% in the pediatric population probably is an overestimate. The prevalence of MVP increases with age. This condition is more common in adults than in children and in females than in males.

B. PATHOLOGY

1. In the primary form of MVP, thick and redundant mitral valve leaflets bulge into the mitral annulus (caused by myxomatous degeneration of the valve leaflets and/or the chordae). The posterior leaflet is more commonly and more severely affected than the anterior leaflet.
2. MVP is associated with several heritable disorders of connective tissue disease, such as Marfan syndrome, Ehlers-Danlos syndrome, osteogenesis imperfecta, and Stickler syndrome, as well as polycystic kidney disease in adults. Nearly all patients with Marfan syndrome have MVP.
3. A CHD is present in one-third of patients with MVP. Secundum ASD is most common.

C. CLINICAL MANIFESTATIONS

1. MVP usually is asymptomatic, but a history of nonexertional chest pain, palpitation, and, rarely, syncope may be elicited. There may be a family history of MVP.
2. An asthenic build with a high incidence of thoracic skeletal anomalies (80%), including pectus excavatum (50%), straight back (20%), and scoliosis (10%), is common.
3. The midsystolic click with or without a late systolic murmur audible at the apex is the hallmark of the condition (Fig. 13.4). The presence or absence of the click and murmur, as well as their timing, varies from one examination to the next.
   a. The click and murmur may be brought out by held expiration, left decubitus position, sitting, standing, or leaning forward.
   b. Various maneuvers can alter the timing of the click and the murmur (see Fig. 13.4):
      (1) The click moves toward the S1 and the murmur lengthens with maneuvers that decrease the LV volume, such as standing,

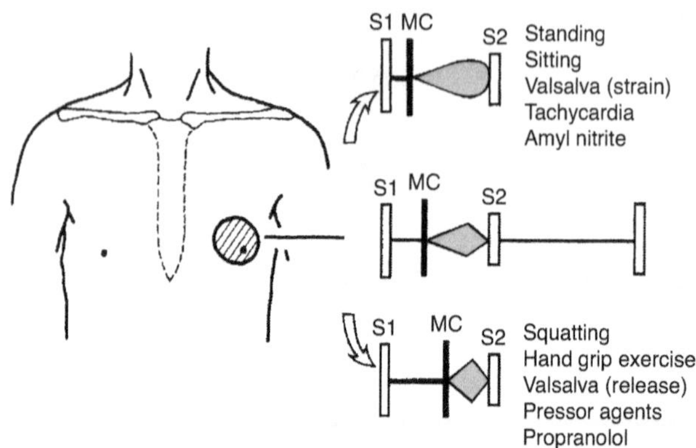

FIG. 13.4

Diagram of auscultatory findings in MVP and the effect of various maneuvers on the timing of the midsystolic click (*MC*) and the murmur. The maneuvers that reduce ventricular volume enhance leaflet redundancy and move the click and murmur earlier in systole. An increase in LV dimension has the opposite effect.

sitting, Valsalva strain phase, tachycardia, and the administration of amyl nitrite.

(2) The click moves toward the S2 and the murmur shortens with maneuvers that increase the LV volume, such as squatting, hand grip exercise, Valsalva release phase, bradycardia, and the administration of pressor agents or propranolol.

4. The ECG is usually normal but may show flat or inverted T waves in II, III, and aVF (in 20% to 60%), and, rarely, SVT, PACs, PVCs, first-degree AV block, or RBBB.
5. Chest radiographs are unremarkable except for LA enlargement seen in patients with severe MR. Thoracic skeletal abnormalities (e.g., straight back, pectus excavatum, and scoliosis) may be present.
6. Two-dimensional echo shows the following.
   a. In adult patients, prolapse of the mitral valve leaflet(s) superior to the plane of the mitral valve seen in the parasternal long-axis view is diagnostic. The superior displacement seen only on the apical four-chamber view is not diagnostic because it occurs in more than 30% of normal individuals due to the “saddle-shaped” mitral valve ring.
   b. In adults with MVP, one or both mitral valve leaflets bulge by at least 2 mm into the LA during systole in the parasternal long-axis view. Thickening of the involved leaflet to more than 5 mm supports the diagnosis.
   c. Some pediatric patients with characteristic body build and auscultatory findings of the condition do not show the adult echo

criterion of MVP; they may only show thickened mitral leaflets with systolic straightening or systolic superior doming and some posterosuperior displacement of the coaptation point of the mitral valve, some with mild MR. It may be because MVP is a progressive disease with the full manifestations occurring in the adult life.

D. NATURAL HISTORY

1. The majority of patients are asymptomatic, particularly during childhood.
2. Rare complications reported in adult patients, although rare in childhood, include infective endocarditis, spontaneous rupture of chordae tendineae, progressive MR, CHF, arrhythmias, conduction disturbances, and sudden death (probably from ventricular arrhythmias).

E. MANAGEMENT

1. Asymptomatic patients require no treatment or restriction of activity.
2. β-Adrenergic blockers (such as propranolol or atenolol) are often used in the following situations. Other drugs, such as calcium channel blockers, quinidine, or procainamide, may prove to be effective in some patients.
   a. Patients who are symptomatic (with palpitation, lightheadedness, dizziness, or syncope) secondary to ventricular arrhythmias. Symptomatic patients suspected to have arrhythmias should undergo ambulatory ECG monitoring and/or treadmill exercise testing.
   b. Patients with self-terminating episodes of SVT.
   c. Patients with chest discomfort may also be treated with propranolol. It is not relieved by nitroglycerine, but may worsen.
3. Antibiotic prophylaxis against infective endocarditis is recommended when significant MR is present.
4. Physical activities such as weight lifting, push-ups, pull-ups, or hanging on a monkey bar should be avoided.
5. Reconstructive surgery or mitral valve replacement rarely may be indicated in patients with severe MR.

Chapter 14

Cardiac Tumors

I. PREVALENCE

1. Cardiac tumors in the pediatric age group are very rare. A large portion of pediatric primary heart tumors (about 70%) are seen in patients younger than 1 year.
2. Relative frequency of cardiac tumors in the pediatric age group is shown in Table 14.1.
   a. In infants younger than 1 year, more than 50% are rhabdomyomas, followed by fibromas (25%).
   b. In children 1 to 16 years, nearly 40% are fibromas and myxomas.
3. More than 90% of primary tumors are benign in infants.

II. PATHOLOGY

Description of three common cardiac tumors follows.

A. RHABDOMYOMA

1. The most common location of rhabdomyoma is in the ventricular septum or free wall.
2. The size ranges from several millimeters to several centimeters.
3. More than 50% of the cases have tuberous sclerosis (e.g., with adenoma of the sebaceous glands, mental retardation, seizures).
4. Tumors regress in size or number or both in most patients younger than 4 years. Spontaneous complete regression may occur.
5. They may produce symptoms of obstruction to blood flow, ventricular arrhythmias, SVT associated with WPW preexcitation, or sudden death.

B. FIBROMA

1. It usually occurs as a single solid tumor, most commonly in the ventricular septum and less commonly in the wall of any cardiac chamber.
2. The size of the tumor varies from several millimeters to centimeters.
3. The tumor may obstruct blood flow, disturb atrioventricular or intraventricular conduction, or cause arrhythmias.

C. MYXOMA

1. It is the most common cardiac tumor in adults (30% of all primary cardiac tumors) but rare in infants and children.

TABLE 14.1

RELATIVE INCIDENCE OF CARDIAC TUMORS IN INFANTS AND CHILDREN

TUMORS	INCIDENCE (%)	TUMORS	INCIDENCE (%)
INFANT (LESS THAN 12 MONTHS) (N = 52)		**CHILDREN (1-16 YEARS OF AGE) (N = 25)**	
BENIGN TUMORS (94%)		**BENIGN TUMORS (58%)**	
Rhabdomyoma	52	Rhabdomyoma	8
Fibroma	25	Fibroma	21
Hemangioma/angioma	6	Myxoma	17
Teratoma	2	Hemangioma/angioma	4
Others	8	Teratoma	0
		Others	8
Malignant Tumors (6%)		Malignant Tumors (43%)	
Rhabdomyosarcoma	2	Rhabdomyosarcoma	8
Leiomyosarcoma	4	Leiomyosarcoma	2
Others	0	Others	33

Adapted from Becker, A. E. (2000). Primary heart tumors in the pediatric age group: a review of salient pathologic features relevant for clinicians. *Pediatric Cardiolology, 21*(4), 317-323.

2. The majority arises in the LA, 25% arise in the RA, and they very rarely arise in the ventricles.
3. Pedunculated myxomas commonly interfere with mitral valve function (due to intermittent protrusion through the valve) or produce thromboembolic phenomenon.

III. CLINICAL MANIFESTATIONS

1. Cardiac tumors usually are found on routine echo studies when the diagnosis is not suspected.
2. Syncope or chest pain may be a presenting complaint in older children. Sudden unexpected death may be the first manifestation. Rarely, symptoms vary with posture in cases of pedunculated tumors (such as myxoma).
3. Cardiac findings are nonspecific and vary primarily with the location and the size of the tumor.
   a. Tumors near cardiac valves may produce heart murmurs of stenosis or regurgitation of valves.
   b. Tumors involving the conduction tissue (such as seen with fibromas) may cause arrhythmias or conduction disturbances.
   c. Intracavitary tumors (such as rhabdomyoma) may produce inflow or outflow obstruction.
   d. Mural tumors may result in heart failure or cardiac arrhythmias.

   e. Pericardial tumors, which may signal malignancy, can produce pericardial effusion and cardiac tamponade.
   f. Fragmentation of intracavitary tumors may lead to embolism of the pulmonary or systemic circulations (as seen with myxoma).
4. The electrocardiogram may show nonspecific ST-T changes, an infarct-like pattern, low-voltage QRS complexes, or WPW preexcitation. Various arrhythmias and conduction disturbances have been reported.
5. Chest radiographs may reveal altered contour of the heart with or without changes in pulmonary vascular markings.

IV. DIAGNOSTIC PROCEDURES

1. Two-dimensional echo is the primary diagnostic tool. Transesophageal echocardiography (TEE) can provide more precise delineation of the tumor.
   a. Multiple intraventricular tumors are most likely rhabdomyomas.
   b. A solitary tumor of varying size, arising from the ventricular septum or the ventricular wall, is likely to be a fibroma.
   c. Left atrial tumors, especially when pedunculated, usually are myxomas.
   d. An intrapericardial tumor arising near the great arteries most likely is a teratoma.
   e. Pericardial effusion suggests a secondary malignant tumor.
2. TEE can provide more precise delineation of the tumor.
3. Magnetic resonance imaging (MRI) also provides the same information as the two-dimensional echo study does. MRI techniques have certain advantages over the echo study.
   a. MRI provides high-resolution images of cardiac cavitary, valvular, myocardial, pericardial, and extracardiac masses, in addition to its relationship with mediastinal and other intrathoracic structures.
   b. It can provide spatial relationship of the tumor mass to the coronary arteries, which may help guide surgical management.
   c. MRI allows differentiation of tumors from myocardium and differentiation of the type of tumor; for example, cardiac hemangiomas from rhabdomyomas and fibromas.
   d. MRI is better than echo in detecting apical tumors.
4. Cardiac catheterization and angiography are usually not necessary. Attempts at tissue diagnosis can be risky due to possible embolization of tumor fragment.

V. MANAGEMENT

Surgery is indicated in patients with inlet or outlet obstruction and in patients with symptoms of cardiac failure or ventricular arrhythmias refractory to medical treatment.

1. Rhabdomyomas: Spontaneous regression of these tumors has been well established so that surgical intervention is no longer indicated unless

the tumors produce obstruction or arrhythmias refractory to medical treatment.

2. Fibromas: A successful complete resection of a fibroma is possible. In some cases, the tumor intermingles with myocardial tissue so that complete resection is not possible without causing damage to the myocardium or conduction tissues.
3. Surgical removal is a standard procedure for myxomas and has a favorable outcome. The stalk of the tumor should be removed completely to prevent recurrence.
4. If myocardial involvement is extensive, surgical treatment is not possible. Cardiac transplantation may be an option in such cases.

Chapter 15

Cardiovascular Involvement in Systemic Diseases

Many systemic diseases may have important cardiovascular (CV) manifestations. The CV manifestations usually are evident when the diagnosis of the primary disease is made, but occasionally CV manifestations may precede evidence of the basic disease. In this chapter, CV manifestations of selected systemic diseases are presented.

I. 22Q11 DELETION SYNDROME (DIGEORGE SYNDROME)

A. DESCRIPTION

This syndrome, formerly known as DiGeorge syndrome, occurs in both males and females. These patients have a deletion of the long arm of chromosome 22 (22q11.2) detectable with the fluorescence in situ hybridization (FISH) technique.

B. CLINICAL MANIFESTATIONS

Clinical features of the syndrome are collectively grouped under the acronym of CATCH-22 (*c*ardiac, *a*bnormal facies, *t*hymic hypoplasia, *c*left palate, and *h*ypocalcemia resulting from *22*q11 deletion).

1. ***C***ardiac. The great majority of patients (85%) with the syndrome have serious CHDs. The common ones include TOF (25%), interrupted aortic arch (15%), VSD (15%), persistent truncus arteriosus (9%), and isolated aortic arch anomalies (5%).
2. ***A***bnormal facies: hypertelorism, micrognathia, short philtrum with fish mouth appearance, antimongoloid slant, telecanthus with short palpebral fissures, and low-set ears, often with defective pinna.
3. ***T***hymic hypoplasia or aplasia, with mild to moderate decrease in T-cell number.
4. ***C***left: anomalies in the palate (70% to 80%) with speech and feeding disorders.
5. ***H***ypocalcemia (60%) is due to hypoparathyroidism.
6. General. Short stature, mental retardation, and hypotonia in infancy are frequent. Occasionally, psychiatric disorders (e.g., schizophrenia and bipolar disorder) develop.

C. MANAGEMENT

1. Correction of cardiac malformation is required; cardiac defects are major causes of early death.

2. Irradiated, cytomegalovirus-negative blood products must be administered because of the risk of graft-versus-host disease with nonirradiated products.
3. Monitoring of serum calcium levels and supplementation of calcium and vitamin D are important.
   a. Calcium gluconate, 500 to 750 mg/kg/day, PO, every 6 hours, or calcium carbonate, 50 to 150 mg/kg/day, PO, every 6 hours.
   b. Ergocalciferol (vitamin D_2), 25,000 to 200,000 U PO QD.
4. Live vaccines are contraindicated in patients with 22q11 deletion syndrome and in household members because of the risk of shedding live organisms.
5. Early thymus transplantation may promote successful immune reconstitution.

II. FRIEDREICH ATAXIA

A. DESCRIPTION

This autosomal recessive disease manifests with the onset of ataxia usually before age 10 years and progresses slowly, involving the lower extremities to a greater extent than the upper extremities. Explosive dysarthric speech and nystagmus are characteristic, but intelligence is preserved.

B. CARDIOVASCULAR MANIFESTATIONS

1. Cardiomyopathy is found in approximately 30% of the cases. Hypertrophic cardiomyopathy with normal LV systolic function is the most common finding. In advanced stage, the LV enlarges, the LV wall thickness decreases, and LV systolic function decreases. CHF is the terminal event, with most patients dying before age 40 years.
2. The electrocardiogram (ECG) may show the T vector change in the limb leads or left precordial leads. Occasionally, LVH, RVH, abnormal Q waves, or short PR intervals are found.

C. MANAGEMENT

The same as described for cardiomyopathy.

III. HYPERTHYROIDISM: CONGENITAL AND ACQUIRED

A. DESCRIPTION

1. Hyperthyroidism results from excess production of T_3 (triiodothyronine), T_4 (thyroxine), or both. The level of thyroid-stimulating hormone (TSH) is suppressed.
2. The actions of thyroid hormone on the CV system include (a) increasing heart rate, cardiac contractility, and cardiac output; (b) increasing systolic pressure and decreasing diastolic pressure, with mean pressure unchanged; and (c) increasing myocardial sensitivity to catecholamines.

B. CLINICAL MANIFESTATIONS

1. Congenital hyperthyroidism (neonatal Graves disease): an anxious, irritable, and unusually alert baby with widely open eyes (exophthalmic). Many of the infants are premature and most have goiters.
2. Children with juvenile hyperthyroidism (Graves disease) are hyperactive, irritable, and excitable. The patients have exophthalmos and a goiter. There is a 5:1 female-to-male ratio.
3. Cardiovascular manifestations include tachycardia, full and bounding pulses, and increased systolic and pulse pressures. Bruits may be audible over the enlarged thyroid in children but not in newborns. In severely affected patients, cardiac enlargement and cardiac failure may develop.
4. Chest radiographs usually are normal unless CHF develops.
5. The ECG may show sinus tachycardia, peaked P waves, various arrhythmias (SVT, junctional rhythm), complete heart block, RVH, LVH, or biventricular hypertrophy.
6. Echo studies reveal a hyperkinetic LV with increased fractional shortening.

C. MANAGEMENT

1. In severely affected patients, a β-adrenergic blocker such as propranolol is indicated to reduce the effect of catecholamines.
2. Treatment of hyperthyroidism consist of oral administration of antithyroid drugs, propylthiouracil or methimazole (Tapazole).
3. If CHF develops, treatment with anticongestive medications is indicated.

IV. HYPOTHYROIDISM: CONGENITAL AND ACQUIRED

A. DESCRIPTION

1. **Congenital type.** Clinical signs may not appear until 3 months of age. A protuberant tongue, cool and mottled skin, subnormal temperature, carotenemia, and myxedema are typical. Untreated children become mentally retarded and slow in physical development.
2. **Acquired type.** It may be caused by lymphocytic thyroiditis (Hashimoto disease or autoimmune thyroiditis), subtotal or complete thyroidectomy, or protracted ingestion of goitrogens, iodides, or cobalt medications. Rarely, amiodarone can cause hypothyroidism. Serum T_3 and T_4 are low or borderline and TSH is high. Hypercholesterolemia is common.

B. CARDIOVASCULAR MANIFESTATIONS

1. Significant bradycardia, weak arterial pulse, hypotension, and nonpitting facial and peripheral edema may be present.
2. The ECG abnormalities may include some or all of the following: low QRS voltages, especially in the limb leads; low T-wave amplitude;

prolongation of PR and QT intervals; and dome-shaped T wave with an absent ST segment ("mosque" sign).

3. Echo studies may show pericardial effusion, hypertrophic cardiomyopathy, or asymmetric septal hypertrophy.
4. In congenital type, PDA and PS are frequently found.
5. There is an increased occurrence of hypercholesterolemia in acquired type.

C. MANAGEMENT

1. L-thyroxine given orally is the treatment of choice. Monitor T_4 and TSH frequently.
2. In acquired type, treatment of hypercholesterolemia, if present.

V. INFANTS OF DIABETIC MOTHERS

A. DESCRIPTION

1. In general, infants of diabetic mothers (IDM) have higher prevalence of congenital malformations of multiple organ systems, occurring at three to four times the rate seen in the general population. Common ones include neural tube defects (anencephaly, myelomeningocele), CHDs (such as ASD, VSD, TGA, tricuspid atresia, COA, etc.), and sacral dysgenesis or agenesis.
2. In addition to the high prevalence of congenital anomalies, IDMs have a high prevalence of cardiomyopathy and persistent pulmonary hypertension of newborn (PPHN).
   a. Hypertrophic cardiomyopathy (either concentric or asymmetric septal hypertrophy) with or without obstruction is seen in 10% to 20% of the patients.
   b. An increased risk of PPHN may be due to conditions that promote the persistence of pulmonary hypertension, such as hypoglycemia, perinatal asphyxia, respiratory distress, and polycythemia.

B. CLINICAL FINDINGS OF CARDIOMYOPATHY

1. Signs of CHF with gallop rhythm may be found in 5% to 10% of these babies.
2. Chest radiographs may show varying degrees of cardiomegaly with normal or increased PVM.
3. The ECG may show a long QT interval (caused by hypocalcemia) and occasional RVH, LVH, or BVH.
4. Echo findings of cardiomyopathy in IDMs may include the following.
   a. An increase in the LV wall thickness, often with asymmetric septal hypertrophy, and supernormal contractility of the LV.
   b. Evidence of LVOT obstruction (seen in about 50% of cases).
   c. Rarely, the LV is dilated with decreased contractility (dilated cardiomyopathy).

C. MANAGEMENT

1. Hypoglycemia and hypocalcemia should be corrected, if present.
2. In most cases, the hypertrophy spontaneously resolves within the first 6 to 12 months of life. β-Adrenergic blockers, such as propranolol, may help reduce the LVOT obstruction, but treatment usually is not necessary.
3. Digitalis and other inotropic agents are contraindicated because they may worsen the obstruction.
4. If CHF develops, the usual anticongestive measures are indicated.

VI. MARFAN SYNDROME

A. DESCRIPTION

Marfan syndrome is a generalized connective tissue disease involving skeletal, cardiovascular, and ocular systems. Mutation in the *FBN1* gene located on chromosome 15 is the cause of Marfan syndrome. It is inherited as an autosomal dominant pattern with variable expressivity. New mutations are the cause of at least 25% of Marfan syndrome cases.

1. Skeletal: tall stature with long slim limbs, arachnodactyly, muscle hypotonia, joint laxity with scoliosis and kyphosis, pectus excavatum or carinatum, and narrow facies.
2. Cardiovascular involvement occurs in 50% by the age of 21 (see next section).
3. Eye manifestations may include lens subluxation, increased axial global length, myopia, and retinal detachment.

B. CARDIOVASCULAR INVOLVEMENT

1. The CV abnormalities may include the following:
   a. Dilatation of the sinus of Valsalva, dilatation of the ascending aorta, and AR are common.
   b. Mitral valve abnormalities are more common than aortic lesions in children, including MR and MVP.
   c. Aneurysm of the PA is less frequently seen.
   d. Rarely, rupture of chordae tendineae, aneurysm of the abdominal aorta, and aneurysmal dilatation of the proximal coronary arteries may occur.
2. The ECG may show LVH; T-wave inversion in leads II and III, aVF, and left precordial leads; and first-degree AV block.
3. Chest radiographs may show a prominence of the ascending aorta, aortic knob, or main PA segment, and rarely cardiomegaly.
4. Echo studies show:
   a. Increased dimension of the aortic root with or without AR.
   b. "Redundant" mitral valve or MVP with thickened valve leaflets and MR.
   c. In children, adult echo diagnostic criteria of MVP are rarely met, because MVP is a progressive disease. Systolic straightening or convex superior bowing of the leaflets or superior displacement of

the mitral coaptation point may be an important sign of early MVP in this age group.

5. Early death is commonly precipitated by aortic dissection, chronic AR, or severe MR.

C. MANAGEMENT

Use of β-blockers, angiotensin-converting enzyme (ACE) inhibitors, or angiotensin II receptor blockers (ARBs) has significantly diminished the progression of aortic root dilatation, thus delaying surgical intervention. Timely and improved surgery has significantly increased the life expectancy of these patients in recent years.

1. Periodic examination of the aortic root dimension and the status of the MR and MVP is important.
2. β-Blockers (atenolol, propranolol) are effective in slowing the rate of aortic dilatation and reducing the development of aortic complications. In addition to traditional -blocker treatment, over the last decade, enalapril (an ACE inhibitor) and losartan (ARB) have been added to the medical regimen to treat dilated aortic root in Marfan syndrome patients. The role of prophylactic medical treatment in children with Marfan syndrome remains controversial; some physicians choose to start medications at the time of diagnosis of Marfan syndrome even without aortic root dilatation.
3. Discourage certain physical activities, such as weight lifting, rowing, push-ups, pull-ups, sit-ups, and hanging on a monkey bar, which may increase damage to the aortic root and aortic and mitral valves.
4. Surgery should be considered when the diameter of the aortic root increases significantly. However, there is controversy as to what is considered significant enlargement of the aortic root to require surgery. Current general recommendation for surgery is an aortic root diameter of ≥50 mm or rapid growth of more than 5 mm/year in Marfan patients. Normal two-dimensional (2D) echo dimensions of the aortic root and the aorta are presented in Table D.3, in Appendix D.
5. Valve-sparing aortic root reconstruction appears to be preferable to composite graft surgery.

15

VII. MUCOPOLYSACCHARIDOSES

A. DESCRIPTION

1. In mucopolysaccharidoses (MPS), excessive amounts of glycosaminoglycans (previously called mucopolysaccharides) accumulate in various tissues, including the myocardium, cardiac valves, and coronary arteries. Hurler (type IH), Hunter (II), Scheie (IS), Sanfilippo (III), and Morquio (IV) are well-known eponyms.
2. A wide variety of clinical manifestations occur, including growth and mental retardation, skeletal abnormalities, clouded cornea, upper airway obstruction, and cardiac abnormalities (see following text).
3. In most cases the cause of death is cardiorespiratory failure secondary to cardiac involvement and upper airway obstruction.

B. CARDIAC MANIFESTATIONS

1. Echo studies show involvement of cardiac valves and myocardium.
   a. MR is present in about 30% of the patients. It is more frequent in types IH (38%) than other types (24% in type II and 20% in type III). Thickening of the mitral valve is common.
   b. AR is present in about 15% of the cases, often with thickened aortic valve. It is more common in type II (56%) and type IV (24%).
   c. Myocardial abnormalities, such as asymmetric septal hypertrophy, hypertrophic cardiomyopathy, dilated cardiomyopathy, and endocardial thickening, are present in about 25% of the cases.
2. The ECG may show a prolonged QTc interval, RVH, LVH, or LAH.
3. Chest radiographs may show cardiomegaly in severe cases of valve regurgitation.

C. MANAGEMENT

Treatment depends on the abnormalities present.

VIII. MUSCULAR DYSTROPHY

A. DESCRIPTION

1. Duchenne muscular dystrophy (MD), a sex-linked recessive disease, involves the pelvic muscles and leads to lordosis, waddling gait, and difficulty rising.
2. Becker MD is the same fundamental disease as Duchenne MD, but it follows a milder and more protracted course.

B. CARDIAC INVOLVEMENT

1. Dilated cardiomyopathy is most common. MR and MVP may rarely develop.
2. The ECG abnormalities occur in 90% of the patients. RVH and RBBB are the most common abnormalities. Other abnormalities may include deep Q waves (in V5, V6), short PR interval, and T-wave inversion (in the limb leads or V5 and V6). Holter monitoring may show atrial tachycardia or frequent ventricular ectopies, especially in patients with low LV ejection fraction.
3. Echo studies show dilated cardiomyopathy in both Duchenne and Becker types. In early stages, only diastolic dysfunction (of reduced diastolic relaxation pattern) may be present. Systolic dysfunction appears later in the disease process. Cardiac magnetic resonance imaging (MRI) can quantify ventricular function as well as extent of myocardial fibrosis in patients with MD.

C. MANAGEMENT

1. Treatment is the same as that described for dilated cardiomyopathy (see Chapter 11).

2. Recent reports suggest ACE inhibitors (e.g., perindopril) may lead to improved LV function and possible delay of progression of the disease.
3. Addition of carvedilol (0.5 to 1 mg/kg, twice daily) may have additional benefits. Carvedilol may be added if average heart rate exceeds 100 beats/min (on a 24-hr Holter monitor).

IX. MYOTONIC DYSTROPHY

A. DESCRIPTION

This autosomal dominant disease is characterized by myotonia (increased muscular irritability and contractility with decreased power of relaxation) combined with muscular weakness.

B. CARDIAC INVOLVEMENT

1. Involvement of the AV conduction and myocardial abnormalities are frequent (due to fatty infiltration).
2. The ECG may show first-degree AV block and intraventricular conduction delay. Second-degree and complete heart block may develop. In addition, atrial fibrillation and flutter and ventricular arrhythmias may develop.
3. Echo studies may show MVP and LV systolic dysfunction with advancing age.
4. Sudden death is frequent, attributable to conduction abnormalities and/or arrhythmias.

C. MANAGEMENT

1. Patients with symptoms or evidence of arrhythmias should be considered for antiarrhythmic agents and/or pacemaker treatment.
2. LV dysfunction, if present, should be treated.

X. NOONAN SYNDROME

A. DESCRIPTION

1. This autosomal dominant genetic disorder occurs in both males and females. Mutations in the *PTPN11* gene located on chromosome 12 have been found in about 50% of the patients with Noonan syndrome. It was first described by Dr. Jacqueline A. Noonan, a pediatric cardiologist, in the early 1960s.
2. Characteristic findings include distinctive facial features (large head, wide-spaced eyes, epicanthal folds, low-set ears, and short and broad nose with depressed root), short webbed neck with low posterior hairline, cubitus valgus, chest deformity (pectus excavatum or carinatum), scoliosis, short stature, and CHD.
3. Although some clinical features are similar to Turner syndrome, patients with Noonan syndrome are often mentally retarded and normal sexual maturation usually occurs, although delayed.

B. CARDIOVASCULAR ABNORMALITIES

1. Cardiovascular abnormalities are seen in more than 80% of the patients.
2. Pulmonary valve stenosis, often dysplastic, is the most common one (occurring in 25% to 35%). Secundum ASD is often associated with PS.
3. Hypertrophic cardiomyopathy is present in approximately 20% of patients.

C. MANAGEMENT

1. For significant PS, initial treatment is usually pulmonary balloon valvuloplasty, but it may be unsuccessful as the valve is at times extremely dysplastic. With severe dysplasia, a pulmonary valvectomy or pulmonary homograft may be needed in childhood.
2. Hypertrophic cardiomyopathy may be treated with β-blockers or surgical myomectomy.
3. Individuals without heart disease on their initial evaluation should be followed every 5 years because of possible late appearance of cardiac problems.
4. The patients should be followed by endocrinologists for possible need of growth hormone therapy, thyroid hormone replacement, or pubertal induction with estrogen (for females) or testosterone (for males).

XI. RHEUMATOID ARTHRITIS

A. DESCRIPTION

The synovium is the principal target of inappropriate immune attack in this condition. Irregular nodular thickening may be seen on cardiac valves (granulomatous valvulitis). Inflammatory cells may infiltrate the myocardium.

B. CARDIAC INVOLVEMENT

1. Pericarditis is the most common finding (occurring in about 50% of cases). It is most frequent in systemic-onset juvenile rheumatoid arthritis (JRA), occasionally in patients with polyarticular-onset JRA. Small pericardial effusion occurs without symptoms, but large effusion may cause chest pain.
2. Myocarditis occurs infrequently (1% to 10%) but can cause CHF and arrhythmias.
3. Rarely, MR and AR with thickening of these valves occur.
4. Occasionally, LV is dilated with systolic dysfunction.
5. The ECG may show nonspecific ST-T changes (in 20% of cases). Rarely, heart block can occur.

C. MANAGEMENT

1. Nonsteroidal antiinflammatory agents such as naproxen (15 mg/kg/day in 2 divided doses) may be used for mild pericarditis.

2. For symptomatic or severe pericarditis, corticosteroids are used. Prednisone 0.5 to 2 mg/kg/day (given TID or QID) for more than 1 week is gradually reduced by approximately 20% each week (given as a single dose).
3. Tamponade is treated with pericardiocentesis.

XII. SYSTEMIC LUPUS ERYTHEMATOSUS

A. DESCRIPTION

1. Girls older than 8 years of age are most commonly affected (78%), with a female-to-male ratio of 6:1.
2. Varying degrees of immune-mediated changes occur in all layers of the heart: pericarditis, myocarditis, and classic verrucous Libman-Sacks lesion (on the cardiac valves).

B. CARDIOVASCULAR MANIFESTATIONS

1. Pericarditis with pericardial effusion is the most common manifestation (occurring in about 25%) and is often asymptomatic.
2. Myocarditis occurs in 2% to 25%, with resting tachycardia.
3. Echo studies show the following:
   a. Irregular vegetations, 2 to 4 mm in diameter (Libman-Sacks endocarditis), are seen most commonly on the mitral valve and less commonly on the aortic valve.
   b. Diffuse thickening of the mitral or aortic valve (with or without regurgitation) is a more frequent finding than the verrucous lesion.

C. MANAGEMENT

1. If active valvulitis is suspected, corticosteroid therapy may be warranted.
2. Anticoagulation therapy should also be considered.

XIII. TURNER SYNDROME

A. DESCRIPTION

1. Standard karyotyping shows 45,X (in more than 50%); others have a combination of monosomy X and normal cells (45,X/46,XX) (mosaic Turner syndrome).
2. Edema of the dorsa of the hands and feet and loose skin folds at the nape of the neck in a female neonate are characteristic.
3. In childhood, webbing of the neck, broad chest with wide-spaced nipples, cubitus valgus, and small stature are characteristic.

B. CARDIAC FINDINGS

1. Cardiovascular abnormalities are found in about 35% of the patients.
2. Bicuspid aortic valve (BAV), COA, and aortic wall abnormalities (ascending aortic dilatation, aneurysm formation, and aortic dissection) are more commonly found in patients with webbing of the neck.

3. Less common anomalies include elongated transverse arch, PAPVR involving the left upper PV (13%), and persistent left SVC (13%).

C. MANAGEMENT

1. Cardiac follow-up is required with attention to the following:
   a. Aortic dimension should be determined on a regular basis (by MRI every 5 to 10 years). If the aorta is enlarged, treat it with β-blockers.
   b. Monitor blood pressure (BP) for hypertension.
   c. Exercise restriction. Highly competitive strenuous sports and isometric exercises are not recommended in patients with a dilated aortic root.
2. Follow-up by pediatric endocrinologists for the need of growth hormone and puberty induction with estrogen therapy.
3. Follow-up by an obstetrics and gynecology specialist because natural pregnancy occurs in 2% to 5% of the patients. Pregnancy carries a high risk because of possible aortic dissection during pregnancy and the postpartum period. History of surgically repaired CV defect, BAV, aortic dilatation, or systemic hypertension is relative contraindications of pregnancy.

XIV. WILLIAMS SYNDROME

A. DESCRIPTION

A microdeletion in the chromosomal region 7q11.23 near the elastin gene (*ELN*) is responsible. Elastin is protein that allows blood vessels and other tissues to stretch. Males and females are equally affected.

Patients with Williams syndrome have multisystem manifestations, including CV disease, developmental delay, learning disability, mental retardation, hearing loss, severe dental disease, ocular problems, nephrolithiasis, and bowel and bladder diverticula.

1. Many children have a history of failure to thrive, poor weight gain, colic, and delayed motor development during early life.
2. Most children with the syndrome have similar characteristic features. These features include a small upturned nose, long philtrum (upper lip length), wide mouth, full lips, small chin, a stellate pattern in the iris (seen in 50%), and puffiness around the eyes.
3. Affected children have personality trait of being very friendly, trusting strangers, fearing loud sounds, and being interested in music. They are also hyperactive, inattentive, easily distracted (attention deficit disorder).
4. Other findings include hoarse voice, joint hyperelasticity, contractures, kyphoscoliosis, and lordosis.

B. CARDIOVASCULAR PATHOLOGY

1. Elastin arteriopathy (with stenosis) most commonly affects the ascending aorta and the pulmonary arteries (supravalvular AS and PA stenosis), occurring singly or together in 55% to 80%.

2. Less common cardiac anomalies include COA, hypoplastic aortic arch, ASD, VSD, TOF, complete AV canal, and hypertrophic cardiomyopathy.
3. Systemic hypertension may be present or develop in approximately 50% of the patients.
4. High pressure in the sinus of Valsalva may lead to coronary ostial narrowing and coronary artery stenosis, resulting in increased risk for sudden death.
5. There may also be renal artery stenosis with resulting hypertension. Renal ultrasonography may find anatomic abnormalities (found in 15% to 20%) or nephrolithiasis (caused by hypercalcemia).
6. Hypercalcemia, which is noted in approximately 15% of infants with Williams syndrome, is frequently asymptomatic and resolves in the first few years of life but can be lifelong.
7. The ECG may show LVH in severe cases of supravalvar AS. BVH or RVH may be present with severe PA stenosis.
8. Sudden deaths with no apparent instigating event have been reported after the use of anesthesia, after sedation, or during invasive procedures (such as cardiac catheterization and heart surgery).
9. Higher frequency of prolonged QTc interval has been found in patients with the syndrome than in the control group; this has been raised as a possible cause of sudden death. Prolonged QTc interval (≥460 msec) is found in 13.6% of the patients (compared with 2.0% in controls). JTc prolongation (>340 msec) is found in 11.7% of the patients (compared with 1.8% in controls).

C. MANAGEMENT

1. Annual cardiology evaluation with assessment of the cardiac conditions, measurement of blood pressure, and check of the QTc interval.
2. Hypercalcemia should be treated, if present. Avoid taking extra calcium and vitamin D.
3. When planning a procedure, history should be evaluated carefully for syncope, angina, fatigue or dyspnea, and hemodynamic instability during previous anesthesia or sedation.
   a. Avoid medications that are known to prolong the QTc interval.

PART V

ARRHYTHMIAS AND ATRIOVENTRICULAR CONDUCTION DISTURBANCES

This part discusses cardiac arrhythmias, atrioventricular conduction disturbances, cardiac pacemakers, and implantable cardioverter defibrillators.

Chapter 16

Cardiac Arrhythmias

Normal heart rate varies with age: the younger the child, the faster the heart rate. Therefore the definitions used for adults of bradycardia (fewer than 60 beats/min) and tachycardia (above 100 beats/min) have little significance for children. A child has tachycardia when the heart rate is beyond the upper limit of normal for age and bradycardia when the heart rate is slower than the lower limit of normal (see Table 2.1).

I. RHYTHMS ORIGINATING IN THE SINUS NODE

All rhythms that originate in the sinoatrial (SA) node (sinus rhythm) have two important characteristics.

1. A P wave is present in front of each QRS complex with a regular PR interval. (The PR interval may be prolonged, as in first-degree AV block).
2. The P axis is between 0 and +90 degrees, often a neglected criterion. This produces upright P waves in lead II and inverted P waves in aVR (see Figs. 2.6 and 2.7).

A. REGULAR SINUS RHYTHM

1. **Description:** The rhythm is regular and the rate is normal for age. Two characteristics of sinus rhythm (as described previously) are present (Fig. 16.1).
2. **Significance:** This rhythm is normal at any age.
3. **Treatment:** No treatment is required.

B. SINUS TACHYCARDIA

1. **Description:** The characteristics of sinus rhythm are present. A rate above 140 beats/min in children and above 170 beats/min in infants may be significant. In sinus tachycardia, the heart rate is usually lower than 200 beats/min (see Fig. 16.1).
2. **Causes:** Anxiety, fever, hypovolemia, circulatory shock, anemia, CHF, catecholamines, thyrotoxicosis, and myocardial disease are possible causes.
3. **Significance:** Increased cardiac work is well tolerated by the healthy myocardium.
4. **Treatment:** The underlying cause is treated.

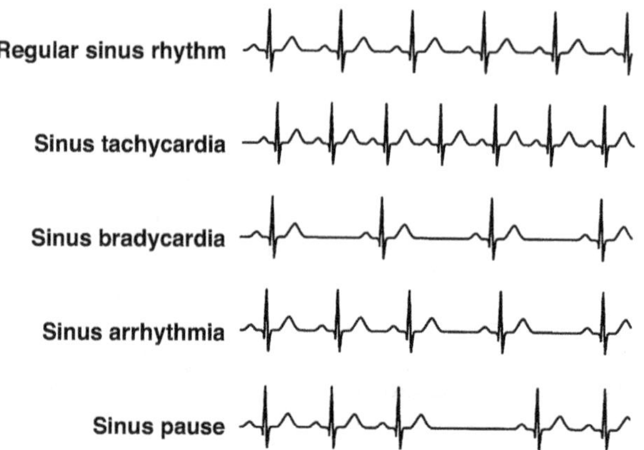

FIG. 16.1
Normal and abnormal rhythms originating in the sinoatrial node. *(From Park, M. K., & Guntheroth, W. G. (2006).* How to read pediatric ECGs *(4th ed.). Philadelphia: Mosby.)*

C. SINUS BRADYCARDIA

1. **Description:** The characteristics of sinus rhythm are present. A rate below 80 beats/min in newborn infants and below 60 beats/min in older children may be significant (see Fig. 16.1).
2. **Causes:** Sinus bradycardia may occur in trained athletes. Vagal stimulation, increased intracranial pressure, hypothyroidism, hypothermia, hypoxia, and drugs such as digitalis and β-adrenergic blockers are possible causes.
3. **Significance:** Some patients with marked bradycardia do not maintain normal cardiac output.
4. **Treatment:** The underlying cause is treated.

D. SINUS ARRHYTHMIA

1. **Description:** There is a phasic variation in the heart rate, increasing during inspiration and decreasing during expiration, and the two characteristics of sinus rhythm are maintained (see Fig. 16.1).
2. **Causes:** This normal phenomenon is due to a phasic variation in the firing rate of cardiac autonomic nerves with the phase of respiration.
3. **Significance:** There is no hemodynamic significance.
4. **Treatment:** No treatment is indicated.

E. SINUS PAUSE

1. **Description:** In *sinus pause*, there is a momentary cessation of sinus node pacemaker activity, resulting in the absence of the P wave and

QRS complex for a relatively short duration (see Fig. 16.1). *Sinus arrest* lasts longer and usually results in an escape beat (such as junctional escape beat).

2. **Causes:** Increased vagal tone, hypoxia, digitalis toxicity, and sick sinus syndrome (see next section). Well-conditioned athletes may have bradycardia and sinus pause of greater than 2 seconds due to prominent vagal influence.
3. **Significance:** Sinus pause of less than 2 seconds is normal in young children and adolescents. Sinus pause usually has no hemodynamic significance.
4. **Treatment:** Treatment is rarely indicated except in sick sinus syndrome and digitalis toxicity.

F. SINOATRIAL EXIT BLOCK

1. **Description:** A P wave is absent from the normally expected P wave, resulting in a long RR interval. The duration of the pause is a multiple of the basic PP interval. An impulse formed within the sinus node fails to propagate normally to the atria.
2. **Causes:** Excessive vagal stimulation, myocarditis or fibrosis involving the atrium, and drugs such as quinidine, procainamide, or digitalis.
3. **Significance:** It is usually transient and has no hemodynamic significance.
4. **Treatment:** The underlying cause is treated.

G. SINUS NODE DYSFUNCTION (SICK SINUS SYNDROME)

1. **Description:** The sinus node fails to function as the dominant pacemaker of the heart or performs abnormally slowly, producing a variety of arrhythmias. The arrhythmias may include profound sinus bradycardia, sinus arrest with junctional (or nodal) escape, and ectopic atrial or nodal rhythm. When these arrhythmias are accompanied by symptoms such as dizziness or syncope, sinus node dysfunction is referred to as sick sinus syndrome. Long-term electrocardiogram (ECG) recording (such as Holter) is usually required in documenting overall heart rate variation and the prevalence of abnormally slow or fast rhythm.
2. **Causes:** Extensive cardiac surgery involving the atria (e.g., the Fontan operation), myocarditis, pericarditis, antiarrhythmic drugs, hypothyroidism, CHD (such as sinus venosus ASD, Ebstein anomaly), and occasionally idiopathic occurring in an otherwise normal heart.
3. **Significance:** Bradytachyarrhythmia is the most worrisome rhythm. Profound bradycardia following a period of tachycardia (overdrive suppression) can cause syncope and even death.
4. **Treatment:**
   a. For severe bradycardia:
   (1) Acute symptomatic bradycardia is treated with intravenous (IV) atropine (0.04 mg/kg IV every 2 to 4 hours) or isoproterenol (0.05 to

0.5 μg/kg IV) or transcutaneous pacing. Temporary transvenous or transesophageal pacing can be used until a permanent pacing system can be implanted.

(2) Permanent implantation of pacemaker is the treatment of choice in symptomatic patients, especially those with syncope. Most patients receive atrial demand pacing. Patients with any degree of AV nodal dysfunction receive dual-chamber pacemakers. Ventricular demand pacemakers may be used.

(3) Asymptomatic patients with heart rate under 40 beats/min or pauses longer than 3 seconds are less clear indications for permanent pacing.

b. For symptomatic tachycardia:

(1) Antiarrhythmic drugs, such as propranolol or quinidine, may be given to suppress tachycardia, but they are often unsuccessful.

(2) Digoxin or amiodarone may help to decrease AV conduction of rapid tachycardia.

(3) Catheter ablation of arrhythmia substrates (often requiring concomitant surgical revision of previous surgeries) may be indicated.

(4) Patients with tachycardia–bradycardia syndrome may benefit from antitachycardia pacemakers.

II. RHYTHMS ORIGINATING IN THE ATRIUM

Atrial arrhythmias (Fig. 16.2) are characterized by the following:

1. P waves of unusual contour (abnormal P axis) and/or an abnormal number of P waves per QRS complex.
2. QRS complexes of normal duration (but with occasional wide QRS duration caused by aberrancy).

A. PREMATURE ATRIAL CONTRACTION

1. Description
   a. In PAC the QRS complex occurs prematurely with abnormal P wave morphology. There is an incomplete compensatory pause—that is, the length of two cycles including one premature beat is less than the length of two normal cycles.
   b. An occasional PAC is not followed by a QRS complex (i.e., a nonconducted PAC) (see Fig. 16.2).
   c. A *nonconducted* PAC is differentiated from a second-degree AV block by the prematurity of the nonconducted P wave (P′ in Fig. 16.2). The P′ wave occurs earlier than the anticipated normal P rate, and the resulting PP′ interval is shorter than the normal PP interval for that individual. In second-degree AV block, the P wave that is not followed by the QRS complex occurs at the anticipated time, maintaining a regular PP interval.

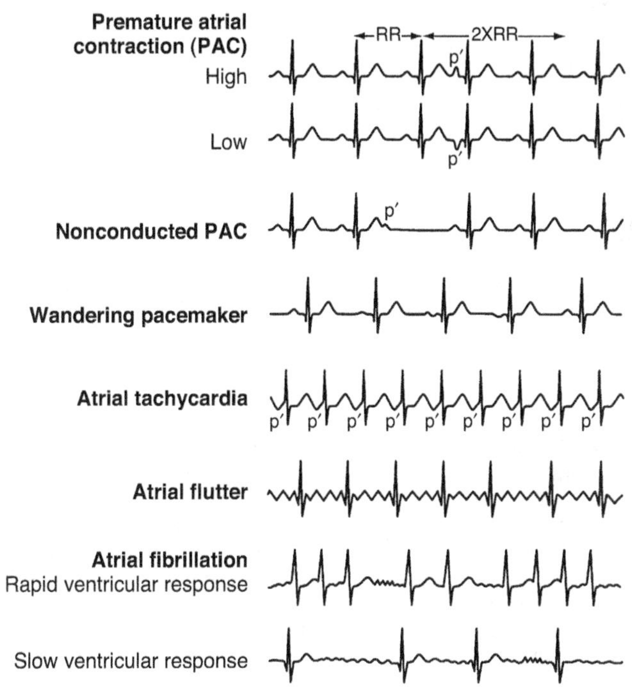

FIG. 16.2
Arrhythmias originating in the atrium. *(From Park, M. K., & Guntheroth, W. G. (2006).* How to read pediatric ECGs *(4th ed.). Philadelphia: Mosby.)*

2. **Causes:** PAC appears in healthy children, including newborns. It also may appear after cardiac surgery and with digitalis toxicity.
3. **Significance:** Isolated PAC has no hemodynamic significance.
4. **Treatment:** Usually no treatment is indicated except in cases of digitalis toxicity.

B. WANDERING ATRIAL PACEMAKER

1. **Description:** Gradual changes in the shape of P waves and PR intervals occur. The QRS complex is normal (see Fig. 16.2).
2. **Causes:** This is seen in otherwise healthy children. It is the result of a gradual shift of impulse formation in the atria through several cardiac cycles.
3. **Significance:** There is no clinical significance.
4. **Treatment:** No treatment is indicated.

C. ECTOPIC (OR AUTONOMIC) ATRIAL TACHYCARDIA

1. Description
   a. There is a narrow QRS complex tachycardia (in the absence of aberrancy or preexisting bundle branch block) with visible P waves at an inappropriately rapid rate.
   b. The P axis is different from that of sinus rhythm (see Fig. 16.2). When the ectopic focus is near the sinus node, the P axis may be the same as in sinus rhythm.
   c. The usual heart rate in older children is between 110 and 160 beats/min, but the tachycardia rate varies substantially during the course of a day, reaching 200 beats/min with sympathetic stimuli. Holter monitoring may demonstrate a characteristic gradual acceleration of the heart rate, the so-called warming up period, rather than abrupt onset and termination seen with re-entrant AV tachycardia.
   d. It represents about 20% of SVT. This arrhythmia is sometimes difficult to distinguish from the re-entrant AV tachycardia and thus it is included under the "Supraventricular Tachycardia" section later.
2. **Causes**: This arrhythmia originates from a single focus in the atrium. It is believed to be secondary to increased automaticity of nonsinus atrial focus or foci. Myocarditis, cardiomyopathies, atrial dilatation, atrial tumors, and previous cardiac surgery involving atria (such as Fontan procedure) may be the cause. Most patients have a structurally normal heart (idiopathic).
3. **Significance**: CHF is common with chronic cases. There is a high association with tachycardia-induced cardiomyopathy.
4. **Treatment**: It is refractory to medical therapy and cardioversion. Drugs that are effective in re-entrant atrial tachycardia (such as adenosine) do not terminate the tachycardia. Cardioversion is ineffective because the ectopic rhythm resumes immediately.
   a. The goal may be to slow the ventricular rate (using digoxin or β-blockers) rather than to try to convert the arrhythmia to sinus rhythm.
   b. Long-term oral antiarrhythmic drugs (such as flecainide or amiodarone) are the mainstay of therapy in patients not undergoing radiofrequency ablation.
   c. Radiofrequency ablation may prove to be effective in nearly 90% of cases. In children, the foci are found in the LA near the pulmonary veins and the atrial appendage (in contrast to the RA found in adults).

D. MULTIFOCAL (OR CHAOTIC) ATRIAL TACHYCARDIA

1. **Description:** There are three or more distinct P-wave morphologies. The PP and RR intervals are irregular with variable PR intervals. The arrhythmia may be misdiagnosed as atrial fibrillation.

2. **Causes:** Most patients with the condition are infants; it is very rare after 5 years of age. Thirty percent to 50% have respiratory illness. Myocarditis and birth asphyxia have been described. This arrhythmia may occur with or without CHDs. The mechanism of this arrhythmia has been poorly defined.
3. **Significance:** CHF may develop. Sudden death has been reported in up to 17% while receiving therapy. Long duration of the arrhythmia may cause LV systolic dysfunction. Spontaneous resolution frequently occurs.
4. Treatment
   a. Adenosine is ineffective in terminating the tachycardia (this is a useful diagnostic sign of the condition). This arrhythmia is also refractory to cardiac pacing and cardioversion.
   b. Drugs that slow AV conduction (propranolol or digoxin) and those that decrease automaticity (such as class IA or IC or class III) have not been very effective. However, they may control the heart rate.
   c. Amiodarone (IV followed by oral [PO]) appears to be the current treatment of choice.

E. ATRIAL FLUTTER

1. **Description:** Atrial flutter is characterized by a fast atrial rate (F waves with saw-tooth configuration) of about 300 (ranges 240 to 360) beats/min, the ventricle responding with varying degrees of block (e.g., 2:1, 3:1, 4:1), and normal QRS complexes (see Fig. 16.2).
2. **Causes:** Structural heart disease with dilated atria, myocarditis, thyrotoxicosis, and previous surgery involving atria (such as Senning or Fontan operation) are possible causes. However, most fetuses and neonates with atrial flutter have a normal heart.
3. **Significance:** The ventricular rate determines the eventual cardiac output; a too-rapid ventricular rate may decrease the cardiac output. Thrombus formation may lead to embolic events. Uncontrolled atrial flutter may lead to heart failure.
4. Treatment
   a. In acute situations, synchronized cardioversion is the treatment of choice. Adenosine is not effective.
   b. For long-standing atrial flutter or fibrillation (of 24 to 48 hours) or those with unknown duration, it is important to rule out intracardiac thrombus by echo (preferably transesophageal echo) before cardioversion because it may lead to cerebral embolization. If a thrombus is found or suspected, anticoagulation with warfarin (with international normalized ratio [INR] 2 to 3) is started and cardioversion delayed for 2 to 3 weeks. After conversion to sinus rhythm, warfarin is continued for an additional 3 to 4 weeks.
   c. For control of the ventricular rate, calcium channel blockers, propranolol, or digoxin may be used.

d. For prevention of recurrence, class I (quinidine) and class III (amiodarone) antiarrhythmic agents may be effective in some cases.
e. For refractory cases, antitachycardia pacing or radiofrequency ablation may be indicated.

F. ATRIAL FIBRILLATION

1. **Description:** Atrial fibrillation (AF) is characterized by an extremely fast atrial rate (F wave at 350 to 600 beats/min) and an irregular ventricular response with narrow QRS complexes (see Fig. 16.2).
2. **Causes:** AF usually is associated with structural heart diseases with dilated atria, such as seen with mitral stenosis and regurgitation, Ebstein anomaly, tricuspid atresia, ASD, or previous intraatrial surgery. Thyrotoxicosis, pulmonary emboli, and pericarditis should be suspected in a previously normal child who develops AF.
3. **Significance:** AF usually suggests a significant pathology. Rapid ventricular rate and the loss of coordinated contraction of the atria and ventricles decrease cardiac output. Atrial thrombus formation is quite common.
4. **Treatment:** Treatment of AF is similar to that described under the "Atrial Flutter section.
   a. If AF has been present more than 48 hours, the patient should receive anticoagulation with warfarin for 3 to 4 weeks to prevent systemic embolization of atrial thrombus, if the conversion can be delayed. Anticoagulation is continued for 4 weeks after restoration of sinus rhythm. If cardioversion cannot be delayed, heparin should be started, and cardioversion performed when activated partial thromboplastin time (aPTT) reaches 1.5 to 2.5 times control (in 5 to 10 days), with subsequent oral anticoagulation with warfarin.
   b. Propranolol or digoxin may be used to slow the ventricular rate.
   c. Class I antiarrhythmic agents (e.g., quinidine, procainamide, flecainide) and the class III agent amiodarone may be used but the success rate in rhythm conversion is disappointingly low. These agents may prevent recurrence.
   d. In patients with chronic AF, anticoagulation with warfarin should be used to reduce the incidence of thromboembolism.
   e. In the Cox maze procedure (or the "cut-and-sew-maze"), multiple surgical incisions are made in the right and left atria that are then repaired in an attempt to minimize the formation of a re-entrant loop. The procedure showed greater than a 96% cure rate 10 years after the surgery in adult patients.
   f. Radiofrequency ablation to electrically isolate the pulmonary veins from the left atrium or directly ablating the ectopic focus within the pulmonary veins has shown better results than pharmacologic agents in rhythm control in adults. Stenosis of the PV(s) is a significant complication of the procedure.

III. RHYTHMS ORIGINATING IN THE AV NODE

Rhythms originating in the AV node (Fig. 16.3) are characterized by the following:

1. The P wave may be absent, or inverted P waves may follow the QRS complex.
2. The QRS complex is usually normal in duration and configuration.

Junctional rhythm describes an abnormal heart rhythm resulting from impulses coming from a locus of tissue in the area of the AV node, the "junction" between atria and ventricles. Since the node-His (NH) region of the AV node is the only part of the AV node with demonstrable ability to pace the heart, some authorities prefer the term "nodal" over "junctional."

A. JUNCTIONAL (OR NODAL) PREMATURE BEATS

1. **Description:** A normal QRS complex occurs prematurely. P waves are usually absent, but inverted P waves may follow QRS complexes. The compensatory pause may be complete or incomplete (see Fig. 16.3).
2. **Causes:** Usually idiopathic in an otherwise normal heart but may result from cardiac surgery or digitalis toxicity.
3. **Significance:** Usually no hemodynamic significance.
4. **Treatment:** Treatment is not indicated unless caused by digitalis toxicity.

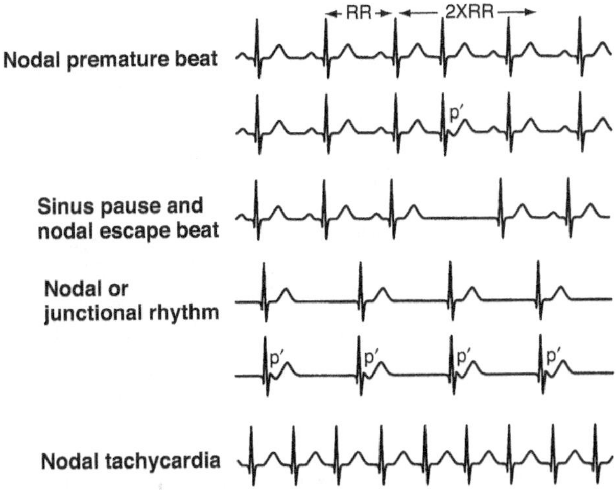

FIG. 16.3

Arrhythmias originating in the atrioventricular node. *(From Park, M. K. (2014).* Park's pediatric cardiology for practitioners *(6th ed.). Philadelphia: Mosby.)*

16

B. JUNCTIONAL (OR NODAL) ESCAPE BEAT

1. **Description:** When the sinus node impulse fails to reach the AV node, the NH region of the AV node will initiate an impulse (nodal or junctional escape beat). The QRS complex occurs later than the anticipated normal beat. The P wave may be absent (see Fig. 16.3), or an inverted P wave may follow the QRS complex.
2. **Causes:** It may follow cardiac surgery involving the atria (e.g., the Fontan operation) or may be seen in otherwise healthy children.
3. **Significance:** Little hemodynamic significance.
4. **Treatment**: Generally no specific treatment is required.

C. JUNCTIONAL (OR NODAL) RHYTHM

1. **Description:** If there is a persistent failure of the sinus node, the AV node may function as the main pacemaker of the heart with a relatively slow rate (40 to 60 beats/min). P waves are absent or inverted P waves follow QRS complexes (see Fig. 16.3).
2. **Causes:** It may be seen in an otherwise normal heart, after cardiac surgery, in conditions of an increased vagal tone (e.g., increased intracranial pressure, pharyngeal stimulation), and with digitalis toxicity. Rarely, it may be seen in children with polysplenia syndrome.
3. **Significance:** The slow heart rate may significantly decrease the cardiac output and produce symptoms.
4. **Treatment:** No treatment is indicated if the patient is asymptomatic. Atropine or electric pacing is indicated for symptoms. Treatment is directed to digitalis toxicity if caused by digitalis.

D. ACCELERATED JUNCTIONAL (OR NODAL) RHYTHM

1. **Description:** In the presence of normal sinus rate and AV conduction, if the AV node (NH region) with enhanced automaticity captures the pacemaker function (60 to 120 beats/min), the rhythm is called accelerated nodal (or AV junctional) rhythm. P waves are absent or inverted P waves follow the normal QRS complexes.
2. **Causes:** Idiopathic, digitalis toxicity, myocarditis, or previous cardiac surgery.
3. **Significance:** Little hemodynamic significance.
4. **Treatment:** No treatment is necessary unless caused by digitalis toxicity.

E. JUNCTIONAL ECTOPIC TACHYCARDIA (NODAL TACHYCARDIA)

1. **Description:** The ventricular rates vary from 120 to 200 beats/min. P waves are absent (see Fig. 16.3) or inverted P waves follow the QRS complexes. The QRS complex is usually normal, but aberration may occur. Junctional tachycardia is difficult to separate from other types of SVT. Therefore the arrhythmia is grouped under SVT.

2. **Causes:** Enhanced automaticity of the junctional area is the suspected mechanism. There are two types: postoperative and congenital.
   a. The postoperative type is more common than the congenital type. This transient disorder is seen after open heart surgery, and lasts 24 to 48 hours. Trauma, stretch, or ischemia to the AV node and electrolyte imbalance may be responsible for the rhythm disorder.
   b. The rare congenital type may occur with or without associated CHDs.
3. Significance
   a. In the postoperative type, a loss of AV synchrony in the presence of a fast rate (nearly 200 beats/min) compromises cardiac output, leading to a fall in blood pressure (BP). Increased endogenous catecholamine levels and administered inotropic support (to maintain adequate BP and renal perfusion) may result in peripheral vasoconstriction, leading to a rise in the core temperature. The rising core temperature exacerbates the tachycardia, worsening ventricular performance.
   b. In the congenital form, most patients present before 6 months of age, usually with CHF (with overall mortality rate of 35%).
4. Treatment
   a. For the postoperative type: Heart rate <170 beats/min is well tolerated but rates >170 to 190 beats/min need to be slowed.
      (1) Atrial overdrive pacing (typically 10 beats/min higher than the rate) often restores AV synchrony.
      (2) Mild systemic hypothermia is induced, usually a core temperature of 34°C to 35°C. At a core temperature below 32°C, ventricular function may be impaired.
      (3) Cardiac output is maximized by carefully titrating fluid and electrolyte balance, inotropic support, and pain management.
      (4) IV amiodarone appears to be the drug of choice as antiarrhythmic therapy. In the past, procainamide IV drip was widely used with good success. Digoxin is no longer used in this situation.
      (5) Extracorporeal membrane oxygenation (ECMO) can be used as an alternative in selected patients.
   b. For the congenital type, amiodarone appears to be the drug of choice. Amiodarone in high dose was effective in 85% of the patients with almost 75% survival rate. If amiodarone is not effective, ablation therapy may be tried.

IV. SUPRAVENTRICULAR TACHYCARDIA

SVT refers to any rapid heart rhythm originating above the ventricular tissue, including atrial and junctional tachycardias. SVTs are caused by two mechanisms: re-entry and automaticity.

1. Re-entry: Most cases of SVTs are due to re-entrant (or reciprocating) AV tachycardia. Only re-entry AV tachycardia is discussed in this section.

2. Automaticity: SVTs caused by increased automaticity of a single focus in the atria or the AV node are infrequent. Examples of this entity include atrial ectopic tachycardia and junctional (or nodal) ectopic tachycardia (as discussed in earlier sections).

A. MECHANISM OF RE-ENTRY TACHYCARDIAS

In SVT caused by reentry, two pathways are involved:

1. The anatomic accessory pathway, such as the bundle of Kent, produces AV re-entry tachycardia (AVRT) (Fig. 16.4A, B). WPW preexcitation is frequently present on the ECG.
2. A functionally separate bypass tract, such as a dual AV node pathway, produces AV nodal re-entry tachycardia (AVNRT) (Fig. 16.4C, D).

   Fig. 16.4 shows four different reentry mechanisms with resulting ECG rhythm strips.

   a. AVRT
      (1) If a PAC occurs, the prematurity of the extrasystole may find the bundle of Kent refractory, but the AV node may conduct (in orthodromic direction), producing a normal QRS complex. When the impulse reaches the bundle of Kent from the ventricular side, the bundle will have recovered and allows re-entry into the atrium retrogradely, producing a superiorly directed P wave. In turn, the cycle is maintained by re-entry into the AV node, with a very fast heart rate. When there is an antegrade conduction through the AV node (slow pathway); the rhythm is called orthodromic AVRT (see Fig. 16.4A). The resulting ECG rhythm will show narrow QRS complexes followed by inverted P waves (that are difficult to detect)
      (2) Less common is a widened QRS complex with antegrade conduction into the ventricle via the accessory (fast) pathway and retrograde conduction (antidromic) through the (slower) AV node (see Fig. 16.4B). A PVC could initiate this arrhythmia if the recovery time of the two limbs is ideal for the initiation of the reentry. The resulting tachycardia demonstrates inverted P waves followed by wide QRS complexes.

   b. AVNRT

   Functional dual pathways in the AV node are more common than anatomic accessory bundles, at least as functional entities. For SVT to occur, the two pathways would have to have, at least temporarily, different conduction and recovery rates, creating the substrate for a reentry tachycardia.

   (1) When the normal, slow pathway through the AV node is used in antegrade conduction to the bundle of His (orthodromic), the resulting QRS complex is normal with an abnormal P vector, but the latter is unrecognizable because it is superimposed on the QRS complex (see Fig. 16.4C). The resulting tachycardia could be the same as that seen with SVT associated with WPW syndrome. The

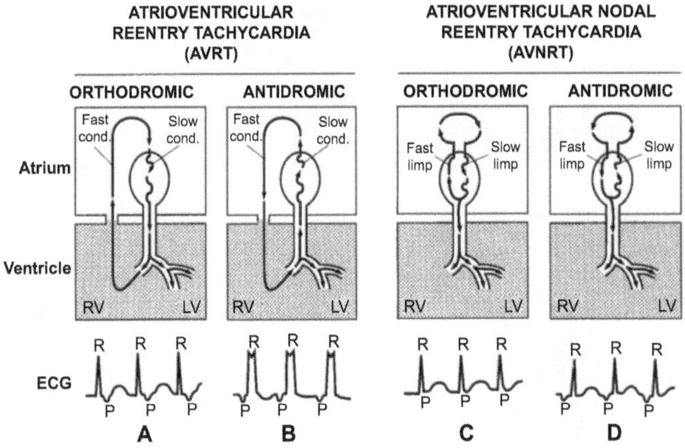

FIG. 16.4

Diagram showing the mechanism of re-entry type of supraventricular tachycardia in relation to ECG findings. (A) Orthodromic atrioventricular reentry tachycardia (AVRT) (B) Antidromic AVRT (C) Orthodromic atrioventricular nodal reentry tachycardia (AVNRT). (D) Antidromic AVNRT. See text for explanation. *(Modified from (From Park, M. K., & Guntheroth, W. G. (2006).* How to read pediatric ECGs *(4th ed.). Philadelphia: Mosby.)*

two can be differentiated only after conversion from the SVT; after conversion, the patient with accessory bundle would have WPW preexcitation.

(2) In antidromic AVNRT (see Fig. 16.4D), which is uncommon, the fast tract of the AV node transmits the antegrade impulse to the bundle of His, and the normal, slow pathway of the AV node transmits the impulse retrogradely. The resulting SVT demonstrates normal QRS duration, a short PR interval, and an inverted P wave.

1. Description

1. The heart rate is extremely rapid and regular (usually 240 ± 40 beats/min) (Fig. 16.5). The P wave is usually invisible, but when it is visible, it has an abnormal P axis and either precedes or follows the QRS complex. The QRS duration is usually normal, but occasionally aberrancy will prolong the QRS, making differentiation of this arrhythmia from ventricular tachycardia difficult. It used to be called PAT because its onset and termination were characteristically abrupt.
2. Some characteristics of AVRT and AVNRT are as follows.
   a. Sympathetic tone: AVNRT is more influenced by increased sympathetic tone than AVRT. Thus it is more likely triggered by

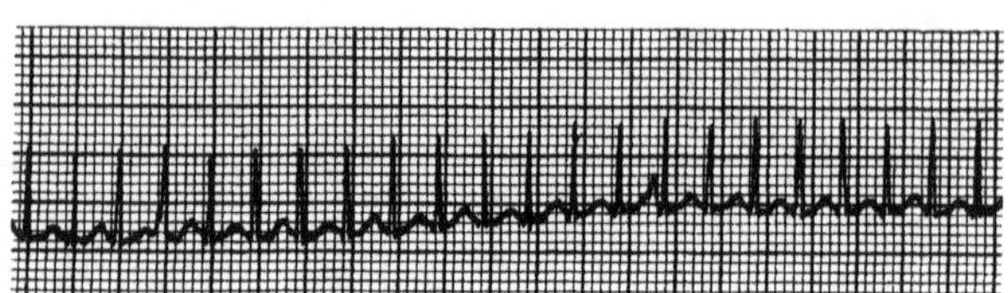

FIG. 16.5

Rhythm strip of SVT. The heart rate is 300 beats/min. *(From Park, M. K., & Guntheroth, W. G. (2006).* How to read pediatric ECGs *(4th ed.). Philadelphia: Mosby.)*

physical activity, emotional stress, or abrupt changes in body position.

b. AVNRT is less likely to be incessant (and therefore rarely causes tachycardia-induced cardiomyopathy).
c. Age of onset: SVT seen in the first year of life is more likely to be AVRT with accessory pathways. An adolescent who has first SVT is more likely to have AVNRT.

3. Any type of AV block is incompatible with re-entrant tachycardia; AV block would abruptly terminate the tachycardia, at least temporarily. This is why adenosine, which transiently blocks AV conduction, works well for this type of arrhythmia.

2. Causes

1. WPW preexcitation is present in 10% to 20% of SVT cases, which is evident only after conversion to sinus rhythm.
2. No heart disease is found in about half of patients. This idiopathic type of SVT occurs more commonly in young infants than in older children.
3. Some congenital heart defects (e.g., Ebstein anomaly, single ventricle, L-TGA) are more prone to this arrhythmia.
4. SVT may occur following cardiac surgeries.

3. Significance

1. Many infants tolerate SVT well. However, if the tachycardia is sustained for 6 to 12 hours, signs of CHF usually develop in infants (with irritability, tachypnea, poor feeding, and pallor).
2. Older children may complain of chest pain, palpitation, shortness of breath, lightheadedness, and fatigue (and seek medical care).
3. A pounding sensation in the neck (i.e., neck pulsation) is fairly unique to the re-entrant–type SVT and considered to be the result of cannon waves when the atrium contracts against a simultaneously contracting ventricle.

4. Management

a. Acute Treatment of SVT

1. Vagal stimulatory maneuvers (unilateral carotid sinus massage, gagging, or pressure on an eyeball) may be effective in older children, but rarely effective in infants. Placing an ice water bag on the face (for up to 10 seconds) is often effective in infants (by diving reflex). In children, a headstand often successfully interrupts the SVT.
2. If the vagal maneuver is ineffective, adenosine is considered the drug of choice. Adenosine has negative chronotropic and inotropic actions of a very short duration (half-life <10 seconds) and minimal hemodynamic consequences. Adenosine is effective for almost all re-entrant–type SVT (in which the AV node forms part of the re-entry circuit) of both narrow and wide QRS complex *regular* tachycardia. It is not effective for irregular tachycardias. It is not effective for non–re-entrant atrial tachycardia, atrial flutter/fibrillation, and VT.

   Adenosine is given by rapid intravenous bolus followed by a saline flush, starting at 50 μg/kg, increasing in increments of 50 μg/kg, every 1 to 2 min. The usual effective dose is 100 to 150 μg/kg with maximum dose of 250 μg/kg. Adenosine is 90% to 100% effective. If patient is hemodynamically stable but not responsive to adenosine, amiodarone (2.5 mg IV over 30 min) could be given and adenosine could be repeated with higher success rate.
3. If the infant is in severe CHF and adenosine is not readily available, immediate cardioversion is indicated.
4. IV administration of propranolol may be used to treat SVT in the presence of WPW syndrome. IV verapamil should be avoided in infants younger than 12 months because it may produce extreme bradycardia and hypotension in infants. Esmolol, other β-adrenergic blockers, verapamil, and digoxin also have been used with some success.
5. Overdrive suppression (by transesophageal pacing or by atrial pacing) may be effective in children who have been digitalized.

b. Prevention of Recurrence of SVT

1. In infants without WPW preexcitation, oral propranolol for 12 months is effective. In children beyond infancy, verapamil can also be used.
2. Children with breakthrough SVT while receiving β-blocker or not responsive to β-blockers will benefit from amiodarone orally.
3. In infants or children with/without WPW preexcitation, β-blockers such as atenolol or nadolol are often the medication of choice in the long-term management. In the presence of WPW preexcitation, digoxin or verapamil may increase the rate of antegrade conduction of the impulse through the accessory pathway, and therefore should be avoided.
4. For children who have infrequent episodes of SVT that result in little hemodynamic compromise, observation is indicated. They should be taught how to apply vagal maneuvers (such as gagging, headstands).

5. Recently intranasal etripamil, a short-acting L-type calcium channel blocker, was successfully used to terminate SVT in adult patients.
6. In adolescent patients, catheter ablation may be an effective alternative to long-term drug therapy. Ablation therapy is controversial for asymptomatic patients with WPW preexcitation. Ablation is not recommended in infants 1 to 2 years of age because of a possibility of spontaneous resolution of SVT. Risk of complication is 3% to 4%, including heart block.

V. RHYTHMS ORIGINATING IN THE VENTRICLE

Ventricular arrhythmias (Fig. 16.6) are characterized by the following:

1. Bizarre and wide QRS complexes with T waves pointing in the opposite directions.
2. QRS complexes randomly related to P waves, if visible.

A. PREMATURE VENTRICULAR CONTRACTION

1. Description

1. A bizarre, wide QRS complex appears earlier than anticipated, and the T wave points in the opposite direction. A full compensatory pause usually appears; that is, the length of two cycles, including the premature beat, is the same as that of two normal cycles (see Fig. 16.6).
2. PVCs may be classified into several types, depending on their interrelationship and similarities.
   a. By interrelationship of PVCs
      (1) Ventricular *bigeminy or coupling:* Each abnormal QRS complex alternates with a normal QRS complex regularly.
      (2) Ventricular *trigeminy:* Each abnormal QRS complex follows two normal QRS complexes regularly.
      (3) *Couplets:* Two abnormal QRS complexes come in sequence.

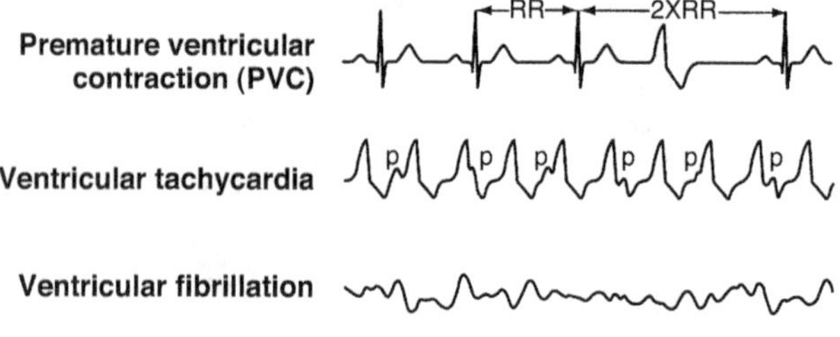

FIG. 16.6

Ventricular arrhythmias. *(From Park, M. K., & Guntheroth, W. G. (2006).* How to read pediatric ECGs *(4th ed.). Philadelphia: Mosby.)*

(4) *Triplets:* Three abnormal QRS complexes come in sequence. Three or more successive PVCs arbitrarily are termed VT.

b. By similarity among abnormal QRS complexes
   (1) Uniform (monomorphic or unifocal) PVCs: Abnormal QRS complexes have the same configuration in a single lead. It is assumed that they originate from a single focus.
   (2) Multiform (polymorphic or multifocal) PVCs: Abnormal QRS complexes have different configurations in a single lead. It is assumed that they originate from different foci.

2. Causes

a. PVCs may be seen in otherwise healthy children. Up to 50% to 70% of normal children may show PVCs on 24-hour Holter monitoring.
b. Myocarditis, myocardial injury or infarction, cardiomyopathy (dilated or hypertrophic), cardiac tumors, false tendon, and mitral valve prolapse are possible causes.
c. Arrhythmogenic RV dysplasia (RV cardiomyopathy), long QT syndrome, and Brugada syndrome may cause PVCs.
d. Congenital or acquired heart disease, preoperative or postoperative.
e. Drugs such as catecholamines, theophylline, caffeine, amphetamines, digitalis toxicity, and some anesthetic agents are possible causes.

3. Significance

1. Occasional PVCs are benign in children, particularly if they are uniform and disappear or decrease in frequency with exercise.
2. PVCs are more likely to be significant if:
   a. They are associated with underlying heart disease (e.g., preoperative or postoperative status, MVP, cardiomyopathy).
   b. There is a history of syncope or a family history of sudden death.
   c. They are precipitated by or increase in frequency with activity.
   d. They are multiform, particularly couplets.
   e. There are runs of PVC with symptoms.
   f. There are incessant or frequent episodes of paroxysmal VT.

4. Management

1. Some or all of the following tools are used in the investigation of PVCs and other ventricular arrhythmias:
   a. ECGs are used to detect QTc prolongation or ST-T changes.
   b. Echo studies detect structural heart disease or functional abnormalities.
   c. 24-hour Holter monitoring or event recorder detects the frequency and severity of the arrhythmia.

d. Exercise stress testing: Arrhythmias that are potentially related to exercise are significant and require documentation of the relationship. The induction or exacerbation of arrhythmia with exercise may be an indication of underlying heart disease. In children, PVCs characteristically are reduced or eliminated by exercise.
e. Cardiac catheterization and/or cardiac MRI, if arrhythmogenic RV dysplasia is suspected.
f. Electrophysiologic studies and endomyocardial biopsy.

2. In children with otherwise normal hearts, occasional isolated uniform PVCs that are suppressed by exercise do not require extensive investigation or treatment. ECG, echo studies, and 24-hour Holter monitoring suffice.
3. Asymptomatic children with multiform PVCs and ventricular couplets should have 24-hour Hotter monitoring, even if they have structurally normal hearts, to detect the severity and extent of ventricular arrhythmias.
4. Children with uniform PVCs, including ventricular bigeminy and trigeminy, do not need to be treated if the echo and exercise stress tests are normal.
5. All children with symptomatic ventricular arrhythmias and those with complex PVCs (multiform PVCs, ventricular couplets, unsustained ventricular tachycardia) should be treated. Tables A.4 and A.5 in Appendix A provide a quick review of antiarrhythmic drugs.
   a. β-Blockers (such as atenolol, 1 to 2 mg/kg orally in a single daily dose) are effective for cardiomyopathy and occasionally for RV dysplasia.
   b. Other antiarrhythmic drugs, such as mexiletine, may be effective.
   c. Antiarrhythmic agents that prolong the QT interval, such as those of class IA (quinidine, procainamide), class IC (encainide, flecainide), and class III (amiodarone, bretylium), should be avoided.
6. For patients with symptomatic ventricular arrhythmias or sustained ventricular tachycardia and seemingly normal hearts, magnetic resonance imaging (MRI) (preferable) or cardiac catheterization may be indicated to investigate for RV dysplasia. Occasionally, invasive electrophysiologic studies and RV endomyocardial biopsy may be indicated.
7. Children with multiform PVCs and runs of PVCs (VT) with or without symptoms need to be evaluated by an electrophysiologist.

B. ACCELERATED VENTRICULAR RHYTHM (AVR)

1. **Description:** AVR is also known by many other names, such as slow VT, idioventricular tachycardia, slow ventricular rhythm, and nonparoxysmal VT. There is a wide QRS complex rhythm of short duration (usually

several beats but can be longer than 100 beats). The QRS morphology is LBBB pattern in the great majority. The ventricular rate approximates the patient's sinus rate, within ± 10% to 15% of the sinus rate (isochronicity). The isochronicity with sinus rhythm is more important than the rate per minute. The ventricular rate is usually ≤ 120 beats/min in children and 140 to 180 beats/min in newborns.

2. **Causes:** AVR is usually an isolated finding. Rarely, it may be associated with underlying heart disease, such as CHD, myocarditis, digitalis toxicity, hypertension, cardiomyopathy, metabolic abnormalities, postoperative state, or myocardial infarction (MI) (in adults). The mechanism of AVR is unknown; ectopic ventricular focus may accelerate its rate enough to overcome sinus rate.
3. **Significance:** Usually asymptomatic and hemodynamically insignificant. Exertional sinus tachycardia usually converts it to sinus rhythm. Rarely seen in patients with syncope, presyncope, or palpitation or found in routine ECG or Holter monitoring
4. **Treatment:** In children, AVR is generally considered benign. AVR is notably resistant to antiarrhythmic agents (no treatment is required).

C. VENTRICULAR TACHYCARDIA

1. Description

1. VT is a series of three or more PVCs with a heart rate of 120 to 200 beats/min. QRS complexes are wide and bizarre, with T waves pointing in opposite directions.
2. By duration, VT may be classified as (a) a salvo of VT—a few beats in a row; (b) nonsustained VT—duration of less than 30 seconds; (c) sustained VT—longer than 30 seconds; and (d) incessant VT—refers to lengthy sustained VT that dominates the cardiac rhythm.
3. By morphology, VT may be classified as (a) monomorphic, referring to one dominant QRS form; (b) polymorphic, referring to a beat-to-beat change in the QRS shape; or (c) bidirectional, which is a specific form of polymorphic VT in which the QRS axis shifts across the baseline.
4. Torsades de pointes (meaning "twisting of the points") is a distinct form of polymorphic VT characterized by a paroxysm of VT during which there are progressive changes in the amplitude and polarity of QRS complexes separated by a narrow transition QRS complex. They occur in patients with marked QT prolongation.
5. VT is sometimes difficult to differentiate from SVT with aberrant conduction. However, wide QRS tachycardia in an infant or child must be considered VT until proven otherwise.

2. Causes

1. Structural heart diseases (such as TOF, AS, cardiomyopathies, or MVP).
2. Postoperative CHDs (such as TOF, D-TGA, or DORV).

3. Myocarditis, Chagas disease (trypanosomiasis, in South America), myocardial tumors, myocardial ischemia or MI, and pulmonary hypertension.
4. Genetic disorders, such as Brugada syndrome or arrhythmogenic RV dysplasia.
5. Torsades de pointes may be seen in patients with long QT syndrome. A partial list of drugs that may prolong the QT interval is shown in Box 16.1. Classes IA, IC, and III antiarrhythmic drugs prolong the QTc interval, but classes II and IV agents do not.
6. Metabolic causes (hypoxia, acidosis, hyperkalemia, hypokalemia, and hypomagnesemia).
7. Mechanical irritation—intraventricular catheter.
8. Pharmacologic or chemical causes (catecholamine infusion, digitalis toxicity, cocaine, and organophosphate insecticides). Most antiarrhythmic drugs (especially classes IA, IC, and III) are also proarrhythmic.
9. Benign VT may occur in healthy children who have structurally and functionally normal hearts. This group is discussed under a separate heading (see following).

3. Significance

1. VT usually signifies a serious myocardial pathology or dysfunction and can cause sudden death. Cardiac output may decrease notably and may deteriorate to ventricular fibrillation.
2. Polymorphic VTs are more significant than monomorphic ones.
3. Those associated with abnormal cardiac structure (preoperative and postoperative) and/or function are more significant than those seen with structurally and functionally normal heart.
4. Some VTs are provoked by exercise, whereas others are suppressed by exercise. The former is usually more significant than the latter.
5. VTs associated with certain forms of cardiomyopathy (arrhythmogenic RV dysplasia, hypertrophic or dilated cardiomyopathy) and genetic electrical heart diseases (long QT syndrome; Brugada syndrome) can be a cause of sudden death.

4. Management

1. Most of the tools suggested for the investigation of PVCs are used for VT, including (a) ECGs (for QTc prolongation or ST-T changes), (b) echo studies (for cardiomyopathy and other structural and functional abnormalities), (c) 24-hour Holter monitoring or event recorder, and (d) exercise stress testing (for induction or exacerbation or elimination of arrhythmia with exercise). MRI is useful to rule out arrhythmogenic RV dysplasia. Electrophysiologic studies and possible ablation, and endomyocardial biopsy are required for some patients.

BOX 16.1

ACQUIRED CAUSES OF QT PROLONGATION

DRUGS

Antibiotics—erythromycin, clarithromycin, telithromycin, azithromycin, trimethoprim-sulfamethoxazole
Antifungal agents—fluconazole, itraconazole, ketoconazole
Antiprotozoal agents—pentamidine isethionate
Antihistamines—astemizole, terfenadine (Seldane) [Seldane has been removed from the market for this reason]
Antidepressants—tricyclics such as imipramine (Tofranil), amitriptyline (Elavil), desipramine (Norpramin), and doxepin (Sinequan)
Antipsychotics—haloperidol, risperidone, phenothiazines such as thioridazine (Mellaril) and chlorpromazine (Thorazine)
Antiarrhythmic agents
Class 1A (sodium channel blockers)—quinidine, procainamide, disopyramide
Class III (prolong depolarization)—amiodarone (rare), bretylium, dofetilide, N-acetyl-procainamide, sotalol
Lipid-lowering agents—probucol
Antianginals— befpridil
Diuretics (through potassium loss)—furosemide (Lasix), ethacrynic acid (Edecrin)
Oral hypoglycemic agents—glibenclamide, glyburide
Organophosphate insecticides
Promotility agents—isapride
Vasodilators— prenylamine

ELECTROLYTE DISTURBANCES

Hypokalemia—diuretics, hyperventilation
Hypocalcemia
Hypomagnesemia

UNDERLYING MEDICAL CONDITIONS

Bradycardia—complete atrioventricular block, severe bradycardia, sick sinus syndrome
Myocardial dysfunction—anthracycline cardiotoxicity, congestive heart failure, myocarditis, cardiac tumors
Endocrinopathy—hyperparathyroidism, hypothyroidism, pheochromocytoma
Neurologic—encephalitis, head trauma, stroke, subarachnoid hemorrhage
Nutritional—alcoholism, anorexia nervosa, starvation

A more exhaustive updated list of medications that can prolong the QTc interval is available at crediblemeds.org.

2. Acute therapy may include the following.
   a. Prompt synchronized cardioversion (0.5 to 1.0 joules/kg) if the patient is unconscious or if there is evidence of low cardiac output.
   b. If the patient is conscious, an IV bolus of lidocaine, 1 mg/kg over 1 to 2 min, followed by an IV drip of lidocaine, 20 to 50 μg/kg/min, may be effective.
3. IV amiodarone is used in patients with drug-refractory VT, particularly that seen in postoperative patients.

4. Patients with long QT syndrome are treated with β-blockers, which alleviate symptoms in 75% to 80%. An implantable cardioverter defibrillator (ICD) is sometimes recommended as initial therapy.
5. Recurrence may be prevented with administration of propranolol, atenolol, diphenylhydantoin, or quinidine. A combination of 24-hour Holter monitoring and treadmill exercise testing is the best noninvasive means of evaluating drug effectiveness.
6. Some incessant ventricular tachycardias are amenable to radiofrequency ablation.
7. ICD has become the established standard for treating many, if not most, forms of ventricular tachycardia, which are potentially lethal.

D. VENTRICULAR ARRHYTHMIAS IN CHILDREN WITH NORMAL HEARTS

Although recurrent sustained VT usually signals an organic cause of the arrhythmia, some VTs are seen in healthy adolescents and young adults with structurally and functionally normal hearts. The prognosis is good. RVOT VT and RBBB VT are examples of this group of VT.

1. Right Ventricular Outflow Tract Ventricular Tachycardia

1. **Description:** This special form of VT originates from the RV conal septum and thus has inferior QRS axis and LBBB morphology (Fig. 16.7). This is usually benign tachycardia. It may manifest as frequent PVCs or short runs or salvos of VT, but many children are asymptomatic or minimally symptomatic. Exercise stress may not completely abolish the tachycardia.
2. **Treatment:** β-Blockers are sufficient for treatment. Verapamil and other agents may also prove to be effective. Radiofrequency ablation can be curative.

2. RBBB Ventricular Tachycardia (Belhassen Tachycardia)

1. **Description:** It appears to arise from the septal surface of the LV and is less common than RVOT VT. It is characterized by RBBB morphology and superior QRS axis.
2. **Treatment:** These types of tachycardia may be calcium channel dependent and respond to slow IV push of verapamil. Long-term treatment with verapamil can prevent recurrences. When refractory to medical therapy, radiofrequency ablation or surgery is effective. The long-term outcome is excellent.

E. VENTRICULAR FIBRILLATION

1. **Description:** Ventricular fibrillation is characterized by bizarre QRS complexes of varying sizes and configurations. The rate is rapid and irregular (see Fig. 16.6).
2. **Causes:** Postoperative state, severe hypoxia, hyperkalemia, digitalis or quinidine toxicity, myocarditis, myocardial infarction, and drugs (catecholamines, anesthetics, etc.) are possible causes.

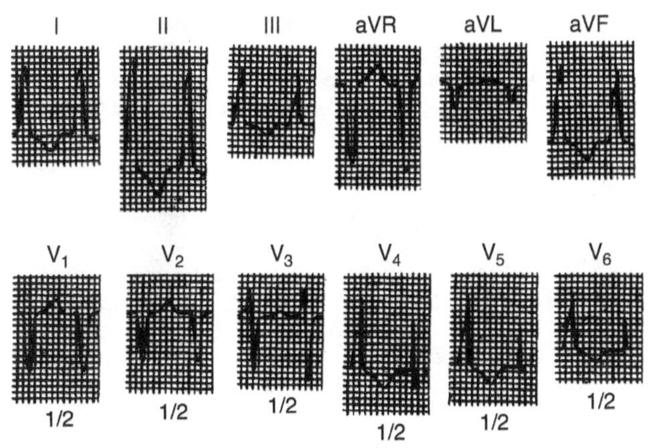

FIG. 16.7

Tracing from a 4-year-old asymptomatic girl with RVOT ventricular tachycardia (and structurally normal heart). The rate of ventricular tachycardia was 160 beats/min. The QRS complexes have LBBB morphology indicating the RV as the ectopic focus and the axis of VT is directed inferiorly. Spontaneous temporary interruption of VT occurred while recording V_4, V_5, and V_6 leads.

3. **Significance:** It is usually fatal because it results in ineffective circulation.
4. **Treatment:** Immediate cardiopulmonary resuscitation, including electric defibrillation at 2 joules/kg, is required. ICDs are often indicated in patients who survived ventricular fibrillation.

F. LONG QT SYNDROME

1. Description

Long QT syndrome (LQTS) is a genetic disorder of ventricular repolarization characterized by a prolonged QT interval on the ECG and ventricular arrhythmias, usually torsades de pointes, that may result in sudden death. Meanwhile, 15 genetic mutations have been identified responsible for LQTS; some are described in the following text.

2. Causes

1. Congenital types: Ion channels that govern the electrical activity of the heart are defective in congenital LQTS.
   a. Jervell and Lange-Nielsen syndrome (autosomal recessive mode) consists of a prolonged QTc interval, congenital deafness, syncopal spells, and a family history of sudden death.

b. Roman-Ward syndrome (autosomal dominant mode) has all the features of Jervell and Lange-Nielsen syndrome except for deafness. A sporadic form of the syndrome with a negative family history also exists.
c. In Anderson-Tawil syndrome, the QU interval (rather than QT interval) is prolonged, along with muscle weakness (periodic paralysis), ventricular arrhythmias, and developmental abnormalities.
d. Timothy syndrome is associated with webbed fingers and toes and a prolonged QTc interval.

2. Acquired type: Prolongation of the QT interval can be caused by a number of drugs, electrolyte disturbances, and other underlying medical conditions (see Box 16.1). A similar ionic mechanism may be involved as in congenital LQTS. Those individuals who manifest acquired LQTS are believed to be genetically predisposed for the condition.

3. Clinical Manifestations

1. Positive family history is present in about 60% and deafness in 5% of patients.
2. Presenting symptoms may be syncope (26%), seizure (10%), cardiac arrest (9%), presyncope, or palpitation (6%).
3. Symptoms usually occur in the setting of intense adrenergic arousal, intense emotion, and during or following rigorous exercise. Swimming appears to be a particular trigger. A loud doorbell, alarm clock, telephone, or security alarm can trigger symptoms.
4. The ECG shows the following:
   a. The QTc interval is prolonged, usually to >0.46 second. The upper limit of normal QTc is 0.44 second.
   b. Abnormal T-wave morphology (bifid, diphasic, or notched) is frequent.
   c. Bradycardia (20%), second-degree AV block, multiform PVCs, and monomorphic or polymorphic VT (10% to 20%) may be present.
5. Echo studies usually show a structurally and functionally normal heart.
6. A treadmill exercise test results in a highly significant prolongation of the QTc interval, with the maximal QTc prolongation present after 1 to 2 minutes of recovery. Ventricular arrhythmias may develop during the test in up to 30% of patients.
7. Holter monitoring reveals prolongation of the QTc interval, major changes in the T-wave configuration (T-wave alternation), and ventricular arrhythmias. The QTc interval on Holter monitor may be longer than that recorded on a standard ECG (see a later section).

4. Diagnosis

A correct diagnosis and proper treatment can save lives, but the diagnosis of this disease should not be made lightly because it implies a high-risk disease with a lifelong commitment to treatment.

1. Accurate measurement of the QTc interval is essential in the diagnosis of LQTS.
   a. Lead II (with q waves) and precordial leads (V1, V3, or V5, with well-defined T waves) are good leads in measuring the QT interval.
   b. In patients with sinus arrhythmia, the QT interval immediately following the shortest RR interval has been recommended to use in calculating the QTc interval. However, the QTc measurement during sinus arrhythmia may not be reliable because the Bazett formula is reliable only for the steady state and sinus arrhythmia is not a steady state.
   c. In patients with wide QRS complexes (such as BBB), the JTc interval may be a more sensitive predictor of repolarization abnormalities than the QTc. Rate correction is accomplished by the use of Bazett formula. Normal JTc interval (mean $\pm$ SD) is 0.32 ± 0.02 second (with the upper limit of normal 0.34 second).
2. **Schwartz diagnostic criteria:** The diagnosis of LQTS is clear-cut when there is a marked prolongation of the QTc interval with positive family history of the syndrome. However, many cases are borderline, making it difficult to make or reject the diagnosis. Schwartz et al. refined diagnostic criteria (2012) using a point system (Table 16.1) as follows.
   a. ≤ 1 point = low probability of LQTS
   b. 1.5 to 3 points = intermediate probability of LQTS
   c. ≥ 3.5 points = high probability LQTS
3. **Initial diagnostic strategy:** The following steps are considered in making the diagnosis of LQTS.
   a. History of presyncope, syncope, seizure, or palpitation and family history are carefully examined.
   b. Causes of acquired LQTS are excluded.
   c. The ECG is examined for the QTc interval and morphology of the T waves. ECGs are also obtained from immediate family members.
   d. The LQTS score is calculated using the Schwartz updated diagnostic criteria (see Table 16.1) and the diagnostic possibility is graded as described earlier.
4. **Exercise testing:** Some centers routinely perform exercise testing. In most normal children and young adults, the QT interval shortens with exercise with increasing heart rate. However, in patients with LQTS, the QT interval may fail to shorten or may lengthen at higher heart rates and with exertion. A lack of appropriate shortening of the QTc interval as well as abnormal T-wave morphology is most often seen in LQTS patients. The QTc of ≥ 480 ms at 4 minutes of recovery after the exercise stress may be significant.
5. For borderline cases, some centers carry out additional testing, such as Holter monitoring, pharmacologic testing, or electrophysiology study. However, the interpretation and significance of these tests are controversial.
6. Genetic testing may identify genotypes of the LQTS. The commercially available genetic tests can identify the five most common gene mutations,

TABLE 16.1

SCHWARTZ UPDATED DIAGNOSTIC CRITERIA FOR LONG QT SYNDROME

ECG FINDINGS **(in the absence of medications or disorders known to prolong the QTc interval)**	
QTc Interval (ms)	Points
>480	3
460–470	2
450–459	1
≥480 ms at 4 minutes of recovery from exercise stress test	1
Torsades de pointes	2
T-wave alternans	1
Notched T waves in three leads	1
Low heart rate for age (<2nd percentile)	0.5
Clinical History	
Syncope	
With stress	2
Without stress	1
Congenital deafness	0.5
Family History	
Family members with definite LQTS	1
Unexplained sudden cardiac death younger than 30 yr among immediate family members	0.5

LQTS, long QT syndrome.

Adapted from Schwartz, P. J., Crotti, L., & Insolia, R. (2012): Long QT syndrome: from genetics to management. *Circulation Arrhythmia and Electrophysiology*, 5(4), 868-877.

all in Romano-Ward syndrome (including *KCNQ1, KCNE1, KCNH2, KCNE2*, and *SCN5A*). The genetic testing has limitations, though. It is important to realize that the testing can identify a particular mutation but it cannot rule out LQTS; a negative genetic test does not rule out LQTS.

5. Management

1. The following are known risk factors for sudden death and should be considered when making a treatment plan.
   a. Bradycardia for age (sinus bradycardia, junctional escape rhythm, or second-degree AV block).
   b. An extremely long QTc interval (>0.55 second).
   c. Symptoms at presentation (syncope, seizure, cardiac arrest).
   d. Young age at presentation (<1 month).
   e. Documented torsades de pointes or ventricular fibrillation.
   f. T-wave alternans (major changes in T-wave morphology) is a relative risk factor.

2. General measures
   a. Physicians should avoid prescribing medications that prolong the QT interval, including some commonly used antibiotics and catecholamines. See Box 16.1 and check on updated Internet sources such as www.sads.org or www.crediblemeds.org.
   b. No competitive sports are allowed. Swimming is not advised.
   c. Alarm clocks or bedside telephones should be removed because these are known triggers of VT in patients with LQTS.
   d. The patients and the parents should be educated about the importance of being compliant with their medication, because noncompliance can result in sudden death.
3. Treatment of congenital LQTS

   For congenital LQTS, the initial treatment is aimed at interrupting sympathetic input to the myocardium with β-blockers. An ICD may be needed in some patients who continue to have symptoms while receiving β-blockers.
   a. β-blockers. β-Blockers are the current treatment of choice. They reduce both syncope and sudden cardiac death, but cardiac events continue to occur while β-blocker therapy is used.
      (1) There is a consensus that all symptomatic children with long QT syndrome should be treated with propranolol, atenolol, or metoprolol.
      (2) Whether to start β-blockers on asymptomatic children with QTc prolongation is controversial. Any patients who score 3.5 or greater on the Schwartz diagnostic criteria should be treated regardless of symptoms. However, it may be prudent to follow those asymptomatic children with borderline scores.
      In addition, β-blockers may be dangerous, because they tend to produce bradycardia, a known risk factor for sudden death.
      (3) Schwartz (1997) has suggested definitive treatment of asymptomatic patients with congenital LQTS in the following circumstances: (a) newborns and infants, (b) patients with deafness, (c) affected siblings with LQTS and sudden cardiac death, (d) extremely long QTc (>0.60 sec) or T-wave alternans, and (e) to prevent family or patient anxiety.
   b. The ICD appears to be the most effective therapy for high-risk patients, defined as those with aborted cardiac arrests or recurrent cardiac events despite conventional therapy (with β-blockers), and those with extremely prolonged QTc intervals (e.g., >0.60 second). Patients with ICD should continue with βblocker therapy.

   The Schwartz group recommends ICD implantation in the following situations.
   (1) All those who survived a cardiac arrest during therapy
   (2) Most of those who survived a cardiac arrest off therapy, except those with a reversible/preventable cause
   (3) Those with syncope despite a full dose of β-blockers therapy, whenever the option of left cardiac sympathetic denervation (LCSD)

is either not available or discarded after discussion with the patients

(4) All patients with syncope, despite a full dose of β-blockers and LCSD, and

(5) Exceptionally, the rare asymptomatic patients with a QTc >550 msec, who also manifest signs of high electric instability (e.g., T-wave alternans) or other evidence of being at high risk (e.g., long sinus pauses followed by abnormal T-wave morphologies), despite β-blockers and LCSD.

c. Left cardiac sympathetic denervation. Because of the availability of other options, such as ICD, this procedure is rarely performed.

d. Targeted pharmacologic therapy. The sodium channel blocker mexiletine was used in patients with mutation in the sodium channel gene *SCN5A* (*LQT3*) with significant shortening of the QTc. Gene or *gene-specific* therapy, or more accurately mutation-specific therapy, has not gained wide clinical application at this time.

6. Prognosis

The prognosis is very poor in untreated patients, with annual mortality as high as 20% and 10-year mortality of 50%. β-Blockers may reduce mortality to some extent, but they do not completely protect patients from sudden death. The ICD appears promising in improving prognosis.

G. SHORT QT SYNDROME

1. Description

Short QT syndrome (SQTS) is a cardiac channelopathy associated with a predisposition to AF and sudden cardiac death, first described by Gassak et al. in 2000. The cause of death is believed to be ventricular fibrillation. Mutations in the *KCNH2, KCNJ2,* and *KCNQ1* genes appear to be the cause of SQTS. It is transmitted in an autosomal dominant manner.

2. Clinical Manifestations

1. The ECG shows a short QTc (usually ≤360 msec) with tall, symmetric, peaked T waves on the ECG.
2. These patients present with sudden death, symptoms of palpitation, dizziness, or syncope, and sometimes, paroxysmal AF. Most patients have easily inducible ventricular fibrillation.
3. Most patients have a family history of sudden death.
4. Although it usually occur in the adult (median age 30 years), a sudden cardiac death was also observed in early infancy. Some infants and neonates present with AF and a slow ventricular response; it may present in utero as persistent bradycardia.
5. Recently diagnostic criteria for SQTS have been proposed by Gollob et al. (2011) (Table 16.2), based on a point system similar to Schwartz's

TABLE 16.2

SHORT QT SYNDROME DIAGNOSTIC CRITERIA

ECG FINDINGS	
QTc interval (ms)	Points
<370	1
<350	2
<330	3
J point to T peak interval <120 msec	1
Clinical History	
Sudden cardiac arrest	2
Polymorphic VT or VF	2
Unexplained syncope	1
Atrial fibrillation	1
Family History	
First- and second-degree relative with SQTS	2
First- and second-degree relative with sudden death	1
Sudden infant death syndrome	1
Genotype	
Genotype positive	2
Mutation of undetermined significance in a culprit gene	1

ECG, electrocardiogram; *SQTS*, short QT syndrome; *VF*, ventricular fibrillation; *VT*, ventricular tachycardia.
Adapted from Gollob, M., Redpath, C., & Roberts, J. (2011). The short QT syndrome: proposed diagnostic criteria. *Journal of the American College of Cardiology, 57*(7), 802-812.

criteria for LQTS. According to these criteria, the scoring of the probability of SQTS is done as follows:

≤2 points = low probability of SQTS
3 points = intermediate probability of SQTS
≥4 points = high probability SQTS

3. Treatment

1. The therapy of choice is the ICD.
2. Certain antiarrhythmic agents, such as quinidine, propafenone, or sotalol, help prolong the QT interval and decrease the potential for VF.

H. BRUGADA SYNDROME

1. Description

This inherited arrhythmogenic disorder with a high risk of sudden cardiac death from ventricular tachyarrhythmia, occurring during sleep, appears to be inherited as an autosomal dominant pattern. It is primarily a disease of adult males, seen most commonly in Southeast Asian men (with mean age of 40 years). However, this syndrome has been demonstrated in children and infants. No male preponderance is observed in children, raising the possibility of a high level of androgen in the occurrence of the fatal event. Mutations in the sodium channel (*SCN5A*) appear to be the cause of the condition, at least in 20% of the patients.

2. Clinical Manifestations

1. Cardiac examination is usually normal. There is no demonstrable structural abnormality of the heart.
2. The ECG changes are characteristic of the condition.
   a. The ECG typically shows cove-type ST-segment elevation (type 1 Brugada ECG pattern) or saddle-back ST-segment elevation (type 2 Brugada ECG pattern) with J point elevation, followed by a negative T wave in the right precordial leads (V1-V3) with or without RBBB appearance.
   b. Prolonged PR interval, AF, and SVT are also frequently found.
3. **Diagnosis:** Only type 1 ECG pattern can be used to confirm the diagnosis of Brugada syndrome because type 2 patterns are frequently seen in persons without the disease. This so-called type 1 ECG pattern may be present either spontaneously or after provocation with ajmaline or flecainide.
4. Most syncope takes place at rest (90%). Fever is an important precipitating factor of syncope.
5. The condition can carry a poor prognosis (i.e., at least a 10% death rate per year), particularly in those who are symptomatic.

3. Treatment

1. β-Blockers do not appear to reduce the risk of death in these patients.
2. In many centers, ICD is standard practice for all symptomatic patients (either aborted cardiac arrest or arrhythmic syncope) to prevent sudden cardiac death.
3. Hydroquinidine has been shown to be a good alternative to ICD implantation in adult patients, and it appears to be effective in preventing syncope in children also.

Chapter 17

Atrioventricular Conduction Disturbances

AV block is a disturbance in conduction between the normal sinus impulse and the eventual ventricular response. The block is assigned to one of three classes, according to the severity of the conduction disturbance.

1. First-degree AV block is a simple prolongation of the PR interval but all P waves are conducted to the ventricle.
2. In second-degree AV block, some atrial impulses are not conducted into the ventricle.
3. In third-degree AV block (or complete heart block), none of the atrial impulses is conducted into the ventricle (Fig. 17.1).

I. FIRST-DEGREE AV BLOCK

1. **Description:** There is a prolongation of the PR interval beyond the upper limits of normal (see Table 2.3) due to an abnormal delay in conduction through the AV node (see Fig. 17.1).
2. **Causes**
   a. In otherwise healthy children and young adults, particularly athletes, mediated through excessive parasympathetic tone.
   b. CHDs (such as endocardial cushion defect, ASD, Ebstein anomaly).
   c. Other causes, including infectious disease, inflammatory conditions (rheumatic fever), cardiac surgery, and certain drugs (such as digitalis, calcium channel blockers).
3. **Significance**
   a. Usually no hemodynamic disturbance results. Exercise, both recreational and during stress testing, induces parasympathetic withdrawal resulting in normalization of AV conduction and the PR interval.
   b. Sometimes it may progress to a more advanced AV block.
4. **Treatment:** No treatment is indicated except in digitalis toxicity.

II. SECOND-DEGREE AV BLOCK

In second-degree AV block, some but not all P waves are followed by QRS complexes (dropped beats). There are three types: Mobitz type I (Wenckebach phenomenon), Mobitz type II, and high-grade (or advanced) second-degree AV block.

A. MOBITZ TYPE I (WENCKEBACH PHENOMENON)

1. **Description:** The PR interval becomes progressively prolonged until one QRS complex is dropped completely (see Fig. 17.1).
2. **Causes:** In otherwise healthy children, myocarditis, cardiomyopathy, myocardial infarction, CHD, cardiac surgery, and digitalis toxicity.
3. **Significance**
   a. The block is at the level of the AV node (with prolonged atrio-His interval).
   b. It occurs in individuals with vagal dominance.
   c. It usually does not progress to complete heart block.
4. **Treatment:** The underlying cause is treated.

B. MOBITZ TYPE II

1. **Description:** The AV conduction is "all or none." AV conduction is either normal or completely blocked (see Fig. 17.1).
2. **Causes:** Same as for Mobitz type I.
3. **Significance**
   a. The block usually occurs below the AV node (at the level of the bundle of His).
   b. It is more serious than type I block because it may progress to complete heart block, resulting in Stokes-Adams attacks.
4. **Treatment:** The underlying cause is treated. Prophylactic pacemaker therapy may be indicated.

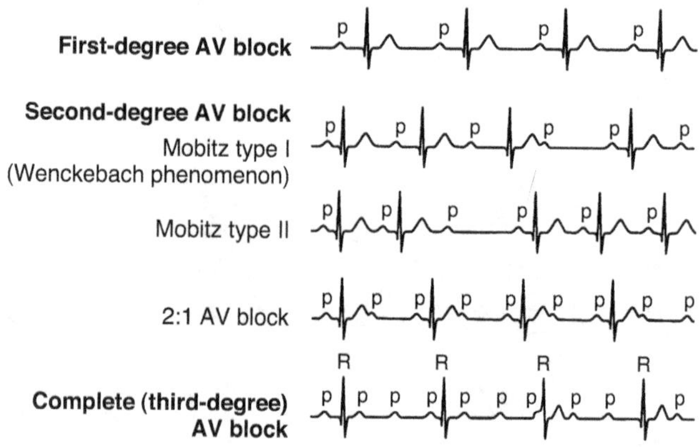

FIG. 17.1
Atrioventricular (AV) block. *(From Park, M. K., & Guntheroth, W. G. (2006).* How to read pediatric ECGs *(4th ed.). Philadelphia: Mosby.)*

C. TWO-TO-ONE (OR HIGHER) AV BLOCK

1. **Description**
   a. A QRS complex follows every second (third or fourth) P wave, resulting in 2:1 (3:1 or 4:1, respectively) AV block (see Fig. 17.1). In contrast to third-degree complete AV block, some P waves continue to be conducted to the ventricle and the PR interval of conducted beats is constant.
   b. When two or more consecutive P waves are nonconducted, the rhythm is called advanced or high-grade second-degree AV block.
2. **Causes:** Similar to those of other second-degree AV blocks.
3. **Significance**
   a. The block is usually at the bundle of His, alone or in combination with the AV nodal block.
   b. It may occasionally progress to complete heart block.
   c. Higher-grade second-degree AV block should always be regarded as abnormal. The implications of high-grade AV block appear to be similar to those of complete AV block.
4. **Treatment:** The underlying cause is treated. Electrophysiologic studies may be necessary to determine the level of the block. Pacemaker therapy is indicated for symptomatic advanced second-degree AV block.

III. THIRD-DEGREE AV BLOCK (COMPLETE HEART BLOCK)

1. **Description**
   a. In third-degree AV block, the atrial and ventricular activities are entirely independent of each other (see Fig. 17.1). The P waves are regular (with regular PP interval) with a rate comparable to the heart rate of the patient's age. The QRS complexes are also quite regular (with regular RR interval) but with a rate much slower than the P rate.
   b. The third-degree AV block is either congenital or acquired.
      i. In *congenital* complete heart block, the duration of the QRS complex is normal, since the pacemaker for the QRS complex is at a level higher than the bifurcation of the bundle of His. The ventricular rate is faster (50 to 80 beats/min) than in the acquired type.
      ii. In surgically induced or *acquired* (from postmyocardial infarction) complete heart block, the QRS duration is prolonged, and the ventricular rate is in the range of 40 to 50 beats/min (idioventricular rhythm). The pacemaker for the wide QRS complex is at a level below the bifurcation of the bundle of His.
2. **Causes**
   a. Congenital heart block
      i. In 60% to 90% of cases, it is caused by neonatal lupus erythematosus. Maternal antibodies to the intracellular ribonucleoprotein Ro (SS-A) and La (SS-B) for autoimmune

connective tissue diseases cross the placenta to the fetus causing the heart block.
   - ii. In 25% to 33%, it is associated with CHDs, most commonly with L-TGA, single ventricle, or polysplenia syndrome.
   - iii. Neonatal myocarditis and several genetic disorders such as familial ASD and Kearns-Sayre syndrome have been identified.
- b. The acquired type
   - i. It occurs as a complication of cardiac surgery in children.
   - ii. Rarely, severe myocarditis, Lyme carditis, acute rheumatic fever, mumps, diphtheria, cardiomyopathies, tumors in the conduction system, or overdose of certain drugs causes the block.
   - iii. It may also follow myocardial infarction.
   - iv. These causes produce either temporary or permanent heart block.

3. **Significance**
   - a. Complete heart block can be diagnosed by fetal bradycardia during fetal echo study between 18 and 28 weeks of gestation. Complications in utero may include hydrops fetalis, myocarditis, and fetal death.
   - b. CHF may develop in infancy, particularly when there are associated CHDs.
   - c. Patients with isolated congenital heart block are usually asymptomatic during childhood and achieve normal growth and development.
   - d. Syncopal attacks (Stokes-Adams attack) or sudden death may occur with the heart rate below 40 to 45 beats/min.
4. **Treatment**
   - a. When detected *in utero*, steroid therapy may be applied if associated with anti-Ro/SS-A and anti-La/SS-B.
   - b. Asymptomatic children with congenital complete heart block with acceptable heart rate, narrow QRS complex, and normal ventricular function may not need to be treated.
   - c. In symptomatic children and adults, atropine or isoproterenol is indicated until temporary ventricular pacing is secured.
   - d. A temporary transvenous or epicardial ventricular pacemaker is indicated in patients with heart block, or it may be given prophylactically in patients who might develop heart block.
   - e. Permanent pacemaker therapy is indicated in patients with congenital heart block under the following situations (see Box 18.1 for detailed indications).
      - i. If the patient is symptomatic or develops CHF.
      - ii. Dizziness or lightheadedness may be an early warning sign of the need for a pacemaker.
      - iii. If an infant has a ventricular rate <50 to 55 beats/min or if the infant has a CHD with a ventricular rate <70 beats/min.

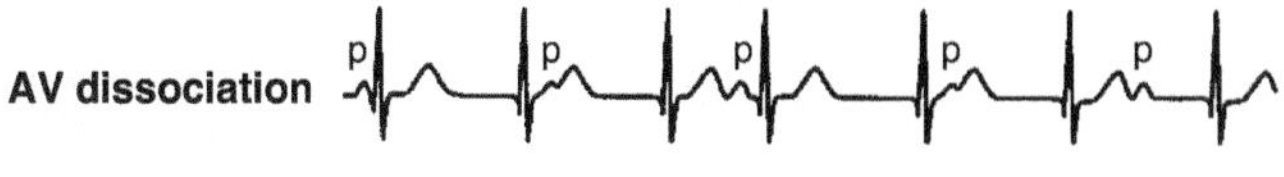

AV dissociation

FIG. 17.2

Diagram of AV dissociation owing to either marked slowing of the sinus node or acceleration of the AV node. The fourth complex is conducted, changing the rhythm (called "interference").

iv. If the patient has a wide QRS escape rhythm, complex ventricular ectopy, or ventricular dysfunction.

v. In patients with surgically induced heart block that is not expected to resolve or that persist at least 7 day after cardiac surgery.

f. A variety of problems may arise after a pacemaker is placed in children. Stress placed on the lead system by the linear growth of the child, fracture of the lead system in a physically active child, electrode malfunction (scarring of the myocardium around the electrode, especially in infants), and the limited life span of the pulse generator require follow-up of children with artificial pacemakers.

IV. ATRIOVENTRICULAR DISSOCIATION

AV dissociation should not be confused with complete heart block (third-degree AV block).

1. AV dissociation results from a marked slowing of the sinus node activity, atrial bradycardia, or acceleration of the AV node.
2. In AV dissociation the atrial rate is slower than the ventricular rate, whereas in complete heart block the ventricular rate is usually slower than the atrial rate.
3. In AV dissociation an atrial impulse may conduct to the AV node if it comes at the right time (Fig. 17.2).

The conducted beat can be recognized by its relative prematurity.

Chapter 18

Pacemakers and Implantable Cardioverter Defibrillators

A pacemaker is a device that delivers battery-supplied electrical stimuli over leads to electrodes that are in contact with the heart. It primarily treats bradycardia. An implantable cardioverter defibrillator (ICD) is a multiprogrammable antiarrhythmic device for treating ventricular tachycardia and ventricular fibrillation. ICDs also possess pacemaking capability to treat bradycardia.

I. PACEMAKERS IN CHILDREN

For pacemakers, the electrical leads are inserted either directly over the epicardium or transvenously; the latter is the method of choice. Electronic circuitry regulates the timing and characteristics of the stimuli. The power source usually is a lithium-iodine battery. Battery life varies from 3 years to 15 years depending on the type of the device, which determines the amount of battery use. New pacemakers are capable of closely mimicking normal cardiac rhythm (physiologic pacemakers), and most of them are small enough to be implanted in an infant.

Physicians encounter an increasing number of children with either temporary or permanent pacemakers. Basic knowledge about the pacemaker and the pacemaker rhythm strip is essential in taking care of these children.

A. ECGS OF ARTIFICIAL CARDIAC PACEMAKERS

1. **Rhythm strips of artificial pacemakers:** The need to recognize rhythm strips of artificial pacemakers has increased in recent years, especially in intensive care and emergency room settings. The position and number of the pacemaker spikes on the electrocardiogram (ECG) rhythm strip are used to recognize different types of pacemakers.
   a. When the pacemaker stimulates the atrium, a P wave follows an electronic spike. The resulting P wave demonstrates an abnormal P axis.
   b. When the pacemaker stimulates the ventricle, a wide QRS complex appears after the electronic spike.
   c. The ventricle that is stimulated (or the ventricle on which the pacemaker electrode is placed) can be identified by the morphology of the QRS complexes. With the pacing electrode on the RV, the

QRS complex resembles an LBBB pattern; with the pacemaker placed on the LV, an RBBB pattern results.

2. **Examples of pacemaker ECGs:** Three examples of pacemaker ECGs are shown in Fig. 18.1.
   a. Ventricular pacemaker (ventricular sensing and pacing). This mode of pacing is recognized by vertical pacemaker spikes that initiate ventricular depolarization with wide QRS complexes (Fig. 18.1A). The electronic spike has no fixed relationship with atrial activity (P wave). The pacemaker rate may be fixed as in the figure, or it may be on a demand (or standby) mode in which the pacemaker fires only after a long pause between the patient's own ventricular beats.
   b. Atrial pacemaker (atrial sensing and pacing). The atrial pacemaker is recognized by a pacemaker spike followed by an atrial complex. When AV conduction is normal, a QRS complex of normal duration follows (see Fig. 18.1B). This type of pacemaker is indicated in patients with sinus node dysfunction with bradycardia. When the patient has high-degree or complete AV block in addition to sinus node dysfunction, an additional ventricular pacemaker may be required

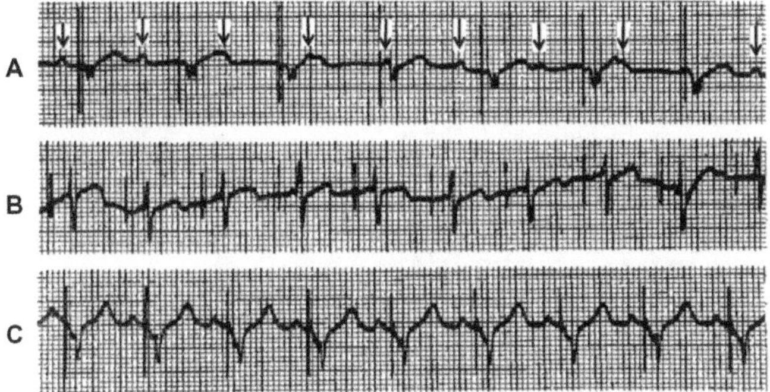

FIG. 18.1
Examples of some artificial pacemakers. (A) Fixed-rate ventricular pacemaker. The tall spikes (~20 mm) are pacemaker firings and they are followed by low-voltage, wide QRS complexes with predominantly S wave (as seen in BBB). Note the regular rate of the electronic spikes with no relationship to the P waves, which are indicated by *arrows*. (B) Atrial pacemaker. This tracing is from a 2-year-old child in whom extreme symptomatic bradycardia developed after the Mustard operation. Pacemaker spikes (~10 mm) are followed by nearly flat atrial activities and by QRS complexes of normal duration. (C) P-wave–triggered pacemaker. This tracing is from a child in whom complete heart block developed after surgical repair of tetralogy of Fallot. *(From Park, M. K., & Guntheroth, W. G. (2006).* How to read pediatric ECGs *(4th ed.). Philadelphia: Mosby.)*

(AV sequential pacemaker, not illustrated in the figure). The AV sequential pacemaker is recognized by two sets of electronic spikes, one before the P wave and another before the wide QRS complex.

c. P-wave–triggered ventricular pacemaker (atrial sensing, ventricular pacing). This type of pacemaker can be recognized by pacemaker spikes that follow the patient's own P waves at regular PR intervals and with wide QRS complexes (see Fig. 18.1C). The patient's own P waves are sensed and trigger a ventricular pacemaker after an electronically preset PR interval. This type of pacemaker is the most physiologic and is indicated when the patient has advanced AV block but a normal sinus mechanism. Advantages of this type of pacemaker are that the heart rate varies with physiologic need and the atrial contraction contributes to ventricular filling and improves cardiac output.

B. INDICATIONS

Box 18.1 lists conditions for which pacemaker therapy is or is not indicated, based on the 2012 American College of Cardiology Foundation/American Heart Association/Heart Rhythm Society (ACCF/AHA/HRS) focused update incorporated into the ACCF/AHA/HRS 2008 guidelines for device-based therapy of cardiac rhythm abnormalities (Epstein et al., 2013).

1. In general, the most common indications for permanent pacemaker implantation in children, adolescents, and patients with CHD fit into one of three categories:
   a. Symptomatic bradycardia (with symptoms of syncope, dizziness, exercise intolerance, or congestive heart failure). In children, significant bradycardia with syncope or near syncope results most commonly from extensive surgery involving the atria (such as the Fontan operation).
   b. The bradycardia-tachycardia syndrome (due to overdrive suppression after a period of tachycardia).
   c. Advanced second- or third-degree AV block, either congenital or postsurgical.
2. Another noncontroversial indication is surgically acquired heart block that lasts more than 7 days after surgery.
3. Temporary pacing is indicated for (a) patients with advanced second-degree or complete heart block secondary to overdose of certain drugs, myocarditis, or myocardial infarction and (b) certain patients immediately after cardiac surgery.

C. TYPES OF PACING DEVICES

The North American Society of Pacing and Electrophysiology (NASPE) and the British Pacing and Electrophysiology Group (BPEG) devised a generic letter code to describe the types and functions of pacemakers (Table 18.1).

1. The letter in the first position identifies the chamber paced (A, atrium; V, ventricle; D, dual) and the second is the chamber sensed (A, atrium; V, ventricle; D, dual; O, none). The third letter corresponds to the

BOX 18.1

RECOMMENDATIONS FOR PERMANENT PACING IN CHILDREN, ADOLESCENTS, AND PATIENTS WITH CONGENITAL HEART DISEASE

CLASS I (IS INDICATED)

1. For advanced second- or third-degree AV block associated with symptomatic bradycardia, ventricular dysfunction, or low cardiac output. *(Level of Evidence: C)*
2. For sinus node dysfunction with correlation of symptoms during age-inappropriate bradycardia. The definition of bradycardia varies with the patient's age and expected heart rate. *(Level of Evidence: B)*
3. For postoperative advanced second- or third-degree AV block that is not expected to resolve or that persists at least 7 days after cardiac surgery. *(Level of Evidence: B)*
4. For congenital third-degree AV block with a wide QRS escape rhythm, complex ventricular ectopy, or ventricular dysfunction. *(Level of Evidence: B)*
5. For congenital third-degree AV block in the infant with a ventricular rate less than 55 beats/min or with congenital heart disease and a ventricular rate less than 70 beats/min *(Level of Evidence: C)*

CLASS IIA (IS REASONABLE)

1. For patients with congenital heart disease and sinus bradycardia for the prevention of recurrent episodes of intraatrial reentrant tachycardia; sinus node dysfunction may be intrinsic or secondary to antiarrhythmic treatment. *(Level of Evidence: C)*
2. For congenital third-degree AV block beyond the first year of life with an average heart rate less than 50 beats/min, abrupt pauses in ventricular rate that are two or three times the basic cycle length, or associated with symptoms due to chronotropic incompetence. *(Level of Evidence: B)*
3. For sinus bradycardia with complex congenital heart disease with a resting heart rate less than 40 beats/min or pauses in ventricular rate longer than 3 seconds. *(Level of Evidence: C)*
4. For patients with congenital heart disease and impaired hemodynamics due to sinus bradycardia or loss of AV synchrony. *(Level of Evidence: C)*
5. For unexplained syncope in the patient with prior congenital heart surgery complicated by transient complete heart block with residual fascicular block after a careful evaluation to exclude other causes of syncope. *(Level of Evidence: B)*

CLASS IIB (MAY BE REASONABLE)

1. For transient postoperative third-degree AV block that reverts to sinus rhythm with residual bifascicular block. *(Level of Evidence: C)*
2. For congenital third-degree AV block in asymptomatic children or adolescents with an acceptable rate, a narrow QRS complex, and normal ventricular function. *(Level of Evidence: B)*
3. For asymptomatic sinus bradycardia after biventricular repair of congenital heart disease with a resting heart rate less than 40 beats/min or pauses in ventricular rate longer than 3 seconds. *(Level of Evidence: C)*

CLASS III (IS NOT INDICATED)

1. For transient postoperative AV block with return of normal AV conduction in the otherwise asymptomatic patient. *(Level of Evidence: B)*
2. For asymptomatic bifascicular block with or without first-degree AV block after surgery for congenital heart disease in the absence of prior transient complete AV block. *(Level of Evidence: C)*

3. For asymptomatic type I second-degree AV block. *(Level of Evidence: C)*
4. For asymptomatic sinus bradycardia with the longest relative risk interval less than 3 seconds and a minimum heart rate more than 40 beats/min. *(Level of Evidence: C)*

Adapted from Epstein, A. E., DiMario, J. P., Ellenbogen, K. A., et al. (2013) 2012 ACCF/AHA/HRS focused update incorporated into the ACCF/AHA/HRS 2008 guidelines for device-based therapy of cardiac rhythm abnormalities: a report of American College of Cardiology Foundation/American Heart Association Task Force on Practice Guidelines and the Heart Rhythm Society. *Journal of the American College of Cardiology*, 61(3)e6-e75.

TABLE 18.1

REVISED NASPE/BPEG GENERIC CODE FOR ANTIBRADYCARDIA PACING

I: CHAMBER(S) PACED	II: CHAMBER(S) SENSED	III: RESPONSE TO SENSING	IV: PROGRAMMABILITY, RATE MODULATION	V: ANTIARRHYTHMIA FUNCTION
0, None	0, None	0, None	0, None	0, None
A, Atrium	A, Atrium	T, Triggered	R, Rate modulation	A, Atrium
V, Ventricle	V, Ventricle	I, Inhibited		V, Ventricle
D, Dual (A + V)	D, Dual (A + V)	D, Dual (T + I)		D, Dual (A + V)

NASPE, North American Society of Pacing and Electrophysiology; *BPEG*, British Pacing and Electrophysiology Group. Adapted from Bernstein AD, Daubert AC, Fletcher RD, et al. (2002). The revised NASPE/BPEG generic code for antibradycardia, adaptive-rate, and multisite pacing. North American Society of Pacing and Electrophysiology/British Pacing and Electrophysiology Group. *Pacing and Clinical Electrophysiology: PACE, 25*(2), 260-264.

response of the pacemaker to an intrinsic cardiac event (I, inhibited; T, triggered; D, dual). For example:

a. A VOO device provides ventricular pacing, no sensing, and no response. This type of pacemaker is commonly used for emergency pacing.
b. A VVI device is ventricle stimulated and ventricle sensed; it inhibits paced output if endogenous ventricular activity occurs (thus preventing competition with native QRS activity). This type is commonly used for episodic AV block or bradycardia in small infants.
c. An AAI device paces and senses the atrium and is inhibited by atrial activity. This type is commonly used in patients with sinus node dysfunction with intact AV conduction.
d. A DDD device is a dual-chamber pacemaker that is capable of pacing either chamber, sensing activity in either chamber, and either triggering or inhibiting paced output (with resulting AV synchrony). This type is used in AV block where AV synchrony is important.

2. The pacemaker choice is based on several factors, including the presence or absence of underlying cardiac disease, the size of the patient, and the relevant hemodynamic factors (including the need for atrial contribution in cardiac output).

II. IMPLANTABLE CARDIOVERTER DEFIBRILLATOR

A. DESCRIPTION

1. An ICD is used in patients at risk for recurrent, sustained ventricular tachycardia or fibrillation. The efficacy of ICD therapy in saving lives of patients at high risk of sudden death has been shown convincingly. All ICDs also have a built-in pacemaker.
2. The ICD automatically detects, recognizes, and treats tachyarrhythmias and bradyarrhythmias using tiered therapy (i.e., bradycardia pacing, overdrive tachycardia pacing, low-energy cardioversion, high-energy shock defibrillation). ICDs can discharge voltages ranging from less than 1 V for pacing to 750 V for defibrillation.
3. The ICD is implanted beneath the skin over the left chest (for right-handed persons) pectoralis muscle and the leads are connected to the ICD. Virtually all ICD systems are implanted transvenously.
4. The longevity of the ICD depends on the frequency of shock delivery, the degree of pacemaker dependency, and other programmable options, but most are expected to last from 5 to 10 years.
5. The most common problem with the ICD is inappropriate shocks, which are usually the result of detection of an SVT, most commonly atrial fibrillation. In adult patients, inappropriate shock has been reported in up to 20% of patients within the first year and 40% by 2 years after implantation, causing pain and anxiety generated by this complication.

B. INDICATIONS

Box 18.2 lists recommendations for ICD therapy according to the 2012 revised guidelines by ACCF/AHA/HRS (Epstein et al., 2013).

1. The two most common indications for ICD implantation in children are hypertrophic cardiomyopathy and long QT syndrome.
2. Other potential indications include idiopathic dilated cardiomyopathy, Brugada syndrome, and arrhythmogenic RV dysplasia.
3. A family history of sudden death may influence the decision to use an ICD in a pediatric patient.
4. Some postoperative CHDs with ventricular tachycardia, such as TOF and TGA, are rare indications for ICD implantation.

III. LIVING WITH A PACEMAKER OR ICD

Electromagnetic interference (EMI) can cause malfunction of the pacemaker or ICD by rate alteration, sensing abnormalities, reprogramming, and other functions, which may result in malfunction of the device or even damage to the pulse generator. Patients should be educated to avoid situations that may cause malfunction or damages to the device. EMI can occur within or outside the hospital. Patients with pacemakers should wear medical identification bracelets or necklaces in case of emergency to show that they have the pacemaker or ICD.

BOX 18.2

RECOMMENDATIONS FOR IMPLANTABLE CARDIOVERTER-DEFIBRILLATORS IN PEDIATRIC PATIENTS AND PATIENTS WITH CONGENITAL HEART DISEASE

CLASS I (IS INDICATED)

1. In the survivors of cardiac arrest after evaluation to define the cause of the event and to exclude any reversible causes. *(Level of Evidence: B)*
2. For patients with symptomatic sustained VT in association with congenital heart disease who have undergone hemodynamic and electrophysiological evaluation. Catheter ablation or surgical repair may offer possible alternatives in carefully selected patients. *(Level of Evidence: C)*

CLASS IIA (IS REASONABLE)

1. For patients with congenital heart disease with recurrent syncope of undetermined origin in the presence of either ventricular dysfunction or inducible ventricular arrhythmias at electrophysiological study. *(Level of Evidence: B)*

CLASS IIB (MAY BE CONSIDERED)

1. For patients with recurrent syncope associated with complex congenital heart disease and advanced systemic ventricular dysfunction when thorough invasive and noninvasive investigations have failed to define a cause. *(Level of Evidence: C)*

CLASS III (IS NOT INDICATED)

1. For patients who do not have a reasonable expectation of survival with an acceptable functional status for at least 1 year, even if they meet ICD implantation criteria specified in Class I, IIa, and IIb recommendation above. *(Level of Evidence: C)*
2. For patients with incessant VT or VF. *(Level of Evidence: C)*
3. In patients with significant psychiatric illness that may be aggravated by device implantation or that may preclude systemic follow-up. *(Level of Evidence: C)*
4. For NYHA Class IV patients with drug-refractory congestive heart failure who are not candidates for cardiac transplantation or CTR-D. *(Level of Evidence: C)*
5. For syncope of undetermined cause in a patient without inducible ventricular tachycardias and without structural heart disease. *(Level of Evidence: C)*
6. When VF or VT is amenable to surgical or catheter ablation (e.g., atrial arrhythmias associated with the Wolff-Parkinson-White syndrome, RV or LV outflow tract VT, idiopathic VT, or fascicular VT in the absence of structural heart disease. *(Level of Evidence: C)*
7. For patients with ventricular tachyarrhythmias due to a completely reversible disorder in the absence of structural heart disease (e.g., electrolyte imbalance, drugs, or trauma). *(Level of Evidence: B)*

CRT-D, cardiac resynchronization therapy device incorporating both pacing and defibrillation capabilities; *NYHA*, New York Heart Association; *VF*, ventricular fibrillation; *VT*, ventricular tachycardia.

Adapted from Epstein, A. E., DiMario, J. P., Ellenbogen, K. A., et al. (2013) 2012 ACCF/AHA/HRS focused update incorporated into the ACCF/AHA/HRS 2008 guidelines for device-based therapy of cardiac rhythm abnormalities: a report of American College of Cardiology Foundation/American Heart Association Task Force on Practice Guidelines and the Heart Rhythm Society. *Journal of the American College of Cardiology, 61(3)e6-e75.*

A. POTENTIAL SOURCES OF ELECTROMAGNETIC INTERFERENCE

The following are some common situations that may or may not affect pacemakers or ICDs.

1. Most home appliances in the following list will NOT interfere with the pacemaker signal.
   a. Kitchen appliances (microwave ovens, blenders, toaster ovens, electric knives)
   b. Televisions, stereos, FM and AM radios, ham radios, CB radios
   c. Electric blankets, heating pads
   d. Electric shavers, hair dryers, curling irons
   e. Garage door openers, gardening electric trimmers
   f. Computers, copying and fax machines
   g. Properly grounded shop tools (except power generator or arc welding equipment)
2. The patient must use caution in the following situations.
   a. Security detectors at airport and government buildings such as courthouses. The patient should not stay near the electronic article surveillance system longer than is necessary and should not lean against the system.
   b. Cellular phones; the patient should not carry a cell phone in the breast pocket when the ICD is implanted in the left upper chest. Keep the cell phone at least 6 inches away from the ICD. When talking on the cell phone, hold it on the opposite side of the body from the ICD.
   c. Avoid working with, holding, or carrying magnets near the pacemaker.
   d. Turn off large motors, such as cars or boats, when working on them. Do not use a chain saw.
   e. Avoid industrial welding equipment. Most welding equipment used for "hobby" welding should not cause any significant problem.
   f. Avoid high-tension wires, radar installations, smelting furnaces, electric steel furnaces, and other high-current industrial equipment.
   g. Abstain from diathermy (the use of heat to treat muscles).
   h. Contact sports are not recommended for children with a pacemaker or ICD.
3. Hospital sources of potentially significant EMI are as follows.
   a. Electrocautery during surgical procedures. Notify surgeon or dentist so that electrocautery will not be used to control bleeding. ICD therapy should be deactivated before surgery and reinitiated after surgery by a qualified professional. Alternatively, a magnet can be placed over the pacemaker throughout the procedure.
   b. For cardioversion or defibrillation. Paddles should be placed in the anteroposterior position, keeping the paddles at least 4 inches from the pulse generator. A qualified pacemaker programmer should be available.

c. Magnetic resonance imaging (MRI) is considered a relative contraindication in patients with a pacemaker or ICD.

B. FOLLOW-UP FOR PACEMAKER AND ICD

1. Patients with pacemakers and ICDs must be followed on a regular schedule because a variety of problems may arise after a pacemaker is placed in children. Problems may arise from stress placed on the lead system by the linear growth of the child, fracture of the lead system in a physically active child, electrode malfunction (scarring of the myocardium around the electrode, especially in infants), and the limited life span of the pulse generator. Many of the same considerations are relevant to both pacemaker and ICD follow-up.
2. Some physicians prefer regular office assessment, others prefer transtelephonic follow-up, and still others prefer a combination of the two techniques. The frequency of clinic follow-up and pacemaker interrogation by the pacemaker manufacturer varies between 3 and 12 months. Monthly transtelephonic evaluation is simple, convenient, and inexpensive.

PART VI

SPECIAL PROBLEMS

This part explores common pediatric cardiac problems not discussed in previous chapters. The topics include (1) congestive heart failure, (2) child with chest pain, (3) syncope, (4) palpitation, (5) systemic hypertension, (6) pulmonary hypertension, (7) athletes with cardiac problems, (8) dyslipidemia, and (9) preventive cardiology.

Chapter 19

Congestive Heart Failure

CHF is a clinical syndrome in which the heart is unable to pump enough blood to the body to meet its needs, to dispose of systemic or pulmonary venous return adequately, or a combination of the two.

A. CAUSES

The heart failure syndrome may arise from diverse causes. By far the most common causes of CHF in infancy are CHDs. Beyond infancy, myocardial dysfunction of various etiologies is an important cause of CHF. Tachyarrhythmias and heart block can also cause heart failure at any age.

1. **Congenital heart disease**
   a. Volume overload lesions such as VSD, PDA, and ECD are the most common causes of CHF in the first 6 months of life.
   b. In infancy, the time of the onset of CHF varies predictably with the type of defect. Table 19.1 lists common defects according to the age at which CHF develops.
   c. Large L-R shunt lesions, such as VSD and PDA, do not cause CHF before 6 to 8 weeks of age because the PVR does not fall low enough to cause a large shunt until this age. CHF may occur earlier in premature infants (within the first month) because of an earlier fall in the PVR.
   d. Note that children with TOF do not develop CHF and that ASDs rarely cause CHF in the pediatric age group, although they can cause CHF in adulthood.
2. **Acquired heart disease.** Acquired heart disease of various etiologies can lead to CHF. Common entities (with the approximate time of onset of CHF) are as follows.
   a. Viral myocarditis (in toddlers, occasionally in neonates with fulminating course).
   b. Myocarditis associated with Kawasaki disease (1 to 4 years of age).
   c. Acute rheumatic carditis (in school-age children).
   d. Rheumatic valvular heart diseases, such as MR or AR (older children and adults).
   e. Dilated cardiomyopathy (at any age during childhood and adolescence).
   f. Doxorubicin cardiomyopathy (months to years after chemotherapy).
   g. Cardiomyopathies associated with muscular dystrophy and Friedreich ataxia (in older children and adolescents).
3. **Miscellaneous causes**
   a. Metabolic abnormalities (severe hypoxia, acidosis, hypoglycemia, hypocalcemia) (in newborns)

TABLE 19.1

CAUSES OF CONGESTIVE HEART FAILURE RESULTING FROM CONGENITAL HEART DISEASE

AGE OF ONSET	CAUSE
At birth	HLHS
	Volume overload lesions
	Severe tricuspid or pulmonary insufficiency
	Large systemic arteriovenous fistula
First wk	TGA
	PDA in small premature infants
	HLHS (with more favorable anatomy)
	TAPVR with pulmonary venous obstruction
	Critical AS or PS
	Systemic arteriovenous fistula
1-4 wk	COA with associated anomalies
	Critical AS
	Large left-to-right shunt lesions (VSD, PDA) in premature infants
	All other lesions previously listed
4-6 wk	Some left-to-right shunt lesions such as ECD
6 wk-4 mo	Large VSD
	Large PDA
	Others such as anomalous left coronary artery from the PA

AS, aortic stenosis; *COA*, coarctation of the aorta; *ECD*, endocardial cushion defect; *HLHS*, hypoplastic left heart syndrome; *PA*, pulmonary artery; *PDA*, patent ductus arteriosus; *PS*, pulmonary stenosis; *TAPVR*, total anomalous pulmonary venous return; *TGA*, transposition of the great arteries; *VSD*, ventricular septal defect.

b. Hyperthyroidism (at any age)
c. SVT (in early infancy)
d. Complete heart block associated with CHDs (in the newborn period or early infancy)
e. Severe anemia (at any age), hydrops fetalis (neonates), and sicklemia (childhood and adolescence)
f. Bronchopulmonary dysplasia (BPD) with right-sided failure (the first few months of life)
g. Primary carnitine deficiency (2 to 4 years)
h. Acute cor pulmonary caused by acute airway obstruction (during early childhood)
i. Acute systemic hypertension with glomerulonephritis (school-age children)

B. DIAGNOSIS OF CHF

The diagnosis of CHF relies on several sources of clinical findings, including history, physical examination, chest radiographs, and echo studies. There is no single laboratory test that is diagnostic of CHF in pediatric patients.

1. Poor feeding of recent onset, tachypnea, poor weight gain, and cold sweat on the forehead suggest CHF in infants. In older children, shortness of breath, especially with activities, easy fatigability, puffy eyelids, or swollen feet, may be presenting complaints.
2. Physical findings can be divided by pathophysiologic subgroups.
   a. Compensatory responses to impaired cardiac function.
      (1) Tachycardia, gallop rhythm, weak and thready pulse, and cardiomegaly on chest radiographs.
      (2) Signs of increased sympathetic discharges (growth failure, perspiration, and cold wet skin).
   b. Signs of pulmonary venous congestion (left-sided failure) include tachypnea, dyspnea on exertion (or poor feeding in small infants), orthopnea in older children, and rarely wheezing and pulmonary crackles.
   c. Signs of systemic venous congestion (right-sided failure) include hepatomegaly and puffy eyelids. Distended neck veins and ankle edema are not seen in infants.
3. Cardiomegaly on chest radiograph is almost always present, except when the pulmonary venous return is obstructed; in that case pulmonary edema or venous congestion will be present.
4. The electrocardiogram (ECG) is not helpful in deciding whether the patient is in CHF, although it may be helpful in determining the cause.
5. Echo studies confirm the presence of chamber enlargement or impaired LV function and help determine the cause of CHF.
6. Increased levels of plasma natriuretic peptides (atrial natriuretic peptide [ANP] and B-type natriuretic peptide [BNP]) are helpful in differentiating causes of dyspnea (lungs vs. heart) in adult patients, but the usefulness of the levels of these peptides is limited in pediatric use. Plasma levels of these peptides are normally elevated in the first weeks of life.
7. Endomyocardial biopsy obtained during cardiac catheterization offers a new approach to specific diagnosis of the cause of CHF, such as inflammatory disease, infectious process, or metabolic disorder.

C. MANAGEMENT

The treatment of CHF consists of (1) elimination of the underlying causes or correction of precipitating or contributing causes (e.g., infection, anemia, arrhythmias, fever, hypertension), (2) general supportive measures, and (3) control of heart failure state by use of drugs, such as inotropic agents, diuretics, and afterload-reducing agents.

1. **Treatment of underlying causes or contributing factors.**

a. Treatment or surgery of underlying CHDs or valvular heart disease when feasible (the best approach for complete cure).
b. Antihypertensive treatment for hypertension.
c. Antiarrhythmic agents or cardiac pacemaker therapy for arrhythmias or heart block.
d. Treatment of hyperthyroidism if it is the cause of CHF.
e. Antipyretics for fever.
f. Antibiotics for a concomitant infection.
g. Packed cell transfusion for anemia (to raise the hematocrit to ≥35%).

2. **General measures.**
   a. Nutritional supports are important. Infants in CHF need significantly higher caloric intakes than recommended for average children. The required calorie intakes may be as high as 150 to 160 kcal/kg/day for infants in CHF.
   b. Increasing caloric density of feeding may be required and it may be accomplished with fortification of feeding (Box 19.1). Frequent small feedings are better tolerated than large feedings in infants.
   c. If oral feedings are not well tolerated, intermittent or continuous nasogastric (NG) feeding is indicated. To promote normal development of oral-motor function, infants may be allowed to take calorie-dense oral feeds throughout the day and then be given continuous NG feeds overnight.
   d. For older children with heart failure, salt restriction (<0.5 g/day) and avoidance of salty snacks (chips, pretzels) and table salt are recommended. Bed rest remains an important component of management. The availability of a television and computer games for entertainment assures bed rest in older children.

BOX 19.1

INCREASING CALORIC DENSITY OF FEEDINGS.

1. Human milk fortifier (Enfamil, Mead Johnson), 1 packet per 25 ml of breast milk = 24 kcal/oz
2. Formula concentration to 24 kcal/oz by:
   a. 1 cup powdered formula + 3 cups water or
   b. 4 oz ready-to-feed + {1/2} scoop powdered formula
3. Supplementation of formula to 26-30 kcal/oz is accomplished in the following manner.
   a. Fat modular products
   b. Medium chain triglycerides (MCT) oil (Mead Johnson), 8 kcal/mL
   c. Microlipid (safflower oil emulsion, Mead Johnson), 4.5 kcal/mL
   d. Low-osmolality polymers
   e. Polycose (Ross), 23 kcal/tablespoon
   f. Moducal (Mead Johnson), 30 kcal/tablespoon
4. Pediasure (Ross), 30 kcal/oz ready-to-feed (for children older than 1 year)

From Wright, G. E., & Rochini, A. P. (2002). Primary and general care of the child with congenital heart disease, *ACC Current Journal Review*, 11(2), 89-93.

3. **Drug therapy**. Three major classes of drugs are commonly used in the treatment of CHF in children: inotropic agents, diuretics, and afterload-reducing agents.
   a. **Effects of angicongestive drugs on the Frank-Starling relationship**. Fig. 19.1 shows the Frank-Starling curve as related to the preload and afterload in normal heart. As the preload (or left ventricular filling pressure) is increased, stroke volume (or cardiac output) increases. If the filling pressure is reduced (as seen in hemorrhage or dehydration), the stroke volume decreases. When the afterload is reduced, cardiac output increases even without increase in preload, as shown in Fig. 19.1, by shifting the Frank-Starling curve upward and to the left. This occurs without increasing oxygen consumption of the heart. An increase in preload (LV filling pressure) increases stroke volume or cardiac output for a given afterload. Thus there are two ways to increase stroke volume or cardiac output: one by increasing preload and the other by reducing afterload.

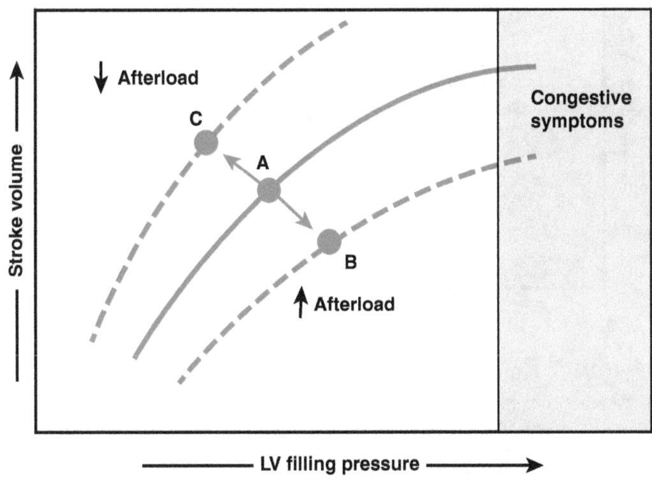

FIG. 19.1
The relationship between the levels of afterload and the Frank-Starling curve. An increase in afterload shifts the Frank-Starling curve down and to the right (from point A to B), which decreases stroke volume and at the same time increases LV end-diastolic pressure (preload). In contrast, a decrease in afterload shifts the Frank-Starling curve up and to the left (from point A to C) and increases stroke volume and at the same time reduces LV end-diastolic pressure. In the treatment of heart failure; vasodilator drugs augment stroke volume by decreasing arterial pressure (afterload) and at the same time reduces the LV preload (moving point A to C).

Effects of anticongestive medications on the Frank-Starling relationship are illustrated in Fig. 19.2. In patients with heart failure (the lower curve), the normal relationship between cardiac outputs (stroke volume) and filling pressure (preload) is shifted downward and to the right so that a low-output state and congestive symptoms may coexist. If the filling pressure reaches a certain point, congestive symptoms (dyspnea, tachypnea) may appear even in a normal heart.

All drugs used in the treatment of heart failure tend to shift the Frank-Starling curve upward and to the left. The effects of three classes of drug used in the treatment of CHF are shown in Fig. 19.2.

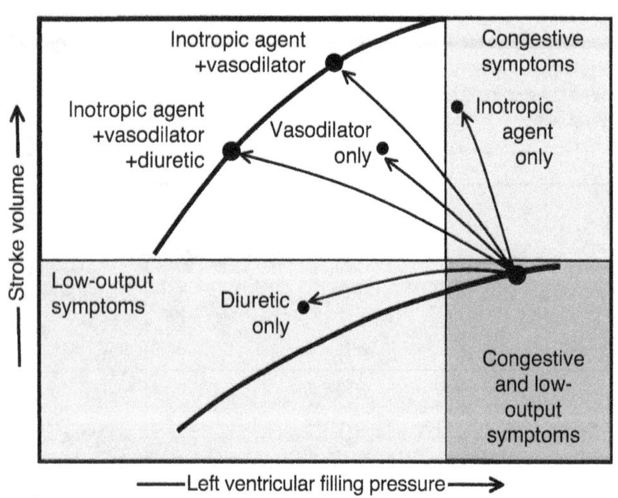

FIG. 19.2

Effects of anticongestive medications on the Frank-Starling relationship for ventricular function. The upper curve shows the Frank-Starling curve for normal heart. In patients with heart failure, the curve is shifted lower and to the right such that a low-output state and congestive symptoms may coincide. The addition of a pure inotropic agent, such as digoxin, primarily increases the stroke volume with minimal impact on LV filling pressure (so that the patient may still have congestive symptoms). Conversely, the addition of a diuretic primarily decreases the LV filling pressure (with improved congestive symptoms) but without improving cardiac output. The addition of vasodilators reduces afterload and moves the curve up and to the left, thus relieving congestive symptoms and increasing stroke volume. Clinically, it is common to use multiple classes of agents (usually a combination of inotropric agents, diuretics, and vasodilators) to produce both increased cardiac output and decreased LV filling pressure. *(Adapted from Cohn, J.N., & Franciosa, J. S. (1977). Vasodilator therapy of cardiac failure [first of two parts].* New England Journal of Medicine, *297(1), 27-31.)*

(1) Inotropic agents, such as digoxin, primarily shift the Frank-Starling curve upward (with minimal impact on filling pressure) (see "Inotropic agent only" in Fig. 19.2).
(2) Diuretics primarily decrease the filling pressure (with improved congestive symptoms) but without improving stroke volume (see "Diuretic only" in Fig. 19.2).
(3) Afterload reducing agents (vasodilators) move the Starling curve upward and to the left and improve cardiac output (stroke volume) and reduce the filling pressure (see "Vasodilator only" in Fig. 19.2).
(4) Clinically, it is common to use multiple classes of agents (usually a combination of inotropic agents, diuretics, and vasodilators) to produce both increased cardiac output and decreased filling pressure.

b. **Diuretics**.

Diuretics remain the principal therapeutic agent to control pulmonary and systemic venous congestion. Diuretics only reduce preload and improve congestive symptoms, but they do not improve myocardial contractility or cardiac output (see Fig. 19.2). Three classes of diuretics are available.

(1) Thiazide diuretics (e.g., chlorothiazide, hydrochlorothiazide), which act at the proximal and distal tubules, are no longer popular.
(2) Rapid-acting diuretics (e.g., furosemide, ethacrynic acid) are the drugs of choice. They act primarily at the loop of Henle ("loop diuretics").
(3) Aldosterone antagonist (e.g., spironolactone) acts on the distal tubule to inhibit sodium-potassium exchange. These drugs have value in preventing hypokalemia produced by thiazide diuretics and thus are used in conjunction with a loop diuretic. However, when ACE inhibitors are used, spironolactone should be discontinued to avoid hyperkalemia.

The main side effects of diuretic therapy are hypokalemia (except when used with spironolactone) and hypochloremic alkalosis. Table 19.2 shows dosages of commonly available diuretic preparations.

c. **Afterload-reducing agents**.

Afterload reducing agents augment the stroke volume without much change in the contractile state of the heart (Figs. 19.1 and 19.2). Combined use of an inotropic agent, a vasodilator, and a diuretic produces most improvement in both inotropic state and congestive symptoms (Fig. 19.2).

Afterload-reducing agents may be divided into three groups based on the site of action: (a) arteriolar vasodilators (hydralazine), (b) venodilators (nitroglycerin, isosorbide dinitrate), and (c) mixed vasodilators (angiotensin-converting enzyme [ACE] inhibitors (captopril, enalapril), nitroprusside, and prazosin. ACE inhibitors are popular in children with chronic severe CHF. Dosages of these agents are presented in Table 19.3.

TABLE 19.2

DIURETIC AGENTS AND DOSAGES

PREPARATION	ROUTE	DOSAGE
Thiazide Diuretics		
Chlorothiazide (Diuril)	Oral	20-40 mg/kg/day in 2 to 3 divided doses
Hydrochlorothiazide (Hydrodiuril)	Oral	2-4 mg/kg/day in 2 to 3 divided doses
Loop Diuretics		
Furosemide (Lasix)	Intravenous	1 mg/kg/dose
	Oral	2-3 mg/kg/day in 2 to 3 divided doses
Ethacrynic acid (Edecrin)	Intravenous	1 mg/kg/dose
	Oral	2-3 mg/kg/day in 2 to 3 divided doses
Aldosterone Antagonist		
Spironolactone (Aldactone)	Oral	1-3 mg/kg/day in 2 to 3 divided doses

(1) Infants with large L-R shunt lesions (e.g., VSD, PDA) have been shown to benefit from captopril and hydralazine.

(2) ACE inhibitors have also shown beneficial effects in patients with dilated cardiomyopathy, adriamycin-induced cardiomyopathy, myocardial ischemia, postoperative cardiac status, and severe MR or AR.

(3) Sodium nitroprusside is used primarily in acute situation such as following cardiac surgery, including pulmonary hypertension after cardiac surgery.

d. **Rapidly acting inotropic agents**

In critically ill infants with CHF or in postoperative cardiac patients with heart failure, rapidly acting catecholamines with a short duration of action are preferable (to digoxin). Dosages for intravenous drip of these catecholamines are suggested in Table 19.4.

(1) This class of agents includes dopamine, dobutamine, isoproterenol, and epinephrine. They also possess vasodilator actions and thus are useful in acute situation.

(2) Milrinone and amrinone are phosphodiesterase-3 inhibitors with lusitropic (myocardial relaxation), and vasodilatory as well as some mild inotropic effects. It improves the cardiac output by augmenting the contractility as well as decreasing the afterload. Thrombocytopenia is a side effect of amrinone; the drug should be discontinued if the platelet count falls below 150,000/mm^3 (see Appendix E, Table E.2 for dosage).

e. **Digitalis glycosides**.

(1) Digoxin, one of the oldest medications used in the treatment of heart failure, increases the cardiac output (or contractile state of the myocardium). Use of digoxin in infants with large L-R shunt lesions

TABLE 19.3

DOSAGES OF VASODILATORS

DRUG	ROUTE AND DOSAGE	COMMENTS
Arteriolar Vasodilator		
Hydralazine (Apresoline)	Intravenous: 0.15-0.2 mg/kg/dose, every 4 to 6 hr (maximum 20 mg/dose)	May cause tachycardia; may be used with propranolol
	Oral: 0.75-3 mg/kg/day, in 2 to 4 doses (maximum 200 mg/day)	May cause gastrointestinal symptoms, neutropenia, and lupus-like syndrome
Venodilators		
Nitroglycerin	IV: 0.5-1 μg/kg/min (maximum 6 μg/kg/min)	Start with small dose and titrate based on effects
Mixed Vasodilators		
Captopril (Capoten)	Oral: Newborn: 0.1-0.4 mg/kg, TID-QID Infant: Initially 0.15-0.3 mg/kg, QD-QID. Titrate upward if needed. Maximum dose 6 mg/kg/24 hr. Child: Initially 0.3-0.5 mg/kg, BID-TID. Titrate upward if needed. Maximum dose 6 mg/kg/24 hr. Adolescents and adults: Initially 12.5-25 mg, BID-TID. Increase weekly if needed by 25 mg/dose to maximum dose 450 mg/24 hr.	May cause hypotension, dizziness, neutropenia, and proteinuria Dose should be reduced in patients with impaired renal function
Enalapril (Vasotec)	Oral: 0.1 mg/kg, once or twice daily	Patient may develop hypotension, dizziness, or syncope
Nitroprusside (Nipride)	Intravenous: 0.3-0.5 μg/kg/min. Titrate to effects. (Maximum dose 10 μg/kg/min)	May cause thiocyanate or cyanide toxicity (e.g., fatigue, nausea, disorientation), hepatic dysfunction, or light sensitivity

(e.g., large VSD) is controversial because ventricular contractility is normal in this situation. However, studies have shown that digoxin improves symptoms in these infants, perhaps because of other actions of digoxin, such as parasympathomimetic action and diuretic action.

(2) **Dosage of digoxin.** The total digitalizing dose (TDD) and maintenance dosage of digoxin by oral and intravenous routes are

TABLE 19.4

SUGGESTED STARTING DOSAGES OF CATECHOLAMINES

DRUG	DOSAGE AND ROUTE	SIDE EFFECTS
Epinephrine (Adrenalin)	0.01-1 μg/kg/min IV	Hypertension, arrhythmias
Isoproterenol (Isuprel)	0.1-0.5 μg/kg/min IV	Peripheral and pulmonary vasodilatation
Dobutamine (Dobutrex)	2-8 μg/kg/min IV	Tachycardia and vasodilatation, arrhythmias
Dopamine (Intropin)	5-10 μg/kg/min IV	Tachycardia, arrhythmias, hypertension or hypotension Dose-related cardiovascular effects (μg/kg/min): Renal vasodilatation: 2-5 Inotropic: 5-8 Tachycardia: >8 Mild vasoconstriction: >10 Vasoconstriction: 15-20

shown in Table 19.5. The maintenance dose is more closely related to the serum digoxin level than is the digitalizing dose, which is given to build a sufficient body store of the drug and to shorten the time required to reach the pharmacokinetic steady state.

(3) **How to digitalize.**

(a) One-half the total digitalizing dose is followed by one-fourth and then the final one-fourth of the total digitalizing dose at 6- to 8-hour intervals. The maintenance dose is given 12 hours after the final total digitalizing dose. This results in a pharmacokinetic steady state in 3 to 5 days.

(b) When an infant is in mild heart failure, the maintenance dose may be administered orally without loading doses; this results in a steady state in 5 to 8 days.

(c) A baseline ECG (rhythm and PR interval) and serum electrolytes are recommended. Hypokalemia and hypercalcemia predispose to digitalis toxicity.

(4) **Monitoring for digitalis toxicity.**

(a) With the relatively low dosage recommended in Table 19.5, digitalis toxicity is unlikely unless there are predisposing factors for the toxicity. Predisposing factors for digitalis toxicity may include renal disease, premature infants, hypothyroidism, myocarditis, electrolyte imbalance (hypokalemia and hypercalcemia), alkalosis, and catecholamine administration.

(b) Serum digoxin levels obtained during the first 3 to 5 days after digitalization tend to be higher than those obtained when the pharmacokinetic steady state is reached. Therefore detection of digitalis toxicity is best accomplished by monitoring with ECGs, not by serum digoxin levels during this period.

TABLE 19.5

ORAL DIGOXIN DOSAGE FOR CONGESTIVE HEART FAILURE

AGE	TOTAL DIGITALIZING DOSE (μg/kg)	MAINTENANCE DOSE[a] (μg/kg/day)
Premature	20	5
Newborns	30	8
<2 yr	40-50	10-12
>2 yr	30-40	8-10

[a]The maintenance dose is 25% of the total digitalizing dose in two divided doses. The intravenous dose is 75% of the oral dose.

Adapted from Park, M. K. (1986). The use of digoxin in infants and children with specific emphasis on dosage. *Journal of Pediatrics, 108*(6), 871-877.

(c) ECG signs of digitalis toxicity involve disturbances in the formation and conduction of the impulse, whereas those of digitalis effect are confined to ventricular repolarization. First-degree (or second-degree) AV block, profound sinus bradycardia or sinoatrial block, supraventricular arrhythmias (atrial or junctional ectopic beats and tachycardias), and, rarely, ventricular arrhythmias are all possible signs of toxicity. Shortening of QTc and diminished amplitude of the T wave are the signs of digitalis effect.

(5) **Serum digoxin levels**. Therapeutic ranges of serum digoxin levels for treating CHF are 0.8 to 2.0 ng/mL. Blood for serum digoxin levels should be drawn just before a scheduled dose or at least 6 hours after the last dose; samples obtained earlier than 6 hours after the last dose will give a falsely elevated level.

(6) **Digitalis toxicity**. The diagnosis of digitalis toxicity is based on the following clinical and laboratory findings.

(a) A history of accidental ingestion.

(b) Noncardiac symptoms in digitalized children: anorexia, nausea, vomiting, diarrhea, restlessness, drowsiness, fatigue, and visual disturbances in older children.

(c) ECG signs of toxicity (as described previously).

(d) An elevated serum level of digoxin (>2 ng/mL) in the presence of clinical findings suggestive of digitalis toxicity.

f. Other drugs.

(1) **β-Adrenergic blockers**

(a) As reported in adults, β-adrenergic blockers have been shown to be beneficial in some pediatric patients with chronic CHF, who were treated with standard anticongestive drugs. Adrenergic overstimulation, often seen in patients with chronic CHF, may have detrimental effects on the failing heart by inducing myocyte injury and necrosis. However, β-adrenergic blockers should not be given to those with decompensated heart failure.

(b) When added to standard medical therapy for CHF, carvedilol (a nonselective β-adrenergic blocker with additional α1-antagonist activities) has been shown to be beneficial in children with idiopathic dilated cardiomyopathy, chemotherapy-induced cardiomyopathy, postmyocarditis myopathy, muscular dystrophy, or postsurgical heart failure (e.g., Fontan operation).
(c) Metoprolol was also beneficial in dilated cardiomyopathy.
(d) Propranolol added to conventional treatment for CHF was also beneficial in a small number of infants with large L-R shunts at the dose of 1.6 mg/kg/day.

(2) **Carnitine**. Carnitine, which is an essential cofactor for transport of long-chain fatty acids into mitochondria for oxidation, has been shown to be beneficial in some cases of dilated cardiomyopathy. The dosage of L-carnitine used was 50 to 100 mg/kg/day, given BID or TID orally (maximum daily dose 3 g).

4. **Surgical management**. If medical treatment as outlined previously does not improve CHF caused by CHD within a few weeks to months, one should consider either palliative or corrective cardiac surgery for the underlying cardiac defect when technically feasible.

Chapter 20
Child With Chest Pain

Although chest pain does not indicate serious disease of the heart or other systems in most pediatric patients, in a society with a high prevalence of atherosclerotic heart disease, it can be alarming to the child and parents. Physicians should be aware of the differential diagnosis of chest pain in children and should make every effort to find a specific cause before making a referral to a specialist or reassuring the child and the parents of the benign nature of the complaint.

I. CAUSE AND PREVALENCE

1. Cardiac causes of chest pain are found in less than 5% of children with complaint of chest pain. Noncardiac causes of chest pain are found in 56% to 86% of reported cases.
2. Among 3700 patients who presented to a large children's hospital with a complaint of chest pain, cardiac pathology or arrhythmias was found in only 1% of these patients, of whom 38% had SVT and 27% had pericarditis (Saleeb et al., 2011).
3. Table 20.1 lists the frequency of the causes of chest pain in children according to organ systems based on published data from six pediatric emergency departments and four pediatric cardiology clinics. According to the table, the three most common causes of chest pain in children are (a) costochondritis, (b) chest wall trauma or muscle strain, and (c) respiratory diseases, especially those associated with coughing.
4. Gastrointestinal and psychogenic causes are identified in fewer than 10% of cases.
5. Even after a moderately extensive investigation, no cause can be found in up to 50% of patients (idiopathic chest pain).
6. In children with chronic chest pain, a cardiac cause is less likely to be found.
7. Box 20.1 is a partial list of *possible* causes of noncardiac and cardiac chest pain in children.

A. NONCARDIAC CAUSES OF CHEST PAIN

1. **Costochondritis**
   a. Costochondritis is found in up to 80% of children with chest pain. It is more common in girls than boys and may persist for several months. It is characterized by mild to moderate anterior chest pain, usually unilateral but occasionally bilateral. The pain may radiate to the remainder of the chest and back, and may be exaggerated by breathing or physical activities. Physical examination is diagnostic;

TABLE 20.1

FREQUENCY OF CAUSES OF CHEST PAIN IN CHILDREN

CAUSES	PEDIATRIC EMERGENCY DEPARTMENT OR PEDIATRIC CLINIC (DATA FROM 6 REPORTS) (%)	CARDIOLOGY CLINIC (DATA FROM 4 REPORTS) (%)
Idiopathic/cause unknown	12-61	37-54
Musculoskeletal/costochondritis	7-69	1-89
Respiratory/asthma	13-24	1-12
Gastrointestinal/gastroesophageal reflux disease	3-7	3-12
Psychogenic	5-9	4-19
Cardiac	2-5	3-7

From Thull-Freedman, J. (2010). Evaluation of chest pain in the pediatric patients. *Medical Clinics of North America, 94 (2)*:327-347.

BOX 20.1

SELECTED CAUSES OF CHEST PAIN

NONCARDIAC CAUSES

Musculoskeletal

Costochondritis
Trauma to chest wall (from sports, fights, or accident)
Muscle strains (pectoral, shoulder, or back muscles)
Overused chest wall muscle (from coughing)
Abnormalities of the rib cage or thoracic spine
Tietze syndrome
Slipping rib syndrome
Precordial catch (Texidor's twinge or stitch in the side)

Respiratory

Reactive airway disease (exercise-induced asthma)
Pneumonia (viral, bacterial, mycobacterium, fungal, or parasitic)
Pleural irritation (pleural effusion)
Pneumothorax or pneumomediastinum
Pleurodynia (devil's grip)
Pulmonary embolism
Foreign bodies in the airway

Gastrointestinal

Gastroesophageal reflux
Peptic ulcer disease
Esophagitis
Gastritis

Esophageal diverticulum
Hiatal hernia
Foreign bodies (such as coins)
Cholecystitis
Pancreatitis

Psychogenic

Life stressor (death in family, family discord, divorce, failure in school, nonacceptance from peers, or sexual molestation)
Hyperventilation
Conversion symptoms
Somatization disorder
Depression
Bulimia nervosa (esophagitis, esophageal tear)

Miscellaneous

Sickle cell disease (vaso-occlusive crisis)
Mastalgia
Herpes zoster

CARDIAC CAUSES

Ischemic Ventricular Dysfunction

Structural abnormalities of the heart (severe AS or PS, hypertrophic obstructive cardiomyopathy, Eisenmenger syndrome)
Mitral valve prolapse
Coronary artery abnormalities (previous Kawasaki disease, congenital anomaly, coronary heart disease, hypertension, sickle cell disease)
Cocaine abuse
Aortic dissection and aortic aneurysm (Turner, Marfan, or Noonan syndromes)

Inflammatory Conditions

Pericarditis (viral, bacterial, or rheumatic)
Postpericardiotomy syndrome
Myocarditis (acute or chronic)
Kawasaki disease

Arrhythmias (and Palpitations)

Supraventricular tachycardia
Frequent PVCs or ventricular tachycardia (possible)

the clinician finds a reproducible tenderness on palpation over the chondrosternal or costochondral junctions. It is a benign condition.

b. *Tietze syndrome* is a rare form of costochondritis characterized by a large, tender fusiform (spindle-shaped), nonsuppurative swelling at the chondrosternal junction. It usually affects the second and third costochondral junctions.

2. **Musculoskeletal**. There is a history of vigorous exercise, weight lifting, acute or chronic trauma to the chest wall from sports, fights, or

accidents as well as continuous muscle strain from video gaming. Physical examination reveals tenderness of the chest wall or pectoralis muscles.

3. **Respiratory**. Lung pathology, pleural irritation, or pneumothorax account for 10% to 20% of the cases. A history of severe cough, tenderness of intercostal or abdominal muscles, and crackles or wheezing on examination suggests a respiratory cause of chest pain.
4. **Exercise-induced asthma**. Exercise-induced asthma is not that uncommon. The response of the asthmatic patient to exercise is quite characteristic. The intensity of exercise is important. Strenuous exercise for 3 to 8 minutes' duration causes bronchoconstriction in virtually all asthmatic subjects, especially when the heart rate rises to 180 beats/min. On the other hand, jogging or slow running for 1 to 2 minutes often causes bronchodilatation. Symptoms range from mild to severe and may include coughing, wheezing, dyspnea, and chest congestion, constriction, or pain. Patients also complain of limited endurance during exercise. Environmental factors, such as cold temperature, pollen, and air pollution, as well as viral respiratory infection can worsen exercise-induced asthma. Exercise-induced bronchospasm provocation test is diagnostic (discussed under "Stress Tests" in Chapter 5).
5. **Gastrointestinal**
   a. Gastroesophageal reflux disease (GERD) may cause chest pain. In addition to chest pain, children with GERD may complain of abdominal pain, frequent sore throat, gagging or choking, frequent respiratory problems (such as bronchitis, wheezing, asthma), and poor weight gain. The onset and relief of pain in relation to eating and diet may help clarify the diagnosis.
   b. In young children, ingested foreign bodies (such as coins or caustic substances) may cause chest pain.
   c. Cholecystitis presents with postprandial pain referred to the right upper quadrant of the abdomen and part of the chest.
6. **Psychogenic**. Psychogenic disturbances account for 5% to 17% of cases and are seen in both boys and girls at equal rates. Psychogenic causes are less likely to be found in children younger than 12 years. Often a recent stressful situation parallels the onset of the chest pain: a death or separation in the family, a serious illness, a disability, a recent move, failure in school, or sexual molestation. However, a psychological cause of chest pain should not be lightly assigned without a thorough history taking and a follow-up evaluation. Psychological or psychiatric consultation may be indicated.
7. **Miscellaneous**
   a. The precordial catch (Texidor's twinge or stitch in the side), a one-sided chest pain, lasts a few seconds or minutes and is associated with bending or slouching.
   b. Slipping rib syndrome (resulting from excess mobility of the eighth to tenth ribs, which do not directly insert into the sternum). In many

cases, the ligaments that hold these ribs to the upper ribs are weak, resulting in slippage of the ribs, causing pain.

c. Mastalgia in some male and female adolescents.
d. Pleurodynia (devil's-grip) is an unusual cause of chest pain caused by coxsackievirus infection.
e. Herpes zoster is another unusual cause of chest pain.
f. Spontaneous pneumothorax and pneumomediastinum are rare respiratory causes of acute chest pain. Children with asthma, cystic fibrosis, or Marfan syndrome are at risk. Inhalation of cocaine can provoke pneumomediastinum and pneumothorax.
g. Hyperventilation can produce chest discomfort and is often associated with paresthesia and lightheadedness.

B. CARDIAC CAUSES OF CHEST PAIN

Cardiac chest pain may be caused by ischemic ventricular dysfunction, pericardial or myocardial inflammatory processes, or arrhythmias, occurring in less than 5% of cases (Box 20.1). A typical *anginal pain* in adults is located in the precordial or substernal area and radiates to the neck, jaw, either or both arms, back, or abdomen. The patient describes the pain as a deep, heavy pressure; the feeling of choking; or a squeezing sensation. Older adolescents are expected to describe the pain as above but young children may not. Exercise, cold stress, emotional upset, or a large meal typically precipitates anginal pain. Table 20.2 summarizes important clinical findings of cardiac causes of chest pain in children.

1. **Ischemic myocardial dysfunction**
   a. Congenital heart defects. Severe AS, subaortic stenosis, severe PS, and pulmonary hypertension (Eisenmenger syndrome) may cause ischemic chest pain. The pain is usually associated with exercise and is a typical anginal pain.
   b. MVP. Chest pain associated with MVP is usually a vague, nonexertional pain of short duration, located at the apex, without a constant relationship to effort or emotion. Occasionally, supraventricular or ventricular arrhythmias may result in cardiac symptoms, including chest discomfort. Nearly all patients with Marfan syndrome have MVP. A midsystolic click with or without a late systolic murmur is the hallmark of the condition.
   c. Cardiomyopathy. Hypertrophic and dilated cardiomyopathies can cause chest pain from ischemia, with or without exercise, or from rhythm disturbances.
   d. CAD. Coronary artery anomalies, either congenital (aberrant or single coronary artery, coronary artery fistula) or acquired (aneurysm or stenosis of the coronary arteries as a result of Kawasaki disease or as a result of previous cardiac surgery involving the coronary arteries) can rarely cause chest pain.
   e. Cocaine abuse. Even children with normal hearts are at risk of ischemia and myocardial infarction if cocaine is used. Cocaine

TABLE 20.2

IMPORTANT CLINICAL FINDINGS OF CARDIAC CAUSES OF CHEST PAIN

CONDITIONS	HISTORY	PHYSICAL FINDINGS	ECG	CHEST RADIOGRAPHY
Severe AS	History of CHD (+)	Loud (> grade 3/6 SEM at URSB with radiation to neck)	LVH with or without strain	Prominent ascending aorta and aortic knob
Severe PS	History of CHD (+)	Loud (grade >3/6) SEM at ULSB	RVH with or without strain	Prominent PA segment
HOCM	Positive FH in one-third of cases	Variable heart murmurs Brisk brachial pulses (±)	LVH Deep Q/small R or QS pattern in LPLs	Mild cardiomegaly with globular-shaped heart
MVP	Positive FH (±)	Midsystolic click with or without late systolic murmur Thin body build Thoracic skeletal anomalies (80%)	Inverted T waves in aVF (±)	Normal heart size Straight back (±) Narrow anteroposterior diameter (±)
Eisenmenger syndrome	History of CHD (+)	Cyanosis and clubbing RV impulse Loud and single S2 Soft or no heart murmur	RVH	Markedly prominent PA with normal heart size
Anomalous origin of left coronary artery	Recurrent episodes of distress in early infancy	Soft or no heart murmur	Anterolateral MI pattern	Moderate to marked cardiomegaly

Sequelae of Kawasaki or other coronary artery diseases	History of Kawasaki disease () Typical exercise-related anginal pain	Usually negative Continuous murmur in coronary fistula	ST-segment elevation (±) Old MI pattern (±)	Normal heart size or mild cardiomegaly
Cocaine abuse	History of substance abuse (±)	Hypertension Nonspecific heart murmur (±)	ST-segment elevation (±)	Normal heart size in acute cases
Pericarditis and myocarditis	History of URI (±) Sharp chest pain	Friction rub Muffled heart sounds Nonspecific heart murmur (±)	Low QRS voltages ST-segment shift Arrhythmias (±)	Cardiomegaly of varying degree
Postpericardiotomy syndrome	Hx of recent heart surgery, pain, and dyspnea	Muffled heart sounds (±) Friction rub	Persistent ST-segment elevation	Cardiomegaly of varying degree
Arrhythmias (and palpitation)	History of WPW syndrome (±) FH of long QT syndrome (±)	May be negative Irregular rhythm (±)	Arrhythmias (±) WPW preexcitation (±) Long QTc interval (> 0.46 sec)	Normal heart size

AS, aortic stenosis; *CHD*, congenital heart disease; *ECG*, electrocardiogram; *FH*, family history; *HOCM*, hypertrophic obstructive cardiomyopathy; *LPLs*, left precordial leads; *LVH*, left ventricular hypertrophy; *MI*, myocardial infarction; *MVP*, mitral valve prolapse; *PA*, pulmonary artery; *PS*, pulmonary stenosis; *RV*, right ventricle; *RVH*, right ventricular hypertrophy; *SEM*, systolic ejection murmur; *ULSB*, upper left sternal border; *URI*, upper respiratory tract infection; *URSB*, upper right sternal border; *WPW*, Wolff-Parkinson-White; (+), positive; (±), may be present.

blocks the reuptake of norepinephrine with an increase in circulating levels of catecholamines causing coronary vasoconstriction. Cocaine also induces the activation of platelets, increases endothelin production, and decreases nitric oxide production. These effects collectively produce anginal pain, infarction, arrhythmias, or sudden death. History and drug screening help physicians in the diagnosis of cocaine-induced chest pain.

2. **Pericardial or myocardial disease**
   a. Pericarditis. Older children with pericarditis may complain of a sharp, stabbing precordial pain that worsens when lying down and improves after sitting and leaning forward. Echo examination is usually diagnostic.
   b. Myocarditis. Acute myocarditis often involves the pericardium to a certain extent and can cause chest pain.
3. **Arrhythmias**. Chest pain may result from a variety of arrhythmias, especially with sustained tachycardia resulting in myocardial ischemia. Even without ischemia, children may consider palpitation or forceful heartbeats as chest pain. In this situation, chest pain may be associated with dizziness and palpitation.

II. DIAGNOSTIC APPROACH

Careful history taking and careful physical examination will suffice to rule out cardiac causes of chest pain and often to find a specific cause of the pain. To rule out cardiac causes of chest pain, physicians will need chest radiographic films and an electrocardiogram (ECG). (Cardiologists may, in addition, obtain an echocardiogram to accomplish the same). Cardiac causes of chest pain can be ruled out by nonexertional nature of pain, negative cardiac examination, and normal results of other investigations, with exception of cardiac arrhythmia as the cause of the pain. Even if physicians cannot find a specific cause of chest pain, it is relatively easy to rule out cardiac causes of chest pain by following the steps outlined below.

1. **History of present illness**

History taking should ask about the nature of the pain, in terms of its association with exertion or physical activities, the intensity, character, frequency, duration, and points of radiation. The following are some examples of questions used in determining the nature of chest pain.

   a. What seems to bring on the pain (e.g., exercise, eating, trauma, emotional stress)?
   b. Do you get the same type of pain while you watch TV or sit in class?
   c. What is the pain like (e.g., sharp, pressure sensation, squeezing)?
   d. What are the location (e.g., specific point, localized or diffuse), severity, radiation, and duration (seconds, minutes) of the pain?
   e. Does the pain get worse with deep breathing? (If so, the pain may be caused by pleural irritation or chest wall pathology.) Does the pain improve with certain body positions? (This is sometimes seen with pericarditis.)

f. Does the pain have any relationship with your meals?
g. How often and how long have you had similar pain (frequency and chronicity)?
h. Have you been hurt while playing, or have you used your arms excessively for any reason?
i. Are there any associated symptoms, such as presyncope, syncope, dizziness, palpitation, or tingling in hands and feet? (History of tingling could be suggestive of hyperventilation.)
j. Have you been coughing a lot lately?

2. **Past and family histories**
   a. Past history of congenital or acquired heart disease, cardiac surgery, asthma, sickle cell disease, Kawasaki disease, or Marfan syndrome (or other connective tissue disease)
   b. Medications, such as asthma medicines or birth control pills
   c. Family history of recent chest pain, heart attack, or a cardiac death
   d. Family history of long QT syndrome, cardiomyopathies, or unexpected sudden death
   e. History of exposure to drugs (cocaine) or cigarettes
3. **Physical examination**
   a. The chest wall should be carefully examined for trauma, asymmetry, and costochondritis.
      (1) For costochondritis, use the soft part of the terminal phalanx of a middle finger (not the palm of a hand) to palpate each costochondral *and* chondrosternal junction. Physical examination is all that is needed for the diagnosis of costochondritis.
      (2) Pectoralis muscles and shoulder muscles should be examined for tenderness.
      (3) Chest wall deformities (scoliosis, kyphosis, or pectus) can be a cause of chronic chest pain.
   b. The abdomen should be carefully examined, because it may be the source of pain referred to the chest.
   c. The heart and lungs should be auscultated for arrhythmias, heart murmurs, rubs, muffled heart sounds, gallop rhythm, crackles, wheezes, or decreased breath sounds. One must be careful not to interpret commonly occurring innocent murmurs as pathologic.
4. **Other investigations**
   a. Chest radiographs (for pulmonary pathology, cardiac size and silhouette, and pulmonary vascularity) may be obtained.
   b. An ECG (for arrhythmias, hypertrophy, conduction disturbances, WPW preexcitation, and prolonged QT intervals) may be obtained.
   c. Drug screening is ordered when cocaine-induced chest pain is suspected.

III. STEPPED APPROACH TO DIAGNOSIS

The stepped approach to diagnosis as described in the following section may be used in dealing with children with a complaint of chest pain.

1. The first step is to search for three common noncardiac causes of chest pain: costochondritis, musculoskeletal causes, and respiratory diseases. History and physical examination frequently uncover one of these conditions as the cause of chest pain in about two-thirds of patients.
2. The second step is to evaluate for possible cardiac causes of the pain. Even if a noncardiac cause of the pain is found, cardiac causes of pain should still be looked into because the final goal is to rule out cardiac causes of chest pain. It is relatively easy to rule out cardiac causes of chest pain by history and physical examination (see Table 20.2). The following lists some relevant facts about chest pain of cardiac origin.
    a. Cardiac cause of chest pain is usually typical anginal pain.
        (1) The patient describes the pain as a deep, heavy pressure; the feeling of choking; or a squeezing sensation. It is not sharp pain of short duration. The pain is located in the precordial or substernal area and may radiate to the neck, jaw, either or both arms, back, or abdomen.
        (2) Exercise, heavy physical activities, or emotional stress typically precipitates the cardiac pain. Nonexertional pain is unlikely of cardiac origin, with the exception of pleural pain (which changes with position of the body and respiration).
        (3) Associated symptoms such as syncope, dizziness, or palpitation suggest potential cardiac origin of the pain.
    b. Chest pain of noncardiac origin is likely when
        (1) Nonexertional pain, occurring while watching TV or sitting in class.
        (2) Sharp pain of short duration.
        (3) Pain of chronic nature.
        (4) Negative past history for heart disease or Kawasaki disease.
        (5) Negative family history for hereditary heart disease (such as long QT syndrome, cardiomyopathies, unexpected sudden death).
        (6) No associated symptoms such as syncope, dizziness, or palpitation.
        (7) Unremarkable cardiac examination.
        (8) Normal ECG and chest radiographs.

        Many of the following are found.
3. If none of the three common noncardiac causes of chest pain is found and history and physical examination suggest a noncardiac cause of chest pain, the clinician can reassure the patient and family of the probable benign nature of the chest pain.
4. At this point, the physician may decide either to do a simple follow-up or to consider a condition in other systems, such as gastrointestinal (such as gastroesophageal reflux, peptic ulcer), pulmonary (including

exercise-induced asthma), or psychogenic origin. Simple follow-up often clarifies the cause or the pain may subside without recurrence.

5. Drug screening for cocaine may be worthwhile in adolescents who have acute, severe chest pain and distress with an unclear cause.
6. An appropriate referral to a specialist may be considered at this stage.

IV. REFERRAL TO A CARDIOLOGIST

The following are some of the indications for referral to a cardiologist for cardiac evaluation of chest pain:

1. When chest pain is triggered or worsened by physical activities or is accompanied by other symptoms, such as palpitation, dizziness, or syncope.
2. When there are abnormal findings in the cardiac examination, or when abnormalities occur in the chest radiographs or ECG.
3. When there is a family history of cardiomyopathy, long QT syndrome, sudden unexpected death, or other hereditary diseases commonly associated with cardiac abnormalities.
4. High levels of anxiety in the family and patient and a chronic, recurring nature of the pain are also important reasons for referral to a cardiologist.

V. TREATMENT

When a specific cause of chest pain is identified, treatment is directed at correcting or improving the cause.

1. Costochondritis can be treated by reassurance and occasionally by nonsteroidal antiinflammatory agents (such as ibuprofen) or acetaminophen. Ibuprofen is a better choice because it is an antiinflammatory as well as analgesic agent.
   a. Ibuprofen, 5 to 10 mg/kg/dose, 3 to 4 times a day, for 7 days, often improves the pain. The same course may be repeated 2 to 3 times with an intervening 1-week period of no medication. Alternatively, for more compliance (due to twice-daily dosing), naproxen could be given for 5 to 7 days.
   b. Physical activities requiring the use of shoulder and arm muscles should be avoided, including sports using arms, push-ups, pull-ups, certain household chores, and others.
   c. Weight of backpacks should be reduced to a minimum.
2. Most musculoskeletal and nonorganic causes of chest pain can be treated with rest, nonsteroidal antiinflammatory agents, or acetaminophen.
3. Exercise-induced asthma is most effectively prevented by inhalation of a β_2-agonist 10 to 15 minutes before exercise. Inhaled albuterol usually affords protection for 4 hours.
4. If gastritis, gastroesophageal reflux, or peptic ulcer disease is suspected, trials of antacids, hydrogen ion blockers, or prokinetic agents (such as metoclopramide [Reglan]) are helpful therapeutically (as well as diagnostically).

5. If organic causes of chest pain are not found and psychogenic etiology is suspected, psychological consultation may be considered.
6. When or if cocaine-associated chest pain is suspected, physicians should arrange a referral to appropriate specialists for confirmation of the diagnosis and management of the problem.

Cocaine's pharmacologic action is through inhibition of the reuptake of norepinephrine, dopamine, and serotonin, and thus it produces signs of heightened sympathetic nervous system. Cocaine produces chest pain through powerful coronary vasoconstriction with decreased oxygen supply to the myocardium. Cocaine leads to increased heart rate, high blood pressure, dilated pupils, and reduced skin temperature. Cocaine also increases the possibility of thrombus formation (by inhibition of endogenous fibrinolysis, increasing thrombogenicity, and enhancing platelet aggregation via increased production of thromboxane).

The following are several points recommended by the American Heart Association guideline on treatment for cocaine abuse patients (McCord et al., 2008)

a. If cocaine intoxication is suspected, benzodiazepines are recommended as the primary treatment for anxiety, tachycardia, and hypertension.
b. Aspirin and nitrates continue to be strongly recommended.
c. However, α-blockers (including agents with mixed α-adrenergic antagonist effects, such as labetalol) are considered contraindicated because the unopposed α-adrenergic effect leads to worsening coronary vasoconstriction and increasing blood pressure.
d. Calcium channel blockers are not recommended because they may increase mortality rates.
e. Early percutaneous coronary intervention is indicated if myocardial infarction is likely the diagnosis.

Chapter 21

Syncope

I. DEFINITION

The brain depends on a constant supply of oxygen and glucose for normal function. Significant alterations in the supply of oxygen and glucose to the brain may result in a transient loss of consciousness.

1. Syncope is a transient loss of consciousness and muscle tone with a fall.
2. Presyncope is the feeling that one is about to pass out but remains conscious with a transient loss of postural tone.
3. Dizziness is the most common prodromal symptom of syncope. It is a nonspecific symptom that may include vertigo and light-headedness. Vertigo is a feeling that you or your surroundings are spinning or whirling, a manifestation of vestibular disorder. Light-headedness is a feeling that you are about to faint, but you do not feel as if you or your surroundings are moving.

II. PREVALENCE AND CAUSES

1. As many as 15% of children and adolescents are estimated to have a syncopal event between the ages of 8 and 18 years.
2. Syncope may be due to noncardiac causes (usually autonomic dysfunction), cardiac conditions, neuropsychiatric disorders, and metabolic disorders. Box 21.1 lists possible causes of syncope.
3. In adults, most cases of syncope are caused by cardiac problems.
4. In children and adolescents, most incidents of syncope are benign, resulting from vasovagal episodes (probably the most common cause), other orthostatic intolerance entities, hyperventilation, and breath holding.
5. Before age 6 years, syncope is likely caused by a seizure disorder, breath holding, or cardiac arrhythmias.

III. DESCRIPTION OF DIFFERENT CAUSES OF SYNCOPE

Only autonomic dysfunction (or noncardiac circulatory) and cardiac causes of syncope are presented; neurologic and metabolic causes are not discussed.

A. NONCARDIAC CAUSES (AUTONOMIC DYSFUNCTION)

1. **Orthostatic intolerance** encompasses disorders of blood flow, heart rate (HR), and blood pressure (BP) regulation that are most easily demonstrable during orthostatic stress. The recently popularized head-up

BOX 21.1

CAUSES OF SYNCOPE

AUTONOMIC (NONCARDIAC)

Orthostatic intolerance group
- Vasovagal syncope (also known as simple, neurocardiogenic, or neurally mediated syncope)
- Orthostatic (postural) hypotension (dysautonomia)
- Postural orthostatic tachycardia syndrome (POTS)

Exercise-related syncope (see further discussion in text)

Situational syncope
- Breath holding, cough, micturition, defecation, etc.
- Carotid sinus hypersensitivity
- Excess vagal tone

CARDIAC

Arrhythmias
- Tachycardias: SVT, atrial flutter/fibrillation, ventricular tachycardia (seen with long QT syndrome, arrhythmogenic RV dysplasia)
- Bradycardias: Sinus bradycardia, asystole, complete heart block, pacemaker malfunction

Obstructive lesions
- Outflow obstruction: AS, PS, hypertrophic cardiomyopathy, pulmonary hypertension
- Inflow obstruction: MS, tamponade, constrictive pericarditis, atrial myxoma

Myocardial
- Coronary artery anomalies, hypertrophic cardiomyopathy, dilated cardiomyopathy, MVP, arrhythmogenic RV dysplasia

NEUROPSYCHIATRIC

Hyperventilation
Seizure
Migraine
Tumors
Hysteria

METABOLIC

Hypoglycemia
Electrolyte disorders
Anorexia nervosa
Drugs/toxins

tilt test has identified three entities: vasovagal syncope, orthostatic hypotension, and postural orthostatic tachycardia syndrome (POTS).

a. **Vasovagal syncope** (also called simple fainting or neurocardiogenic syncope).
   (1) This is the most common type of syncope seen in otherwise healthy children and adolescents. It is uncommon before ages 10 to 12 but quite prevalent in adolescents, especially girls. It is

characterized by a prodrome lasting a few seconds to a minute. The prodrome may include dizziness, nausea, pallor, diaphoresis, palpitation, blurred vision, headache, and/or hyperventilation. The prodrome may be followed by the loss of consciousness and muscle tone with a fall. The unconsciousness does not last more than a minute. The syncope may occur after rising in the morning or in association with prolonged standing, anxiety or fright, pain, blood drawing or the sight of blood, fasting, hot and humid conditions, or crowded places. Typical response of patients with vasovagal syncope to the head-up tilt table test is precipitous drops in both the HR and BP (Fig. 21.1). History is most important in establishing the diagnosis of vasovagal syncope.

(2) **Proposed pathophysiology of vasovagal syncope**. The normal responses to assuming an upright posture are a reduced cardiac output, an increase in heart rate, and an unchanged or slightly diminished systolic pressure with about 6% decrease in cerebral blood flow.

In susceptible individuals, a sudden decrease in venous return to the ventricle produces a large increase in the force of ventricular contraction, which causes activation of the LV mechanoreceptors. A sudden increase in neural traffic to the brainstem somehow mimics the conditions seen in hypertension and thereby produces a paradoxical

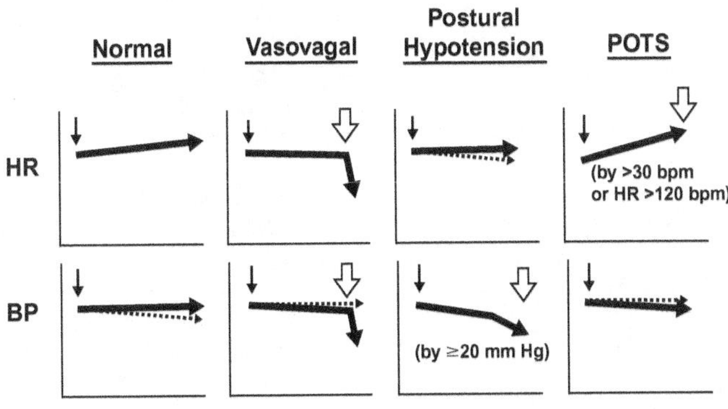

FIG. 21.1

Schematic drawing of changes in heart rate *(HR)* and blood pressure *(BP)* observed during the head-up tilt test. *Thin arrows* mark the start of orthostatic stress. *Large unfilled arrows* indicate appearance of symptoms with changes seen in HR and BP. *POTS*, postural orthostatic tachycardia syndrome. *(From Park, M. K., & Salamat, M. (2020).* Park's pediatric cardiology for practitioners *(7th ed.). Philadelphia: Mosby.)*

21

withdrawal of sympathetic activity. This results in peripheral vasodilatation, hypotension, bradycardia, and subsequent decrease in cerebral perfusion, leading to either presyncope or syncope (with loss of consciousness). Vasovagal syncope always occurs while the patient is in standing position. Hypovolemia (or dehydration) is often a predisposing factor; a dehydrated person is more likely to have syncope.

b. **Orthostatic hypotension (dysautonomia)**
   (1) The normal response to standing is reflex arterial and venous constriction and a slight increase in HR. In orthostatic hypotension, the normal adrenergic vasoconstriction of the arterioles and veins in the upright position is absent or inadequate, resulting in hypotension without a reflex increase in HR (see Fig. 21.1). Unlike the prodrome seen with vasovagal syncope, patients experience only light-headedness in orthostatic hypotension. They do not display the autonomic nervous system signs seen with vasovagal syncope, such as pallor, diaphoresis, and hyperventilation. Prolonged bed rest, prolonged standing, dehydration, medications that interfere with the sympathetic vasomotor response (e.g., calcium channel blockers, antihypertensive drugs, vasodilators, phenothiazines), and diuretics may exacerbate orthostatic hypotension.
   (2) In patients suspected of having orthostatic hypotension, BPs should be measured in the supine and standing positions. In adults, the American Autonomic Society has defined orthostatic hypotension as a persistent fall in systolic/diastolic pressure of more than 20/10 mm Hg within 3 minutes of assuming the upright position without moving their arms or legs, with no increase in the HR but without fainting. Orthostatic hypotension may only be demonstrable in the presence of dehydration. In a well-hydrated state when seen in an office setting, orthostatic hypotension may not occur.

c. **Postural orthostatic tachycardia syndrome (POTS)**
   (1) This syndrome, most often observed in young women, is a form of autonomic neuropathy that predominantly affects the lower extremities. Venous pooling associated with assuming a standing position leads to a reduced venous return and a resulting increase in sympathetic discharge with a significant degree of tachycardia. An increased level of adrenomedullin, a potent vasodilator with natriuric and diuretic effects, has been observed in some children with the syndrome. Affected patients often complain of chronic fatigue, exercise intolerance, palpitation, light-headedness, nausea, and recurrent near syncope (and sometimes syncope). These symptoms may be related to *chronic fatigue syndrome* and may be misdiagnosed as panic attacks or chronic anxiety. Occasional patients develop swelling

of the lower extremities with purplish discoloration of the dorsum of the foot and ankle.

(2) For the diagnosis of POTS, HR and BP are measured in the supine, sitting, and standing positions. POTS is defined as the development of orthostatic symptoms that are associated with at least a 30-beat/min increase in HR (or a HR of ≥ 120 beats/min) that occurs within the first 10 minutes of standing or upright tilt, with occurrence of symptoms described previously (see Fig. 21.1).

2. **Exercise-related syncope**. Athletic adolescents may experience syncope or presyncope during or after strenuous physical activities. This may signal serious cardiac problems, but in most cases it occurs due to a combination of venous pooling in vasodilated leg muscles, inadequate hydration, and high ambient temperature. To prevent venous pooling, athletes should keep moving after running competitions. Secondary hyperventilation from exercise activities with resulting hypocapnia may also contribute to this form of syncope. Tingling or numbness of extremities may occur with hypocapnia.
3. **Situational syncope**.
   a. Micturition syncope is a rare form of orthostatic hypotension. In this condition, rapid bladder decompression results in decreased total peripheral vascular resistance with splanchnic stasis and reduced venous return to the heart, resulting in postural hypotension.
   b. Cough syncope follows paroxysmal nocturnal coughing in asthmatic children. Paroxysmal coughing produces a marked increase in intrapleural pressure with a reduced venous return and reduced cardiac output, resulting in altered cerebral blood flow and loss of consciousness.

B. CARDIAC CAUSES OF SYNCOPE

Cardiac causes of syncope may include obstructive lesions, myocardial dysfunction, and arrhythmias (see Box 21.1).

1. **Obstructive lesions**. Patients with severe AS, PS, or hypertrophic obstructive cardiomyopathy (HOCM), as well as those with pulmonary hypertension, may have syncope. Exercise often precipitates syncope associated with these conditions. These patients may also complain of chest pain, dyspnea, and palpitation.
2. **Myocardial dysfunction**. Although rare, myocardial ischemia or infarction secondary to congenital anomalies of the coronary arteries or acquired disease of the coronary arteries (such as Kawasaki disease, postsurgical, or atherosclerotic heart disease) may cause syncope.
3. **Arrhythmias**. Either extreme tachycardia or bradycardia can cause syncope. Commonly encountered rhythm disturbances include SVT, VT, sick sinus syndrome, and complete heart block. Imaging studies may or may not show structural abnormalities.

a. No identifiable structural defect is present in long QT syndrome, WPW syndrome, RV dysplasia, and Brugada syndrome.
b. Identifiable structural heart defects are imaged for the following conditions.
   (1) Preoperative CHDs (such as Ebstein anomaly, MS, or MR, and L-TGA).
   (2) Postoperative CHDs (such as TOF, TGA, after Fontan operation) may cause sinus node dysfunction, SVT, VT, or complete heart block.
   (3) Dilated cardiomyopathy can cause sinus bradycardia, SVT, or VT.
   (4) Hypertrophic cardiomyopathy is a rare cause of VT and syncope.

IV. EVALUATION OF A CHILD WITH SYNCOPE

A. HISTORY

Accurate history taking is most important in determining cost-effective diagnostic strategies.

1. About the syncopal event
   a. The time of day: Syncope occurring after rising in the morning suggests vasovagal syncope. Hypoglycemia is a very rare cause of syncope.
   b. The patient's position: Syncope while sitting or recumbent suggests arrhythmias or seizures. Syncope after standing for some time suggests vasovagal syncope or other orthostatic intolerance group.
   c. Relationship to exercise
      (1) Syncope occurring during exercise suggests arrhythmias.
      (2) Syncope occurring immediately after cessation of strenuous physical activities (such as football practice or game) may be due to venous pooling in the leg, and rarely due to arrhythmias. Vigorousness and duration of the activity, relative hydration status, and ambient temperature are important.
   d. Associated symptoms
      (1) Palpitation or racing HR suggests arrhythmia or tachycardia.
      (2) Chest pain suggests possible myocardial ischemia (due to obstructive lesions, cardiomyopathy, carditis, etc.).
      (3) Shortness of breath or tingling or numbness of extremities suggests hyperventilation.
      (4) Nausea, epigastric discomfort, and diaphoresis suggest vasovagal syncope.
      (5) Headache or visual changes also suggest vasovagal syncope.
   e. The duration of syncope
      (1) Syncopal duration less than 1 minute suggests vasovagal syncope, hyperventilation, or syncope due to other orthostatic mechanism.

(2) A longer duration of syncope suggests convulsive disorders, migraine, or cardiac arrhythmias.

f. The patient's appearance during and immediately following the episode.
   (1) Pallor indicates hypotension.
   (2) Abnormal movement or posturing, confusion, focal neurologic signs, amnesia, or muscle soreness suggests the possibility of seizure.

2. Past history of cardiac, endocrine, neurologic, or psychological disorders may suggest a disorder in that system.
3. Medications, including prescribed, over-the-counter, and recreational drugs, should be checked.
4. Family history should include the following data:
   a. Myocardial infarction in family members younger than 30 years of age.
   b. Cardiac arrhythmia, CHD, cardiomyopathies, long QT syndrome, seizures, and metabolic and psychological disorders.
   c. Positive family history of fainting is common in patients with vasovagal syncope.
5. Social history is important in assessing whether there is a possibility of substance abuse, pregnancy, or factors leading to a conversion reaction.

B. PHYSICAL EXAMINATION

Although physical examination is usually normal, it should always be performed, focusing on the cardiac and neurologic systems.

1. Careful auscultation includes heart murmurs or abnormally loud second heart sounds.
2. If orthostatic intolerance group is suspected, the HR and BP should be measured repeatedly while the patient is supine and after standing without moving for up to 10 minutes.
3. Neurologic examination should include a fundoscopic examination, test for Romberg sign, gait evaluation, deep tendon reflexes, and cerebellar function.

C. DIAGNOSTIC STUDIES

History and physical examinations guide practitioners in choosing the diagnostic tests that apply to a given syncopal patient.

1. Serum glucose and electrolytes are of limited value, because patients are seen hours or days after the episode.
2. When an arrhythmia is suspected as the cause of syncope:
   a. The electrocardiogram (ECG) should be inspected for HR (bradycardia), arrhythmias, WPW preexcitation, heart block, long QTc interval, and abnormalities suggestive of cardiomyopathies and myocarditis.
   b. Ambulatory ECG monitoring (24-hour Holter monitor or event recorder) is usually obtained.

3. Echo studies are performed to rule out CHDs, pulmonary hypertension, and cardiomyopathies and to check on the status of postoperative CHDs.
4. Exercise stress test is indicated if the syncopal event is associated with exercise.
5. Rarely cardiac catheterization and electrophysiologic study may be indicated in some equivocal cases.
6. Head-up tilt table test. If patients with positional syncope have autonomic symptoms (such as pallor, diaphoresis, or hyperventilation), tilt table testing is sometimes performed by some centers (see following section).
7. Neurologic consultation. Patients who faint while sitting or recumbent and those who exhibit prolonged loss of consciousness, seizure activity, and a postictal phase with lethargy or confusion should be referred for neurologic consultation.

D. HEAD-UP TILT TABLE TEST

The goal of the test is to provoke the patient's symptoms during an orthostatic stress while closely monitoring the patient's cardiac rhythm, HR, and BP responses associated with symptoms. Orthostatic stress is created by a tilting table with the patient placed in an upright position for a certain period of time. Various protocols are available.

Positive responses commonly include light-headedness, dizziness, nausea, visual changes, and frank syncope. Sinus bradycardia, junctional bradycardia, and asystole for as long as 30 seconds are common. Hypotension generally is manifested by systolic BPs of less than 70 mm Hg. Returning the patient to the supine position produces resolution of symptoms rapidly, usually with a reactive tachycardia.

Although several distinct abnormal patterns have been identified during the head-up tilt table tests (as shown in Fig. 21.1), there are serious questions about the sensitivity, specificity, diagnostic yield, and day-to-day reproducibility of the tilt test. In adults, the overall reproducibility of syncope by the tilt test is disappointingly low (62%). About 25% of adolescents with no prior fainting history fainted during the tilt test. Moreover, among habitual fainters, 25% to 30% did not faint during the test on a given day.

V. TREATMENT

1. Orthostatic intolerance group. Regardless of the type, the same preventive measures are used for all orthostatic intolerance groups. Beginning the therapy empirically without performing a head-up tilt table test is not unreasonable.
   a. Placing the patient in a supine position until the circulatory crisis resolves may be all that is indicated.
   b. The patient is advised to lie down with the feet raised above the chest, if he or she feels the prodrome to a faint. The patient is also advised to avoid extreme heat and dehydration and to increase salt and fluid intake.

c. β-Blocker therapy is used commonly, especially in adolescents and young adults, to modify the feedback loop. Atenolol (1 to 1.2 mg/kg/day PO QD, maximum dose 2 mg/kg/day) or metoprolol (1.5 mg/kg/day given PO in two or three doses) is most commonly used.
d. α-Agonist therapy using pseudoephedrine (60 mg, PO, BID) or an ephedrine-theophylline combination (Marax) stimulates the HR and increases the peripheral vascular tone, preventing reflex bradycardia and vasodilation. Midodrine, an α_1-agonist, (given 2.5 to 10 mg PO TID) may be used.
e. Fludrocortisone (Florinef), a mineralocortisone, 0.1 mg PO, QD, or BID for children; 0.2 mg/day for adults, with increased salt intake or a salt tablet (1 g daily) may be tried. Average children commonly gain 1 kg or 2 kg water weight into their circulating volume within 2 or 3 weeks.

2. Cardiac arrhythmias presenting as syncopal events require antiarrhythmic therapy or radiofrequency ablation (see treatment for specific arrhythmias in Chapter 16).

VI. DIFFERENTIAL DIAGNOSIS OF SYNCOPE

1. **Epilepsy.** Patients with epilepsy may have incontinence, marked confusion in the postictal state, and abnormal electroencephalograms (EEGs). Patients are rigid rather than limp and may have sustained injuries. Patients do not experience the prodromal symptoms of syncope (e.g., dizziness, pallor, palpitation, and diaphoresis). The duration of unconsciousness is longer than that typically seen with syncope (<1 minute).
2. **Hypoglycemia.** Hypoglycemic attacks differ from syncope in that the onset and recovery occur more gradually, and they do not occur during or shortly after meals.
3. **Hyperventilation.** Hyperventilation produces hypocapnia, which in turn produces intense cerebral vasoconstriction, causing syncope. It may also have a psychological component. The patient often experiences air hunger, shortness of breath, chest tightness, abdominal discomfort, palpitations, dizziness, and numbness or tingling of the face and extremities, and rarely loss of consciousness. The syncopal episode can be reproduced in the office when the patient hyperventilates.
4. **Hysteria.** Syncope resulting from hysteria is not associated with injury and occurs only in the presence of an audience. During these attacks, the patient does not experience the pallor and hypotension that characterize true syncope. The attacks may last longer (up to an hour) than a brief syncopal spell. Episodes usually occur in an emotionally charged setting and are rare before 10 years of age.

Chapter 22

Palpitation

I. DEFINITION

Palpitation is one of the most common cardiac symptoms encountered in medical practice but it poorly corresponds to demonstrable abnormalities. The term *palpitation* is used loosely to describe an unpleasant subjective awareness of one's own heartbeats. This usually occurs as a sensation in the chest of rapid, irregular, or unusually strong heartbeats.

II. CAUSES

Many palpitations are often not serious, but they may indicate the possible presence of serious cardiac arrhythmias. Box 22.1 lists causes of palpitation.

1. A high percentage of patients with palpitation have no etiology that can be established.
2. Certain stimulants, such as caffeine, can be identified as a cause of palpitation. Caffeine is found in many foods and drinks, such as coffee, tea, hot cocoa, soda, and chocolate, as well as in some medicines. Most energy drinks (such as Venom, Whoopass, Red Bull, Adrenalin Rush) contain large doses of caffeine and other legal stimulants, including ephedrine, guarana, taurine, and ginseng.
3. Certain drugs, prescription or over-the-counter, can be identified as a cause of palpitation.
4. Some medical conditions, such as hyperthyroidism, anemia, and hypoglycemia, may be the cause of palpitation.
5. Rarely, slow heart rates may cause palpitation.
6. Some patients report palpitation while having sinus tachycardia.
7. Rarely, cardiac arrhythmias should be looked into as a cause of palpitation, although most arrhythmias are not perceived and reported as palpitations.
8. Occasionally, a psychogenic or psychiatric cause for the symptoms can be suspected. Some adult patients with palpitations have panic disorder or panic attack.

III. EVALUATION

A. HISTORY

1. The nature and onset of palpitation may suggest causes.
   a. Isolated "jumps" or "skips" suggest premature beats.
   b. Sudden start and stop of rapid heartbeat or a pounding of the chest suggests SVT. Some children with SVT will appear sweaty or pale.
   c. A gradual onset and cessation of palpitation suggest sinus tachycardia or anxiety state.

BOX 22.1
CAUSES OF PALPITATION.

Normal physiologic event
- Exercise, excitement, fever

Psychogenic or psychiatric
- Fear, anger, stress, anxiety disorders, panic attack or panic disorder

Certain drugs and substances
- Stimulants: caffeine (coffee, tea, soda, chocolate), some energy drinks, smoking
- Over-the-counter drugs: decongestants, diet pills, etc.
- Drugs that cause tachycardia: catecholamines, theophylline, hydralazine, minoxidil, cocaine
- Drugs that cause bradycardia: β-blockers, antihypertensive drugs, calcium channel blockers
- Drugs that cause arrhythmias: antiarrhythmics (some of which are proarrhythmic), tricyclic antidepressants, phenothiazines

Certain medical conditions
- Anemia
- Hyperthyroidism
- Hypertension
- Pheochromocytoma (with catecholamine excess)
- Hypoglycemia
- Hyperventilation
- Poor physical condition

Heart diseases
- Certain CHDs that are prone to arrhythmias or result in poor physical condition
- Following surgeries for CHD: Fontan connection, Senning operation
- Mitral valve prolapse
- Hypertrophic cardiomyopathy
- Dilated cardiomyopathy
- Cardiac tumors or infiltrative diseases

Cardiac arrhythmias
- Tachycardias: sinus tachycardia, SVT, VT
- Bradycardia
- Premature beats: PACs, PVCs
- Atrial fibrillation
- Sick sinus syndrome

CHD, congenital heart defect; *PACs*, premature atrial contractions; *PVCs*, premature ventricular contractions; *SVT*, supraventricular tachycardia; *VT*, ventricular tachycardia.

d. Palpitation characterized by slow heart rate may be due to atrioventricular (AV) block or sinus node dysfunction.

2. Relationship to exertion
   a. A history of palpitation during strenuous physical activity may be a normal phenomenon (due to sinus tachycardia), although it could be due to exercise-induced arrhythmias.
   b. Nonexertional palpitation may suggest atrial flutter/fibrillation, febrile state, thyrotoxicosis, hypoglycemia, or anxiety state.
   c. Palpitation on standing suggests postural hypotension.

3. Associated symptoms
   a. Symptoms of dizziness or fainting associated with palpitation may indicate VT.
   b. The presence of other symptoms, such as chest pain, sweating, nausea, or shortness of breath, may increase the likelihood of identifiable causes of palpitation.
4. Personal and family history may help identify the cause.
   a. Ask about eating and drinking habits, such as sodas, coffee, tea, hot cocoa, chocolates, which contain caffeine.
   b. Ask if the patient is using energy drinks.
   c. Ask about prescription and over-the-counter medications that could cause palpitation.
   d. Ask about medical or heart conditions that may cause tachycardia or palpitation.
   e. Ask about family history of syncope, sudden death, or arrhythmias.

B. PHYSICAL EXAMINATION

1. Most children with palpitation have normal physical examinations, except for those with hyperthyroidism.
2. Cardiac examination may reveal findings of MVP, obstructive lesions, or possibly cardiomyopathy.

C. RECORDING OF ECG RHYTHM

Recording of the electrocardiogram (ECG) rhythm that coincides with the timing of the patient's complaint of palpitation is a certain way of making diagnosis of arrhythmia or ruling it out as the cause of palpitation. A number of ECG recording techniques are available.

1. Routine ECG may show prolonged QTc interval, delta waves (WPW preexcitation), or AV block.
2. When palpitation occurs almost daily, a 24-hour Holter monitoring is usually most helpful in making the diagnosis of the rhythm abnormality. Some children actually complain of palpitation during sinus tachycardia.
3. When palpitation occurs infrequently, long-term event monitor recording (up to 30 days) is indicated. With infrequent palpitations that are fairly long-lasting, handheld or patient-activated nonlooping memory event recorders are indicated. However, with infrequent short-lasting palpitation, external loop recorders are indicated.
4. Implantable loop recorders (inserted under the skin at about the second rib on the left front of the chest) can be used to monitor for a period longer than 1 month (the period may be up to a year). These can be worn during swimming or other vigorous exercises.
5. Continuous outpatient telemetry monitoring is a new monitoring modality available at most tertiary care facilities. The patient is fitted with a transmitter that sends the ECG data to the area of the hospital where the

telemetry monitoring occurs. The patient can move around within the device's transmitting range.

6. If the symptoms occur during exercise, an exercise stress test may be helpful in making the diagnosis.
7. If there is a high suspicion of VT, sometimes provocative electrophysiologic studies may be indicated.
8. When all other means have been exhausted and Holter and/or event monitoring have shown sinus tachycardias at unexpected times and the heart rate is unusually high for the state of activity, the diagnosis of inappropriate sinus tachycardia (IST) is a possibility. (This diagnosis is more common in female adult patients than children and adolescents. The mechanism of this tachycardia is not clearly understood. Although it is a benign condition, it can cause significant disturbance to patient's daily life, and its management is at times frustrating to the family and to the physician.)

D. ECHOCARDIOGRAPHY

Echo studies help identify structural heart disease, such as cardiomyopathies, cardiac tumors, MVP, and other structural abnormalities of the heart.

E. EXERCISE STRESS TEST

If the symptoms occur during exercise, an exercise stress test may be helpful in making the diagnosis.

F. LABORATORY STUDIES

When other medical conditions are suspected as a cause of palpitation, full blood count (for anemia), electrolytes, blood glucose, and thyroid function testing may be indicated. When pheochromocytoma is suspected, free metanephrines could be measured in blood plasma.

G. ELECTROPHYSIOLOGY

If there is a high suspicion of VT, sometimes provocative electrophysiologic studies may be indicated.

IV. MANAGEMENT

1. If the rhythm recorded on the 24-hour Holter monitoring shows sinus tachycardia at the time of the complaint of palpitation, reassure the parent and child of the normal, benign nature of palpitation.
2. Stimulant-containing drinks (coffee, tea, hot cocoa, chocolate, sodas, and energy drinks) should be reduced or eliminated.
3. Treat medical causes of palpitation (such as hyperthyroidism) if present.
4. Examination of all medications that the patient is taking may be helpful in the diagnosis, in modifying the dosage or schedule, or changing to other medications.

5. For isolated PACs or PVCs, nothing needs to be done except avoidance of stimulants such as those listed previously.
6. If a significant cardiac arrhythmia or an AV conduction disturbance is found, appropriate therapy should be given for the conditions found.
7. If palpitation is associated with symptoms, such as fainting, dizziness, chest pain, pallor, or diaphoresis, further evaluation is guided as described under syncope or chest pain.
8. In adult patients suspected to have inappropriate sinus tachycardia, a variety of medications have been tried with different levels of success. β-Blockers are often tried first; calcium-channel blockers are alternatives.

Chapter 23

Systemic Hypertension

I. DEFINITION

For adults, the 2017 Guidelines by the American College of Cardiology, American Heart Association, and several other organizations jointly revised the earlier definition and classification of hypertension (HTN) of 2003. The following are the new classification (Whelton et al., 2018). Table 23.1 shows different levels of blood pressure (BP) readings by the new definition of elevated BP.

1. Normal BP is defined as <120 mm Hg systolic pressure (SP) and <80 mm Hg diastolic pressures (DP).
2. SP between 120 and 129 mm Hg and DP <80 mm Hg are now called "elevated blood pressure," formerly called "prehypertension."
3. Hypertension is classified as stage 1 and stage 2, depending on the level of abnormalities.
   a. Stage 1 HTN is defined as SP 130 to 139 systolic mm Hg *or* DP 80 to 89 mm Hg.
   b. Stage 2 HTN is defined as SP ≥140 mm Hg *or* DP ≥90 mm Hg.

In children, hypertension is defined statistically, because BP levels vary with age and gender and because outcome-based data are not available for children. Following the new definition of hypertension in adults, the American Academy of Pediatrics updated the earlier guidelines of 2004 (Flynn et al., 2017) (see Table 23.1). In the new guidelines, the term "prehypertension" has been replaced with "elevated blood pressure" for children as in the adults.

1. *Normal BP* is defined as systolic and diastolic pressure <90th percentile.
2. *Elevated BP* is defined as an average systolic and diastolic pressure between the 90th and 95th percentiles for age and gender.
3. *HTN* is defined as systolic or diastolic pressure levels that are greater than the 95th percentile for age and gender. As in adults, adolescents with BP levels ≥120/80 mm Hg by auscultatory method are considered hypertensive even if they are <95th percentile. HTN is further classified into stage 1 and stage 2.
   a. Stage 1 HTN is present when BP readings are between 95th percentile and 99th percentiles + 12 mm Hg.
   b. Stage 2 HTN is present when BP readings higher than 95th percentile + 12 mm Hg.
4. *White coat HTN* is present when BP readings in health care facilities are greater than the 95th percentile but are normotensive outside a clinical setting. This condition may not be as benign as once thought to be and

TABLE 23.1

CLASSIFICATION OF BLOOD PRESSURE FOR ADULTS AND CHILDREN

	ADULTS[a] AND ADOLESCENT >13 YEARS[b]			
	SP (MM HG)		DP (MM HG)	CHILDREN AND ADOLESCENTS <13 YEARS[b]
Normal BP	<120	and	<80	<90th %
Elevated BP	120-129	and	<80	≥ 90th% to <95th% or ≥ 120/80 mm Hg, whichever is lower
Stage 1 HTN	130-139	or	80–89	≥ 95th% to 95th% + 12 mm Hg or 130/80 to 139/89 mm Hg (whichever is lower)
Stage 2 HTN	≥ 140	or	≥ 90	Higher than 95th% + 12 mm Hg or ≥ 140/90 mm Hg (whichever is lower)

Blood pressure levels are based on an average of ≥ 2 careful readings or ≥ 2 occasions. Individuals with systolic and diastolic pressure in two different categories should be designated to the higher BP category. BP, *blood pressure;* DP, *diastolic pressure;* HTN, *hypertension;* SP, *systolic pressure;* %, *percentile.*

[a]Adapted from Whelton, P. K., Carey, R. M., Aronow, W. S., et al, (2018). ACC/AHA/AAPA/ABC/ACPM/AGS/APhA/ASH/ASPC/NMA/PCNA guidelines for the prevention, detection, evaluation, and management of high blood pressure in adults: a report of the American College of Cardiology/American Heart Association Task Force on Clinical Practice Guidelines. *Journal of the American College of Cardiology, 71*(10), e127-e248.

[b]Adapted from Flynn, J. T., Kaelber, D. C., Barker-Smith, C. M., et al. (2018). Clinical practice guideline for screening and management of high blood pressure in children and adolescents. *Pediatrics, 140*(3), e20171904.

regular follow-up is now recommended. This topic is discussed further later in this chapter.

II. NORMATIVE BP STANDARDS

1. The BP tables provided by the Working Group of the National High Blood Pressure Education Program (NHBPEP) are not acceptable standards because they are obtained by a methodology currently unacceptable and are discordant from their own recommendations, statistically unsound, and impractical for practitioners (as discussed in Chapter 1).
2. Normative BP standards from the San Antonio Children's Blood Pressure Study (SACBPS) are the most reliable sets; they are the only large sets of BP standards obtained using the currently recommended methodology. In that study, both auscultatory and oscillometric (Dinamap 800) methods were used.
   a. The auscultatory BP standards for children 5 to 17 years old are shown in Tables B.3 and B.4 in Appendix B.
   b. A different set of BP standards is needed for the oscillometric method because BP readings by Dinamap monitor model 8100, a popular oscillometric device, are significantly different from those obtained by the auscultatory method. Dinamap readings are on

average 10 mm Hg higher for the SP and 5 mm Hg higher for the DP than readings using the auscultatory method.

(1) Normative oscillometric BP standards for children 5 to 17 years old from the SACBPS are presented in Tables B.5 and B.6 in Appendix B.

(2) Oscillometric BP standards for neonates and small children up to 5 years of age are presented in Table 1.3.

3. Kaelber et al. (2009) have recommended a simplified table of BP levels according to age and gender (without height percentiles), above which further evaluation should be carried out for possible HTN. This approach is well justified and more practical because one does not need to use the unscientific normative standards of the NHBPEP and because height is not measured at some BP screening sites (as discussed in Chapter 2). Table 23.2 shows the 90th percentile BP values by both methods side-by-side. Table 23.2 is replication of Table 1.4 in Chapter 1. It is interesting to note that the auscultatory BP levels recommended by Kaelbert et al. are almost the same as the 90th percentile of BP levels by the San Antonio study (Park et al., 2005).

III. CAUSES OF HYPERTENSION

1. With the increasing prevalence of obesity in recent decades, overweight and obesity have become the most common causes of pediatric HTN.
2. More than 90% of secondary HTN in nonobese children is caused by three conditions: renal parenchymal disease, renal artery disease, and COA.
3. In general, children with essential HTN are older than 10 years, have mild HTN, and often are obese.
4. Children with secondary HTN are generally younger than 10 years and have higher levels of BP. Children with secondary HTN rarely are obese and often are less than normal height.
5. Table 23.3 lists the common causes of HTN by age group in (nonobese) children. Box 23.1 lists causes of secondary HTN.

IV. DIAGNOSIS OF HYPERTENSION

A. STEPS IN DIAGNOSIS OF HYPERTENSION

Diagnosis of HTN is not simple and easy. There are many factors that contribute to the erroneous diagnosis of HTN in children and in adults. Careless, erroneous diagnosis of HTN can lead to costly investigation and even treatment using drugs, some of which may have irreversible side effects. The following issues must be considered in making the diagnosis of HTN. After the diagnosis is confirmed, the clinician must proceed with workups to find the cause of HTN: primary or secondary.

1. One must use correct BP measurement techniques and compare the reading with reliable BP standards. BP obtained by a wrist BP device

TABLE 23.2

THE 90TH PERCENTILES OF BLOOD PRESSURE BY AUSCULTATORY AND OSCILLOMETRIC METHODS FROM THE SAN ANTONIO STUDY

	AUSCULTATORY[a,b]					OSCILLOMETRIC[c]			
AGE (YR)	MALE		FEMALE		AGE (YR)	MALE		FEMALE	
	SP	DP	SP	DP		SP	DP	SP	DP
5	103	60	102	60	5	115	68	114	68
6	105	64	103	63	6	117	68	115	68
7	107	66	104	65	7	118	69	116	69
8	108	68	106	67	8	119	70	118	70
9	109	68	108	67	9	121	70	119	70
10	111	68	110	68	10	122	71	121	71
11	113	68	112	68	11	124	71	122	71
12	116	68	113	68	12	126	71	123	71
13	118	68	115	68	13	129	71	125	71
14	120	68	116	68	14	131	72	125	72
15	120	69	117	69	15	133	72	126	72
16	120	71	117	69	16	134	72	126	72
17	120	73	118	70	17	134	72	126	72
≥18	120	73	120	70					

SP, *systolic pressure*; DP, *diastolic pressure.*

[a]The 90th percentile of systolic pressure for males 14 years and older are higher than 120 mm Hg, but 120 mm Hg is listed in the table to be consistent with the definition of "elevated blood pressure" in adults.

[b]Data from Park, M. K., Menard, S. W., & Yuan, C. (2001). Comparison of blood pressure in children from three ethnic groups. *American Journal of Cardiology, 87*(11), 1305-1308.

[c]Data from Park, M. K., Menard, S. W., & Schoolfield, J. (2005). Oscillometric blood pressure standards for children. *Pediatric Cardiology, 26*(5), 601-607. These values were obtained by Dinamap model 8100 and in general fall between the 90th and 95th percentiles of blood pressure (prehypertension range).

should not be used because the readings are likely to be high due to the peripheral amplification of SP (as discussed in Chapter1).

2. BP readings measured by the auscultatory and oscillometric methods are significantly different and thus not interchangeable; one must use BP standards specific for the method used.
3. White coat HTN further complicates the issue as the prevalence of white coat HTN in children and adolescents is estimated to be about 30% to 50%. Therefore one must make efforts to confirm elevated BP readings outside the health care facilities.
4. In addition, one must confirm *persistently* elevated BP levels at least on three consecutive examinations.

TABLE 23.3

COMMON CAUSES OF CHRONIC HYPERTENSION ACCORDING TO AGE

AGE GROUP	CAUSES
Newborns	Renal artery thrombosis, renal artery stenosis, congenital renal malformation, COA, bronchopulmonary dysplasia (transient)
<6 yr	Renal parenchymal disease, COA, renal artery stenosis
6-10 yr	Renal artery stenosis, renal parenchymal disease, COA
>10 yr	Primary hypertension, renal parenchymal disease

COA, *coarctation of the aorta.*
Adapted from Task Force on Blood Pressure Control in Children. National Heart, Lung, and Blood Institute. (1987). Report of the second task force on blood pressure control in children. *Pediatrics, 79*(1), 1-25.

BOX 23.1

CAUSES OF SECONDARY HYPERTENSION.

RENAL

- Renal parenchymal disease
    - Glomerulonephritis, acute and chronic
    - Pyelonephritis, acute and chronic
    - Congenital anomalies (polycystic or dysplastic kidneys)
    - Obstructive uropathies (hydronephrosis)
    - Hemolytic-uremic syndrome
    - Collagen disease (periarteritis, lupus)
    - Renal damage from nephrotoxic medications, trauma, or radiation
- Renovascular disease
    - Renal artery disorders (e.g., stenosis, polyarteritis, thrombosis)
    - Renal vein thrombosis

CARDIOVASCULAR

- Coarctation of the aorta
- Conditions with large stroke volume (patent ductus arteriosus, aortic insufficiency, systemic arteriovenous fistula, complete heart block) (these conditions cause only systolic hypertension)

ENDOCRINE

- Hyperthyroidism (systolic hypertension)
- Excessive catecholamine levels
    - Pheochromocytoma
    - Neuroblastoma
- Adrenal dysfunction
    - Congenital adrenal hyperplasia
        - 11β-hydroxylase deficiency
        - 17-hydroxylase deficiency
    - Cushing syndrome

Hyperaldosteronism
- Primary
  Conn syndrome
  Idiopathic nodular hyperplasia
  Dexamethasone-suppressible hyperaldosteronism
- Secondary
  Renovascular hypertension
  Renin-producing tumor (juxtaglomerular cell tumor)

Hyperparathyroidism (and hypercalcemia)

NEUROGENIC

Increased intracranial pressure (any cause, especially tumors, infections, trauma)
Poliomyelitis
Guillain-Barré syndrome
Dysautonomia (Riley-Day syndrome)

DRUGS AND CHEMICALS

Sympathomimetic drugs (nose drops, cough medications, cold preparations, theophylline)
Amphetamines
Corticosteroids
Nonsteroidal antiinflammatory drugs
Oral contraceptives
Heavy metal poisoning (mercury, lead)
Cocaine, acute or chronic use
Cyclosporine
Thyroxine
Tacrolimus

MISCELLANEOUS

Hypervolemia and hypernatremia
Stevens-Johnson syndrome
Bronchopulmonary dysplasia (newborns)

B. WHAT TO DO WHEN A HIGH BP READING IS OBTAINED IN THE OFFICE

The following is one way of handling a case of high BP readings in the office setting.

1. If an abnormal reading is the result of single reading, obtain two additional readings.
2. If BP is still high, a repeat set of three readings is obtained at the end of the office visit, and readings are compared with a reliable BP standard, such as those from the SACBPS (see Tables B.3 through B.6 in Appendix B).
3. Even if BP readings are still high at the end of the office visit, a possibility of white coat HTN still exists. Consider ways to identify cases of white coat HTN by measuring BPs outside the health care facility.
   a. Having reliable school nurses take daily BP for 2 to 4 weeks may be a cost-effective way to get the same information.

b. Home BP monitoring can be an option. It is reasonable to try home BP measurement in children under certain circumstances. However, objectivity and conflict of interest of the patient and/or parents should be considered before using this approach. An average of two (or three) BP readings taken in the morning and at night for 1 week (with a total of at least 12 readings) is recommended. For home BP monitoring, the monitor should be checked for its accuracy and the patient should be taught correct measurement technique and correct BP cuff size. Wrist monitors are not acceptable because the readings are expected to be higher due to peripheral amplification of SP. In evaluating home BP readings, it may be more reasonable to use the oscillometric BP standards, because most home BP devices use the oscillometric method rather than the auscultatory standards.
c. If a reliable BP measurement outside the doctor's office cannot be arranged, serial BP measurements (more than 10) can be obtained in the doctor's office by the same friendly staff to minimize the white coat effect.
d. The American Academy of Pediatrics (AAP) guidelines (Flynn et al., 2017) recommend routine use of ambulatory BP measurement (ABPM) to confirm the diagnosis of HTN in children and adolescents older than 5 years of age for technical reasons. It is recommended (1) in patients with office BP measurements in the elevated BP category for 1 year or more or (2) in patients with stage 1 HTN over three clinic visits, and (3) in patients suspected to have white coat HTN. Normative ABPM data are available in Tables B.8 and B.9 in Appendix B.

4. If multiple BP readings obtained outside the health care facility or in the doctor's office show persistently elevated BP levels above the 95th percentile most of the time, or the results of AMBP measurement confirm the finding, a tentative diagnosis of HTN may be made, and initial investigation begun for the cause HTN (as described in the following section).
5. If the repeated BP measurements or ABPM results fall between the 90th and 95th percentiles (elevated BP), the patient should be followed on a regular basis (every 3 to 6 months) with repeat BP measurements.
6. Even with the diagnosis of white coat HTN the patient should not be dismissed from follow-up. White coat HTN may not be as benign as it was once thought to be. Several recent studies in adults and children suggest that about 30% to 40% of patients with white coat HTN spontaneously evolve into HTN, with accompanying end-organ damage. Thus white coat HTN can be considered a prehypertension and patients should have several follow-ups before they are labeled as hypertensive or dismissed as normotensives. Some of these patients may need additional investigations as described for patients with established HTN (see the following section).

V. EVALUATION FOR CAUSES OF HYPERTENSION

Evaluate the history (present, past, and family), perform a careful physical examination, and proceed with the initial investigation to look for the cause of HTN, as outlined in the section to follow. In general, children younger than 10 years with sustained HTN require extensive evaluation, because identifiable and potentially curable causes are more likely to be found. Adolescents with mild HTN and a positive family history of HTN are more likely to have essential HTN, and extensive studies are not indicated.

A. HISTORY

1. Neonatal: use of umbilical artery catheters or bronchopulmonary dysplasia.
2. History of palpitation, headache, and excessive sweating (signs of excessive catecholamine levels).
3. Renal: history of obstructive uropathies, urinary tract infection, and radiation, trauma, or surgery to the kidney area.
4. Cardiovascular: history of COA or surgery for it.
5. Endocrine: weakness and muscle cramps (hypokalemia seen with hyperaldosteronism).
6. Medications: corticosteroids, amphetamines, antiasthmatic drugs, cold medications, oral contraceptives, nephrotoxic antibiotics, cyclosporine, cocaine use.
7. Family history of essential HTN, atherosclerotic heart disease, and stroke.
8. Familial or hereditary renal disease (polycystic kidney, cystinuria, familial nephritis).

B. PHYSICAL EXAMINATION

1. Accurate measurement of BP is essential.
2. Physical examination should focus on delayed growth (renal disease), bounding peripheral pulse (PDA or AR), weak or absent femoral pulses, or BP differential between the arms and legs (COA), abdominal bruits (renovascular), and tenderness over the kidney (renal infection).
3. Children's weight and body mass index (BMI) percentile (for obesity-related HTN).

C. LABORATORY AND OTHER INVESTIGATIONS

1. Initial laboratory tests should be directed toward detecting renal parenchymal disease, renovascular disease, COA, endocrine diseases, and CV risk factors for obesity-related HTN. Therefore tests should include urinalysis; urine culture; and serum electrolyte, blood urea nitrogen, creatinine, lipid profile. The electrocardiogram (ECG), chest radiographs, and possibly echo study may be useful. Initial screening tests and relevant populations are suggested in Table 23.4.

TABLE 23.4

SCREENING TESTS AND RELEVANT POPULATIONS

PATIENT POPULATION	SCREENING TESTS
All patients	Urinalysis Chemistry panel (electrolytes BUN, creatinine) Lipid profile, fasting or nonfasting (total cholesterol, HDL) Renal ultrasonography in those <6 yr of age or those with abnormal urinalysis or renal function
Obese (BMI >95th percentile) child or adolescent	Hemoglobin A1c AST and ALT (screen for fatty liver) Fasting lipid panel (dyslipidemia)
Optional tests to be obtained on the basis of history, physical examination, and initial studies	Fasting glucose for those at high risk for diabetes mellitus Thyroid-stimulating hormone Drug screen Sleep study (if found snoring, daytime sleepiness, or reported history of apnea) CBC (those with growth delay or abnormal renal function)

AST, *aspartate transaminase (formerly serum glutamic-oxaloacetic transaminase [SGOT]);* ALT, *alanine transaminase (formerly serum glutamic-pyruvic transaminase [SGPT]);* BMI, *body mass index;* BUN, *blood urea nitrogen;* CBC, *complete blood cell count;* HDL, *high-density lipoprotein.*

From Flynn, J. T., Kaelber, D. C., Barker-Smith, C. M., et al. (2018). Clinical practice guideline for screening and management of high blood pressure in children and adolescents. *Pediatrics, 140*(3), e20171904.

a. Urinalysis: Abnormal urinalysis suggests nephritis or infectious processes. Urinalysis is normal in essential HTN, renovascular HTN, and endocrine HTN.
b. Serum electrolytes: Low potassium levels suggest aldosterone excess. Hypokalemia may be seen in Cushing syndrome or certain (not all) types of congenital adrenal hyperplasias. Hypercalcemia suggests hyperparathyroidism.
c. Blood urea nitrogen (BUN) and creatinine: Abnormal values suggest renal parenchymal or renovascular disease.
d. Uric acid level: Uric acid level above 5.5 mg/dL was found in 89% of subjects with primary HTN, 30% of children with secondary HTN, and 0% of children with white coat HTN and normal control participants.

2. Renal ultrasonography is indicated in children younger than 6 years and those with abnormal urinalysis or renal function test. Renal ultrasonography adds very little in obese children.

   When obesity is the likely cause of HTN, metabolic aspects of risk factors should be evaluated (including fasting lipid profile, liver function test, blood glucose, etc).

3. Thyroid function test (TSH, T_4) may be indicated when rapid heart rate and HTN coexist.

D. SPECIALIZED STUDIES

Depending on the results of the initial laboratory tests, more specialized tests have been used in the diagnosis of secondary HTN. When COA is suspected, echocardiographic diagnosis and follow-up is indicated. When renovascular or renoparenchymal HTN is a possibility, nephrology consultation is indicated because most of the specialized tests belong to the domain of nephrology. Consultation with endocrinology should be obtained when endocrine disorders are suspected to be the cause of HTN.

1. Echocardiography

   Echocardiogram is not only a diagnostic tool for COA, but it also measures and follows LV target organ injury.

   a. The following three measurements (LV mass, LV wall thickness, and LV ejection fraction) are checked to assess LV target organ injury:
   b. Repeat echo study is done to monitor improvement or progression of target organ damage at 6 to 12 months intervals
2. Images for renovascular disease
   a. *Doppler renal ultrasonography* may be used in evaluation of possible renal artery stenosis in normal-weight children and adolescent.
   b. In addition, computed tomographic angiography or magnetic resonance angiography may be used to investigate renal artery stenosis.
3. Specialized chemistries
   a. Peripheral plasma rennin activity (PRA): An elevated value suggests renal parenchymal or renovascular diseases. A suppressed value suggests excess mineralocorticoid effects such as seen with hyperaldosteronism.
   b. PRA in blood collected from both renal veins and the inferior vena cava, at the time of angiography, is helpful in diagnosing unilateral or bilateral kidney disease.
   c. Aldosterone levels in serum and urine is indicated in patients with hypokalemia for possible hyperaldosteronism.
   d. Twenty-four-hour urine collection for catecholamine levels and their metabolites (metanephrine, normetanephrine, and vanillylmadelic acid [VMA]) is indicated when a catecholamine-secreting tumor (such as pheochromocytoma, neuroblastoma) is suspected.
   e. Twenty-four-hour urine collection for free cortisol and 17-ketosteroid. The former is elevated in Cushing syndrome and the latter is elevated in congenital adrenal hyperplasia (adrenogenital syndrome).

VI. MANAGEMENT OF ESSENTIAL HYPERTENSION

A. NONPHARMACOLOGIC INTERVENTION

When the diagnosis of HTN is established, nonpharmacologic intervention should be started as an initial treatment, as outlined in the following.

1. Counseling on weight reduction, if indicated
2. Low-salt (and potassium-rich) foods
3. Regular aerobic exercise and
4. Avoidance of smoking and oral contraceptives.

B. PHARMACOLOGIC INTERVENTION

1. **Indications for drug therapy**. There are no clear guidelines for identifying those who should be treated with antihypertensive drugs. However, based on the recent AAP guidelines (Flynn et al., 2017) and other recommendations, the following are generally considered indications for initiating antihypertensive drug therapy in children.
   a. Severe symptomatic HTN should be treated with intravenous (IV) antihypertensive medications initially).
   b. Persistent HTN despite a trial of lifestyle modification.
   c. Symptomatic HTN.
   d. Stage 2 HTN without clearly modifiable factor (e.g., obesity).
   e. Any stage of HTN associated with renovascular and renoparenchymal disease or diabetes.
   f. Hypertensive target-organ damage: LV hypertrophy or increased LV mass may be used (normal 2-dimensional echocardiograph-drived M-mode measurements of the LV dimensions and wall thickness based on body surface area are available in table D.1, Appendix D).
   g. Family history of early complications of HTN,
   h. Child who has dyslipidemia and other coronary artery risk factors.
2. **The choice of drug**. Recent studies in adults suggest that β-blockers are not as effective as other classes of antihypertensive agents. Currently, many adult cardiologists, especially those from European countries, strongly favor using angiotensin-converting enzyme (ACE) inhibitors, angiotensin receptor blockers (ARBs), or calcium channel blockers (CCBs) as the drugs of choice for initial therapy.

   Most pediatric cardiologists now recommend ACE inhibitors (or ARBs), CCBs, and possibly thiazide diuretics, as the initial drug for treatment of HTN in children and adolescents. β-Blockers are not recommended as initial treatment in children.
   a. Diuretics and β-blockers are known to raise blood glucose levels. Thus CCBs and ACE inhibitors appear preferable to β-blockers and diuretics, especially for overweight patients at risk of developing diabetes.
   b. ACE inhibitors and ARBs are good choices in patients with diabetes or renal disease because they are especially renoprotective.

c. African American children do not show as robust a response to ACE inhibitors, and thus CCBs appear to be better choice for them.
d. For adolescent males:
    (1) ACE inhibitors (or ARBs) and CCBs, alone or in combination, are equally good, especially in obese children with high glucose and triglyceride levels.
    (2) ACE inhibitors + diuretics is a good combination because diuretics enhance the effects of ACE inhibitors. However, this combination is not recommended in obese patients with acanthosis nigricans because it could cause diabetes.
e. For adolescent females or childbearing-age women.
    (1) CCBs (such as amlodipine [Norvasc] or extended release nifedipine) are good choices in females because they lack teratogenic effects.
    (2) ACE inhibitors or ARBs should not be used in female adolescents because they are known teratogens.
    (3) Diuretics or β-blockers are probably safe. However, blood glucose levels should be checked regularly because they raise glucose levels.
f. Coexisting conditions. The choice of initial therapy is influenced by other conditions that frequently coexist with HTN. Preferences, contraindications, and side effects of different classes of antihypertensive agents are summarized in Table 23.5, based on the information derived from adult experiences.
    (1) Migraine patients: β-blockers or CCBs are preferred. β-blockers appear to be more effective than CCBs in prevention of migraines.
    (2) Asthma: CCBs may be the drugs of first choice. ARBs and diuretics may work well. ACE inhibitors may cause persistent dry cough in 10% of 20% of patients with asthma and this may possibly cause bronchospasm. Nonselective β-blockers are contraindicated in patients with asthma because they may cause bronchospasm.
    (3) Hyperthyroidism or hyperdynamic HTN with fast heart rates: β-blockers are preferred.
    (4) Diabetic patients: ACE inhibitors or ARBs are preferred. Thiazide diuretics or β-blockers should not be used because they increase blood glucose levels.
    (5) Renal failure: CCBs or ACE inhibitors are preferred.

C. FOLLOW-UP

1. Once the most appropriate agent for initial therapy has been selected, a relatively small dose of a single drug should be started, aiming for BP reduction of 5 to 10 mm Hg at each step of the dosage, until the full dosage or the target BP is reached (see following).

TABLE 23.5

CLASSES OF ANTIHYPERTENSIVE AGENTS: PREFERENCES, CONTRAINDICATIONS, AND SIDE EFFECTS

DRUG CLASSES	PREFERRED	CONTRAINDICATED (NOT TO USE IN)	ADVERSE EFFECTS
Thiazide diuretics	Asthma (±)	*Not to use in:* Diabetic or prediabetic (It increases glucose level.)	Hypokalemia, hyponatremia (±) May increase glucose May increase uric acid
β-blockers	Migraine Hyperthyroidism Hyperdynamic hypertension Coarctation of the aorta	*Contraindicated in:* Asthma and diabetes *Not to use in:* Prediabetic patients	Increases glucose Increases triglycerides Rarely hypoglycemia
ACE inhibitors	Male adolescents Diabetic or prediabetic Obese males (may be used in combination with CCB Lotrel) Renal failure	*Contraindicated in:* Pregnancy (due to teratogenic effects) *Not to use in:* Childbearing-aged females Patients with asthma (can cause cough)	Hyperkalemia Azotemia Angioedema Dry cough Rash, loss of taste, and leukopenia
Angiotensin receptor blockers	Male adolescents Diabetic or prediabetic Renal failure	*Contraindicated in:* Pregnancy (due to teratogenic effects) *Not to use in:* Childbearing-aged females	Angioedema rarely (but no cough)
Calcium channel blockers (CCBs)	Female adolescents Male adolescents African Americans Migraine Asthma Renal failure	*Contraindicated in:* Heart block	Occasional headache, flushing, ankle edema

ACE, *angiotensin-converting enzyme.*

2. If the first drug is not effective, a second drug may be added to, or substituted for, the first drug.
3. In many situations, however, more than one drug is needed to control severely elevated BPs like those seen in patients with renal disease, and thus starting with a combination of two drugs from classes with complementary mechanisms of action may be acceptable.
4. Single daily dose of a long-acting agent improves adherence to the medication. Long-acting preparations are available within each class of antihypertensive drug. Table 23.6 shows the dosage of antihypertensive drugs for children.

TABLE 23.6

ORAL DOSAGES OF SELECTED ANTIHYPERTENSIVE DRUGS FOR CHILDREN

DRUGS	INITIAL DOSE	TIMES/DAY
Angiotensin-Converting Enzyme Inhibitors		
Captopril (Capoten)	0.3-0.5 mg/kg/dose (max. 6 mg/kg/day)	3
Enalapril (Vasotec)	0.08 mg/kg/day up to 5 mg/day (max.. 0.6 mg/kg/day up to 40 mg/day) Adult: 2.5-5 mg (max. 40 mg daily)	1-2
Lisinopril (Zestril, Prinivil)	0.07 mg/kg/day up to 5 mg/day (max. 0.6 mg/kg/day up to 40 mg/day) Adult: 10 mg (max. 80 mg daily)	1
Angiotensin-Receptor Blocker		
Losartan (Cozaar)	0.7 mg/kg/day up to 50 mg/day (max. 1.4 mg/kg/day up to 100 mg/day) Adult: 50 mg (max. 100 mg daily)	1
Calcium Channel Blockers		
Amlodipine (Norvasc)	6-17 yr: 2.5-5 mg/day Adult: 5-10 mg (max. 10 mg/24 hr)	1
Isradipine (DynaCirc)	0.15-0.2 mg/kg/day (max. 0.8 mg/kg/day up to 20 mg/day)	3-4
Diuretics		
Hydrochlorothiazide (Hydrodiuril)	1 mg/kg/day (max. 3 mg/kg/day up to 50 mg/day) Adult: 25-100 mg	1
Chlorthalidone	0.3 mg/kg/day (max. 2 mg/kg/day up to 50 mg/day) Adult: 12.5-25 mg	1
Furosemide (Lasix)	0.5-2 mg/kg/dose (max. 6 mg/kg/day)	1-2
Spironolactone (Aldactone)	1 mg/kg/day (max. 3.3 mg/kg/day up to 100 mg/day)	1-2
Triamtrene (Dyrenium)	1-2 mg/kg/day (max. 3-4 mg/kg/day up to 300 mg/day)	2
Adrenergic Inhibitors		
Propranolol (Inderal)	1-2 mg/kg/day (max. 4 mg/kg/day up to 640 mg/day)	2-3
Metoprolol (Lopressor)	1-2 mg/kg/day (Max. 6 mg/kg/day up to 200 mg/day)	2

TABLE 23.6 *(continued)*

ORAL DOSAGES OF SELECTED ANTIHYPERTENSIVE DRUGS FOR CHILDREN

DRUGS	INITIAL DOSE	TIMES/DAY
Atenolol (Tenormin)	0.5-1 mg/kg/day (max. 2 mg/kg/day up to 100 mg/day)	1-2
Vasodilators, Direct Acting		
Hydralazine (Apresoline)	0.75 mg/kg/day (max. 7.5 mg/kg/day up to 200 mg/day)	4
Minoxidil (Loniten)	>12 yr: 5 mg/day (max. 100 mg/day)	1-3

max., *maximum.*

Modified from National High Blood Pressure Education Program Working Group on High Blood Pressure in Children and Adolescents. (2004). The fourth report on the diagnosis, evaluation, and treatment of high blood pressure in children and adolescents. *Pediatrics, 114*(2 Suppl 4th Report), 555-576.

5. The goal of the treatment.
   a. For children with uncomplicated primary HTN without hypertensive end-organ damage, the goal of the treatment is reduction of BP to <95th percentile.
   b. For children with chronic renal disease, diabetes, or hypertensive target organ damage, the goal is reduction of BP to <90th percentile.
6. A *"step-down" therapy* or cessation of therapy may be considered in selected patients who had uncomplicated primary HTN that is well under control, especially overweight children who successfully lose weight. Such patients require ongoing follow-up of their BP levels and their weight status.
7. Follow-up examinations should include ongoing monitoring of BP levels, target organ damage, periodic serum electrolyte determination in children treated with ACE inhibitors or diuretics, counseling regarding other CV risk factors, and adherence to newly adopted healthy lifestyle.

VII. TREATMENT OF SECONDARY HYPERTENSION

Treatment of secondary HTN should be aimed at removing the cause of HTN whenever possible.

1. Coarctation. Surgical or catheter interventional correction is indicated for coarctation of the aorta.
2. Renal parenchymal disease. The same therapy as discussed for essential HTN is given. Salt restriction and antihypertensive drug therapy can control HTN caused by most renal parenchymal diseases. If HTN is difficult to control and the disease is unilateral, unilateral nephrectomy may be considered.

3. Renovascular disease may be treated by interventional catheterization (balloon or stent angioplasty) or successful surgery, such as reconstruction of a stenotic renal artery or autotransplantation.
4. HTNs caused by tumors that secrete vasoactive substances, such as pheochromocytoma, neuroblastoma, and juxtaglomerular cell tumor, are treated primarily by surgery.

Chapter 24

Pulmonary Hypertension

I. DEFINITION

Thirty 30 mm Hg has been used as the normal upper limit for systolic PA pressure and 25 mm Hg as the normal upper limit for mean PA pressure when measured directly by cardiac catheterization in adults and children older than 3 months of age at sea level. Thus a diagnosis of pulmonary hypertension (PH) was made when mean PA pressure was $\geq$25 mm Hg.

However, at the 2018 Sixth World Symposium on PH, consensus was reached to define PH in adults when mean PA pressure is $\geq$20 mm Hg and to include pulmonary vascular resistance of $\geq$3 Woods units to identify precapillary PH. The pediatric task force chose to follow the same recommendations. Of note is that the PA pressure is higher at high elevations. There is a wide range of severity in PH; in some, it reaches or surpasses the systemic pressure.

II. CAUSES

PH is a group of conditions with multiple causes rather than a single one. Pathogenesis and management differ among entities. Box 24.1 shows five groups of conditions that cause PH according to the pathogenesis and examples of the diseases belonging to each group.

III. PATHOPHYSIOLOGY

1. The endothelial cells and lung tissues normally synthesize and/or activate some vasoactive hormones and inactivate others. Three endothelium signaling cascades are known: (a) nitric oxide–cyclic guanosine monophosphate (cGMP) cascade, (b) prostanoids, and (c) endothelin-1 (ET-1). Balance among the vasoactive substances maintains vascular tone in normal and pathologic situations.
   a. Normally, balanced release of nitric oxide (NO, a vasodilator) and ET-1, a potent vasoconstrictor, by endothelial cells is a key factor in the regulation of the pulmonary vascular tone.
   b. Prostanoids: Arachidonic acid metabolism within vascular endothelial cells results in the production of prostaglandin I_2 (PGI_2 or prostacyclin) and thromboxane (TXA_2). PGI_2 is a vasodilator and TXA_2 is a vasoconstrictor.
2. Reduced alveolar oxygen tension (*alveolar hypoxia*) induces vasoconstriction (by reducing NO production and increasing endothelin production).
   a. Acidosis significantly increases PVR, acting synergistically with hypoxia.

BOX 24.1

CAUSES OF PULMONARY HYPERTENSION

1. Large L-R shunt lesions (hyperkinetic pulmonary hypertension): VSD, PDA, ECD
2. Alveolar hypoxia
   a. Pulmonary parenchymal disease
      i. Extensive pneumonia
      ii. Hypoplasia of lungs (primary or secondary, such as that seen in diaphragmatic hernia)
      iii. Bronchopulmonary dysplasia
      iv. Interstitial lung disease (Hamman-Rich syndrome)
      v. Wilson-Mikity syndrome
   b. Airway obstruction
      i. Upper airway obstruction (large tonsils, macroglossia, micrognathia, laryngotracheomalacia, sleep-disordered breathing)
      ii. Lower airway obstruction (bronchial asthma, cystic fibrosis)
   c. Inadequate ventilatory drive (central nervous system diseases, obesity hypoventilation syndrome)
   d. Disorders of chest wall or respiratory muscles
      i. Kyphoscoliosis
      ii. Weakening or paralysis of skeletal muscle
   e. High altitude (in certain hyperreactors)
3. Pulmonary venous hypertension: MS, cor triatriatum, TAPVR with obstruction, chronic left heart failure. Rarely, congenital pulmonary vein stenosis causes incurable pulmonary hypertension.
4. Primary pulmonary vascular disease
   a. Persistent pulmonary hypertension of the newborn
   b. Primary pulmonary hypertension—rare, fatal form of pulmonary hypertension with obscure cause
5. Other diseases that involve pulmonary parenchyma or pulmonary vasculature, directly or indirectly
   a. Thromboembolism: ventriculoatrial shunt for hydrocephalus, sickle cell anemia, thrombophlebitis
   b. Connective tissue disease: scleroderma, systemic lupus erythematosus, mixed connective tissue disease, dermatomyositis, rheumatoid arthritis
   c. Disorders directly affecting the pulmonary vasculature: schistosomiasis, sarcoidosis, histiocytosis X
   d. Portal hypertension (hepatopulmonary syndrome)
   e. HIV infection

   b. High altitude (with low alveolar oxygen tension) is associated with pulmonary vasoconstriction (and pulmonary hypertension), for which large species and individual variations exist.
3. Other agents or conditions that affect pulmonary vascular tones include the following.
   a. Angiotensin II, a vasoconstrictor, is activated from angiotensin I in the lungs by angiotensin-converting enzyme (ACE).
   b. Serotonin is a vasoconstrictor that promotes smooth muscle cell hypertrophy.

c. Stimulation of α- and β-adrenoceptors produces vasoconstriction and vasodilation, respectively.

4. Pressure (P) is related to both flow (F) and vascular resistance (R), as shown in the following formula:

$$P = F \times R$$

An increase in pulmonary blood flow, pulmonary vascular resistance, or both can result in PH. Regardless of its cause, PH eventually involves constriction of the pulmonary arterioles, resulting in an increase in PVR and hypertrophy of the RV.

5. The normally thin RV cannot sustain sudden increase in the PA pressure over 40 to 50 mm Hg and results in right-sided heart failure. Examples of this include infants who develop acute upper airway obstruction and adult patients who develop massive pulmonary thromboembolism.
6. However, if PH develops slowly, the RV hypertrophies and can tolerate mild PH (with a systolic pressure of about 50 mm Hg) without producing clinical problems. The RV pressure rises gradually with accompanying RV hypertrophy, and the PA pressure may eventually exceed the systemic pressure.

IV. PATHOGENESIS OF PULMONARY HYPERTENSION

Pathogenesis of PH is presented in the following text according to the (first four) general categories of causes, because they are distinctly different from each other.

A. HYPERKINETIC PULMONARY HYPERTENSION

1. PH associated with large L-R shunt lesions (e.g., VSD, PDA) is called *hyperkinetic PH*. It is the result of an increase in pulmonary blood flow, a direct transmission of the systemic pressure to the PA, and compensatory pulmonary vasoconstriction. Endothelial cell dysfunction with overproduction of ET-1 and reduced NO production result.
2. Hyperkinetic PH is usually reversible if the cause is eliminated before permanent changes occur in the pulmonary arterioles (see later section). If large L-R shunt lesions are left untreated, irreversible changes take place in the pulmonary vascular bed, with severe PH and cyanosis due to a reversal of the L-R shunt. This stage is called Eisenmenger syndrome or PVOD. Surgical correction is not possible at this stage.

B. ALVEOLAR HYPOXIA

1. An acute or chronic reduction in the oxygen tension (Po_2) in the alveolar capillary region (alveolar hypoxia) elicits a strong pulmonary

vasoconstrictor response, which may be augmented by acidosis. Although the exact mechanisms of the pulmonary vasoconstrictor response to alveolar hypoxia are not completely understood, ET-1 and NO are the strongest candidates responsible for the response.
2. Alveolar hypoxia may be an important basic mechanism of many forms of PH, including that seen in pulmonary parenchymal disease, airway obstruction, inadequate ventilatory drive (central nervous system diseases), disorders of chest wall or respiratory muscles, and high altitude.

C. PULMONARY VENOUS HYPERTENSION

1. Increased pressures in the pulmonary veins produce reflex vasoconstriction of the pulmonary arterioles and raise the PA pressure to maintain a high enough pressure gradient between the PA and the pulmonary vein. The mechanism for the vasoconstriction is not entirely clear, but a neuronal component may be present. Moreover, an elevated pulmonary venous pressure may also close small airways, resulting in alveolar hypoxia, which may contribute to the vasoconstriction. Mitral stenosis, TAPVR with obstruction (of pulmonary venous return to the LA), and chronic left-sided heart failure are examples of this entity.
2. PH with increased pulmonary venous pressure is usually reversible when the cause is eliminated.

D. PRIMARY PULMONARY HYPERTENSION

1. Primary pulmonary hypertension is characterized by progressive, irreversible vascular changes similar to those seen in Eisenmenger syndrome but without intracardiac lesions. The pathogenesis of primary PH is not fully understood, but endothelial dysfunction of the pulmonary vascular bed (with overproduction of ET-1) and enhanced platelet activities may be important factors. Overproduction of ET-1 is associated with not only vasoconstriction but also cell proliferation, inflammation, medial hypertrophy, and fibrosis.
2. This condition is rare in pediatric patients; it is a condition of adulthood and is more prevalent in women. It has a poor prognosis.

E. OTHER DISEASE STATES

PH associated with other disease states has similar pathogenesis to that described in the earlier four categories, singly or in combination.

V. PATHOLOGY

1. Heath and Edwards classified the changes into six grades.
   a. Grade 1: hypertrophy of the medial wall of the small muscular arteries
   b. Grade 2: hyperplasia of the intima

c. Grade 3: hyperplasia and fibrosis of the intima with narrowing of the vascular lumen
d. Grades 4 to 6: dilatation and plexiform lesions, angiomatous and cavernous lesions, hyalinization of intimal fibrosis, and necrotizing arteritis

2. Changes up to grade 3 are considered reversible if the cause is eliminated. Changes seen in grades 4 through 6 are considered irreversible and preclude surgical repair of CHDs.
3. The progressive vascular changes that occur in primary PH are identical to those that occur with CHDs.
4. With pulmonary venous hypertension, pulmonary arteries may show severe medial hypertrophy and intimal fibrosis. However, the changes are limited to grades 1 through 3 of Heath and Edwards' classification and they are often reversible when the cause is eliminated.

VI. CLINICAL MANIFESTATIONS

1. With significant PH, exertional dyspnea and fatigue may manifest. Some patients complain of headache. Syncope, presyncope, or chest pain also occurs on exertion.
2. On physical examination, cyanosis with or without clubbing may be present. The neck veins are distended, and a right ventricular lift or tap occurs on palpation. The S2 is loud and single. An ejection click and an early diastolic decrescendo murmur of PR are usually present along the MLSB. A holosystolic murmur of TR may be audible at the LLSB. Signs of right-sided heart failure (e.g., hepatomegaly, ankle edema) may be present.
3. The electrocardiogram (ECG) shows RAD and RVH with or without "strain." RAH is frequently seen. Arrhythmias occur in the late stage.
4. Chest radiographs show either normal or slightly enlarged heart. A prominent PA segment and dilated hilar vessels with clear lung fields are characteristic.
5. Echo studies usually demonstrate the following:
   a. Enlargement of the RA and RV, with normal or small LV dimensions.
   b. With an elevated RV pressure, the interventricular septum shifts toward the LV and appears flattened at the end of systole.
   c. PA pressure can be estimated by a Doppler study (see Chapter 4 for detailed discussion).
      (1) Using the peak TR velocity, the RV systolic pressure (P) can be estimated by the simplified Bernoulli equation ($\Delta P = 4V^2$) and adding estimated RA pressure. Using estimated RA pressure is often unreliable and error prone. Therefore, recently the European Society of Echocardiography guidelines (2015) suggested just using the TR_{max} without adding estimated RA pressure, and suggested the following probabilities of PH (Galie N et al., 2016):
         $TR_{max} \leq 2.8$ m/sec: Low probability of PH
         TR_{max} 2.9 to 3.4 m/sec: Intermediate probability of PH
         $TR_{max} > 3.4$ m/sec: High probability of PH

(2) With a shunt lesion, such as VSD or PDA, the peak systolic velocity across the shunt is used to estimate the RV pressure.
(3) The end-diastolic velocity of PR can be used to estimate the *diastolic* pressure in the PA.

6. Exercise testing: A symptom-limited exercise test, such as the 6-minute walk test, may be useful in children for following disease progression or measuring the response to medical interventions.
7. Natural history and prognosis
   a. PH secondary to the upper airway obstruction is usually reversible when the cause is eliminated.
   b. PH associated with large L-R shunt lesions or that associated with pulmonary venous hypertension improves or disappears after surgical removal of the cause, if performed early.
   c. Chronic pulmonary conditions that produce alveolar hypoxia have a relatively poor prognosis.
   d. Primary PH is progressive and has a fatal outcome, usually 2 to 3 years after the onset of symptoms.
   e. PH associated with Eisenmenger syndrome, collagen disease, and chronic thromboembolism is usually irreversible and has a poor prognosis but may be stable for two to three decades.
   f. Right-sided heart failure and cardiac arrhythmias occur in the late stage. Chest pain, hemoptysis, and syncope are ominous signs.

VII. DIAGNOSIS

1. Noninvasive tools (ECG, chest radiographs, and echo) are used to detect and estimate the severity of PH. Collectively, they are reasonably accurate in assessing severity.
2. Cardiac catheterization is performed to confirm the diagnosis and severity of PH and to determine whether the elevated PVR is due to active vasoconstriction ("responders") or to permanent changes in the pulmonary arterioles ("nonresponders"). Protocol for vasodilator testing varies from center to center.
   a. NO inhalation (20 ppm) with or without increased oxygen concentration for 10 minutes is commonly used. One may also use 100% oxygen, inhaled or intravenous (IV) prostacyclin, or IV adenosine.
   b. "Acute responders" should show (1) a decrease of at least 10 mm Hg in the mean PA pressure to $<$40 mm Hg (with a normal or increase in cardiac output) or (2) a decrease of $\geq$20% in the mean PA pressure or PVR with an unchanged or increased cardiac output.
3. Lung biopsies have been used in an attempt to evaluate the "operability" of patients with PH and CHD. Unfortunately, pulmonary vascular changes are not uniformly distributed and the biopsy findings correlated poorly with the natural history of the disease and operability.

Hemodynamic data appear to predict survival better than biopsy findings.

VIII. MANAGEMENT

A. TREATING UNDERLYING CAUSES

Measures to remove or treat the underlying cause should be the primary emphasis whenever possible.

1. Timely corrective surgery for CHDs (such as large-shunt VSD, ECD, or PDA).
2. Tonsillectomy and adenoidectomy when the cause of PH is the upper airway obstruction.
3. Treatment of underlying diseases, such as cystic fibrosis, asthma, pneumonia, or bronchopulmonary dysplasia.

B. GENERAL MEASURES

General measures are aimed at preventing further elevation of PA pressure or treating its complications.

1. The patient should avoid or limit strenuous exertion, isometric activities (weight lifting), and trips to high altitude.
2. Oxygen supplementation is provided as needed.
3. The patient should avoid vasoconstrictor drugs, including decongestants with α-adrenergic properties.
4. Patients should be strongly advised to avoid pregnancy. Pregnancy may increase the risk of pulmonary embolism from deep vein thrombosis or amniotic fluid, and may cause syncope and cardiac arrest.
5. Oral contraceptives should not be used because they worsen PH (surgical contraception is preferred).
6. CHF is treated with ACE inhibitors, digoxin, and diuretics and a low-salt diet.
7. Cardiac arrhythmias are treated with antiarrhythmic agents.
8. Partial erythropheresis is performed for polycythemia and headache.
9. Annual flu shots are recommended.

C. ANTICOAGULATION AND ANTIPLATELET AGENTS

1. Anticoagulation with warfarin (with the international normalized ratio of 2.0 to 2.5) is widely recommended in patients with thromboembolic disease. It may be beneficial in patients with PH from other causes.
2. Some recommend antiplatelet drugs (aspirin) instead of warfarin to prevent microembolism in the pulmonary circulation.

D. PHARMACOLOGIC TREATMENT OF CHRONIC PULMONARY HYPERTENSION

The pulmonary vasodilators are used in responders. For nonresponders, vasodilators have limited success. Vasodilators should not be used without testing first in the catheterization laboratory.

Drugs that are used to relieve pulmonary vasoconstriction can be divided into endothelial-based and smooth muscle-based drugs (Oishi et al., 2011).

- Endothelial-based drugs act on endothelial mechanisms and cause vasodilatation:
  - NO inhalation
  - Phosphodiesterase type 5 inhibitors (PDE5i) (sildenafil, tadalafil)
  - Prostacyclin analogues (epoprostenol, treprostinil, iloprost, beraprost)
  - Endothelin receptor antagonists (bosentan, sitaxsentan, ambrisentan)
- Smooth muscle–based drugs act directly on the smooth muscle.
  - Calcium channel blockers (nifedipine)

1. **For acute responders**. The following vasodilators are used in acute responders. Most of the experiences are based on adult trials. Some vasodilators may lower the systemic vascular resistance more than the PVR and thus are not suitable.
   a. **Calcium channel blockers (CCBs)**. For acute responders with primary PH treated with CCBs, survival was 97% and 81% at 1 and 10 years, respectively. Children who were not acute responders but were still treated with CCBs had survival rates of 45% and 29% at 1 and 4 years. Hypotension is a side effect of the medication. Nifedipine (at a dose of 0.2 mg/kg PO q8h) is one of the oldest drugs used with beneficial effects seen in 40% of children with primary PH. The dosages of other CCBs are diltiazem (3 to 5 mg/kg/day) and amlopidine (2.5 to 10 mg/day). Diltiazem lowers heart rate and therefore is used more frequently in younger children with higher heart rate. Verapamil is contraindicated because of its negative inotropic effects.
   b. **Prostacyclins**. Continuous IV infusion of epoprostenol (PGI_2) has been shown to improve quality of life and survival in patients with primary PH, Eisenmenger syndrome, or chronic lung disease. The starting dose of epoprostenol was 2 ng/kg/min, with increments of 1 to 2 ng/kg/min every 15 min, until desired effects appeared; the average final dose was 9 to 11 ng/kg/min. Prostacyclins are administered by an ambulatory IV system because of a very short half-life (1 to 2 minutes).
   c. Endothelin receptor antagonists, **bosentan** and **sitaxsenton**, have been used in both primary PH and Eisenmenger syndrome. Side effects of ET antagonists include elevation of hepatic aminotransferase levels, teratogenicity, anemia, and peripheral edema, decreased effectiveness of oral contraceptive agents, and effects on male fertility.
      (1) In children with primary pulmonary hypertension or Eisenmenger syndrome, oral bosentan, a nonselective endothelin receptor blocker, in the dose of 31.25 mg BID for children <20 kg, 62.5 mg BID for children 20 to 40 kg, and 125 mg BID for children >40 kg (with or without concomitant IV prostacyclin therapy) for median duration of 14 months, resulted in a significant functional improvement in about 50% of the cases.

(2) Sitaxsentan, a selective endothelin-A (ET_A) receptor antagonist, given orally once daily at a dose of 100 mg (for mostly adult patients and children older than 12 years), resulted in improved exercise capacity after 18 weeks of treatment.

d. Sildenafil, a phosphodiesterase inhibitor, prevents the breakdown of cGMP resulting in pulmonary vasodilatation. Oral dose of 0.25 to 1 mg/kg, four times daily for 12 months' duration, has resulted in improvement in hemodynamics and exercise capacity. Adverse effects include headache, flushing, exacerbation of nosebleed, and rare systemic hypotension or erection.

e. NO inhalation is effective in lowering PA pressure in adult respiratory distress syndrome, primary PH, and persistent PH of the newborn. NO can be administered only by inhalation because it is inactivated by hemoglobin. Rebound PH is problematic.

2. **For nonresponders**. The following measures can be used in nonresponders.
   a. NO inhalation and continuous IV or possibly nebulized prostacyclin (PGI_2) may provide selective pulmonary vasodilatation.
   b. Atrial septectomy (either by catheter or surgery) improves survival rates and abolishes syncope by providing a R-L atrial shunt, thereby helping to maintain cardiac output but with increased hypoxemia.
   c. Potts shunt placed between the LPA and descending aorta providing R-L shunting has shown improvement in functional status and midterm transplant free survival of patients with suprasystemic PH (Aggarwal, 2018).
   d. Lung or heart-lung transplantation remains the only available treatment for patients unresponsive to vasodilator treatment. Bilateral lung transplantation is preferred at most centers, but some centers prefer single lung transplantation.

Chapter 25

Athletes With Cardiac Problems

Almost all states in the United States require some type of preparticipation screening of participants in organized sports. The major reason for this screening is to help prevent sudden unexpected death. Most physicians encounter this issue in association with high school and college sports, and therefore physicians should have a general understanding of the eligibility guidelines and the participation eligibility for patients with specific CV conditions. Athletic competitions substantially increase the sympathetic drive. The resulting increase in catecholamine levels increases blood pressure (BP), heart rate (HR), and myocardial contractility and increases oxygen demand. The increase in sympathetic tone can cause arrhythmias and may aggravate existing myocardial ischemia.

The recommendations presented are mostly from American Heart Association (AHA) and American College of Cardiology (ACC) Scientific Statement (2015) and some are from the 36th Bethesda conference (2005). The following areas are presented.

1. Causes of sudden unexpected death
2. AHA/ACC) 14-element screening procedure (of 2014)
3. Classification of sports according to the type and intensity to help physicians select allowable types of sports
4. Overview of participation eligibility for athletes with different types of CV problems
5. Guidelines for athletes with hypertension

I. SUDDEN CARDIAC DEATH IN YOUNG ATHLETES

A. STATISTICS OF SUDDEN UNEXPECTED DEATH

1. Sudden cardiac death (SCD) occurs in about 1 per 200,000 high school sports participants per academic year. It is far more common in boys than in girls. In the United States, football and basketball are the sports most frequently associated with SCD.
2. The two most important groups of heart disease that cause SCD are hypertrophic cardiomyopathy (HCM) and coronary artery anomalies or diseases, accounting for nearly 70% of the cases (see Table 25.1).

B. COMMON CAUSES OF SCD

1. HCM (up to 36%) and its variant (8%) account for nearly half of the unexpected SCD cases (see Table 25.1).
2. Anomalies of the coronary arteries, both congenital and acquired (atherosclerotic or the result of Kawasaki disease), is the next important group of causes of SCD, accounting for 23%.

TABLE 25.1

CARDIOVASCULAR CAUSES OF SUDDEN DEATH IN YOUNG ATHLETES (N = 690)[a]

CAUSE	PERCENT
Hypertrophic cardiomyopathy	36
Coronary artery anomalies, congenital and acquired	23
Possible hypertrophic cardiomyopathy	8
Myocarditis	6
Arrhythmogenic right ventricular cardiomyopathy	4
Ion channel disease	4
Mitral valve prolapse	3
Aortic rupture	3
Aortic stenosis	2
Dilated cardiomyopathy	2
Wolff-Parkinson-White syndrome	2
Others	5

[a]Original data from Maron, B. J., Doerer, J. J., Haas, T. S., Tierney, D. M., & Mueller, F. E. (2009). Sudden deaths in young competitive athletes: analysis of 1866 deaths in the United States, 1980-2006. *Circulation, 119*(8), 1085-1092. Modified from Balady, G. J., & Ades PA. (2012). Exercise and sports cardiology. In O. Bonow, D. Mann, D. Zipes, & P. Libby (Eds.) *Braunwald's heart disease: A textbook of cardiovascular medicine* (9th ed.). Philadelphia: Saunders.

3. Myocarditis and dilated cardiomyopathy are found in up to 8% of SCDs.
4. Cardiac arrhythmias (caused by long QT syndrome, WPW syndrome, sinus node dysfunction, arrhythmogenic right ventricular dysplasia [ARVD]) account for 10% of SCD.
5. Other rare causes of SCD in athletes include severe AS or PS, Marfan syndrome (from ruptured aortic aneurysm), MVP, dilated cardiomyopathy, primary pulmonary hypertension, "commotio cordis," sarcoidosis, and sickle cell trait.

C. PREPARTICIPATION SCREENING

The most important reason for the screening is to detect "silent" CVD that can cause SCD. Detailed prospective CV screening of a large athletic population is impractical, because there are 8 to 10 million competitive athletes in the United States. Even with the use of specialized cardiologic tools, complete prevention of SCD is nearly impossible. Thus, medical clearance for sports does not necessarily imply the absence of CVD or complete protection from sudden death.

1. Recommended screening
   a. Recommended screening for U.S. high school and college athletes is confined to history taking and physical examination, which is known to be limited in its power to consistently identify important CV abnormalities. In 2014, the AHA and ACC recommended using a

BOX 25.1

THE 14-ELEMENT AHA RECOMMENDATIONS FOR PREPARTICIPATION CARDIOVASCULAR SCREENING OF COMPETITIVE ATHLETES

MEDICAL HISTORY[a]

Personal History

1. Chest pain/discomfort/tightness/pressure to exertion
2. Unexplained syncope/near syncope[b]
3. Excessive and unexplained dyspnea/fatigue or palpitations, associated with exercise
4. Prior recognition of heart murmur
5. Elevated systemic blood pressure
6. Prior restriction from participation in sports
7. Prior testing for the heart, ordered by a physician

Family History

8. Premature death (sudden and unexpected, or otherwise) before 50 years of age attributable to heart disease in ≥ 1 relative
9. Disability from heart disease in close relative <50 years of age
10. Hypertrophic or dilated cardiomyopathy, long-QT syndrome, or other ion channelopathies, Marfan syndrome, or clinically significant arrhythmias, specific knowledge of genetic cardiac conditions in family members.

Physical Examination

11. Heart murmur[c]
12. Femoral pulse to exclude aortic coarctation
13. Physical stigmata of Marfan syndrome
14. Brachial artery blood pressure (sitting position)[d]

[a] Parental verification is recommended for high school and middle school athletes.
[b] Judged not to be of neurocardiogenic (vasovagal) origin, of particular concern when occurring during or after physical exertion.
[c] Refers to heart murmurs judged likely to be organic and unlikely to be innocent; auscultation should be performed with the patient in both the supine and standing positions (or with Valsalva maneuver), specifically to identify murmurs of dynamic left ventricular outflow tract obstruction.
[d] Preferably taken in both arms.

Modified by American Heart Association with permission from Maron, B. J., Friedman, R. A., Kligfield, P., et al. (2014). Assessment of the 12-lead ECG as a screening test for detection of cardiovascular disease in healthy general populations of young people (12-25 years of age): a scientific statement from the American Heart Association and the American Collee of Cardiology. *Circulation, 64*(14):1479-514.

14-element screening procedure (formerly a 12-point screening) as shown in Box 25.1. Ten of the 14 points are related to the history and the remaining 4 to physical examination.

b. Although the European Society of Cardiology has recommended an electrocardiogram (ECG) with each evaluation, the AHA/ACC does not recommend it. The ECG may detect most cases of HCM, but the cost of obtaining ECGs versus the yield is prohibitive, and the cost of evaluating false-positive results is too great to make this practice cost-effective. The ECG is used only for those patients in whom a potentially lethal CVD is suspected based on the 14-element screening.

2. Screening tools
   a. History and physical examination. Although simple history and physical examination can raise suspicion of CVD in some at-risk athletes, they do not have sufficient power to guarantee detection of many critical CV abnormalities. However, the AHA's screening method has the capability of raising the clinical suspicion of several CV abnormalities.

      Personal history

      (1) History of chest pain, discomfort, tightness, or pressure to exertion.
      (2) Unexplained syncope or near syncope, except for vasovagal syncope.
      (3) Excessive and unexplained dyspnea or fatigue or palpitation, associated with exercise.
      (4) Prior recognition of heart murmur.
      (5) Elevated systemic blood pressure.
      (6) Prior restriction from participation in sports.
      (7) Prior testing for the heart, ordered by a physician.

      Family history

      (8) Premature death (sudden and unexpected, or otherwise) before 50 years of age attributable to heart disease in one or more relative.
      (9) Disability from heart disease in close relative younger than 50 years.
      (10) Hypertrophic or dilated cardiomyopathy, long QT syndrome, or other ion channelopathies, Marfan syndrome, or clinically significant arrhythmias, specific knowledge of genetic cardiac conditions in family members.

      Physical examination

      (11) Heart murmur (likely to be organic, not likely to be innocent).
      (12) Femoral pulse to exclude aortic coarctation.
      (13) Physical stigmata of Marfan syndrome.
      (14) Brachial artery BP (sitting position).

   If CV abnormalities are suspected by the AHA's screening procedure, a physician should request specialty consultation or order additional testing. The athlete should be temporarily withdrawn from activities until the issue can be resolved. The utility of ECG and an echocardiographic study are briefly outlined in the following text, although they are not routinely recommended by the AHA.

3. Electrocardiography

   The 12-lead ECG is indicated in patients suspicious of serious CVD raised by the 14-element AHA screening history and physical examination. The ECG is a practical and cost-effective alternative to routine echocardiography. Table 25.2 lists examples of normal and abnormal findings in the ECG screen.

TABLE 25.2

NORMAL AND ABNORMAL FINDINGS IN ECG SCREENING IN ATHLETES

NORMAL ECG FINDINGS	ABNORMAL ECG FINDINGS

• Sinus bradycardia (HR >30 beats/min)
• Ectopic atrial rhythm
• Junctional escape
• First-degree AV block
• Mobitz type I second-degree AV block (Wenckebach)
• Isolated incomplete RBBB
• Early repolarization
• Isolated voltage criteria for LVH in the absence of:
  • Left-axis deviation
  • LAH
  • ST depression
  • T-wave inversion
  • Pathologic Q waves
	• T-wave inversion (in two or more leads V1-V6, II, aVF, or I and aVL)
	• ST depression (≥0.5 mm in 2 or more leads)
	• Pathologic Q waves (>3 mm in depth or >4 msec in duration in 2 or more leads except III and aVR)
	• Left bundle branch block
	• Left-axis deviation (−30° to −90°)
	• LAH
	• RVH
	• LVH voltage criteria in association with:
	  • LAH (or enlargement)
	  • ST depression
	  • T-wave inversion
	• Ventricular preexcitation
	• Sinus bradycardia (HR <30 beats/min)
	• Supraventricular tachycardia
	• Brugada-like ECG pattern
	• Frequent PVC's (≥ two PVCs per 10-second tracing or non-sustained ventricular tachycardia)

AV, *atrioventricular;* ECG, *electrocardiogram;* HR, *heart rate;* LAH, *left atrial hypertrophy (or enlargement);* LVH, *left ventricular hypertrophy;* PVC, *premature ventricular contraction;* RAH, *right atrial hypertrophy;* RBBB, *right bundle branch block;* RVH, *right ventricular hypertrophy.*

Modified from Lisman KA. (2016). Electrocardiographic Evaluation in athletes and use of the Seattle Criteria to improve specificity. *Methodist Debakey Cardiovascular Journal, 2*(2), 81-85.

a. The ECG is abnormal in 75% to 95% of patients with HCM. Abnormalities may include LVH, ST-T changes, and abnormally deep Q waves (owing to septal hypertrophy) with diminished or absent R waves in V5 and V6. Occasionally, "giant" negative T waves are seen in V5 and V6. Cardiac arrhythmias and first-degree AV block may be seen occasionally.
b. Coronary artery abnormalities may show ST-T wave abnormalities or abnormal Q waves.
c. Long QT syndrome (QTc >0.46 sec), Brugada syndrome (RBBB with ST-segment elevation), and other inherited syndromes can be identified by the ECG.
d. The ECG may also raise suspicion of myocarditis (PVCs, ST-T changes) or arrhythmogenic RV cardiomyopathy (by T-wave inversion in leads V1 through V3, tall P waves, decreased RV potentials).
e. However, abnormal ECG findings are seen in about 40% of trained athletes, and this may be the source of confusion. ECG abnormalities seen in trained athletes include (1) increased R- or S-wave voltages, (2) Q-wave and repolarization abnormalities, and (3)

frequent or complex ventricular tachyarrhythmias on Holter ECG monitors.

f. On the other hand, normal ECG does not necessarily rule out significant cardiac abnormalities.

4. Echocardiography. Echocardiographic study is the principal diagnostic imaging modality for clinical identification of HCM and other cardiac abnormalities.
   a. In adults, HCM is diagnosed when diastolic LV wall thickness ≥15 mm (or on occasion, 13 or 14 mm), usually with LV dimension <45 mm, is present. For children, a *z* score of 2 or more relative to body surface area is theoretically compatible with the diagnosis.
   b. Some highly trained athletes may show LVH, making the differentiation between the physiologic hypertrophy and HCM difficult. An LV wall thickness ≥13 mm is very uncommon in highly trained athletes and it is always associated with an enlarged LV cavity (with LV diastolic dimension >54 mm; ranges 55 to 63 mm). Therefore athletes with LV wall thickness >16 mm and a nondilated LV cavity are likely to have HCM.
   c. Echo will detect other CHDs (such as AS, PS), Marfan syndrome (aortic root dilatation, MVP), myocarditis, or dilated cardiomyopathy (LV dysfunction and/or enlargement).
   d. Definitive diagnosis of congenital coronary artery anomalies may not be accomplished by echo studies; it may require other tests such as computed tomography or coronary angiography.

II. CLASSIFICATION OF SPORTS

If CV or other abnormalities are found when evaluating an individual, the next step is to estimate how much physical exercise can be safely tolerated. Depending on the cardiac condition, the athlete may be able to safely engage in less-demanding athletic activities. This requires knowledge of the type of exercise the individual will be doing, how much static and dynamic exertion is required, and how vigorous the training program is.

For the purpose of making recommendations on athletes' participation eligibility, the AHA/ACC in 2015 jointly published the Scientific Statement on Classification of Sports (Fig. 25.1). Sports are divided into two broad types, dynamic and static, and each sport is categorized by the level of intensity (low, medium, high). Most sports activities are a combination of static and dynamic exercises. Sports can also be classified with regard to the danger of bodily injury from collision (*) as well as the consequences of syncope (†).

1. Dynamic (isotonic) exercise
   a. Dynamic exercise involves changes in muscle length and joint movement with rhythmic contractions that develops relatively small intramuscular force.
   b. Dynamic exercise causes a marked increase in oxygen consumption with a substantial increase in cardiac output, HR, and stroke volume

Increasing Static Component →	A. Low (<50%)	B. Moderate (50–75%)	C. High (>75%)
III. High (>30%)	Bobsledding/Luge Field events (throwing) Gymnastics*† Martial arts Rock climbing Sailing Water skiing*† Weight lifting*† Windsurfing*†	Body building*† Downhill skiing Skakeboarding*† Snow boarding*† Wrestling*	Boxing Canoeing Kayaking Cycling*† Decathlon Rowing Speed skating Triathlon*†
II. Moderate (10–20%)	Archery Auto racing*† Diving*† Equestrian*† Motorcycling*†	American football* Field events (jumping) Figure skating Rodeoing*† Rugby Running (spring) Surfing Synchronized swimming† "Ultra" racing	Basketball* Ice hockey* Cross-country skiing (skating technique) Lacrosse* Running (middle distance) Swimming Team handball Tennis
I. Low (<10%)	Bowling Cricket Curling Golf Riflery Yoga	Baseball/Softball Fencing Table tennis Volleyball	Badminton Cross-country skiing (skating technique) Field hockey* Orienteering Race walking Racquetball/Squash Running (long distance) Soccer*

Increasing Dynamic Component →

FIG. 25.1

Classification of sports. Sports in each category are listed in alphabetical order to make them easier to find. *Danger of bodily collision. †Increased risk if syncope occurs. *(Modified from Levine, B. D., Baggish, A. L., Kovacs RJ, et al. (2015). Eligibility and disqualification recommendations for competitive athletes with cardiovascular abnormalities: Task Force 1: classification of sports: dynamic, static, and impact. A scientific statement from the American Heart Association and American College of Cardiology.* Circulation, 132*(22):e262-e266.)*

and a decrease in SVR. Systolic pressure increases, but the diastolic pressure decreases slightly.

c. Thus dynamic exercise primarily causes a volume load on the left ventricle.

2. Static (isometric) exercise
   a. Static exercise involves development of relatively large intramuscular force with little or no change in muscle length or joint movement.
   b. Static exercise causes a marked increase in systolic, diastolic, and mean arterial pressures. It causes only a small increase in oxygen consumption, cardiac output, and HR (and no change in stroke volume).
   c. Thus static exercise causes a pressure load on the LV.

III. ELIGIBILITY DETERMINATION OF ATHLETES WITH CARDIOVASCULAR DISEASES

Most of the following recommendations are excerpts from the AHA/ACC Scientific Statement of 2015. These recommendations apply to athletes in high school and college. For further details on a specific condition, readers are advised to refer to the original articles.

A. ACYANOTIC CONGENITAL HEART DEFECTS

1. **L-R shunt lesions**. Participation eligibility of athletes with L-R shunt lesions is primarily determined by the level of mean pulmonary artery (PA) pressure and the status of left ventricular (LV) systolic function (see Van Hare et al. [2015] for details).
   a. Mean PA pressure:
      (1) Athletes with the mean PA pressure <25 mm Hg can participate in all competitive sports.
      (2) Athletes with the mean PA pressure ≥25 mm Hg, regardless the associated lesions, are restricted from all competitive sports, with the possible exception of low-intensity class IA sports.
   b. LV systolic function
      (1) Athletes with normal or near-normal LV systolic function (ejection fraction [EF] >50%) can participate in all sports.
      (2) Athletes with mildly diminished LV function (EF 40% to 50%) can participate in low- and medium-intensity static and dynamic sports (classes IA, IB and IIA and IIB).
      (3) Athletes with moderate to severely diminished LV function (EF <40%) should be restricted from all competitive sports, with the possible exception of low-intensity class IA sports.
2. **Obstructive lesions** (see Van Hare [2015] for details).
   a. For mild PS (Doppler gradient <30 mm Hg), mild AS (peak Doppler gradient <20 mm Hg), and mild COA (arm-to-leg systolic pressure gradient at rest <20 mm Hg), all competitive sports are allowed.
   b. With moderate PS (peak Doppler gradient 40-60 mm Hg) or moderate AS (Doppler gradient 40-70 mm Hg), classes IA, IB, and possibly IIA are allowed.
   c. Following correction of more severe abnormalities to mild abnormality, appropriate level of sports may be allowed 2 to 4 weeks after balloon procedures or 3 months after surgery.

B. CYANOTIC CONGENITAL HEART DEFECTS

In patients with arterial oxygen desaturation from cyanotic CHD, moderate to severe restriction in sports participation is recommended (see Van Hare GF [2015] for details).

1. Patients with cyanotic CHDs that are unoperated or for which palliative procedures have been done can participate only in low-intensity competitive sports, such as class IA.
2. Most patients with cyanotic CHDs for which surgical repair has been performed can participate only in low-intensity sports.

3. Patients who have received an excellent result from the surgical repair of TOF or arterial switch operation for TGA may participate in all competitive sports.

C. CORONARY ARTERY ABNORMALITIES (SEE GRAHAM ET AL. [2005] FOR DETAILS)

1. For most patients with congenital abnormalities of the coronary arteries or following Kawasaki disease, moderate to severe restriction in sports participation is recommended.
2. Those children who had no coronary artery involvement during the acute phase of Kawasaki disease may participate in all sports 6 to 8 weeks after the illness.
3. Patients with isolated small to medium-sized aneurysms in one or more coronary artery following Kawasaki disease may participate in IA, IB and IIB sports.

D. VALVULAR HEART DISEASES

The severity of the valvular lesion determines eligibility for participation in competitive sports (see Bonow et al. [2015] for details).

1. In patients with mild valvular lesions (such as MS, MR, AS, and AR), participation in all competitive sports is allowed.
2. In patients with moderate valvular lesions, participation is limited to low- to moderate-intensity sports.
3. In patients with severe obstructive lesions such as AS, participation in competitive sports is not permitted.
4. In patients with valvular lesions that produce significant pulmonary hypertension, no participation in competitive sports is permitted.
5. For those patients with prosthetic valves who are taking warfarin, no sports involving the risk of bodily contact are allowed.

E. CARDIOMYOPATHY, PERICARDITIS, AND OTHER MYOCARDIAL DISEASES (SEE GRAHAM ET AL [2005] FOR DETAILS)

1. Athletes who have either confirmed or probable diagnosis of HCM or arrhythmogenic RV dysplasia are excluded from most competitive sports, with the possible exception of class IA sports.
2. Athletes with myocarditis or pericarditis of any etiology should be excluded from all competitive sports during the acute phase. After complete recovery from these illnesses, they may gradually participate in sports.
3. Athletes with Marfan syndrome can participate only in class IA or IB sports
4. Athletes with MVP who have any symptoms or abnormalities in ECG, LV function, or arrhythmias are permitted to participate only in low-intensity sports.

F. CARDIAC ARRHYTHMIAS

The following are general statements regarding participation eligibility for athletes with cardiac arrhythmias who are asymptomatic and do not have underlying structural heart disease (see Zipes et al. [2015] for details).

1. The presence of a symptomatic cardiac arrhythmia requires exclusion from physical activity until this problem can be adequately evaluated and controlled by a cardiologist or an electrophysiologist.
2. Asymptomatic athletes with sinus bradycardia, sinus exit block, sinus pauses, and sinus arrhythmia can participate in all competitive sports.
3. Sinus arrhythmias and PACs are benign if the heart is structurally normal; athletes can participate in all competitive sports.
4. Asymptomatic athletes with atrial flutter or fibrillation and structurally normal heart may participate in competitive sports when the arrhythmias are fully under control either by medication or ablation.
5. Athletes with SVT and structurally normal heart may participate in all competitive sports when the SVT is in full control with medication or following successful ablation.
6. For athletes with a structurally normal heart who have PVCs or more complex arrhythmias, an exercise stress test (EST) is a useful technique. If the PVCs disappear when the HR reaches 140 to 150 beats/min, the PVCs are benign and full participation may be permitted.
7. Athletes with VT who had successful treatment to prevent recurrence of the arrhythmias may participate in sports, provided that VT is not inducible by an EST or EPS.
8. Asymptomatic adult athletes with WPW preexcitation with no history of SVT may participate in all competitive sports after risk stratification by EST, but children with the same diagnosis require more in-depth evaluation.
9. Athletes with long QT syndrome can participate only in class IA sports.
10. Athletes with catecholaminergic polymorphic ventricular tachycardia can participate only in class IA sports.
11. Athletes who had a successful ablation for any of the arrhythmias may participate in all competitive sports after verification of the success by appropriate tests.
12. Athletes with an implantable cardioverter defibrillator may participate in class IA sports if they are free of ventricular flutter or ventricular fibrillation requiring device therapy for 3 months. Participation in sports with a higher component than class IA may be considered if the athlete is free of ventricular flutter or fibrillation requiring device therapy for 3 months.

G. AV BLOCK AND INTRAVENTRICULAR BLOCKS

Athletes with AV block or intraventricular blocks need to be fully investigated and treated before eligibility for participation in sport activities can be decided. Some of them may require pacemaker implantation (see Zipes et al. [2015] for details).

1. Asymptomatic athletes with first-degree AV block and structurally normal heart can participate in all competitive sports.
2. Asymptomatic patients with Wenckebach AV block (Mobitz type 1 second-degree AV block) with improvement in conduction with exercise or recovery can participate in all competitive sports.
3. Athletes with Mobitz type 2 second-degree AV block or complete heart block usually require pacemaker implantation before being permitted to participate in any sports.
4. Asymptomatic athletes without heart disease who have a junctional escape rhythm with normal QRS duration and resting ventricular rate >40 beats/min that increase appropriately with exertion can participate in any competitive sports.
5. Athletes with acquired complete heart block should have a permanent pacemaker placed regardless of symptoms, type of structural heart disease, and exercise capacity.
6. Asymptomatic athletes with RBBB or LBBB who do not have ventricular arrhythmias or develop AV block during exercise can participate in all sports. However, patients with LBBB who have an abnormal prolongation of HV interval on EPS should receive a pacemaker.
7. Athletes with permanent pacemaker
   a. Athletes who are completely pacemaker dependent should not engage in sports in which there is a risk of collision.
   b. Athletes who are not pacemaker dependent may participate in sports with a risk of collision or trauma if they understand and accept the risk of damage to the pacemaker system.
   c. For athletes with permanent pacemakers, protective equipment should be considered for participation in contact sports that have the potential to damage the implanted device.

IV. ATHLETES WITH SYSTEMIC HYPERTENSION

A. BLOOD PRESSURE AND TYPE OF EXERCISE

Reports of cerebrovascular accident during maximal exercise have raised concerns that the rise in BP during strenuous activity may cause harm. However, changes in BP depend on the type of exercise in which athletes are engaged.

1. Dynamic exercise causes a substantial increase in systolic pressure, no significant change in diastolic pressure, and a decrease in mean pressure (with a marked decrease in total peripheral vascular resistance.
2. Static exercise, in contrast, causes a marked increase in systolic, diastolic, and mean arterial pressures with no appreciable change in total peripheral resistance.

B. RECOMMENDATIONS BY 2014 AHA/ACC SCIENTIFIC STATEMENT (SEE BLACK ET AL. [2015])

1. Athletes with elevated BP (formerly prehypertension): BP levels between the 90th and 95th percentiles, or >120/80 mm Hg.

a. May participate in physical activity, but should be encouraged to modify lifestyle.
b. If pre-hypertension persists, echo studies are done to see if there is LVH (beyond that seen with "athlete's heart.")
c. If LVH is present, athletic participation is limited until BP is normalized by appropriate drug therapy.

2. Athletes with stage 1 hypertension (BP levels between the 95th and 95th percentiles + 12; or 130/80 to 139/89 mm Hg) may participate in any competitive sports, in the absence of target organ damage.
3. Athletes with stage 2 hypertension (BP levels higher than 95th percentile + 10 mm Hg or >140/90 mm Hg), even in the absence of target organ damage (such as LVH), should be restricted, particularly from high static sports (such as weight lifting, boxing, and wrestling), until hypertension is controlled by either lifestyle modification or drug therapy.

C. DRUG TREATMENT

1. All drugs being taken must be registered with appropriate governing bodies to obtain a therapeutic exemption.
2. With respect to the treatment of hypertension, β-blockers are not banned for most sports, including football and basketball, but they are not good choices because they reduced athletes' maximum performance. Angiotensin-converting enzyme (ACE) inhibitors and calcium channel blockers are preferred to β-adrenergic blockers. However, one should be aware of potential teratogenic effects of ACE inhibitors if taken during pregnancy.
3. It should be noted that β-blockers that are used to treat hypertension and arrhythmias are expressly banned in sports such as riflery (class IA) and archery (class IIA) in which the athlete would benefit from a slow HR. Therefore β-blockers should not be prescribed for athletes in these sports because it would risk them having a positive drug test result.

Chapter 26

Dyslipidemias

High levels of total cholesterol (TC) and low-density lipoprotein cholesterol (LDL-C) and low levels of high-density lipoprotein cholesterol (HDL-C) are all risk factors for coronary atherosclerosis. A link has been established between increased levels of triglycerides (TGs) and coronary heart disease as well. Cholesterol reduction results in reduced angiographic progression of CAD and even modest regression in some cases. Therefore controlling dyslipidemia has become a primary goal of reducing premature CAD. It has been established that the coronary arteriosclerosis begins to develop during childhood. In 2011, the Expert Panel convened by the National Heart Lung and Blood Institute (NHLBI) made recommendations on screening for dyslipidemia in children in an effort to reduce the prevalence of premature CAD.

I. DIAGNOSIS OF DYSLIPIDEMIA

The diagnosis of dyslipidemia is made by measuring blood lipid, lipoproteins, or apolipoprotein factors.

1. The routine lipid profile typically includes: TC, HDL-C, LDL-C, and triglycerides (TG). A lipoprotein analysis is obtained after an overnight fast of 12 hours. The LDL level is usually estimated by the Friedewald formula:

   $$\text{LDL} = \text{Total cholesterol} - \text{HDL} - (\text{Triglyceride}/5)$$

   This formula is not accurate if the child is not fasting, if the TG level is >400 mg/dL, or if chylomicrons or dysbetalipoproteinemia (type III hyperlipoproteinemia) is present. Methods are currently available to measure LDL-C directly, which does not require a fasting specimen.
2. An extended profile may also include very-low-density lipoprotein cholesterol (VLDL-C), non-HDL cholesterol (non-HDL-C), and the ratio of TC to HDL-C.
3. Non-HDL-C: Serum non-HDL-C (TC − HDL-C) is considered a better screening tool than LDL-C for the assessment of CAD risk because it includes all classes of atherogenic (apolipoprotein B–containing) lipoproteins: VLDL-C, intermediate-density lipoproteins (IDLs), LDL-C, and lipoprotein (a) or Lp(a). Non-HDL-C from a nonfasting lipid profile is recommended in routine lipid screening.
4. The ratio of the TC to HDL cholesterol (TC-to-HDL-C ratio) is a useful parameter for assessing risk for CVD. The usual TC-to-HDL-C ratio in children is approximately 3 (based on TC of 150 mg/dL and an HDL-C of 50 mg/dL). The higher the ratio, the higher is the risk of developing CVD.
5. Small, dense LDL particles: In recent years, small, dense LDL particles have been shown to be more important than the total LDL levels in CAD. The size of LDL particles is not routinely measured because the presence of this

phenotype is predictable. It occurs in association with elevated triglyceride levels (> 140 mg/dL) and a decreased HDL-C level (<40 mg/dL in men; <50 mg/dL in women). Although not routinely measured, small, dense LDL can be measured directly by commercial laboratories.

II. NORMAL LEVELS OF LIPIDS AND LIPOPROTEINS

Table 26.1 shows normal, borderline, and abnormal levels of lipid and lipoprotein levels in children. Table 26.2 shows those values for young adults. In children, TC ≥200 mg/dL; LDL-C ≥130 mg/dL; TGs ≥100 mg/dL for patients younger than 10 years and ≥130 mg/dL for 10- to19-year olds; and HDL-C <40 mg/dL are considered abnormal.

TABLE 26.1

CONCENTRATIONS OF PLASMA LIPID, LIPOPROTEIN, AND APOLIPOPROTEIN IN CHILDREN AND ADOLESCENTS (MG/DL): LOW, ACCEPTABLE, BORDERLINE, AND HIGH

CATEGORY	LOW	ACCEPTABLE	BORDERLINE	HIGH
Total cholesterol	–	<170	170-199	≥200
LDL cholesterol	–	<110	110-129	≥130
Non-HDL cholesterol	–	<120	120-144	≥145
Triglycerides: 0-9 years	–	<75	75-99	≥100
10-19 years	–	<90	90-129	≥130
HDL cholesterol	<40	>45	40-45	–
Apolipoprotein A1	<115	>120	115-120	–
Apolipoprotein B		<90	90-109	≥110

HDL, high-density lipoprotein; *LDL*, low-density lipoprotein.

From Expert Panel on Integrated Guidelines for Cardiovascular Health and Risk Reduction in Children and Adolescent, National Heart, Lung, and Blood Institute. (2011). Expert panel on integrated guidelines for cardiovascular health and risk reduction in children and adolescents: Summary report. *Pediatrics, 128*(suppl 5), S213-S256.

TABLE 26.2

RECOMMENDED CUT POINTS FOR LIPID AND LIPOPROTEIN LEVELS IN YOUNG ADULTS (MG/DL)

CATEGORY	LOW	BORDERLINE-LOW	ACCEPTABLE	BORDERLINE-HIGH	HIGH
Total cholesterol	–	–	<190	190-224	≥225
LDL cholesterol	–	–	<120	120-159	≥160
Non-HDL cholesterol	–	–	<150	150-189	≥190
Triglycerides	–	–	<115	115-149	≥150
HDL cholesterol	<40	40-44	>45	–	–

HDL, high-density lipoprotein; *LDL*, low-density lipoprotein.

From Expert Panel on Integrated Guidelines for Cardiovascular Health and Risk Reduction in Children and Adolescent, National Heart, Lung, and Blood Institute. (2011). Expert panel on integrated guidelines for cardiovascular health and risk reduction in children and adolescents: Summary report. *Pediatrics, 128*(suppl 5), S213-S256.

III. CLASSIFICATION OF DYSLIPIDEMIA

Dyslipidemia can be classified as primary (genetic) or secondary dyslipidemia.

- Primary dyslipidemia is caused by single- or multiple-gene mutations that result in either overproduction or defective clearance of TGs and LDL-C or in underproduction or excessive clearance of HDL-C.
- Secondary dyslipidemia is caused by associated diseases or conditions. The majority of the cases found during screening are secondary forms.

A. SECONDARY DYSLIPIDEMIA

1. Box 26.1 lists causes of secondary dyslipidemia.
   a. The most common cause of pediatric dyslipidemia is obesity.
   b. Medications such as oral contraceptives, isotretinoin (Accutane), anabolic steroids, diuretics, β-blockers, antipsychotics, and estrogens are uncommon causes of dyslipidemia.
   c. Medical conditions including hypothyroidism, renal failure, nephrotic syndrome, and alcohol usage are less common causes of secondary dyslipidemia.
   d. Most secondary causes of dyslipidemia raise TG and often lower HDL-C levels, with the exception of (1) increased levels of HDL-C seen with estrogen and (2) increased LDL-C seen with nephrosis, systemic lupus, primary biliary cirrhosis, protease inhibitors (for treatment of human immunodeficiency virus [HIV]), and hypothyroidism.
   e. Each child with dyslipidemia should have laboratory tests to help rule out secondary causes of dyslipidemia. The tests should include (1) fasting blood glucose or glycated hemoglobin (Hgb A1c), (2) renal function, (3) liver function, and (4) thyroid function.

BOX 26.1

CAUSES OF SECONDARY DYSLIPIDEMIA

Metabolic	Metabolic syndrome, diabetes, lipodystrophies, glycogen storage disorders
Renal disease	Chronic renal failure, nephrotic syndrome, glomerulonephritis, hemolytic uremic syndrome
Hepatic	Biliary atresia, cirrhosis
Hormonal	Estrogen, progesterone, growth hormone, hypothyroidism, corticosteroids
Lifestyle	Obesity, physical inactivity, diets rich in fat and saturated fat, alcohol intake
Medications	Isotretinoin (Accutane), certain oral contraceptives, anabolic steroids, thiazide diuretics, β-adrenergic blockers, antipsychotics, anticonvulsants, glucocorticoids, estrogen, testosterone, immunosuppressive agents (cyclosporine), antiviral agents (HIV protease inhibitor)
Others	Kawasaki disease, anorexia nervosa, post–solid organ transplantation, childhood cancer survivor, progeria, idiopathic hypercalcemia, Klinefelter syndrome, Werner syndrome

HIV, human immunodeficiency virus.

f. When the diagnosis of secondary dyslipidemia is made, one should treat the associated disorder (such as diabetes, obesity, or nephritic syndrome) that is producing the dyslipidemia first and then treat the dyslipidemia using the same guidelines as in primary dyslipidemia.

B. SELECTED PRIMARY DYSLIPIDEMIAS

Primary (genetic) dyslipidemias are far less commonly found in the screening process. Five well-known primary dyslipidemias are presented in summary format in Table 26.3.

TABLE 26.3

SELECTED PRIMARY DYSLIPIDEMIAS

LIPID DISORDERS	CLINICAL INFORMATION
Familial hypercholesterolemia (FH): FH heterozygotes	Fairly common (1 in 500 people) One out of 2 siblings and one parent have ↑TC (>240 mg/dL; Avg. 300 mg/dL) and ↑LDL (>160 mg/dL; Avg. 240 mg/dL). Unaffected are perfectly normal. Xanthomas (of Achilles tendon or extensor tendons of hands) in parents (seen in 10% to 15%) almost confirm the diagnosis. TX: (a) Diet low in fat and cholesterol and high in fiber. (b) Statins are the drugs of choice.
FH homozygotes	One in 1 million children TC and LDL-C are 5 to 6 times higher than normal. (TC average levels 700 mg/dL and may reach ≥1000 mg/dL). Planar xanthomas may be present by age 5 years (flat, orange-colored lesions in the webbing of the hands and over the elbows and buttocks). Tendon xanthomas, arcus corneae, and significant CAD are often present by age 10 years. Atherosclerosis often results in aortic stenosis. TX: (a) High-dose statins and niacin. (b) Will require LDL apheresis (with extracorporeal affinity LDL absorption column and plasma reinfusion) every 2 weeks.
Familial combined hyperlipidemia (FCH)	AD disorder (3 times more frequently than FH) Characterized by variable lipid phenotypic expression: ↑LDL alone, ↑LDL + ↑TG, or normal LDL with ↑TG (difficult to separate it from FH). TC (190-220 mg/dL) and LDL (normal or mildly ↑) are lower than in patients with FH. Diagnosis suspected when a parent or sibling has a different lipoprotein phenotype than the proband. LDL levels fluctuate from time to time, with TG levels fluctuating in the opposite direction.

TABLE 26.3 *(continued)*

SELECTED PRIMARY DYSLIPIDEMIAS

LIPID DISORDERS	CLINICAL INFORMATION
	Usually no tendon xanthomas are present. Often other signs of the metabolic syndrome (e.g., visceral obesity, hyperinsulinemia, glucose intolerance, and hypertension) are present. TX: (a) Low-fat and low-cholesterol diet, (b) low glycemic index foods, and (c) weight control + exercise. (d) Statins are the most effective drugs in lowering LDL. (e) Drug therapy if TG (> 350 mg/dL) to prevent pancreatitis. (f) Metformin (±)
Familial hypertriglyceridemia	AD disorder, caused by lipoprotein lipase (LPL) deficiency, resulting in hepatic overproduction of VLDL-C. TG typically increased (200-1000 mg/dL) but TC is not increased. High TG levels accompany (a) ↓HDL, (b) the production of smaller, denser LDL particles (more atherogenic), and (c) a hypercoagulable state. TX: (a) Diet very low in fat and simple sugar; (b) lifestyle change with exercise; (c) when TG reaches 500-1000 mg/dL, pancreatitis is a major concern (fibrate or niacin may be used).
Dysbetalipoproteinemia (type III hyperlipoproteinemia)	Rare AR disorder, due to a defect in apolipoprotein E, resulting in increased accumulation of chylomicron remnants and VLDL remnants. Both TC and TG increased equally to >300 mg/dL (not usually seen in childhood). (TC: 250-500 mg/dL; TG: 50-600 mg/dL) TX: (a) Low-fat and low glycemic index diet; (b) fibric acid or statin is very effective.
Familial hypoalphalipoproteinemia (low-HDL syndrome)	AD disorder, caused by decreased concentration of apolipoprotein A1 and apolipoprotein AII and absent apolipoprotein CIII. Low HDL-C increases the risk of premature CAD. *Tangier disease:* HDL nearly absent (with markedly enlarged yellow tonsils). TX: (a) Low carbohydrate and low fat diet. (b) Exercise and weight loss are also helpful. (c) Goal is to keep LDL low.

AD, autosomal dominant; *AR*, autosomal recessive; *Avg.*, average; *CAD*, coronary artery disease; *HDL*, high-density lipoprotein; *LDL*, low-density lipoprotein; *VLDL*, very-low-density lipoprotein; *TC*, total cholesterol; *TG*, triglycerides; *TX*, treatment.

IV. LIPID SCREENING

In 2011, the Expert Panel convened by the NHLBI made the following recommendations. These recommendations are major changes from the past recommendations of *selective* screening of children and adolescents with a family history of premature CVD or those with at least one parent with high serum cholesterol levels (by the Expert Panel of 1991).

The new recommendations are as follows.

1. **Universal screening** is recommended for children 9-11 years old and patients 17-21 years old (see Box 26.2).
   a. For universal screening, either nonfasting lipid profile (non-FLP) or fasting lipid panel (FLP) is acceptable.
   b. When non-FLP is obtained, non-HDL-C is calculated (by subtracting HDL-C from TC. Non-HDL-C has been shown to be as powerful a predictor of atherosclerosis as any other lipoprotein cholesterol measurement in children and adolescents.
2. **Selective screening** is recommended for children in other age groups (i.e., ages 2 to 8 years and ages 12 to 16 years) if any of the following applies (see Box 26.2). Measure FLP twice and average the results.
   a. Positive family history (see Box 26.3 for details).
   b. Parent(s) with TC ≥240 mg/dL or known dyslipidemia.

BOX 26.2

RECOMMENDATIONS FOR LIPID ASSESSMENT ACCORDING TO AGE GROUP

AGE GROUP	
<2 years	No lipid screening
2 to 8 years	Selective screening. Measure FLP twice and average the result if any of the following applies: • Positive family history (see below) • Parent with TC ≥240 mg/dL or known dyslipidemia • Child has diabetes, hypertension, BMI ≥95th%, or smokes cigarettes • Child has a moderate- or high-risk medical condition (see Box 26.3) Interpret the results according to Table 26.1.
9 to 11 years	Universal screening (by either non-FLP or FLP) Non-FLP: Calculate non-HDL cholesterol (non-HDL cholesterol = TC − HDL cholesterol). If non-HDL cholesterol ≥145 mg/dL or ± HDL <40 mg/dL, measure FLP twice and average results. OR FLP: If LDL cholesterol ≥130 mg/dL; ± non-HDL cholesterol ≥145 mg/dL; ± HDL cholesterol <40 mg/dL; ± triglycerides ≥100 mg/dL if <10 years; or ≥130 mg/dL if ≥10 years, repeat FLP and average results. Interpret the results according to Table 26.1.

12 to 16 years	Selective screening Measure FLP twice and average results if any of the following applies: • Positive family history (see Box 26.3) • Parent with TC ≥240 mg/dL or known dyslipidemia • Child has diabetes, hypertension, BMI ≥85th percentile, or smokes cigarettes • Child has a moderate- or high-risk medical condition (see following) Interpret the results according to Table 26.1.
17 to 21 years	Universal screening once in this time period (by either non-FLP or FLP) For 17-19 yr: Non-FLP: Calculate non-HDL-cholesterol. If non-HDL cholesterol ≥145 mg/dL or ± HDL <40 mg/dL, measure FLP twice and average results OR FLP: If LDL cholesterol ≥130 mg/dL; or non-HDL-cholesterol ≥145 mg/dL; ± HDL cholesterol <40 mg/dL or ± triglycerides ≥130 mg/dL, repeat FLP and average results. Interpret the results according to Table 26.1. *For 20-21 years:* Non-FLP: Calculate non-HDL cholesterol If non-HDL cholesterol ≥190 mg/dL or ± HDL cholesterol <40 mg/dL, measure FLP twice and average results. OR FLP: If LDL cholesterol ≥160 mg/dL; ± non-HDL cholesterol ≥190 mg/dL; ± HDL cholesterol <40 mg/dL or ± triglycerides ≥150 mg/dL, repeat FLP and average results. Interpret the results according to Table 26.1 or Table 26.2.

BMI, body mass index; *FLP*, fasting lipid panel; *HDL*, high-density lipoprotein; *LDL*, low-density lipoprotein; *Non-FLP*, non-fasting lipid profile; *TC*, total cholesterol.

From Expert Panel on Integrated Guidelines for Cardiovascular Health and Risk Reduction in Children and Adolescent, National Heart, Lung, and Blood Institute. (2011). Expert panel on integrated guidelines for cardiovascular health and risk reduction in children and adolescents: Summary report. *Pediatrics, 128*(suppl 5), S213-S256.

c. Child who has moderate- to high-level **risk factors**, such as diabetes, hypertension, body mass index (BMI) ≥85th percentile, or smokes cigarettes (see Box 26.3).

d. Child who has a moderate- or high-risk **medical condition** (such as diabetes, chronic renal disease, posttransplant patients, Kawasaki disease, HIV infection, nephritic syndrome, and others) (see Box 26.3).

V. WHAT TO DO WITH THE RESULTS OF SCREENING

1. If non-HDL-C is ≥145 mg/dL in non-FLP, the averages of two FLPs are obtained to determine LDL-C and TG levels. The following are abnormal levels (by FLPs):

$$\text{LDL} - \text{C} > 130\ \text{mg/dL}$$

BOX 26.3

CARDIOVASCULAR RISK FACTOR CATEGORIES

Positive Family History

Parent, grandparent, aunt/uncle, or sibling with myocardial infarction, angina, coronary artery bypass graft/stent/angioplasty, or sudden cardiac death, at <55 years for males; <65 years for females.

Risk Factors

High-level risk factors:

- Hypertension that requires drug therapy (BP ≥99th percentile + 5 mm Hg)
- Current cigarette smoker
- BMI ≥97th percentile
- Presence of high-risk conditions, including diabetes mellitus (see following)

Moderate-level risk factors:

- Hypertension that does not require drug therapy
- BMI at the ≥95th percentile, <97th percentile
- HDL cholesterol <40 mg/dL
- Presence of moderate-risk conditions (see following)

Special Risk Conditions

High-risk conditions:

- Type 1 and type 2 diabetes mellitus
- Chronic kidney disease/end-stage renal disease/postrenal transplant
- Postorthotopic heart transplant
- Kawasaki disease with current aneurysm

Moderate-risk conditions:

- Kawasaki disease with regressed coronary aneurysm
- Chronic inflammatory disease (systemic lupus erythematosus, juvenile rheumatoid arthritis)
- HIV infection
- Nephrotic syndrome

BMI, body mass index; *BP*, blood pressure; *HDL*, high-density lipoprotein; *HIV*, human immunodeficiency virus.
From Expert Panel on Integrated Guidelines for Cardiovascular Health and Risk Reduction in Children and Adolescent, National Heart, Lung, and Blood Institute. (2011). Expert panel on integrated guidelines for cardiovascular health and risk reduction in children and adolescents: Summary report. *Pediatrics, 128*(suppl 5), S213-S256.

TGs > 100 mg/dL for children < 19 years

TGs > 130 mg/dL for 10-to 19-year-olds

2. When lipid profiles are abnormal, obtain other laboratory tests to rule out secondary dyslipidemia: fasting blood glucose, renal function, liver function, and thyroid function tests.
3. For children with high LDL-C levels:
   a. Initial dietary management and lifestyle changes are used with the Cardiovascular Health Integrated Lifestyle Diet-1 (CHILD-1) and CHILD-2-LDL (see Table 26.4 for CHILD diets).

TABLE 26.4

NUTRIENT COMPOSITION OF CHILD DIETS

NUTRIENTS (% TOTAL CALORIES)	CHILD-1	CHILD-2-LDL	CHILD-2-TG
Total fat	<30%	25% to 30%	25% to 30%
Saturated fat	7% to 10%	≤7%	≤7%
Cholesterol	300 mg/day	<200 mg/day	<200 mg/day
Mono- and poly-unsaturated fatty acids	20%	≈10%	≈10%
Carbohydrate	50% to 55%		
Protein	15% to 20%		
Others	Reduce *trans* fat intake May add plant sterol or plant sterol esters, or water-soluble fiber psyllium	Avoid *trans* fat as much as possible	Decrease sugar intake Increase intake of complex carbohydrate Increase dietary fish (omega 3-fatty acids)

CHILD, Cardiovascular Health Integrated Lifestyle Diet; *LDL*, low-density lipoprotein; *TG*, triglycerides.

   b. Lipid-lowering drugs ("statins") are considered if the diets are unsuccessful in lowering LDL-C. Indications and dosages of the statins follow.
4. For children with high TG levels:
   a. Dietary therapy and lifestyle changes are used as the primary tools, with CHILD-1 for 3 to 6 months advancing to CHILD-2-TG.
   b. Weight control efforts, reduction of sugar consumption, and increased consumption of fish (or omega-3 fish oil) are used.
   c. Drugs are not recommended to reduce TGs. Further discussion follows in this chapter.
5. Those children with LDL-C ≥250 mg/dL and those with TGs ≥500 mg/dL should be referred to lipid specialists.

VI. MANAGEMENT OF HYPERCHOLESTEROLEMIA

A. DIETARY MANAGEMENT

1. Reduced intake of saturated fat and cholesterol is most basic to the dietary therapy of hypercholesterolemia. Diet therapy is prescribed in two steps that progressively reduce the intake of saturated fats and cholesterol.
   a. The CHILD-1 diet for 3 to 6 months is the first stage in dietary change (see Table 26.4).

b. If this diet fails to lower LDL-C levels to ≤130 mg/dL in 6 months, a more stringent diet, CHILD-2-LDL, is used for an additional 6 months.

2. If the dietary intervention with CHILD-2-LDL fails, one may proceed with drug therapy (see the next section).

B. DRUG THERAPY

1. Lipid-lowering drugs
   a. Five well-known classes of lipid-lowering drugs have been used for adults with dyslipidemia. They are (1) bile acid sequestrants, (2) 3-hydroxy-3-methylglutaryl coenzyme-A (HMG-CoA) reductase inhibitors (statins), (3) cholesterol absorption inhibitors, (4) nicotinic acid (niacin, vitamin B3), and (5) fibric acid derivatives. The mechanisms of action, side effects, and ranges of adult dosages of the lipid-lowering agents are presented in Table 26.5.
   b. The bile acid sequestrants (cholestyramine, colestipol) are not used widely because they have a low compliance rate (due to gritty texture and gastrointestinal complaints) and provide only a modest reduction of LDL cholesterol level. Ezetimibe, a cholesterol absorption inhibitor, is effective in lowering blood cholesterol levels, but pediatric experience is quite limited. Nicotinic acid and fibrates have been shown to lower LDL-C and TG levels and increase HDL-C levels in adults, but they are not frequently used in adolescents because of the limited data available.
2. The statins
   a. The statins (HMG-CoA reductase inhibitors) are the most effective drugs in lowering LDL-C in adults as well as in children and adolescents. The statins inhibit HMG-CoA reductase, which is the rate-limiting step in the endogenous production of cholesterol in the hepatic cells.
   b. Indications for the use of statins:
      (1) The decision to use statins depends not only on the high levels of LDL-C (>130 mg/dL), but also on the presence of a positive family history, and/or the presence of high or moderate risk factors or risk conditions (as listed in Box 26.3). The indications for consideration of drug therapy are detailed in Box 26.4.
      (2) Statin therapy is NOT indicated for children with LDL cholesterol 130-189 mg/dL in a child ≤10 years in the absence of a positive family history and high- or moderate-level risk factor or risk (as outlined in Box 26.3). They should continue with lifestyle changes (CHILD-2-LDL), plus weight management if the BMI is at the ≥85th percentile.
   c. Adverse effects of statins. Adverse effects of statins are infrequent but may include gastrointestinal upset, elevation of liver transaminases, and myopathy, ranging in severity from

TABLE 26.5

SUMMARY OF LIPID-LOWERING DRUGS

DAILY DOSAGE RANGE	MECHANISM OF ACTION	SIDE EFFECTS	DAILY DOSAGE RANGE
Bile Acid Sequestrants: Cholestyramine (Questran), Colestipol (Colestid), Colesevelam (WelChol)	Increases excretion of bile acids in stool; increases LDL receptor activity	Constipation, nausea, bloating, flatulence, transient increase in transaminase and alkaline phosphatase levels, increased triglyceride levels (± ±), possible prevention of absorption of fat-soluble vitamins	Related to levels of cholesterol, not body weight
HMG-CoA Reductase Inhibitors (Statins): Atorvastatin (Lipitor), Fluvastatin (Lescol), Lovastatin (Mevacor), Pravastatin (Pravachol), Rosuvastatin (Crestor), Simvastatin (Zocor)	Inhibits HMG-CoA reductase, with resulting decrease in cholesterol synthesis; increases LDL receptor activity; and reduces LDL and VLDL secretion by the liver	Mild gastrointestinal symptoms, myositis syndrome, elevated hepatic transaminase levels, increased CPK levels Contraindicated during pregnancy because of potential risk to a developing fetus Risk of myopathy is higher with a high dose of simvastatin (80 mg) and is lower with atorvastatin or rosuvastatin	Adult dose ranges: Atorvastatin: 10-80 mg Fluvastatin: 20-80 mg Lovastatin: 20-80 mg Pravastatin: 10-40 mg Simvastatin: 10-40 mg The starting dose for children: Atrovastatin: 10 mg Fluvastatin: 20 mg Lovastatin: 10 mg Pravastatin: 10 mg Simvastatin: 10 mg
Cholesterol Absorption Inhibitors: Ezetimibe (Zetia; Ezetrol)	Selective inhibition of intestinal sterol absorption	Abdominal pain, rhabdomyolysis (±)	*Adults:* 10 mg/day
Nicotinic Acid (Niacin, Vitamin B3)	Decreases plasma levels of free fatty acid; possibly inhibits cholesterol synthesis; decreases hepatic VLDL synthesis	Cutaneous flushing, pruritus, gastrointestinal upset, liver function abnormalities, increased uric acid levels, increased glucose intolerance	*Children+:* only short-term efficacy reported for homozygous FH; not recommended for routine use *Adults:* 1-3 g
Fibric Acid Derivatives: Gemfibrozil (Lopid), Clofibrate	Decreases hepatic VLDL synthesis; increases LPL activity	Increased incidence of gallstones and perhaps gastrointestinal cancer, myositis, diarrhea, nausea, rash, altered liver function, increased CPK levels, potentiation of warfarin	*Children:* not recommended *Adults:* gemfibrozil, 600-1200 mg; clofibrate, 1-2 g

CPK, creatine phosphokinase; *FH,* familial hypercholesterolemia; *HDL,* high-density lipoprotein; *HMG-CoA,* 3-hydroxy-3-methylglutaryl coenzyme A; *LDL,* low-density lipoprotein; *LPL,* lipoprotein lipase; *VLDL,* very-low-density lipoprotein.

BOX 26.4

INDICATIONS FOR DRUG THERAPY FOR HYPERCHOLESTEROLEMIA IN CHILDREN AND ADOLESCENTS

1. Failure of diet therapy and lifestyle management for 6 to 12 months, *plus*
2. Age ≥ 10 years with one of the following lipid profiles and/or risk factors.
   - LDL cholesterol ≥ 190 mg/dL
   - LDL cholesterol 160-189 mg/dL with:
     (1) a positive family history of premature CVD/events in first-degree relatives, or
     (2) at least 1 high-level risk factor or risk condition, or
     (3) at least 2 moderate-level risk factors or risk conditions.
   - LDL cholesterol 130-159 mg/dL with:
     (1) at least 2 high-level risk factors or risk conditions, or
     (2) at least 1 high-level risk factor or risk condition *plus* at least 2 moderate-level risk factors or risk conditions (see Box 26.3).

OR

Children aged 8 or 9 years with LDL-C persistently ≥ 190 mg/dL together with *multiple* first-degree family members with premature CV disease/events, or the presence of at least 1 high-level risk factor or risk condition, or the presence of at least 2 moderate-level risk factors or risk conditions.

CV, cardiovascular; *CVD*, cardiovascular disease; *LDL-C*, low-density lipoprotein cholesterol.

From Expert Panel on Integrated Guidelines for Cardiovascular Health and Risk Reduction in Children and Adolescent, National Heart, Lung, and Blood Institute. (2011). Expert panel on integrated guidelines for cardiovascular health and risk reduction in children and adolescents: Summary report. *Pediatrics, 128*(suppl 5), S213-S256.

asymptomatic increases in creatine kinase (CK), to muscle aches or weakness, to fatal rhabdomyolysis. Myopathy and elevated liver enzymes are main concerns.

(1) More than a 10-time increase in CK levels and more than a 3-time increase in alanine aminotransferase (ALT) or aspartate aminotransferase (AST) levels above the upper limits of normal are worrisome levels. Box 26.5 provides step-by-step instruction on initiation, titration, and monitoring of statin therapy (McGrindle et al., 2007).

(2) It is known that vigorous exercise, particularly contact sports or weightlifting, may result in an increase in CK level.

(3) Myopathy is defined as a serum CK level 10 times the upper limit of normal with or without muscle weakness or pain. Rhabdomyolysis is defined as unexplained muscle pain or weakness with a serum CK level of more than 40 times the upper limit of normal.

(4) Normal ranges of laboratory values are as follows (source: *Nelson textbook of pediatrics*, 18th edition):
   (a) CK: 5-130 U/L (adults)
   (b) ALT: 5-45 U/L (1-19 years)
   (c) AST: 15-55 U/L (1-9 years); 5-45 U/L (10-19 years)

BOX 26.5

SUGGESTED INITIATION, TITRATION, AND MONITORING OF STATIN THERAPY IN CHILDREN AND ADOLESCENTS

1. Measure baseline CK, ALT, and AST levels.
2. Start with lower dose given once orally at bedtime (see text for dosage).
3. Monitoring for potential adverse effects:
   - Instruct the patient to report *immediately* all potential adverse effects, especially myopathy (muscle cramps, weakness, asthenia, and more diffuse symptoms).
   - If myopathy is present, its relation to recent physical activities should be assessed, the medication stopped, and CK assessed.
   - The patient should be monitored for resolution of myopathy and any associated increases in CK.
   - Consideration can be given to restarting the medication once symptoms and laboratory abnormalities have resolved.
   - Advise female patients about concerns with regard to pregnancy and the need for appropriate contraception if warranted.
4. After 4 weeks, measure fasting lipoprotein profile, CK, ALT, and AST.
   - The threshold for worrisome level of CK is 10 times above the upper limit of reported normal; consider impact of physical activity.
   - The threshold for worrisome level of ALT or AST is 3 times above the upper limit of reported normal.
   - Target level for LDL: minimal, <130 mg/dL; ideal, 110 mg/dL.
5. At 4-week follow-up:
   - If target LDL levels achieved; no laboratory abnormalities:
     → Continue therapy and recheck in 8 weeks and then 3 months.
   - If laboratory abnormalities noted or symptoms reported:
     → Temporarily withhold the drug and repeat the blood work in ≈2 weeks.
     → When anomalies return to normal, the drugs may be restarted with close monitoring.
   - If target LDL levels not achieved:
     → Increase the dose by 10 mg and repeat the blood work in 4 weeks.
     → Continue stepped titration up to the maximum recommended dose until target LDL levels are achieved or there is evidence of toxicity.
6. Repeat laboratory tests every 3 to 6 months: fasting lipoprotein profile, CK, ALT, and AST.
7. Continue counseling on:
   - Compliance with medications and reduced-fat diets.
   - Other risk factors, such as weight gain, smoking, and inactivity.
   - Counsel adolescent females about statin contraindication in pregnancy and the need for appropriate contraception. Seek referral to an adolescent medicine or gynecologic specialist as appropriate.

CK, creatine kinase; *ALT*, alanine aminotransferase; *AST*, aspartate aminotransferase; *HDL*, high-density lipoprotein.
Modified from McCrindle, B. W., Urbina, E. M., Dennison, B. A., et al. (2007). Drug therapy of high-risk lipid abnormalities in children and adolescents. *Circulation, 115*(14), 1948-1967

d. Dosages of statins
   (1) The starting dose of the statins is usually 10 mg (with the exception of fluvastatin, 20 mg) given once daily at bedtime (see Table 26.5).
   (2) The dose of statin is increased by 10 mg every 3 months to the 1/2 or even the full adult dosage with periodic measurements of cholesterols. The maintenance dosage of the drug is decided by periodic determinations of cholesterol levels.
   (3) The minimal target level for LDL cholesterol is <130 mg/dL and the ideal target level is 110 mg/dL.

VII. HYPERTRIGLYCERIDEMIA

1. Significance of high TG levels.
   a. Hypertriglyceridemia is an independent risk factor for major coronary events after controlling for LDL-C and HDL-C.
   b. Metabolic consequences of hypertriglyceridemia include (1) lowering of HDL-C, (2) production of smaller, denser LDL particles with more atherogenicity, and (3) a hypercoagulable state.
2. There are different cut-off points for treatment of hypertriglyceridemia in children and adults: (a) 100 mg/dL for children <10 years; (b) 130 mg/dL for ages 10 to 19 years; and (c) 150 mg/dL for young adults (see Tables 26.1 and 26.2).
3. Steps in the management of hypertriglyceridemia is as follows.
   a. Diet therapy is the primary tool in treating high TG levels. Reduction of simple carbohydrate intake (and increased intake of complex carbohydrate), reduced saturated fat intake (such as CHILD-2-TG), and weight loss are associated with reduced levels of TG. It is important to know that both a high-fat diet and a high-carbohydrate diet raise TG levels. In fact, a diet high in carbohydrates, especially a high glycemic index diet, may be a more important source of hypertriglyceridemia than high fat intake. Therefore all refined carbohydrate foods, such as sugary drinks, cookies, ice cream, and after dinner desserts, should be avoided and complex carbohydrates such as whole grain products should be consumed more.
   b. Weight control: Lifestyle changes with increased physical activity (at least 30 minutes of moderate-intensity exercise daily, 5 days a week) and weight control help reduce TG levels. Exercise will also help decrease LDL-C and increase HDL-C.
   c. Fish and fish oil: Increasing dietary fish and administration of fish oil may be effective in lowering TG levels. Omega-3 fatty acids in fish oils lower plasma TG levels by inhibiting the synthesis of VLDL cholesterol and TG in the liver. They also have antithrombotic properties.
      (1) Increasing dietary fish consumption is the first step.
      (2) Fish oil supplementation may be the next step.

(3) A prescription omega-3 fatty acid product (e.g., Omacor) may be used. Most fish oil capsules contain only one-third of the omega-3 fatty content contained in Omacor.

4. Management of mild hypertriglyceridemia (TG level 100-200 mg/dL for children <10 years, and TG 130-200 mg/dL for teenagers).
   a. Dietary therapy with low-carbohydrate diet and reduced saturated fat intake (such as CHILD-2-TG) and weight control efforts are tried.
   b. Increase dietary fish consumption for 6 month and check fasting lipid profile.
5. Management of moderate hypertriglyceridemia (TG level 200 to 499 mg/dL, non-HDL cholesterol level of >145 mg/dL)
   a. Lifestyle/diet management with CHILD-2-TG.
   b. Fish oil supplementation, and consider Omacor 4 g/day.
6. Management of severe hypertriglyceridemia (TG level >500 mg/dL)
   a. They should be treated in conjunction with a lipid specialist.
   b. In addition to the dietary management with CHILD-2-TG and fish oil, use of fibrate or niacin should be considered to prevent pancreatitis.
      (1) Fibrates have the effect of both lowering TG and raising HDL-C. Side effects seen in adults include myalgia, myositis, myopathy, rhabdomyolysis, liver toxicity, gallstones, and glucose intolerance. Safety and efficacy data in children are limited. CK level and liver enzymes should be monitored every 3 months.
      (2) Niacin is the best-known drug that raises HDL-C, but it also reduces TG levels. Adverse effects of niacin include liver toxicity, gastrointestinal tract upset, and facial flushing. Less commonly seen side effects are hyperuricemia and glucose intolerance. Extended-release preparations produce less flushing but are more likely to produce liver toxicity. Niacin is rarely used to treat the pediatric population because of reported poor tolerance and the potential for very serious adverse effects. Liver transaminases should be checked every 3 months.

VIII. LOW HDL LEVEL

1. Significance of low HDL-C level.
   a. Low HDL-C level is defined as <40 mg/dL in adolescent boys and girls. In adults, low HDL level is defined as <40 mg/dL in men and <50 mg/dL in women.
   b. Low levels of HDL-C represent a major CV risk factor. Despite the presence of desirable total TC levels, patients with low HDL-C may be at high risk of developing CV events.
   c. HDL-C has a number of antiatherogenic effects. The best known of these relates to the ability of HDL-C to promote the efflux of cholesterol from macrophages in the arterial wall, through reverse cholesterol transport.
2. Management of low levels of HDL cholesterol.

a. Primary approach in managing low levels of HDL cholesterol is lifestyle change and diet therapy. The following measures have been suggested for adult patients with low levels of HDL-C.
   (1) Lifestyle change with regular exercise (30 minutes of brisk aerobic exercise every day or every other day) is recommended. Weight control (and quitting smoking) is equally important.
   (2) Dietary intervention.
      (a) Diets low in saturated fat and rich in the polyunsaturated fatty acids are recommended because the most effective way to reduce CV risk in patients with low HDL levels is to maintain low LDL-C levels, not to raise HDL levels.
      (b) Consumption of high glycemic index foods should be restricted.
      (c) Omega-3 fatty acids may help raise HDL levels.

b. Current pharmacologic options for adults include nicotinic acid (niacin), fibrates, and statins but none of them are without major adverse effects. The use of drugs should be considered only when all nonpharmacologic measures do not achieve the goal of raising HDL-C level in pediatric patients.
   (1) Niacin (nicotinic acid or vitamin B_3) is the most effective medication for raising HDL-C (raising HDL level by 20% to 35%). However, niacin is rarely used in the pediatric population because of the potential for serious adverse effects. One of the major adverse effects of niacin is severe flushing. A newer extended-release formulation of niacin (Niaspan) may reduce flushing substantially, but it is more likely to increase liver toxicity. Flushing (which may involve prostaglandin D_2) can be blocked by taking aspirin 325 mg 30 minutes before taking niacin.
   (2) Fibrate therapy is also effective, producing an average increase of HDL by 10% to 25%. Statins are the least effective of the three drug classes in raising HDL levels.

Chapter 27

Pediatric Preventive Cardiology

Atherosclerotic CVD is a major cause of morbidity and mortality and is responsible for more than 50% of all deaths in the United States. Although most of the clinical burden of CVD occurs in adulthood, risk factors for CVD develop during childhood and adolescence. In fact, there is now clear evidence that atherosclerosis begins during childhood, with a rapid increase in the prevalence of coronary pathology during adolescence and young adulthood. Studies have found that:

1. Fatty streak, the earliest lesion of the atherosclerosis, occurred by 5 to 8 years of age and fibrous plaque, the advanced lesion, appeared in the coronary arteries in subjects in their late teens.
2. Fibrous plaque was found in over 30% of 16- to 20-year-olds and the prevalence of the lesion reached nearly 70% by age 26 to 39.
3. The extent of pathologic changes in the coronary arteries increased with age and so did the number of known CV risk factors that the individual had at the time of death.

Therefore one strategy of reducing CAD in adults would be to prevent or correct CV risk factors in children and adolescents.

Unfortunately, the importance of preventing heart disease in pediatric population is not well perceived by pediatricians and pediatric cardiologists. Although CHD is associated with the highest mortality of any congenital defects, only 0.4% of deaths from CVDs are caused by CHD. The great majority of CV death is from coronary artery disease (54%), stroke (18%), CHF (6%) and hypertension (5%). Therefore preventive cardiology is and should be pediatric domain.

The primary purpose of this chapter is to raise physicians' attention to the emerging importance of practicing medicine to prevent future CVD (and type 2 diabetes) during childhood. This chapter discusses the topics listed below. Lipid screening for dyslipidemia and its management and hypertension, two other important CV factors, are discussed in earlier chapters (Chapters 26 and 23, respectively).

1. Cardiovascular risk factors
2. Metabolic syndrome in children.
3. Diagnosis and principles of management of childhood obesity
4. Strategies for smoke cessation.
5. The summary table of the American Heart Association (AHA) guidelines on practice of pediatric preventive cardiology.

BOX 27.1

MAJOR RISK FACTORS FOR CORONARY HEART DISEASE

- Family history of premature coronary heart disease, cerebrovascular or occlusive peripheral vascular disease (with onset before age 55 years for men and 65 years for women in parents or grandparents)
- Hypercholesterolemia
- Low levels of high-density lipoprotein (<40 mg/100 mL)
- Hypertension (blood pressure >140/90 mm Hg or taking antihypertensive medication)
- Cigarette smoking
- Diabetes mellitus (regarded as a coronary heart disease risk equivalent)

Adapted from the 2002 Third Report of the National Cholesterol Education Program (NCEP) Expert Panel on Detection, Education, and Treatment of High Blood Cholesterol in Adults (Adult Treatment Panel III) final report. *Circulation, 106* (25), 3143–3421.

I. CARDIOVASCULAR RISK FACTORS

Well-known CV risk factors include positive family history of coronary heart disease, high levels of cholesterol, low levels of high-density lipoprotein cholesterol (HDL-C, hypertension, cigarette smoking, and diabetic or prediabetic states (Box 27.1).

Obesity is now known to be an independent risk factor for CVD. Obese individuals have increased prevalence of clustering of multiple CV risk factors, called the metabolic syndrome, which lead to increased incidence of both type 2 diabetes and CV events (see the following text). Unfortunately, the prevalence of obesity has increased rapidly in recent decades.

II. METABOLIC SYNDROME

Obese individuals often have emerging risk factors, including atherogenic dyslipidemia (also known as *"lipid triad,"* consisting of raised level of triglycerides, and small, dense low-density lipoprotein (LDL) particles, and low levels of HDL cholesterol), insulin resistance (hyperinsulinemia), a proinflammatory state (elevation of serum high-sensitivity C-reactive protein), and a prothrombotic state (increased amount of plasminogen activator inhibitor-1 [PAI-1]). The cluster of the these risk factors occurring in one person is known as "the metabolic syndrome." In the metabolic syndrome, LDL cholesterol (LDL-C) levels may not be elevated but apoprotein B (apoB) and small, dense LDL particles are elevated. The smallest particles in the LDL fraction are known to have the greatest atherogenicity. This syndrome occurs more commonly in individuals with abdominal (visceral) obesity. Hispanics and South Asians seem to be particularly susceptible to the syndrome.

Clinically identifiable components of the metabolic syndrome for adults are listed in Box 27.2. The presence of at least three of the risk factors is required to make the diagnosis of the metabolic syndrome in adults according to the AHA/National Heart, Lung, and Blood Institute (NHLBI scientific statement) (Grundy et al., 2005), but the International Diabetes Federation (IDF)

BOX 27.2

DEFINITIONS OF THE METABOLIC SYNDROME IN ADULTS AND IN CHILDREN AND ADOLESCENTS

	ADULTS[a]	CHILDREN AND ADOLESCENTS[b]
Obesity (WC)	Men: WC ≥40 inches (102 cm) Women: WC ≥35 inches (88 cm)	WC ≥90th percentile or adult cutoff point
Triglycerides	≥150 mg/dL	≥150 mg/dL
HDL cholesterol	Men <40 mg/dL Women <50 mg/dL	≤40 mg/dL
Hypertension	130/85 mm Hg or greater	Systolic BP ≥130 mm Hg; diastolic BP ≥85 mm Hg
Elevated fasting glucose	≥100 mg/dL	≥100 mg/dL
Defining criteria	≥3 criteria (AHA/NHLBI consensus statement)[a] or Obesity + ≥2 remaining 4 criteria[c]	Obesity + ≥2 remaining 4 criteria[b]

BMI, body mass index; *BP*, blood pressure; *HDL*, high-density lipoprotein; *NHLBI*, National Heart, Lung, and Blood Institute; *WC*, waist circumference.

[a]From Grundy, S. M., Cleeman, J. I., Daniels, S. R., et al. (2005). Diagnosis and management of the metabolic syndrome: an American Heart Association/National Heart, Lung, and Blood Institute Scientific Statement. *Circulation, 112*(17), 2735–2752.

[b]From Zimmet, P., Alberti, G., Kaufman, F., et al. (2007). *Lancet, 369*(9579), 2059–2061.

[c]From Alberti, K. G., Zimmet, P., & Shaw, J. (2006). Metabolic syndrome—a new world-wide definition. A Consensus Statement from the International Diabetes Federation. *Diabetic Medicine, 23*(5), 469–480.

recommends obesity plus at least two of the remaining four criteria (Alberti et al., 2006). Evidence has supported that waist circumference (reflecting visceral adiposity) is a better predictor of CVD than body mass index (BMI). Other components of metabolic syndrome, such as proinflammatory and prothrombotic states, are not routinely measured in clinical practice.

For children, the IDF has proposed new cutoff points for triglycerides and fasting glucose different from earlier criteria. The new criteria for children make the definition almost the same as for adults (Box 27.2). Obesity and the presence of at least two of the remaining four criteria are required to make the diagnosis of the metabolic syndrome in children. As in adults, waist circumference is preferable to BMI for children as well, which represents abdominal (visceral or central) obesity. Ethnicity and gender specific waist circumference percentiles are now available for children (Fernandez et al., 2004) as presented in Appendix C (Tables C1 through C3). The prevalence of the metabolic syndrome is 30% to 50% in overweight adolescents.

Comorbidities are frequently found in patients with metabolic syndrome: (1) nonalcoholic fatty liver disease (NAFLD), (2) polycystic ovary syndrome (PCOS) in females, (3) obstructive sleep apnea (OSA), and (4) mental health disorders (Magge et al., 2017).

1. NAFLD can be screened by measuring aspartate aminotransferase (AST) and alanine aminotransferase (ALT) in overweight and obese children.
2. PCOS is characterized by hyperandrogenism, menstrual irregularities and/or ovulatory dysfunction, and polycystic ovaries.
3. OSA occurs because of enlarged soft tissues in and around the airway as well as decreased lung volumes because of increased abdominal fat.

A. MANAGEMENT

1. The mainstay of the treatment of the metabolic syndrome for both adults and children is weight control through dietary intervention and promotion of active lifestyle to achieve and maintain optimum weight, normal blood pressure, and normal lipid profile for age. Reducing obesity results in decreases in insulin resistance and inflammatory markers.
2. In addition, each component of the syndrome present should be treated aggressively, because the presence of the syndrome indicates a higher risk for CVDs and diabetes.
3. Treatment of insulin resistance involves lifestyle modification only (Magge et al., 2017). Although some studies have revealed beneficial effects of metformin on BMI, total cholesterol levels, fasting plasma glucose, and insulin resistance, metformin is not currently recommended for treatment of insulin resistance.
4. Treatment of dyslipidemias is presented in some detail in Chapter 26 (Dyslipidemia). The principles of managing obesity are presented in the section of obesity in this chapter.

B. LIPID SCREENING FOR DYSLIPIDEMIA

Dyslipidemia, including high levels of LDL-C, elevated triglycerides, and low levels of HDL-C, are the best-known, long-established risk factors for CAD. Therefore the most important approach to preventing CV events is to detect and treat patients with dyslipidemia. This topic has been presented in Chapter 26 (Dyslipidemia).

In the past, *selective* screening of children was recommended. In 2011, however, the Expert Panel convened by the NHLBI) made major changes in the recommendation (Pediatrics, 2011) (see Box 27.2).

1. A universal screening for children between the ages of 9 and 11 years (late childhood)
2. An additional universal screening between the ages of 17 and 21 years
3. Selective screening for children in other age groups who have certain CV risk factors (see Chapter 26).

III. OBESITY

Information in this section is provided only to assist health care providers in making the diagnosis of overweight and obesity, recognizing complications of obesity, and providing the basic knowledge needed in patient counseling. This section is not intended to describe in detail treatment of obesity; successful treatment of obesity requires special skills and facilities with availability of a multidisciplinary team consisting of registered dietitians, specialized nurses, psychologists, and exercise specialists.

A. DEFINITION AND CLASSIFICATION

The BMI (weight in kilograms divided by square of the height in meters [kg/m^2]) is a simple, valid measure of relative weight and is recommended in clinical diagnosis of overweight states. A large BMI does not always indicate an increase in body fat; lean muscular individuals may have a large BMI.

1. In adults, obesity is present when BMI is >30 and overweight is present when BMI is between 25.0 and 29.9.
2. For children, the statistical definition of overweight states is used.
   a. Overweight: BMI between the 85th and 95th percentiles
   b. Obese: BMI ≥95th percentile, and
   c. Severely obese: BMI >99th percentile

Age- and gender-specific BMI percentile curves for the U.S. pediatric population are presented in Appendix C (Figs. C1 and C2).

B. PREVALENCE

Obesity is one of the most pressing public health issues today in the United States. Nearly half of all American children and adolescents are either overweight or obese. According to a recent national statistics, 16.9% of children and adolescents (2- to 19-year-olds) and 34.9% of adults in the United States are obese. In addition, approximately 32% of children and adolescents are either overweight or obese (Ogden et al., 2014).

C. PATHOGENESIS

The pathogenesis of obesity may be, in part, inherited, but environmental factors appear importantly related to the recent rise in the prevalence of obesity.

1. Increased consumption of calorie-dense food and a decrease in physical activity and/or an increased time spent on television viewing and video games may be causally related to the increasing prevalence of obesity seen in children and adolescents.
2. In recent decades, the role of high glycemic index (GI) foods has emerged as an important cause of weight gain.

1. Concept of Energy Balance

The concept of energy balance applies to the pathogenesis of obesity (Fig. 27.1).

1. When energy intake exceeds energy expenditure on a chronic basis, obesity results. When energy intake is less than energy expenditure, weight loss may result.
2. All energy intake comes from ingestion of macronutrients. Caloric value of fat is 9 kcal/g, whereas that of protein and carbohydrate is

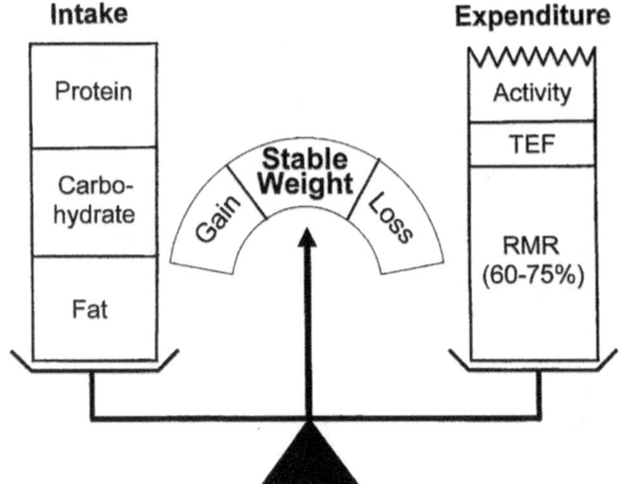

FIG. 27.1
Energy balance. To maintain a stable weight, energy intake (protein, carbohydrate, and fat) of a person should be equal to energy expenditure, which is composed of resting metabolic rate (RMR), the thermic effect of food (TEF), and expenditure associated with physical activities. When intake is greater than expenditure, weight gain will result; when expenditure of energy is greater than the intake, weight loss may result.

4 kcal/g; this is an important reason for recommending reduced-fat intake to control weight.

3. A large portion of energy expenditure is the resting metabolic rate (RMR), accounting 60% to 75% of energy expenditure. Approximately 10% of energy expenditure is dissipated through the thermic effect of food (TEF), which is mainly the result of the energy cost for nutrient absorption, processing, and storage. Energy expenditure resulting from physical activity is relatively small, accounting for only 10% to 15% of the total energy expenditure. This component is least affected by genetics and varies greatly from individual to individual depending on the level of physical activities. The level of energy expenditure from RMR and TEF may be predominantly determined by genetic factors.
4. By measure, 3500 calories is equivalent to 1 lb. A relatively small positive energy balance can lead to significant weight gain over time. For example, an excess intake of only 100 calories per day will lead to a 10-lb weight gain over 1 year.

2. High Glycemic Index Food as a Cause of Obesity and Increased CV Risks

In addition to the traditional concept of energy balance in the pathogenesis of obesity as discussed earlier, the consumption of high-GI food has emerged an important cause of obesity in recent decades.

Several decades ago, the U.S. government and scientific organizations recommended that people eat low-fat diets to reduce weight gain and improve CV health. However, low-fat diets have not had much effect on the obesity rate. Even though mean fat intake in the United States has decreased since the 1960s (from 42% to 34% of dietary energy), the prevalence of obesity has risen over the past several decades. During this period, people were eating low-fat/high-carbohydrate (CHO) diets. On the other hand, low CHO diets (with more protein and fat), such as the Atkins diet, became popular, appearing to be effective in terms of weight reduction.

Researchers started finding out that the high CHO portion in the diet was respondible for weight gain. CHOs consumed by people following low-fat diets were mostly refined and high in sugar content (i.e., high-GI food). Consumption of high-GI food results in hormonal and metabolic changes that can cause weight gain (as discussed later). A brief review of the concept of the GI (and glycemic load [GL]) follows.

The **glycemic index** is the number given to a food based on how quickly a CHO diet is digested and absorbed into the bloodstream (Jenkins et al., 1981). The amount of glucose absorbed into the blood a in 2-hour period after consuming 50 g of CHO in a given food is compared with the glycemic response after the consumption of 50 g of glucose, which is set at 100. The GI is classified into three categories: (1) low (a GI ≤ 55), (2) medium or intermediate (a GI of 55 to 69), and (3) high (a GI ≥ 70).

Here are some general information about the GI of various food:

1. In general, fruits, vegetables (except potatoes), and legumes have a low-GI, whereas sweets, refined-grain products (e.g., white bread), and potatoes have a high-GI.
2. The presence of fat lowers the GI. A baked potato has a GI of 85, but fried potatoes (French fries) have a GI of 75.
3. The presence of soluble dietary fiber lowers the GI. Whole-wheat breads with higher amounts of fiber generally have a lower GI than white breads.
4. The way food is prepared can change its GI. A boiled potato has a GI of 56, steamed potatoes have a GI of 65, and a microwaved potato has a GI of 82.
5. The ripeness of fruit increases the GI. The GI of underripe bananas is 30, whereas that of overripe bananas is 52.

Glycemic load. One criticism of the GI is that it tells only how rapidly 50 g of CHO in a particular food turns into blood sugar, but it does not tell how much of that CHO is in a serving of a particular food. The GL is a new way of assessing the impact of CHO consumption that takes into account serving size. For example, although candies have a high-GI, eating a single piece of candy, which contains a small fraction of 50 g, will result in a relatively small glycemic response. Thus the GL of the candy is not high. A GL of a typical serving of food is the product of the amount of available CHO in that serving and the GI of the food (calculated by the amount of CHO contained in a specified serving size of the food × the GI of that food ÷ 100). The GL is categorized as follows: (1) high (a GL of ≥20 points) (2) medium (a GL of 11 to 19 points) and (3) low (a GL of ≤10 points).

The higher the food's GL, the greater the expected elevation in blood glucose after consumption. A diet with a low GL has been linked to a lower risk of heart disease. A diet low in CHO automatically has a low GL. Almost all food with a low-GI has a low GL. Table 27.1 shows the GI and GL of selected food. As seen in the table, some foods with high GIs turn out to have low GLs. A more complete list of the GI is periodically published by the American Society for Clinical Nutrition (the official website for the GI is http://www.ajcn.org/content/76/1/5.full).

3. How May High-GI Food Contribute to Weight Gain and Increase CV Risk?

Hormonal and metabolic changes following ingestion of high-GI and low-GI diets in adolescents are shown in Fig. 27.2 (modified from Ludwig et al., 1999).

1. Two important differences observed in blood *glucose* and serum *fatty acid* levels may offer partial explanation for weight gain following consumption of high-GI food (see Fig. 27.2).
   a. Much higher and sustained levels of *glucose* and *insulin* may predispose one to the development of diabetes.
   b. Low glucose levels seen 4 hours after eating high-GI food (reactive hypoglycemia) may trigger hunger sensations and lead to overeating, resulting in weight gain.

TABLE 27.1

GLYCEMIC INDEX AND GLYCEMIC LOAD FOR SELECTED FOODS[a]

FOOD	GI	GL[b]	FOOD	GI	GL[b]
Instant rice	91	24.8 (110 g)	Banana	53	13.3 (170 g)
Baked potato	85	20.3 (110 g)	Corn tortilla	52	12 (50 g)
Cornflakes	81	21 (30 g)	Wheat breads	50	10 (30 g)
French fries	75	22 (150 g)	Brown rice	50	16 (150 g)
Bagel, white	72	25 (70 g)	Orange	48	5 (120 g)
Carrot	71	3.6 (55 g)	Spaghetti	41	16.4 (55 g)
White bread	70	21.0 (2 slices)	Apple	36	8.1 (170 g)
Rye bread	65	19.5 (2 slices)	Lentil beans	29	5.7 (110 g)
Coca-Cola	63	16 (250 g)	Milk	27	3.2 (225 mL)
Sweet corn	60	11 (80 g)	Peanuts	14	0.7 (30 g)

GI, *glycemic index;* GL, *glycemic load.*

[a]From various sources.

[b]The numbers in the parentheses indicate the amount of the food consumed.

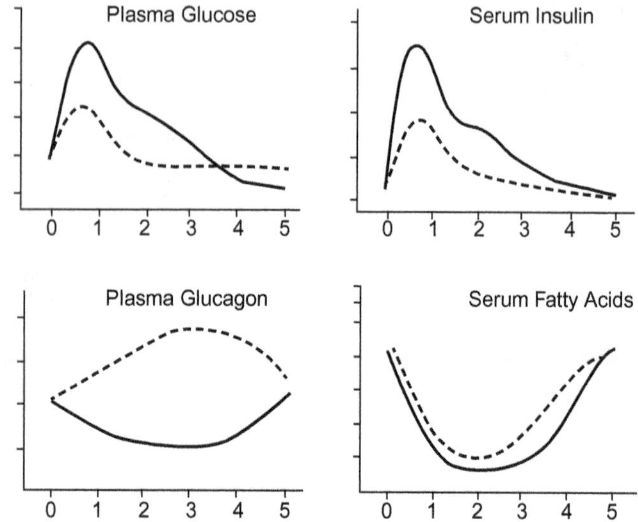

FIG. 27.2

Comparison of hormonal and metabolic changes following ingestion of high glycemic index (GI) and low-GI food in adolescents. The thick lines represent the high-GI food group, and thin broken lines represent the low-GI food group. *(Redrawn from Ludwig, D. S., Majzoub, J. A., Al-Zahrani A., Dallal, G. E., Blanco, I., & Roberts, S. B. (1999). High glycemic index foods, overeating, and obesity.* Pediatrics, 103*(3): E26.)*

   c. Lower levels of serum *fatty acid* seen (2 hours after eating) may mean that insulin forced fat cells to take in fatty acids or a low level of glucagon impaired the breakdown of lipids (lipolysis) in the fat cells. The combined action of high insulin and low glucagon may be fat accumulation and preservation, resulting in weight gain.
2. Consuming high-GI food may also produces the following changes (not shown in Fig. 27.2)
   a. A higher level of growth hormone after eating a high-GI food may also promote weight gain.
   b. Undesirable metabolic effects similar to those seen in metabolic syndrome may result, including raising blood triglyceride (TG) levels, raising LDL-C and lowering HDL-C levels.

4. Why Is Low-GI Food Good for Your Health?

Consumption of low-GI food has been shown to have the following benefits, opposite to those described for high-GI food:

1. No reactive hypoglycemia is seen, and thus people feel fuller and hunger pangs are delayed.

2. The levels of glucose and insulin are much lower, reducing the risk of developing diabetes.
3. Serum fatty acid levels remain higher, which may mean that lipids are not forced into the body cell or that high levels of glucagon made the cells break down fats and made more fatty acids available for the energy system.
4. Serum *growth hormone* levels do not rise after low-GI food, not promoting weight gain.
5. The prevalence of metabolic syndrome is lower in people eating low-GI food, reducing the risk of heart disease and stroke (by reducing TG and LDL-C levels, increasing HDL-C, and reducing plasminogen activator inhibitor).

D. HEALTH CONSEQUENCES OF OBESITY

Obesity in adults is associated with a number of diseases, such as hyperlipidemia, heart disease, hypertension, type 2 diabetes, stroke, osteoarthritis, and so on. Obesity also increases the prevalence of some cancers, gallbladder disease, sleep disorders, gout, and mood disorders. Obesity is also responsible for significant health care costs; approximately 5% of total health care costs (> $100 billions) can be attributed to obesity.

Health consequences of obesity in children differ somewhat from those seen in obese adults (Dietz, 1998) as listed below.

1. Common medical consequences of obesity:
   a. Increased CV risk factors, including hypercholesterolemia (31%), hypertriglyceridemia (64%), and low HDL-C (64%)
   b. Glucose intolerance, which is linked to the recent increase in the prevalence of type 2 diabetes in children.
   c. Hypertension (present in 10% to 30% of overweight children).
   d. Asthma, which is more common in obese children and is more difficult to control than in nonobese children.
   e. Acanthosis nigricans (~25%), an indication of hyperinsulinemia
   f. Hepatic steatosis (fatty degeneration) with elevated liver enzymes (seen in >10% of overweight children), cholelithiasis (due to increased cholesterol synthesis), and cholecystitis (occurring more often with weight reduction).
2. Less common medical consequences of obesity:
   a. Pseudotumor cerebri (with manifestations of headache, visual impairment or blindness, papilledema, occurring before adolescence) requires aggressive treatment. About 50% of children with the condition are obese.
   b. Sleep apnea occurs in <7% of obese children. This requires an aggressive treatment, including tonsillectomy and adenoidectomy or weight reduction.
   c. Orthopedic complications: Blount disease (bowing of the tibia and femur with resulting overgrowth of the medial aspect of the proximal tibial metaphysis) or slipped capital femoral epiphysis.
   d. PCOD: Menstrual abnormalities and hirsutism in association with obesity, acanthosis, hyperinsulinemia, and hyperandrogenemia suggest this condition.

3. Psychosocial consequences:
   a. Early discrimination (in childhood)
   b. Negative self-esteem (in adolescence)
   c. Inappropriate expectation to be more mature because of their large size. This may lead to frustration, a sense of failure, and social isolation.
   d. Learning difficulties
   e. Eating disorders

E. EVALUATION OF OBESE CHILDREN

1. Physicians should consider identifiable underlying causes of obesity, such as genetic or endocrine disorders
   a. Genetic causes: Prader-Willi, Bardet-Biedl, and Alström syndrome all have severe early onset of obesity.
   b. Endocrine abnormalities, such as hypothyroidism, Cushing syndrome, and generalized hypothalamic dysfunction, should be considered.
2. Check for the presence of other risk factors for CVD, diabetes, or metabolic syndrome (see Boxes 27.1 and 27.2), including blood pressure measurement, lipoprotein analysis, fasting insulin, blood glucose, glycosylated hemoglobin (Hb A1C).
3. Search for possible obesity-related complications by history and physical examination, such as those listed below.
   a. Acanthosis nigricans is associated with hyperinsulinemia and a higher risk of developing type 2 diabetes.
   b. Thyroid enlargement may be associated with hypothyroidism.
   c. History of nighttime snoring, breathing difficulties, or daytime somnolence may indicate OSA or obesity hypoventilation syndrome.
   d. Hip or knee pain may be manifestations of slipped capital femoral epiphysis.
   e. Abdominal pain or tenderness may be associated with gallbladder disease
   f. Headaches and blurred optic disc margins may indicate pseudotumor cerebri.
   g. Hepatomegaly may be associated with hepatic steatosis.
   h. Oligomenorrhea, amenorrhea, striae, or hirsutism may indicate PCOD or Cushing syndrome.
   i. Signs of depression, bulimia nervosa, binge-eating disorder, or other serious psychological disorders require further evaluation and treatment by a child psychiatrist or psychologist.

F. MANAGEMENT

All successful pediatric weight management programs include four components: (1) dietary component, (2) exercise, (3) behavior modification, and (4) family. Among these, dietary intervention and regular exercise combined are the cornerstones of the weight management. Only through behavior modification can long-term healthy eating and activity patterns be established; attempts at using diet and exercise for quick weight loss usually fail. Without involvement of the parents and family, behavior modification of children and adolescents is difficult to achieve. Currently there are no pharmacologic agents that are shown to be safe and effective for long-term weight management in children and adolescents. Presently, the U.S. Food and Drug Administration has approved two drugs—sibutramine (Meridia) and orlistat (Xenical)—that may be used for treating severely obese children. Consultations with registered dietitians, psychologists, and/or exercise specialists may be sought or a referral to a multidisciplinary weight management programs may become necessary.

1. Dietary Component

1. The following questions are helpful in assessing dietary habits of the child and family.
   a. How often are vegetables and fruits eaten as a main meal or snack?
   b. How often are high-calorie drinks (soda pops, fruit punches, fruit juices, etc.) consumed?
   c. Number and types of fast food eaten per week?
   d. How often does the child eat fish, chicken, and red meats?
   e. What type of milk, bread, and butter are consumed?
   f. How often are fried foods eaten in a week?
2. The counseling should include at least the following:
   a. The diet of choice is a diet low in saturated fat and cholesterol that includes 5 or more daily servings of vegetables and fruits and 6 to 11 servings of whole-grain and other complex CHO food.
   b. Low-GI diets may be more effective than low-fat diets in reducing weight and improving CV risks (as discussed in earlier sections).
   c. The new Food Guide system—MyPlate—should be introduced. Half of a plate is filled with fruits and vegetables, a quadrant with grains (bread, wheat, rice, etc.), and the last quadrant with protein (meat, poultry, fish, soy, etc.).

2. Physical Activity

Exercise is also an integral part of the management. Without regular exercise, dietary modification alone is insufficient for successful weight management. Physicians should first assess the level of physical activity of overweight children and use their influential position to counsel children and their family to adopt healthy lifestyle.

1. The following topics are useful in assessing physical activity in children:
   a. Amount of time regularly spent walking, bicycling, swimming, and in backyard play.
   b. Use of stairs, playgrounds, and gymnasiums, and interactive physical play with other children.

c. Number of hours per day spent watching television or videotapes and playing video or computer games.
d. Time spent participating in organized sports, lessons, clubs, or league games.
e. Time spent in school physical education that includes a minimum of 30 minutes of exercise.
f. Participation in household chores.
g. Positive role modeling for a physically active lifestyle by parents and other caretakers.

2. Physician counseling and education should include the following areas.
   a. Physicians should formally address the subject of exercise, emphasizing the health benefits of regular physical activity, which include the following:
      (1) Helping weight control by lowering level of weight gain.
      (2) Metabolic benefits including improved glucose tolerance and insulin sensitivity. reduction in very-low-density lipoprotein (VLDL), and rise in HDL-C levels.
      (3) Lowering of blood pressure.
      (4) Improving psychological well-being.
      (5) Predisposition to increased physical activity in adulthood.
   b. Children should participate in at least 30 minutes of moderate physical activity at least 4 or more days of the week, and preferably every day.
   c. Parents should be encouraged to help their children reduce excessive time spent on sedentary behaviors, such as watching television and videotapes, playing on a computer, listening to music, and talking on the phone. The television set should be removed from the child's bedroom.
   d. More physical activity should be part of their lifestyle, such as walking or biking to school instead of driving, skating, stairs instead of elevators, and helping with active chores inside and outside of the house.
   e. Teach parents the importance of being role models for active lifestyle and providing children with opportunities for increased physical activity.

The 5-2-1-0 Message. To help people better understand what constitutes healthy habits for controlling obesity, some simple guidelines have been developed, such as "the 5-2-1-0" message. It was first developed by the New Hampshire Health Department and endorsed by the American Academy of Pediatrics as a basic healthy lifestyle counseling tool. The message is simple to understand and remember and can be given in a few minutes. The 5-2-1-0 message stands for:

5: Eating at least 5 servings of fruits and vegetables most days.
2: Limiting screen time to 2 hours or less daily.
1: Participating in at least one or more hours of physical activity every day.
0: Encouraging no soda and sugar-sweetened drinks. Instead, drink water and low-fat or fat-free milk.

3. Behavior Modification

Behavior modification is essential for permanent changes in dietary and exercise habits. Promotion of long-term permanent changes in behavior patterns, rather than short-term diet or exercise programs for rapid weight loss, should be the goal of the treatment. Emphasis should be on small and gradual behavior changes.

4. Family Involvement

Family involvement is very important in pediatric weight management programs.

1. Willingness on the part of both the child and the family to participate and involvement of the entire family and other caregivers are important.
2. Parents need to learn certain skills and commit themselves to the program.
   a. Parent role modeling of healthful dietary and activity habits.
   b. Understanding the new food guide system MyPlate.
   c. Ability to read food labels.
   d. Understanding the benefits of low-GI food and of reducing consumption of high-GI food and drinks.
   e. Appropriate ways of praising and rewarding good progress.
   f. Changes in family environment, such as removing high-calorie food, reducing the number of meals eaten outside of the home, serving portion-controlled meals to the child, promoting active lifestyles and discouraging sedentary lifestyle, etc.
   g. Inclusion of activities to help families monitor their eating and physical activity behaviors and establishing formal routine exercise program at a scheduled time each day or evening.
   h. Physicians may suggest motivated parents to read books written specifically for them that are available on the market.

The primary emphasis in weight control efforts should be the lifestyle change; the weight loss itself is the secondary importance. Active lifestyle improves risk factors even when weight loss is minimal. When a weight loss goal is set, it should be realistic and should not attempt to fully normalize weight. In children without complications of obesity, maintenance of the current weight or modest weight loss, while children continue to grow in height, reduces their degree of overweight. Children with complications of obesity (e.g., hypertension, hyperlipidemias, insulin resistance, hepatic steatosis) should attempt to lose weight to correct those complications.

IV. CIGARETTE SMOKING

Cigarette smoking is a powerful independent risk factor for myocardial infarction, sudden death, and peripheral vascular disease, in addition to being a major cause of lung cancer. Even passive exposure to smoke causes alterations in the risk factors in children.

A. PREVALENCE

Overall, cigarette smoking among American adults (aged ≥ 18 years) declined from 21% in 2005 to 16% in 2016. Yet nearly 38 million American adults smoke cigarettes. Some recent statistics on the prevalence of smoking among youth are presented below.

1. In 2016, 20% of high school students reported current use of any tobacco product; e-cigarettes were the most commonly used tobacco product (11%) followed by cigarettes (8%) and cigars (7%).
2. Among middle school students, 7% reported current use of any tobacco product; e-cigarettes were the most commonly used tobacco product (4%), followed by cigarettes (3%), and cigars (2%).
3. Among college students, 33% are current users of tobacco products and nearly 50% used tobacco products in the past year.
4. Tobacco use was significantly higher among white students than black students.
5. Nearly 90% of adult smokers began smoking at or before age 18. Two-thirds of adult smokers became everyday smokers at or before age 18.
6. There were smokers in the household in 72% of middle school student smokers and in 58% among high school student smokers.
7. Nearly 50% of middle school student smokers and 62% of high school student smokers reported a desire to stop smoking cigarettes and most of them have made at least one cessation attempt during the past 12 months. On the other hand, among students who have never smoked cigarettes, 21% of middle school students and 23% of high school students were susceptible to initiating cigarette smoking in the next year.

B. PATHOPHYSIOLOGIC EFFECTS OF SMOKING

The following are some pathophysiologic effects of smoking on the cardiovascular system, all of which appear likely to be involved in accelerating atherosclerosis in the coronary artery and peripheral arteries or increasing the probability of thrombosis (with potential for stroke). Physicians could use this information in counseling session with smokers.

1. Smoking causes atherogenic dyslipidemia. It increases levels of LDL and VLDL cholesterols and TGs and lowers HDL-C. Even passive smoking lowers HDL-C.
2. Smoking contributes to a prothrombotic predisposition by (a) increasing levels of fibrinogen, factor VII and decreasing the concentration of plasminogen, and (b) activating platelets to increase their ability to adhere to the vessel wall.
3. Smoking increases blood viscosity by increasing hemoglobin levels (by an increase in carboxyhemoglobin) and by an elevation of plasma fibrinogen levels.
4. Smoking accelerates atherosclerotic process by (a) increasing monocyte adhesion to endothelial cell, (b) decreasing nitric oxide synthesis (with

resulting endothelial dysfunction), and (c) decreasing synthesis of prostacyclin.
5. Smoking causes peripheral arterial disease through endothelial dysfunction.
6. Smoking raises blood pressure transiently, raises heart rate, and increases myocardial contractility and myocardial oxygen consumption (by stimulation of sympathetic nervous system).

C. PSYCHOSOCIOLOGY OF SMOKING

Physicians should be aware of the psychosociology of initiating smoking to help prevent smoking in children.

1. Most smoking starts during adolescence. The high-risk period is transition from elementary school to middle school and the first and second years of middle school. This should be the target age group to counsel individually or through school systems.
2. Known predictors of smoking include peer influence (the most important), family members who smoke (siblings and parents), less educated parents, being a more independent and rebellious child, and having less academic success.
3. Cited reasons for starting to smoke include wanting to fit into a group, to lose weight, and to appear more mature.

D. MANAGEMENT

Physicians and health care professionals should assess the status of smoking, provide smoking prevention messages, help counsel parents and children about smoking cessation, and also encourage school and community anti-smoking efforts.

1. Physicians should assess the status of smoking during office visits.
   a. Smoking history should be obtained in all children older than 8 years during routine health assessments and updated. History regarding any siblings and friends who smoke should also be obtained.
   b. For current smokers, onset of smoking, number and type of cigarettes smoked per day, week or month, and whether they want to quit smoking and need help to quit the habit.
   c. Smoking history should also be obtained for parents and be updated.
2. Parents who smoke should be encouraged to quit. Physicians should emphasize adverse effects of passive smoking on their children and that they should be a role model for their children. Physicians should refer parent smokers to community smoking cessation programs.
3. The physician's office should be nonsmoking environment (without ashtrays), and antismoking posters, pamphlets, and videos in the waiting room may be productive.
4. Counseling techniques may vary with the age of the child.
   a. For elementary school children, antismoking message at each well child assessment may counterbalance any negative prosmoking

TABLE 27.2

SUMMARY GUIDELINES FOR PREVENTIVE PEDIATRIC CARDIOLOGY

RISK IDENTIFICATION	TREATMENT GOALS	RECOMMENDATIONS
Blood Cholesterol Total cholesterol: > 170 mg/dL is borderline: > 200 mg/dL is elevated LDL-C: > 110 mg/dL is borderline > 130 mg/dL is elevated.	LDL-C: < 130 mg/dL (<110 mg/dL is even better) For patients with diabetes, LDL-C <100 mg/dL	If LDL-C is above goals, initiate additional therapeutic lifestyle changes, including diet (<7% of calories from saturated fat; <200 mg cholesterol per day), in conjunction with a trained dietitian. Consider LDL-lowering dietary options (increase soluble fiber by using age [in years] plus 5 to 10 g up to age 15, when the total remains at 25 g per day) in conjunction with a trained dietitian. Emphasize weight management and increased physical activity. If LDL-C is persistently above goals, evaluate for secondary causes (TSH, LFT, renal function tests, urinalysis). Consider pharmacologic therapy for individuals with LDL >190 mg/dL with no other risk factors for CVD; or >160 mg/dL with other risk factors present (BP elevation, diabetes, obesity, strong family history of premature CVD). Pharmacologic intervention for dyslipidemia should be accomplished in collaboration with a physician experienced in treatment of disorders of cholesterol in pediatric patients.
Other Lipids and Lipoprotein TGs: > 100 mg/dL is elevated for <10 yr > 130 mg/dL is elevated for >10 yr HDL-C: < 40 mg/dL is reduced	Fasting TGs: < 75 mg/dL for <10 yr < 90 mg/dL for >10 yr HDL-C >40 mg/dL	Elevated fasting TG and reduced HDL-C are often seen in the context of overweight with insulin resistance. Therapeutic lifestyle change should include weight management with appropriate energy intake and expenditure. Decrease intake of simple sugars. If fasting TGs are persistently elevated, evaluate for secondary causes such as diabetes, thyroid disease, renal disease, and alcohol abuse. No pharmacologic interventions are recommended in children for isolated elevation of fasting TG unless this is very marked. Treatment may be initiated at TG >400 mg/dL to protect against postprandial TG of ≥ 1000 mg/dL, which may be associated with an increased risk of pancreatitis.

TABLE 27.2 *(continued)*

SUMMARY GUIDELINES FOR PREVENTIVE PEDIATRIC CARDIOLOGY

RISK IDENTIFICATION	TREATMENT GOALS	RECOMMENDATIONS
BP Systolic and diastolic pressure >95th percentile for age, sex, and height percentile.	Systolic and diastolic BP <90th percentile for age, sex, and height	Promote achievement of appropriate weight. Reduce sodium in the diet. Emphasize increased consumption of fruits and vegetables. If BP is persistently above the 95th percentile, consider possible secondary causes (e.g., renal disease, coarctation of the aorta). Consider pharmacologic therapy for individuals above the 95th percentile if lifestyle modification brings no improvement and there is evidence of target organ changes (LVH, microalbuminuria, retinal vascular abnormalities). Start BP medication individualized to other patient requirements and characteristics (e.g., age, race, need for drugs with specific benefits). Pharmacologic management of hypertension should be accomplished in collaboration with a physician experienced in pediatric hypertension.
Weight BMI: 85th to 95th percentile is overweight $> 95^{th}$ percentile is obese	Achieve and maintain BMI <95th percentile for age and sex	For children who are overweight (> 85th percentile) or obese (> 95th percentile), a weight management program should be initiated with appropriate energy balance achieved through changes in diet and physical activity. Use the 5-2-1-0 message and MyPlate for education and counseling. For children of normal height, a secondary cause of obesity is unlikely. Weight management should be directed at all family members who are overweight, using a family-centered, behavioral management approach. Weight management should be done in collaboration with a trained dietitian.

27

TABLE 27.2 *(continued)*

SUMMARY GUIDELINES FOR PREVENTIVE PEDIATRIC CARDIOLOGY

RISK IDENTIFICATION	TREATMENT GOALS	RECOMMENDATIONS
Diabetes Fasting plasma glucose: ≥126 mg/dL	Near-normal fasting plasma glucose (<120 mg/dL) Near-normal Hg A1c (<7%)	Management of type 1 and type 2 diabetes in children and adolescents should be accomplished in collaboration with a pediatric endocrinologist. For type 2 diabetes, the first step is weight management with improved diet and exercise. Because of risk for accelerated vascular disease, other risk factors (e.g., BP, lipid abnormalities) should be treated more aggressively in patients with diabetes.
Cigarette Smoking	Complete cessation of smoking for children and parents who smoke	Advise every tobacco user (parents and children) to quit and be prepared to provide assistance with this (counseling/referral to develop a plan for quitting using available community resources to help with smoking cessation).

BMI, body mass index; *BP*, blood pressure; *CVD*, cardiovascular disease; *HDL-C*, high-density lipoprotein cholesterol; *LDL-C*, low-density lipoprotein cholesterol; *LFT*, liver function test; *LVH*, left ventricular hypertrophy; *TGs*, triglycerides; *TSH*, thyroid-stimulating hormone.

Modified from Kavey, R-E. W., Daniels, S. R., Lauer, R. M., et al. (2003). American Heart Association guidelines for primary prevention of atherosclerotic cardiovascular disease beginning in childhood. *Circulation, 107* (11), 1562–1566.

influences exerted by friends or family. Emphasize the harmful physical consequences of smoking and the addictive nature of cigarettes. Parental assistance in the child's cessation of smoking should also be sought.

b. For adolescents, emphasis should be on current negative physiologic and social effects of smoking than long-term health consequence. Adolescents understand the health consequences of smoking but see them as remote and irrelevant. The more immediate negative effects, such as bad breath, smelling like smoke, yellow-stained fingers, smell from clothing and hair, increasing heart rate and blood pressure, lack of stamina for sports, shortness of breath, and so on should be emphasized.

5. Some adolescents will quit smoking on the advice of their physician and a cessation message as brief as 3 minutes may be effective. Many adolescents will require repeated efforts to quit smoking. Physicians should also encourage activities that tend to preclude cigarette smoking, such as regular physical activity and a variety of school and after-school activities.

1. Pharmacologic Approach

Currently there is insufficient evidence for the effectiveness of pharmacologic treatments with young smokers. The available experimental studies of youth cessation intervention find that behavioral interventions increase the chances of young smokers achieving successful cessation.

For established adult smokers, if counseling is ineffective, physicians may try nicotine replacement and bupropion to help them quit smoking.

1. Nicotine replacement (by nitotine polacrilex gum or transdermal patch) delivers less nicotine than does cigarette smoking, which delivers a bolus of nicotine. It also eliminates carbon monoxide inhalation.
2. Bupropion, an antidepressant, stimulates dopamine release and curbs the severe withdrawal symptoms of smoking cessation.
3. Other medications, such as varenicline, clonidine, have mixed reviews on beneficial effects and side effects in adults, but they are not approved for use in children and adolescents.

V. PRACTICE OF PREVENTIVE CARDIOLOGY

The AHA has published a guideline for the prevention of CVD. The guideline is a handy summary that presents goals and recommendations for reducing risks in children and adolescents for future CVD (Table 27.2).

PART VII

CARDIAC SURGICAL PATIENTS

Chapter 28

Pre- and Postoperative Management

The current trend is to carry out total repair of CHDs at an early age whenever such repair is technically possible. Early total repair may obviate the need for palliative procedures. This may also prevent pulmonary vascular disease or permanent damages to the CV system, which is known to develop in certain CHDs. However, recommendations for the timing and type of operation vary from institution to institution. The improved results currently seen with pediatric cardiac surgery are in part attributed to improved operative techniques and cardiopulmonary bypass (CPB) methods. In addition, the coordinated multidisciplinary approach has contributed to significant decrease in perioperative morbidity and mortality.

Open heart procedures use CPB with some degree of hypothermia and a varying duration of low flow or circulatory arrest. Open procedures are required for repair of intracardiac anomalies (e.g., VSD, TOF, TGA). Closed procedures do not require CPB; they are performed for repair of extracardiac anomalies (e.g., COA, PDA) or palliative procedures (e.g., B-T shunt procedures or PA banding). The following sections outline some basic aspects of pre- and postoperative management of cardiac patients for pediatricians.

I. PREOPERATIVE MANAGEMENT

Good preoperative preparation, including complete delineation of cardiac anatomy and assessment of hemodynamics, is mandatory for a smooth operative and postoperative course. Some infants require preoperative stabilization with prostaglandin E_1 (continuous intravenous [IV] drip at 0.01–0.1 μg/kg/min) to maintain ductus arteriosus patency, whereas others may need inotropic and lusitropic support. Patients with TGA and restrictive PFO may require balloon atrial septostomy.

1. All children should have a careful history and physical examination within a few days before the procedure. This is to gain full understanding of chronic medical problems (e.g., renal dysfunction, asthma) and to uncover acute medical problems (e.g., upper and lower respiratory, and urinary tract infections) that would mandate rescheduling of elective surgeries.
2. Laboratory evaluation
   a. Complete blood cell count, urinalysis, and comprehensive metabolic panel, including serum electrolytes and glucose, liver enzymes, blood urea nitrogen (BUN), and serum creatinine, of all cardiac patients are routinely obtained.

   b. Chest radiography and electrocardiogram (ECG) of all patients are obtained.
   c. Cardiac computed tomography angiography (CTA) or magnetic resonance imaging (MRI) if needed to complete the anatomic assessment.
   d. Head and renal ultrasound is performed in most neonates with congenital heart defects. Preoperative brain MRI for patients with complex congenital heart defects is recommended.
   e. For open heart procedures, blood coagulation studies—prothrombin time (PT), activated partial thromboplastin time (aPTT), and platelet count—are obtained.
   f. If necessary, blood should be collected for chromosome studies (karyotyping, fluorescence *in situ* hybridization [e.g., FISH for chromosome 22q11.2 deletion syndrome—DiGeorge syndrome], and DNA microarray) preoperatively.
   g. Check for chromosome 22q11.2 deletion syndrome (DiGeorge syndrome, and DNA microarray) preoperatively.
3. Patients undergoing CPB whose weight is more than 3.5 kg are cross-matched for four units of packed red blood cells (PRBCs) and those weighing less for two units of whole blood. One to two units of PRBCs are cross-matched for those undergoing closed procedures. One to four units of platelets are needed for the procedure additionally. Irradiated blood products will be required for immunocompromised patients (e.g., patients with suspected or confirmed chromosome 22q11.2 deletion).
4. Medications
   a. Angiotensin-converting enzyme (ACE) inhibitors are withheld 24 hours prior to the planned surgery in an effort to minimize anesthesia-induced refractory hypotension during anesthesia induction.
   b. Diuretics are discontinued 8 to 12 hours preoperatively (or this may be individualized).
   c. Digoxin is discontinued after the evening dose.
   d. Antiarrhythmic agents are continued at the same dosage until immediately before the surgery.
   e. Nonsteroidal antiinflammatory drugs (e.g., aspirin, ibuprofen) and antiplatelet drugs (e.g., dipyridamole) are discontinued 7 to 10 days prior to surgery.
   f. Warfarin is discontinued 4 days prior to the planned operation. If the patient is at high risk for thromboembolism, continuous heparin drip is started 2 days prior to the operation and the infusion rate is adjusted to maintain an aPTT of 60 to 85 sec.
5. **Prevention of infection**. Broad-spectrum antibiotics are used to decrease the risk of perioperative infection. Duration of antibiotic regimen is institution dependent but can be individualized based on the patient's age, condition, and comorbidities.

a. Vancomycin, 10–15 mg/kg/dose IV every 6 to 8 hours (maximum dose 4 g/day).
b. Clindamycin, 10 mg/kg/dose (adolescents/adults: 600 mg/dose) IV every 6 to 8 hours, starting immediately prior to surgery, is the recommended regimen at some institutions.
c. Neonates who already receiving ampicillin and gentamicin continue to take these drugs.
d. Thin layer of mupirocin 2% ointment is applied to both nostrils to prevent methicillin-resistant *Staphylococcus aureus* (MRSA) colonization.

6. For older children, the emotional preparation for surgery is as important as the physical preparation.

II. POSTOPERATIVE CARE OF CARDIAC PATIENTS

A high level of vigilance for signs of complications should be maintained during the postoperative period so that appropriate therapy can be initiated early.

A. NORMAL CONVALESCENCE

Physicians should be familiar with the postoperative course of normally recovering patients in order to recognize abnormal convalescence.

1. **General care**. Successful postoperative management requires accurate monitoring and documentation of the patient's vital signs, medication administration, and laboratory results. Vital signs including heart rate, arterial or noninvasive blood pressure (BP), oxygen saturation, and respiratory rate are monitored closely (e.g., every 15 to 60 min). Urine and chest tube outputs, end-tidal or transcutaneous CO_2, central venous pressure, and, at times, right and left atrial and pulmonary arterial pressures are recorded meticulously. All administered medications, enteral or parenteral fluids, and blood products are documented. Fluid balance is monitored continuously. Laboratory results and their trends are charted for review electronically.
2. Pulmonary system
   a. Arterial blood gases are in the acceptable normal range.
   b. Chest radiography shows no evidence of pneumothorax, atelectasis, pleural effusion, or elevation of hemidiaphragm.
3. Cardiovascular system
   a. Warm skin, full peripheral pulses with brisk capillary refill, normal BP, and an adequate urine output (at least 1 mL/kg/hr) are clinical evidence of good cardiac output. Decrease in expected systemic venous saturation is a sensitive predictor of low cardiac output. A normal systemic arterial-to-venous oxygen saturation difference of less than 30% is indicative of good cardiac output.
   b. Mild arterial hypertension is present in the early postoperative period following CPB (due to increased levels of catecholamines, plasma renin, or angiotensin II).

TABLE 28.1

HEART RATE RANGES IN NORMALLY CONVALESCING POSTOPERATIVE PATIENTS

AGE	HEART RATE (BEATS/MIN)
Less than 6 months	110 to 190
6 to 12 months	100 to 170
1 to 3 years	90 to 160
Over 3 years	80 to 150

   c. Cardiac rhythm should be sinus and the heart rate relatively high. Ranges of heart rates in normally convalescing postoperative patients are shown in Table 28.1.
4. **Renal system**. Adequate urine output (i.e., >1 mL/kg/hr) and evidence of adequate solute excretion (e.g., serum K^+ <5 mEq/L; BUN <40 mg/dL; creatinine <1 mg/dL) are signs of normal renal function.
5. Metabolic system
   a. Retention of water and sodium and depletion of whole-body potassium are commonly seen following open heart surgeries. They result in mild hyponatremia and hypokalemia, and a 5% weight gain. In anticipation of fluid overload, mechanical ultrafiltration is performed in selected cases intraoperatively.
   b. Mild metabolic acidosis (with a base deficit of −4 mEq/L) associated with mild lactic acidemia is common in the first few hours after CPB and does not usually require treatment.
   c. Varying degrees of fever are nearly always present during the first few days, and extensive workup for infection is not indicated. Causes of fever include reaction to CPB, reaction to allogenic blood, atelectasis, pleural effusion, low cardiac output, infection, and brainstem damage.
6. **Gastrointestinal (GI) system**. As the splanchnic circulation receives over 25% of total cardiac output, avoidance of low cardiac output syndrome is the principal strategy to avoid GI dysfunction. Feedings are started after the patient becomes hemodynamically stable and are advanced as tolerated. Daily caloric count and its adjustment are crucial. H_2-receptor antagonists (famotidine, 0.25 mg/kg/dose every 12 hours, maximum pediatric dose of 40 mg/day) or protein pump inhibitors (e.g., esomeprazole 0.5–1 mg/kg/dose IV every 24 hours, maximum pediatric dose 20 mg/day) are initiated for gastric protection.
7. **Hematologic system**. Results of clotting studies should be normal, and hemoglobin should be at least 9.5 g/dL or higher depending on the patient's age, cardiac anatomy, and surgical procedure.
8. **Neurologic system**. The patient should respond appropriately for the level of sedation without evidence of neurologic defects (e.g., hemiplegia, visual field defects) or seizures. Near-infrared spectroscopy

(NIRS) for transcranial cerebral oximetry is a noninvasive method to monitor frontal lobe oxygen metabolism. Cerebral oxygen saturation, measured by NIRS, is a composite of the oxygen saturation in combined cerebral arterial and venous vascular bed (arterial and venous blood flow ratio of ≈25:75, with negligible capillary blood). It is a helpful method to detect cerebral hypoxia during low cardiac output states.

B. CARE FOLLOWING UNCOMPLICATED OPERATION

Postoperative care in congenital cardiac surgery is unique due to the complexity and heterogeneity of cardiac defects and the wide age range of patients. Furthermore, the guidelines for postoperative management differ from institution to institution, making this task even more complicated. Although the following recommendations are only one set of these guidelines, one aspect of successful management remains the same: anticipation of possible complications (e.g., decrease of cardiac index 6 to 12 hours postoperatively; pulmonary hypertension in association with particular defects; arrhythmias after specific surgeries, etc.).

1. General care
   a. Fluid replacement: Because of the tendency to retain sodium and water, a minimal amount of dextrose in water without ($D_{10}W$ in infants, D_5W in children) or with only a small amount of sodium (D_{10} {1/4}NS, D_5 {1/4}NS) is administered for approximately 48 hours after surgery. A modest amount of potassium (e.g., KCl, 4 mEq/100 mL IV fluids) is given on the first day of surgery. Recommended fluid volume in the first 24 hours after open procedures is 50% of maintenance volume with gradual increase over the following postoperative days to 60% and then to 75%.
   b. The patient should receive medications for adequate analgesia and sedation. For pain relief fentanyl (IV drip at 1 to 3 μg/kg/hr or 1 to 2 μg/kg/dose IV every 30 to 60 min) or morphine sulfate (IV drip at 0.01 to 0.05 mg/kg/hr or 0.1 to 0.2 mg/kg/dose IV every 2 to 4 hours, maximum dose 15 mg/dose) are commonly used. Sedation is achieved by administration of midazolam (0.05 to 0.15 mg/kg/dose IV every 1 to 2 hours or IV drip at 1 to 2 μg/kg/min) or other benzodiazepams. Another medication used for sedation and/or analgesia includes dexmedetomidine a selective α_2-adrenergic receptor agonist with minimal risk of respiratory depression, which is infused continuously at a rate of 0.2 to 1.5 μg/kg/hr after a loading dose of 0.1 to 1 μg/kg IV over 10 min.
2. Pulmonary system
   a. Extubated patients should show no signs of respiratory distress (grunting, nasal flaring, and retraction). Good chest expansion and evidence of good air exchange to both lungs should be present. Depending on the hemodynamics or cardiopulmonary pathophysiology, patients may be administered supplemental oxygen via nasal cannula or face mask. Pulmonary physiotherapy (consisting of incentive spirometry, coughing and deep breathing

exercise, and chest percussion with postural drainage) is administered as necessary.

b. In intubated patients, chest radiographs are obtained to check the position of chest tubes and central and arterial lines and to check for evidence of pneumothorax, atelectasis, pleural effusion, or main-stem bronchus intubation. Significant degrees of pneumothorax or pleural effusion may require treatment. Widening of the mediastinal shadow suggests accumulation of blood and requires investigation of the function of the mediastinal chest tube.

c. In the first postoperative days, the goal of ventilation is to maintain adequate arterial partial pressure of oxygen (Pao_2) and mild respiratory alkalosis along with an arterial partial pressure of carbon dioxide ($Paco_2$) between 28 and 35 mm Hg (all to decrease PVR). Hyperventilation ($Paco_2$ <28 mm Hg) is corrected by decreasing the ventilator rate, decreasing the tidal volume, and adding dead space (5 to 10 mL at a time) to the airway. Hypoventilation is corrected by the opposite maneuvers. Low Pao_2 is corrected by raising the Fio_2, adding positive-end expiratory pressure (PEEP), or increasing tidal volume. Physiologic PEEP of 3 to 5 cm H_2O is used in children. The use of high mean airway pressure or high levels of PEEP may increase PVR and decrease cardiac output; both should be avoided in a patient who has had atrial switch operation (i.e., Senning, Mustard procedure) or cavopulmonary anastomosis (i.e., Glenn or Fontan operation).

d. Tracheal toilet is carried out through the endotracheal tube every 2 hours, or more often if necessary. It consists of instillation of 0.5 to 5 mL of saline solution and suctioning of both main-stem bronchi and bag ventilation for 1 to 2 min with oxygen (Fio_2 1) immediately before and after suctioning.

e. Extubation is performed as soon as possible, usually in the operating room in children undergoing closed procedures, within 4 to 8 hours after uncomplicated open heart procedures, and the day after complex open procedures. Criteria for extubation include the following:
   (1) The patient should be awake and alert, and should have a favorable nutritional status.
   (2) The patient should be breathing well, with a satisfactory spontaneous respiratory rate for age and no use of accessory respiratory muscles. Ideally, vital capacity should be more than 15 mL/kg. On minimal ventilatory support (Fio_2 no more than 0.4, tidal volume at 8 to 10 mL/kg, and PEEP no more than 5 cm H_2O), there should be adequate Pao_2 and no evidence of acidosis or hypercapnia.
   (3) The patient should be in a reasonable and stable hemodynamic state (normal BP, adequate cardiac output, no significant arrhythmias). There should be no significant pneumothoraces or pleural effusions. The patient should not have important bleeding and should have minimal chest tube drainage.

(4) Postextubation laryngeal edema is treated with racemic epinephrine (2.25% solution; 0.125 to 0.5 mL diluted with 3 mL of water or normal saline solution given via nebulizer).

f. Postoperative *pulmonary hypertensive crisis* leads to decreased cardiac output and, if untreated, may be fatal. The best strategy is prevention. Measures to prevent pulmonary hypertensive crisis are important for patients who had severe pulmonary arterial hypertension preoperatively. The following are recommended:

(1) Adequate analgesia and sedation.

(2) Paralysis by vecuronium bromide (continuous IV drip at 0.05 to 0.15 mg/kg/hr or intermittent IV infusion of 0.05 to 0.1 mg/kg/dose every 60 min) or pancuronium bromide (continuous IV drip at 0.02 to 0.1 mg/kg/hr or intermittent IV infusion of 0.05 to 0.1 mg/kg/dose every 30 to 60 min).

(3) Supplemental oxygen.

(4) Avoidance of hypercapnia.

(5) Low PEEP.

(6) Maintaining alkalotic pH.

(7) Avoidance of deep and vigorous tracheal aspiration.

(8) Administration of inhaled nitric oxide (selective pulmonary vasodilator) at 5 to 40 ppm (usual range 5 to 20 ppm).

(9) Intravenous vasodilators (α-adrenergic antagonists, phosphodiesterase inhibitors, nitrovasodilators, and prostaglandins) may be considered. However, it should be noted that essentially all these agents dilate the systemic vasculature as well, leading to systemic hypotension.

3. **Cardiovascular system**. Complete correction of the intracardiac defect and adequate intraoperative myocardial protection generally will result in good cardiac function. Signs of reduced cardiac output, abnormal BPs, abnormal heart rate, and abnormal rhythm should be monitored continually.

a. *Low cardiac output syndrome* (LCOS) is the most serious condition of abnormal convalescence. Signs of LCOS include systemic vasoconstriction (poor perfusion, cold extremities, weak pulses), resting tachycardia, oliguria, pulmonary venous congestion (rales, rhonchi), and systemic venous congestion (hepatomegaly, anasarca, ascites). Systemic hypotension may be a late result of LCOS and is an ominous sign. Means to evaluate for LCOS include mixed venous oximetry, NIRS, serial lactate levels, and transthoracic or transesophageal echocardiography. Laboratory findings of LCOS may include metabolic acidosis, lactic acidemia, azotemia, reduced creatinine clearance, rising serum K^+, decreased partial central venous pressure of oxygen (Pvo_2) below 30 mm Hg from RA or central venous line, and increased arterial-to-venous oxygen saturation difference of more than 40%.

b. Inadequate cardiac output may be caused by (1) low preload, (2) high afterload, (3) depressed myocardial contractility, (4) cardiac tamponade, (5) arrhythmias including sinus bradycardia or sinus tachycardia, (6) inadequate surgical repair, (7) pulmonary hypertension, and (8) insufficient ventilation. Treatment is directed at the cause.

(1) Low preload may be due to intravascular volume depletion (manifested by decreased RA and LA pressures) or due to diminished blood flow to LV (e.g., pulmonary venous obstruction, PA hypertension, PS, or RV failure in the absence of adequate intraarterial shunting; evident by elevated RA and decreased LA pressure). In the case of MS, which also decreases LV preload, RA and LA pressures are both elevated. Although all these conditions ultimately reduce the LV preload and subsequently the cardiac output, treatment is specific to each condition. Low intravascular volume is treated with IV crystalloid or colloid to increase the intravascular volume to raise central venous pressure to 10 to 15 mm Hg. Other conditions are treated by eliminating the cause.

(2) High afterload (with increased SVR) may be caused by hypoxia, acidosis, hypothermia, or pain. In addition to the correction of the cause, the elevated SVR is treated with afterload reduction.

  (a) Phosphodiesterase inhibitors (e.g., milrinone) play a crucial role in treatment of LCOS. They not only have a vasodilatory effect, but also lusitropic and inotropic effects without being significantly arrhythmogenic. These effects occur without an increase in myocardial oxygen consumption. Milrinone is usually initiated in the operating room and is continued as an IV drip at a rate of 0.1 to 1 μg/kg/min (usual range 0.25 to 0.75 μg/kg/min) postoperatively.

  (b) Nitroprusside (IV drip at 0.3 to 10 μg/kg/min) or nitroglycerin (IV drip at 0.5 to 6 μg/kg/min) can be used to further reduce elevated SVR. Both agents have a favorable effect on PVR. In addition, nitroglycerin is a potent coronary vasodilator, which may be beneficial after arterial switch operation.

  (c) Phenoxybenzamine, a long-acting α-adrenergic blocking agent, is used in selected postoperative patients.

(3) Depressed myocardial contractility (demonstrated by echo) may be treated by optimizing arterial oxygen saturation; by addressing anemia, hypocalcemia, and/or acidemia; and by administration of inotropic agents. The optimal oxygenation is achieved by maintaining a patent airway with good respiratory care, adjusting FIO_2 if necessary, reducing pulmonary shunting by the use of PEEP, and reducing pulmonary edema by the use of diuretics. The following inotropic agents among others may be used:

  (a) Epinephrine (continuous IV drip at a rate of 0.01–0.05 μg/kg/min; low dose to minimize undesirable α-agonist effects).

(b) Dopamine (continuous IV drip, starting at 2.5 μg/kg/min and increasing up to 10 μg/kg/min if necessary).

(c) Milrinone (by inhibition of type III phosphodiesterase increases intracellular cyclic adenosine monophosphate [cAMP], which ultimately augments myocardial contractility) is started with or without a loading dose of 50 μg/kg and is maintained at an infusion rate of 0.1 to 1 μg/kg/min.

(4) Cardiac tamponade is treated with urgent decompression of the pericardial space. Early cardiac tamponade results from persistent surgical bleeding not properly drained by the chest tubes; it may even occur when the pericardium is removed or left widely open. It must be suspected when the chest tube drainage abruptly decreases or stops in a patient with previously significant bleeding. Characteristically, the patient is tachycardic and hypotensive with narrowed pulse pressure. Atrial pressures are elevated. Response to volume administration and inotropic agents is minimal. Chest radiographs show widening of the cardiac silhouette. Echo demonstrates pericardial effusion and diastolic collapse of the RA and RV, sensitive indicators of tamponade. Cardiac tamponade requires prompt pericardiocentesis or surgical exploration for evacuation of the pericardial hematoma or control of bleeding by urgent opening of the sternotomy, often in the intensive care unit.

(5) Sinus bradycardia or tachycardia may be detrimental in a postoperative patient with limited cardiac reserve.

(a) Attention to detail is necessary to unmask secondary causes of sinus bradycardia, such as medication interaction, hypoxia, hypoglycemia, electrolyte imbalance, increased intracranial pressure, and hypothyroidism. Injury to the sinus node or its artery, particularly during Fontan procedure or atrial switch operations (Senning and Mustard), may occur and result in persistent sinus bradycardia. If necessary, patients are treated with atrial and/or ventricular pacing, or chronotropic agents. Atrial and ventricular pacing wires are usually placed at the time of open heart procedures and are left postoperatively until the desired heart rate and AV synchrony are returned, maintained, and verified.

(b) Extreme sinus tachycardia is treated by eliminating causes (e.g., pain, anemia, fever, volume depletion, chronotropic agents). Administration of catecholamines should be minimized, as excessive tachycardia increases myocardial oxygen consumption. Furthermore, tachycardia shortens the diastolic period and consequently reduces coronary blood flow.

(c) Treatments of other arrhythmias are described in a section to follow.

(6) Revision of surgical repair is occasionally indicated when an inadequate repair (such as a large residual L-R shunt or significant residual COA) is the cause of low cardiac output. Echo and, if necessary, cardiac catheterization may reveal a residual defect and its significance.

(7) Pulmonary hypertensive crisis is characterized by an acute rise in PA pressure followed by a reduction in cardiac output and a fall in arterial oxygen saturation. It occurs in neonates and infants who had CHDs with pulmonary hypertension (e.g., complete ECD, persistent truncus arteriosus), often after vigorous suctioning of the endotracheal tube. It is difficult to treat and may be fatal; prevention is critically important (see "General care" earlier in this chapter). Treatment includes sedation, paralysis, supplemental oxygen, and inhaled nitric oxide.

(8) Inadequate ventilation secondary to hemothorax, pleural effusion, or pneumothorax should be searched for and if necessary treated, such as with replacement of chest tube or even return to the operation room to manage possible hemorrhage.

c. Hypotension and hypertension

(1) Hypotension due to low intravascular volume, recognized by low RA (central venous) and LA pressure, is treated as follows:

(a) Volume expanders or PRBCs are given as an IV bolus (initially 5 to 10 mL/kg, up to 20 mL/kg). As transfused citrated blood binds ionized calcium, replacement of calcium is necessary in maintaining BP and cardiac output.

(b) Inotropic agents are used if volume expansion fails to raise BP.

(c) Vasopressin (IV drip at 0.0003 to 0.01 U/kg/min) may be considered in patients with adequate myocardial function but with severe vasodilatory hypotension.

(2) Severe hypertension is treated with vasodilators (see "Low cardiac output syndrome" earlier in this chapter).

d. **Rhythm disorders**. Sinus rhythm and maintenance of AV synchrony are optimal. Junctional rhythm may reduce cardiac output by 10% to 15%. In addition to the specific treatment for arrhythmias, possible causes should be investigated and corrected (e.g., oxygenation status, acid-base status, electrolyte imbalance, arrhythmogenic medications). If the patient is hemodynamically unstable, defibrillation or synchronized cardioversion should not be delayed.

(1) Infrequent and isolated PACs or PVCs are followed without intervention.

(2) Paroxysmal SVT (AV node and accessory pathway re-entry tachycardia) is treated with the drug of choice, adenosine (rapid IV bolus of 0.1 mg/kg/dose followed by rapid saline flush; if unsuccessful subsequent doses can be increased to 0.2 mg/kg). Intermittent episodes of SVT are treated with IV amiodarone (loading dose: 5 to 10 mg/kg over 20 to 60 minutes, followed by IV drip at a rate of 5 to 15 μg/kg/min or IV boluses of 2.5 mg/kg every 6 hours). Persistent SVT may also be treated with overdrive suppression or synchronized cardioversion. In more resistant cases, other medications, such as IV β-receptor blockers, verapamil, procainamide, and digoxin, may be used with caution (taking into account myocardial function, BP stability, ventricular preexcitation, etc.). Oral β-receptor blockers, flecainide, or sotalol can be used in more chronic and stable patients.

(3) Other SVTs (multifocal atrial tachycardia or ectopic atrial tachycardia) are treated by ventricular rate control with medications such as amiodarone, β-receptor blockers, calcium channel blockers, or digoxin.

(4) Atrial flutter is treating with overdrive atrial pacing (through esophageal or intraoperatively placed temporary atrial leads) or synchronized cardioversion. Procainamide (loading dose: 2 to 6 mg/kg, maximum dose 100 mg/dose followed by IV continuous drip at 20 to 80 μg/kg/min, maximum 2 g/day) and/or digoxin is the pharmacologic approach for this condition.

(5) Atrial fibrillation is a rare condition in the acute postoperative pediatric cardiac population; nevertheless, it is treated with amiodarone, sotalol, or flecainide (in stable patients) or cardioversion (in hemodynamically compromised patients). If unsuccessful, ventricular rate control is the management of choice.

(6) Postoperative junctional ectopic tachycardia (JET), the most common significant postoperative tachycardia, is discussed in detail in Chapter 29.

(7) Frequent PVCs, if hemodynamically significant, are managed with avoidance of arrhythmogenic drugs, optimizing homodynamic status, or correction of electrolyte imbalance (especially magnesium), hypoxia, and acidemia, and are suppressed with lidocaine (IV bolus 1 mg/kg followed by continuous drip at 20 to 50 μg/kg/min).

(8) Monomorphic VT with adequate perfusion is treated with amiodarone (loading dose: 5 mg/kg over 20 minutes, followed by IV drip at a rate of 5 to 15 μg/kg/min or IV boluses of 2.5 mg/kg every 6 hours), lidocaine (IV bolus of 1 mg/kg, followed by IV drip at 20 to 50 μg/kg/min), procainamide

(loading dose: 2 to 6 mg/kg, maximum dose 100 mg/dose, followed by IV continuous drip at 20 to 80 μg/kg/min, maximum 2 g/day), esmolol (loading dose of 100 to 500 μg/kg IV over 1 min followed by 50 to 500 μg/kg/min continuous drip), or electrical cardioversion.

(9) Torsades de pointes (uncommon variant of polymorphic VT), which occurs mostly in the setting of prolonged QT, requires a special approach. Amiodarone and procainamide may have a disastrous effect on this type of VT with further prolongation of the QT. Torsades often responds to IV magnesium sulfate (25 to 50 mg/kg, maximum dose 2 g), even when the magnesium level is normal. Esmolol and lidocaine may also be effective.

(10) Postoperative advanced second- or third-degree heart block is treated by temporary pacing and/or isoproterenol (IV drip at 0.05–2 μg/kg/min). Permanent pacemaker implantation may be indicated if advanced AV block persists at least 7 days after the surgery.

4. **Renal system**. Anuria or oliguria (<1 mL/kg/hr) and evidence of solute accumulation (serum K^+ >5 mEq/L, BUN >40 mg/dL, creatinine >1 mg/dL) indicate acute kidney injury. Acute reduction of cardiac output is the most common cause of renal failure. Initial treatment is directed at improving cardiac output and inducing diuresis.
   a. Preload and afterload should be optimized.
   b. Furosemide, 0.5 to 2 mg/kg/dose every 6 to 12 hours IV or as a continuous IV drip at 0.05 to 0.4 mg/kg/hr, is given if the patient is oliguric.
   c. If serum K^+ rises above 6.0 mEq/L, calcium chloride (10 mg/kg/dose, slow central IV push), bicarbonate (1 mEq/kg/dose IV), $D_{25}W$ (2 mL/kg IV; 0.5 g glucose/kg) plus regular insulin (0.1 U/kg IV) solution, and sodium polystyrene sulfonate (Kayexalate; 1 g/kg per rectum or nasogastric tube) are used.
   d. Peritoneal dialysis may be necessary if the above measures are ineffective. Indications for peritoneal dialysis include hypervolemia, azotemia (BUN over 150 mg/dL or lower if rising rapidly), life-threatening hyperkalemia, intractable metabolic acidosis, neurologic complications (secondary to uremia or electrolyte imbalance), calcium-phosphate imbalance, pulmonary compromise, or fluid restrictions limiting caloric intake.
5. Metabolic system
   a. Abnormalities of electrolytes and acid-base balance:
      (1) Metabolic acidosis is treated if the base deficit is >5 mEq/L. Total extracellular base deficit = base deficit (mEq/L) × 0.3 × body weight (kg). The dosage of sodium bicarbonate is half the total extracellular base deficit.
      (2) Lactic acidemia may be caused by LCOS and ensuing poor cerebral and intestinal tissue perfusion. Treatment is directed at improvement of cardiac output.

(3) Mild hyponatremia does not require treatment except for fluid restriction and diuresis. Serum Na^+ <125 mEq/L requires treatment to elevate sodium levels.

(4) Hypernatremia with the serum Na^+ >155 mEq/L requires treatment with sodium restriction and liberalization of fluids.

(5) Hypocalcemia may cause hypotension secondary to decreased myocardial function. It should be followed closely, especially in neonates and patients with DiGeorge syndrome. Ionized calcium level below 1.2 mEq/L should be treated. Central line administration is the ideal route of IV calcium, as extravasation will lead to tissue necrosis.

(6) Hypomagnesemia may lead to arrhythmia and subsequently to low cardiac output. A magnesium level of more than 0.7 mmol/L (1.4 mEq/L) is desirable.

b. Postoperative hypoglycemia (<5 mmol/L or 90 mg/dL) or hyperglycemia (>7.8 mmol/L or 140 mg/dL) has been associated with increased mortality and morbidity. It seems prudent to avoid these conditions. Hypoglycemia is managed with a bolus of dextrose or administration of higher-concentrated glucose in water. Hyperglycemia is treated with restriction of glucose and/or infusion of insulin.

c. Postoperative hypothermia could interfere with hemostasis and exacerbate coagulopathy, necessitating gradual rewarming to control hemorrhage. Shivering should be avoided, as it increases the oxygen consumption. However, management of junctional ectopic tachycardia may include core temperature cooling. Unlike hypothermia, treatment of postoperative fever (>38.5°C) is more urgent. LCOS is one of the causes of postoperative hyperthermia so that management of postoperative fever not only includes antipyretics or cooling, but also optimizing cardiac output with afterload reduction.

6. **GI system**. Adequate caloric intake (120 to 150 kcal/kg/day) is essential in infants recovering from congenital cardiac surgery. Enteral feeding is individualized. When stable hemodynamically, several hours after extubation, oral feeding can be started with clear liquids (e.g., oral rehydration solutions). It is then advanced to an appropriate formula. Nasogastric tube feeding should be used in infants who are too weak to suck. Children with prolonged intubation require gavage feeding or total parenteral nutrition. Gastric protection is achieved with H_2-receptor blockade (e.g., famotidine, 0.25 mg/kg/dose every 12 hours, maximum pediatric dose of 40 mg/day) or protein pump inhibitors (e.g., esomeprazole, 0.5 to 1 mg/kg/dose IV every 24 hours, maximum pediatric dose 20 mg/day). The ranitidine dose needs to be adjusted in patients with renal failure, or alternatively protein pump inhibitors could be used. Enterally fed patients should be examined frequently for any signs of intestinal dysfunction. Evidence of abdominal distention, absence of peristalsis, hyperperistalsis, or hematochezia is sought routinely. If one of these develops, enteral feeding is discontinued,

nasogastric suction is applied, and parenteral nutrition is considered. GI dysfunction may be caused by LCOS, acute pancreatitis, hepatic or intestinal necrosis, ileus, and others.

7. **Hematologic system**. Different thresholds are established for transfusion of PRBCs, fresh frozen plasma, or platelets at different institutions. Transfusion of blood products depends on hemodynamic status and coagulation status of individual patients.
   a. Maintain adequate hemoglobin (Hgb) and a desirable filling pressure (e.g., LA pressure 10 to 15 mm Hg) by infusion of PRBCs or albumin, depending on the patient's Hgb or hematocrit (Hct). Patients with cyanotic CHD or myocardial dysfunction are given PRBCs to maintain Hct above 40%.
   b. Coagulation abnormalities may result from inadequate heparin neutralization (causing prolongation of aPTT), thrombocytopenia (<50,000 platelets/mm^3), or disseminated intravascular coagulation (DIC; secondary to sepsis, low cardiac output, acidosis, hypoxia, or tissue necrosis or as a reaction to blood transfusion).
      (1) Unneutralized heparin is corrected by administration of additional protamine.
      (2) Thrombocytopenia is treated with slow infusion of platelet concentrates with an infusion pump, given over 20 to 30 min; rapid infusion may cause pulmonary hypertension and RV failure.
      (3) DIC (characterized by hemorrhage, tissue necrosis, hemolytic anemia, positive D-dimer test, low platelets and serum fibrinogen, and prolonged PT and aPTT) is managed by prompt and vigorous treatment of the underlying cause. Management may include transfusion of platelets, cryoprecipitates, and/or fresh frozen plasma as well as administration of heparin.
   c. Excessive postoperative bleeding occurs more frequently in severely cyanotic patients, polycythemic patients, and patients who had a reoperation. The necessity to infuse more than 10 to 15 mL/kg of volume requires investigation for excessive blood loss and for a possible surgical exploration. Surgical exploration is indicated (1) if the chest tube drainage in the absence of clotting abnormalities exceeds 3 mL/kg/hr for 3 hours or (2) if there is a sudden marked increase in chest tube drainage of 5 mL/kg/hr in any 1 hour.
   d. Long-term anticoagulation with aspirin or warfarin is indicated in selected patients. Patients with cavopulmonary anastomosis (e.g., Glenn or Fontan procedure) or systemic-to-pulmonary shunts (e.g., modified B-T shunt) are bridged to oral anticoagulation by continuous heparin drip and its dose is adjusted for aPTT of 60 to 85 seconds. Aspirin (3 to 5 mg/kg PO once daily) is started when chest is closed, all major intracardiac lines are removed, and patients are hemodynamically stable and have adequate platelet count without evidence of active bleeding. Alternatively or

additionally, warfarin is given if the patient is in a hypercoagulable state (e.g., factor V Leiden mutation, protein S or C deficiency). Patients with mechanical valve prostheses will require warfarin; the dose is adjusted to maintain adequate anticoagulation (international normalized ratio [INR] 2.5 to 3.5 for mitral valve and INR 2.0 to 3.0 for aortic valve). While patients are maintained on aspirin, cyclooxygenase (COX)-2 inhibitors (e.g., ibuprofen, naproxen) should be avoided as they inhibit the antiplatelet effect of aspirin.

8. **Neurologic system**. The incidence of central nervous system anomalies including brain dysmorphology or neurobehavioral abnormalities is increased in patients with congenital cardiac defects. These may be multifactorial, isolated findings, or in association with particular genetic defects. In addition, pre- and perioperative neurologic events complicate establishing the accurate cause of the neurologic insult.
   a. Localized neurologic defects such as hemiplegia and visual field defects are abnormal and may be due to air or particulate emboli.
   b. Seizures may be caused by hypoxia, metabolic abnormalities, infections, cerebral edema, embolism or hemorrhage, or decreased cerebral perfusion. Early postoperative clinical seizures occur at an incidence rate of 3% to 6%; however, EEG and video monitoring may reveal an incidence of 20% of subclinical seizures. Seizures documented by electroencephalography have been associated with worse neurodevelopmental outcome. Management of seizures includes the following:
      (1) Determine arterial blood gases, serum glucose, calcium, electrolytes, cardiac output, and temperature. Correct any abnormalities.
      (2) Anticonvulsant therapy.
         (a) Lorazepam, 0.05 to 0.1 mg/kg/dose IV over 2 to 5 min (maximum single dose 2 mg; may cause respiratory depression).
         (b) Fosphenytoin, 15 to 20 mg phenytoin equivalent (PE)/kg IV (maximum infusion rate of 150 mg PE/min due to risk of hypotension), followed by a maintenance dose of 5 mg PE/kg/day IV or IM. Therapeutic levels are 10 to 20 mg/L (free and bound phenytoin) or 1 to 2 mg/L (free phenytoin). Fosphenytoin causes less hypotension than traditional phenytoin; however, both medications are contraindicated in patients with heart block or sinus bradycardia.
         (c) Phenobarbital, 10 to 20 mg/kg IV over 5 to 10 min. The full effect may take several hours. Phenobarbital maintenance dose is 5 mg/kg/day given in 1 or 2 daily doses. Therapeutic level is 10 to 40 mg/L. Side effects of phenobarbital include myocardial depression with hypotension, particularly after large and rapid infusion.

c. Choreiform movement and grossly inadequate behavior are major neurologic complications. Pharmacologic control is difficult. These complications usually but not always clear without demonstrable sequelae.

Chapter 29

Selected Postoperative Complications

Selected postoperative complications are discussed briefly in this chapter. Problems that occur in the immediate postoperative period, such as low cardiac output state, minor rhythm disorders, blood pressure abnormalities, and renal, metabolic, and hematologic abnormalities, are discussed in Chapter 28. Postoperative complications that occur frequently with certain types of cardiac defects are discussed under those specific conditions.

I. PLEURAL EFFUSION

A small amount of fluid is present in the pleural cavity. The reabsorption of this pleural fluid is mainly through the venous system and to some degree through the lymphatic system. Any increase in capillary hydrostatic pressure as a result of disrupted systemic venous hemodynamics (e.g., Fontan surgery, right ventricular failure) may result in accumulation of transudates in the pleural cavity. Trauma to the lymphatic system as is caused by cutting large tributaries of the thoracic duct causes buildup of chyle in the pleural space. Both conditions create a management problem.

Duration of *persistent pleural effusion*, as a result of increased systemic venous pressure that is common after Fontan operation, may be shortened by intraoperative creation of baffle fenestration. Symptoms may include fever, tachycardia, tachypnea, increased work of breathing, and, in severe cases, respiratory failure. Diagnosis is usually made by chest radiography (frontal, lateral, and decubitus films). Thoracentesis (with ultrasonographic guidance) may be necessary for determination of etiology and/or for treatment. Transudates can be differentiated by amount of protein (<3 g/100 mL) and lactate dehydrogenase (LDH) (<200 IU/L) from exudates (protein >3 g/100 mL and LDH >200 IU/L), which are caused by increased capillary permeability and may be a sign of infection. In addition, transudates have fewer leukocytes (<10,000/mm3), have more glucose (60 mg/dL), and have a serous appearance compared with exudates, which are cloudy and have significantly more leukocytes (> 50,000/mm^3). Furthermore, fluid-to-serum ratios of LDH (> 0.6) and protein (> 0.5) are further clues to the exudative nature of the fluid.

A small amount of pleural effusion can be tolerated well. It usually responds to medical management with diuresis, afterload reduction, and inotropic support. However, significant and recurrent amounts of pleural effusion will cause cardiorespiratory compromise and will require more aggressive management strategies, including chest tube drainage, now rarely implemented pleurodesis with a sclerosing agent (e.g., talc), and/or Fontan revision. When the drainage is large, appropriate replacement of fluid, electrolytes, and protein is essential.

Chylothorax, an accumulation of chyle in the pleural cavity, may be caused by trauma to peritracheal lymphatics or transmission of increased systemic venous pressure to the thoracic duct, or a combination of both. It may be seen after surgery (up to about 6% of cases) such as COA repair, B-T shunt, or cavopulmonary anastomosis (e.g., Glenn or Fontan operation), or rarely, after ligation of PDA. Occasionally, chylothorax occurs in combination with chylopericardium.

Chyle may or may not have a creamy appearance, depending on the nutritional status of the patient (consumption of fat results in creamy appearance), but a triglyceride level above 110 mg/dL is highly probable for the diagnosis, whereas a triglyceride concentration of less than 50 mg/dL makes the diagnosis of chylothorax extremely unlikely. The fluid is usually sterile and is abundant of lymphocytes (2,000 to 20,000/mm^3). Presence of chylomicrons (triglyceride-rich lipoprotein particles containing some phospholipids and cholesterol) confirms a diagnosis of chylothorax.

Treatment, apart from medical management (i.e., diuresis, improvement of cardiac output) described previously, is directed at drainage of chylothorax (chest tube placement) and reducing the flow of lymph (by limiting physical activity to reduce lymph flow from the extremities).

1. In most cases, chest tube drainage is all that is necessary. If chylothorax develops after chest tube removal, needle aspiration every 3 to 4 days usually constitutes adequate treatment. The drainage slows or stops within 7 days in most cases.
2. Careful attention to the nutrition of the patient is important. Either parenteral hyperalimentation or a diet with medium-chain triglycerides (MCTs) as the fat source is called for. As MCT oil does not contribute in chylomicron formation, it is absorbed by the portal system and not by the lymphatic system. Serum albumin should be followed closely and replaced if necessary.
3. In persistent cases, continuous intravenous (IV) octreotide (0.5 to 10 μg/kg/hr), a somatostatin analog, has been used effectively.
4. If the drainage persists, making the patient's status non per os (NPO) and starting total parenteral nutrition therapy and/or surgical intervention may be considered because continuous loss of chyle results in lymphocyte depletion and subsequent immunocompromise. Indications for the intervention may include (a) average daily loss above 1000 mL, or, in children, chest tube output more than 2 mL/kg/day), (b) the chyle flow not slowing after 2 weeks, or (c) imminent nutritional complications.
5. Thoracic duct ligation with or without chemical pleurodesis has been used successfully. During pleurodesis, the introduced chemicals cause inflammation between the parietal and visceral pleura. This reaction causes adhesions between the layers and prevents further fluid accumulation. The procedure may be painful and cause fever and nausea so that this procedure has become out of favor at most centers.

II. PARALYSIS OF THE DIAPHRAGM

Paralysis or paresis of a hemidiaphragm occurs in about 0.5% to 2% of patients after thoracic surgery, though the incidence may be as high as 10% in young children. It is the result of damage to the phrenic nerve. It may occur after COA repair, PDA ligation, B-T shunt, or open heart surgery and may be due to nerve transection, blunt trauma, stretching during retraction, electrocautery, or hypothermic injury. Infants are more vulnerable to respiratory distress owing to their greater dependence on the diaphragm for respiration.

The diagnosis should be suspected if there is persistent unexplained tachypnea, respiratory distress, hypoxia and/or hypercapnia, atelectasis, inability to wean from the ventilator, or persistent elevation of a hemidiaphragm on serial chest radiographs. Fluoroscopy or sonogram that reveals paradoxical motion of the hemidiaphragms is diagnostic if it is done during spontaneous breathing. When paralysis is not caused by transection, return of function usually occurs in 2 weeks to 6 months. In 20% of the cases the paralysis is permanent.

Management ranges from conservative to surgical intervention.

1. Some investigators recommend ventilator support only for the initial 2 to 6 weeks.
2. Continuous positive airway pressure (CPAP) may be useful in management as well as in identifying patients who may benefit from plication.
3. If respiratory insufficiency persists, surgical plication should be considered. Plication of the diaphragm usually is not necessary as long as the patient can be extubated without developing respiratory insufficiency.

III. POSTPERICARDIOTOMY SYNDROME

Postpericardiotomy syndrome (PPS), a febrile illness with pericardial and pleural inflammatory reactions, develops after surgery involving pericardiotomy. This occurs in about 25% to 30% of patients who undergo pericardiotomy. The etiology remains speculative. Though questioned in more recent studies, an autoimmune response to cardiac antibodies in association with a recent or remote viral infection was postulated in the 1970s. Studied patients who developed PPS had a high titer of antiheart antibodies along with high antibody titers against adenovirus, coxsackievirus B1-6, and cytomegalovirus.

Onset is a few weeks to a few months (median 4 weeks) after pericardiotomy. PPS is characterized by fever, chest pain, irritability, malaise, joint pain, decreased appetite, nausea, and vomiting. Chest pain, which may be severe, is caused by both pericarditis and pleuritis. It may be worse in supine position or with deep inspiration. It is rare in infants younger than 2 years. Physical examination may reveal pericardial and pleural friction rubs and hepatomegaly. Tachycardia, tachypnea, rising venous pressure, falling arterial pressure, and narrow pulse pressure with a paradoxical pulse are signs of cardiac tamponade. Blood laboratory findings include leukocytosis with left shift. Erythrocyte sedimentation rate (ESR) and C-reactive protein (CRP) are usually elevated. Chest radiography shows enlarged cardiac silhouette and pleural effusion. Electrocardiogram (ECG) shows persistent ST-segment elevation and flat or inverted T waves in the limb and left precordial leads. Echo is a reliable test in confirming the presence and amount of pericardial effusion and in evaluating evidence of cardiac tamponade. Although the disease is self-limited, its duration is highly variable; the median duration is 2 to 3 weeks. About 20% of patients have recurrences.

Bed rest is all that is needed for a mild case. A nonsteroidal antiinflammatory agent such as oral aspirin (80 to 100 mg/kg/day divided in 3 or 4 doses) or ibuprofen (20 to 40 mg/kg/day divided in 3 or 4 doses) is effective in most cases. In severe cases, corticosteroids (prednisone, 2 mg/kg/day up to 60 mg/day) tapered over 3 to 4 weeks may be indicated if the diagnosis is secure and infection has been ruled out. Emergency pericardiocentesis or creation of pericardial window may be required if signs of cardiac tamponade are present. Diuretics may be used for pleural effusion.

IV. POSTCOARCTECTOMY HYPERTENSION

Paradoxical hypertension following repair of COA is quite common, particularly in older children. This condition is usually biphasic with mostly systolic hypertension developing within 24 to 48 hours of the procedure, followed by a more delayed phase. The mechanism is believed to be multifactorial, including intraoperative stimulation of sympathetic nerve fibers, postoperative altered baroreceptor activity, and derangement of the renin-angiotensin system. The first phase of hypertension is believed to be the result of increased catecholamine levels and altered baroreceptor response. Elevated levels of renin and angiotensin are believed to be responsible for the later phase hypertension, which is more pronounced in diastole.

Systemic hypertension needs to be treated promptly, as this could increase the risk of postoperative hemorrhage. In addition to pain management and sedation, short-acting IV β-receptor blocker administration (e.g., esmolol, loading dose of 100 to 500 μg/kg IV over 1 minute followed by 50 to 500 μg/kg/min continuous drip) can be used to control the first phase of postcoarctectomy hypertension. Other medications that have been used successfully include longer-acting β-receptor blockers (e.g., propranolol, nadolol), combined α- and β-receptor blockers (e.g., labetalol), and vasodilators (nitroprusside, hydralazine). Long-term management of paradoxical hypertension is achieved with angiotensin-converting enzyme (ACE) inhibitors (e.g., enalapril, captopril) or angiotensin II receptor antagonists (e.g., losartan).

Postcoarctectomy syndrome is a well-described but rare complication of repair of COA. Occurring in up to 5% to 10% of older children, it is characterized by severe, intermittent abdominal pain beginning 2 to 4 days after surgery with accompanying fever, leukocytosis, and vomiting. In severe cases ascites, ileus, melena, ischemic bowel, and even death were reported. Persistent paradoxical hypertension may be present. Abdominal findings are believed to be caused by acute inflammatory changes in mesenteric arteries resulting from sudden increase in pulsatile pressures in arteries distal to the coarctation.

Because of mesenteric arteritis, feeding of solid foods is delayed; some centers advocate NPO status for the first 48 hours following the repair. Treatment includes bowel decompression and treatment of the accompanying hypertension.

V. PROTEIN-LOSING ENTEROPATHY

Protein-losing enteropathy (PLE) is a condition characterized by excessive loss of plasma protein through the intestinal mucosa. Although it can be a primary gastrointestinal disorder with intestinal lymphangiectasia and associated peripheral edema, PLE occurs most frequently as a complication of Fontan procedure. It is believed to be caused by chronically elevated central venous pressure secondary to unfavorable PA anatomy, increased PVR, decreased cardiac output, or loss of electrical AV synchrony. Patients with PLE have been shown to have loss of heparin sulfate and syndecan-1 proteoglycans necessary for maintenance of intestinal epithelial barrier function, thus promoting intestinal protein loss. Additionally, inflammatory mediator release and individual genetic predisposition are postulated in the mechanism of PLE after Fontan operation. PLE in association with Fontan-type surgery has a cumulative 10-year occurrence risk of 13% and a poor 5-year survival rate of about 50%.

Children may present a few weeks, months, or even years after the surgery with symptoms of anasarca, abdominal pain and distention, diarrhea, emesis, and poor weight gain. Patients may be tachycardic if sinus node function is preserved. Tachypnea may be a clue to concurrent pleural effusion. Hepatomegaly is seen frequently. Signs of fluid retention including ascites and anasarca may be found on examination.

Serum albumin, immunoglobulins, and total protein are decreased. In addition, α_1-antitrypsin 24-hour fecal clearance and α_1-antitrypsin random fecal concentration are increased. Electrolyte imbalance is seen, which may be iatrogenic secondary to diuretic therapy. ECG and Holter monitoring need to be obtained to rule out any arrhythmia such as sinus node dysfunction. Chest radiography may reveal cardiomegaly and/or pleural effusion. Echo is performed to evaluate ventricular function or Fontan baffle obstruction. Cardiac catheterization may be needed as a diagnostic but also as a therapeutic tool.

Treatment includes the following:

1. High-protein, low-fat, high-MCT, low-sodium, high-calcium diet
2. Consider vitamin D supplement
3. Diuretics (furosemide, spironolactone)
4. ACE inhibitors (enalapril)
5. Phosphodiesterase type 5 inhibitors (sildenafil, tadalafil)
6. Endothelin receptor antagonists (bosentan)
7. Subcutaneous unfractionated (100 units/kg, maximum 5000 units daily) or low-molecular-weight heparin (enoxaparin, 0.5 to 1.5 mg/kg/dose SC every 12 to 24 hours) to achieve target anti-factor Xa levels of 0.5 to 1 units/mL in a sample taken 4 to 6 hours after SC injection)

8. Corticosteroids (budesonide, 6 mg for children <4 years, 9 mg for children >4 years; dose should be weaned after normalization of albumin [3 mg/dL] to lifelong 3 mg every other day)
9. Trial of octreotide (continuous IV drip 0.5 to 10 μg/kg/hr or subcutaneous injection of 1 to 10 μg/kg/day divided 3 times daily to a maximum of 150 μg per dose)
10. IV albumin

More invasive management apart from interventional cardiac catheterization may include selective lymphatic embolization of pathologic regional lymphatic network, pacemaker insertion, repair of residual defects (e.g., repair of AV valve, repair of residual COA), Fontan revision, or cardiac transplantation.

VI. FONTAN-ASSOCIATED LIVER DISEASE

With improvement in technical aspects of congenital cardiac surgery as well as medical management, more patients with single ventricular physiology survive to adulthood. The number of the patients who have successfully undergone Fontan procedure has increased. This, however, means increased prevalence of medium-term and long-term Fontan-associated complications. One entity that has been of significant concerns is Fontan-associated liver disease (FALD). Derangement in perinatal circulation as well as lifetime hepatic insults by means of medications, frequent cardiac catheterization, and surgical interventions all contribute to an abnormal hepatic physiology. Not surprisingly, nearly all Fontan patients have abnormal liver histology. A detailed FALD pathophysiology and management is beyond the scope of this handbook. However, a short list of studies for FALD evaluation, which should be performed every 1 to 2 years, is provided:

1. Complete blood cell count
2. Prothrombin time (PT), international normalized ratio (INR)
3. Aspartate aminotransferase (AST), alanine aminotransferase (ALT), albumin, total protein, alkaline phosphatase, creatinine
4. Total and direct bilirubin
5. Ultrasound of liver with Doppler and elastography
6. Ultrasound of spleen

In the case of abnormal findings with thrombocytopenia, abnormal liver enzymes, prolonged PT, INR, elevated direct bilirubin, hypoalbuminemia, splenomegaly, or hepatic mass, consider referral to hepatology.

VII. JUNCTIONAL ECTOPIC TACHYCARDIA

Postoperative junctional ectopic tachycardia (JET) occurs in 5% to 10% of pediatric postoperative patients, most frequently following surgeries adjacent to the AV node (e.g., VSD, TOF, ECD repair, Fontan procedure), as well as in patients with prolonged aortic cross-clamp and CPB times. Postoperative JET usually occurs within hours after cardiac surgery and may last for several days. Though it is self-limited, it is a serious and life-threatening arrhythmia owing to its occurrence in a very vulnerable phase of a patient's postoperative course. It is characterized by tachycardia with a ventricular rate usually in excess of 180 beats/min (faster than atrial rate), AV dissociation (unlike re-entrant SVT), and capture beats (occasional antegrade conduction of a normal sinus beat).

Driven by an automatic focus within the proximity of the AV node or bundle of His, JET does not respond to strategies such as electrical or pharmacologic cardioversion. Tachycardia and loss of AV synchrony are responsible for a decrease in cardiac output, especially in an already hemodynamically compromised patient. Treatment is aimed at correcting tachycardia and restoring AV synchrony as well as optimizing cardiac output.

1. Measures to maximize cardiac output include the following:
   a. Treatment of anemia.
   b. Treatment of acidosis.
   c. Inotropic, lusitropic, and vasodilatory support with milrinone without the undesired arrhythmogenic effect.
   d. Measures to decrease oxygen consumption (e.g., pain control, sedation, and, if necessary, paralysis).
2. Attempts to restore AV synchrony include:
   a. Correction of electrolyte imbalance (magnesium^{2+}, calcium^{2+}, and potassium^{+}).
   b. Attempting atrial pacing at a rate higher than the JET rate to achieve AV synchrony, once the ventricular rate is less than 200 beats/min.
3. Attempts to control the ventricular rate, though challenging, may include the following strategies and/or antiarrhythmic medications:
   a. Fever control.
   b. Lowering the infusion rate of catecholamines (proarrhythmogenic).
   c. Antiarrhythmics:
      (1) IV amiodarone (loading dose: 5 mg/kg over 30 to 60 minutes, followed by IV drip at a rate of 5 to 15 μg/kg/min or IV boluses of 2.5 mg/kg every 6 hours).
      (2) Combination of IV procainamide (loading dose: 2 to 6 mg/kg, maximum dose 100 mg/dose, followed by IV drip at 20 to 80 μg/kg/min, maximum 2 g/day) and hypothermia.
      (3) IV esmolol (loading dose: 100 to 500 μg/kg IV over 1 minute, followed by IV drip at 50 to 500 μg/kg/min).
   d. Induced hypothermia (34° to 36°C) using cooling blanket or IV cold saline infusions.
4. If the above efforts to control JET fail and the patient continues to deteriorate, extracorporeal life support (ECLS) may need to be initiated.

APPENDICES

Appendix A Miscellaneous

TABLE A.1

RECURRENCE RISKS GIVEN ONE SIBLING WHO HAS A CARDIOVASCULAR ANOMALY

ANOMALY	SUGGESTED RISK (%)
Ventricular septal defect	3.0
Patent ductus arteriosus	3.0
Atrial septal defect	2.5
Tetralogy of Fallot	2.5
Pulmonary stenosis	2.0
Coarctation of the aorta	2.0
Aortic stenosis	2.0
Transposition of the great arteries	1.5
Atrioventricular canal (complete endocardial cushion defect)	2.0
Endocardial fibroelastosis	4.0
Tricuspid atresia	1.0
Ebstein anomaly	1.0
Persistent truncus arteriosus	1.0
Pulmonary atresia	1.0
Hypoplastic left heart syndrome	2.0

Modified from Nora, J. J., & Nora, A. H. (1978). The evaluation of specific genetic and environmental counseling in congenital heart diseases. *Circulation, 57*(2), 205-213.

TABLE A.2

AFFECTED OFFSPRING GIVEN ONE PARENT WITH A CONGENITAL HEART DEFECT

DEFECT	MOTHER AFFECTED (%)	FATHER AFFECTED (%)
Aortic stenosis	13.0-18.0	3.0
Atrial septal defect	4.0-4.5	1.5
Atrioventricular canal (complete endocardial cushion defect)	14.0	1.0
Coarctation of the aorta	4.0	2.0
Patent ductus arteriosus	3.5-4.0	2.5
Pulmonary stenosis	4.0-6.5	2.0
Tetralogy of Fallot	6.0-10.0	1.5
Ventricular septal defect	6.0	2.0

From Nora J.J., Nora A.H. (1987). Maternal transmission of congenital heart disease: New recurrence risk figures and the questions of cytoplasmic inheritance and vulnerability to teratogens. *Am J Cardiol* 59, 459–463.

TABLE A.3

NEW YORK HEART ASSOCIATION FUNCTIONAL CLASSIFICATION

CLASS	IMPAIRMENT
I	The patient has the disease, but the condition is asymptomatic.
II	The patient experiences symptoms with moderate activity.
III	The patient has symptoms with mild activity.
IV	The patient's condition is symptomatic at rest.

This is a classification of functional impairment in exercise capacity based on symptoms of dyspnea and fatigue. It is simple and useful in the evaluation of cardiac patients.

TABLE A.4

SUMMARY OF ANTIARRHYTHMIC AGENTS

CLASS	MECHANISM OF ACTION	EXAMPLES	REMARKS
I	Sodium channel blockers Delays phase 0 of the action potential and slows conduction velocity in the tissue		Has a significant proarrhythmic effect
IA	Slows the rate of rise of phase 0 and prolongs the refractory period	Quinidine Procainamide	Major effect on QTc and QRS prolongation
IB	Minimal effect on phase 0 and refractory period	Lidocaine Mexiletine	Least proarrhythmic among Class I agents
IC	Marked depression in conduction velocity with minimal effects on refractoriness	Flecainide Propafenone	Major effect on PR and QRS duration
II	β-Blockers	Propranolol ($\beta_1 + \beta_2$) Atenolol (β_1) Nadolol ($\beta_1 + \beta_2$) Esmolol (β_1)	Minor effects on ECG
III	Potassium channel blockers Delays repolarization	Amiodarone Sotalol Dofetilide Ibutilide	Has a significant proarrhythmic effect Major effect on QT prolongation
IV	Calcium channel blockers (slows inward Ca^{2+} current) Slows conduction velocity and increases refractoriness in the AV node	Verapamil Diltiazem	Minor effects on ECG

AV, atrioventricular; *ECG*, electrocardiogram.

TABLE A.5

EFFECTS OF ANTIARRHYTHMIC AGENTS ON THE ECG

		PR	QRS	QT
CLASS I				
IA	Quinidine	±	↑↑	↑↑↑
	Procainamide	±	↑	↑↑
IB	Lidocaine	±	±	±
	Mixiletine	±	±	±
IC	Flecainide	↑↑	↑↑	↑
	Propafenone	↑↑	↑↑	±
CLASS III	Amiodarone	Acu ± Chr ↑	Acu ± Chr ↑	Acu ± Chr ↑↑↑
	Sotalol	↑	±	↑↑↑
	Dofetilide	±	±	↑↑↑
	Ibutilide	±	±	↑↑↑

Acu, acute effect; *Chr*, chronic effect; *ECG*, electrocardiogram.
Modified from Fischbach, P. S. (2010). Pharmacology of antiarrhythmic agents. In D. Macdonald (Ed.). *Clinical cardiac electrophysiology in the young* (2nd ed.) (pp. 267-288). New York: Springer.

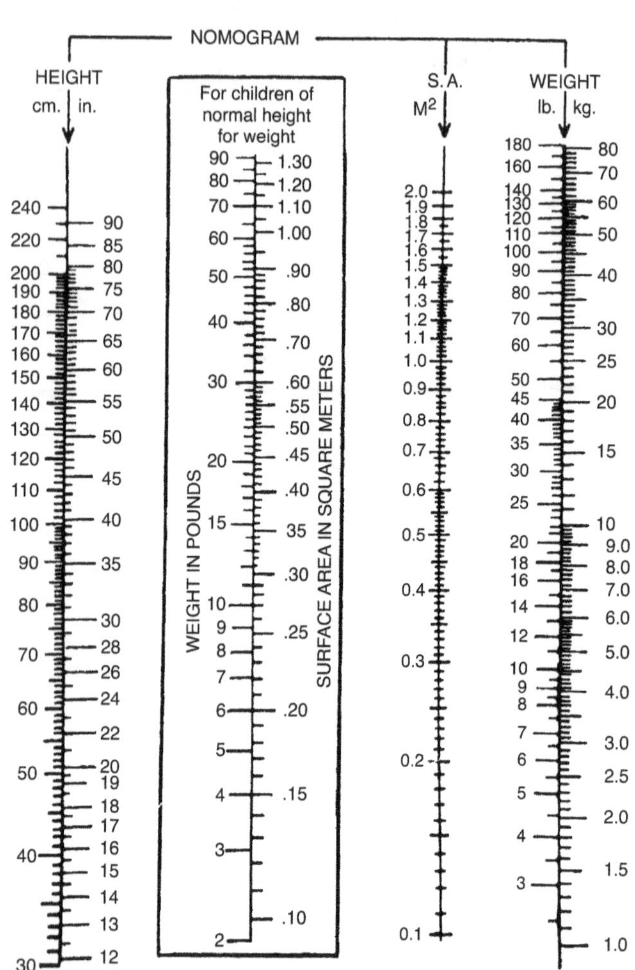

FIG. A.1
Body surface area nomogram.

TABLE A.6

OXYGEN CONSUMPTION PER BODY SURFACE AREA[a]

AGE (YR)	HEART RATE (BEATS/MIN)												
	50	**60**	**70**	**80**	**90**	**100**	**110**	**120**	**130**	**140**	**150**	**160**	**170**
Male Patients													
3				155	159	163	167	171	175	178	182	186	190
4			149	152	156	160	163	168	171	175	179	182	186
6		141	144	148	151	155	159	162	167	171	174	178	181
8		136	141	145	148	152	156	159	163	167	171	175	178
10	130	134	139	142	146	149	153	157	160	165	169	172	176
12	128	132	136	140	144	147	151	155	158	162	167	170	174
14	127	130	134	137	142	146	149	153	157	160	165	169	172
16	125	129	132	136	141	144	148	152	155	159	162	167	
18	124	127	131	135	139	143	147	150	154	157	161	166	
20	123	126	130	134	137	142	145	149	153	156	160	165	
25	120	124	127	131	135	139	143	147	150	154	157		
30	118	122	125	129	133	136	141	145	148	152	155		
35	116	120	124	127	131	135	139	143	147	150			
40	115	119	122	126	130	133	137	141	145	149			

TABLE A.6 *(continued)*

OXYGEN CONSUMPTION PER BODY SURFACE AREA[a]

	HEART RATE (BEATS/MIN)												
AGE (YR)	**50**	**60**	**70**	**80**	**90**	**100**	**110**	**120**	**130**	**140**	**150**	**160**	**170**
Female Patients													
3				150	153	157	161	165	169	172	176	180	183
4			141	145	149	152	156	159	163	168	171	175	179
6		130	134	137	142	146	149	153	156	160	165	168	172
8		125	129	133	136	141	144	148	152	155	159	163	167
10	118	122	125	129	133	136	141	144	148	152	155	159	163
12	115	119	122	126	130	133	137	141	145	149	152	156	160
14	112	116	120	123	127	131	134	133	143	146	150	153	157
16	109	114	118	121	125	128	132	136	140	144	148	151	
18	107	111	116	119	123	127	130	134	137	142	146	149	
20	106	109	114	118	121	125	128	132	136	140	144	148	
25	102	106	109	114	118	121	125	128	132	136	140		
30	99	103	106	110	115	118	122	125	129	133	136		
35	97	100	104	107	111	116	119	123	127	130			
50	94	98	102	105	109	112	117	121	124	128			

[a]In (mL/min)/m^2.

From LaFarge, C. G., & Miettinen, O. S. (1970). The estimation of oxygen consumption. *Cardiovascular Research, 4*(1), 23-30.

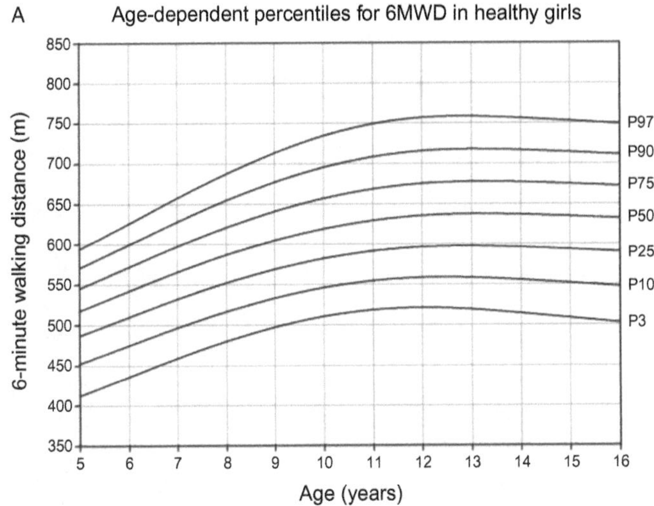

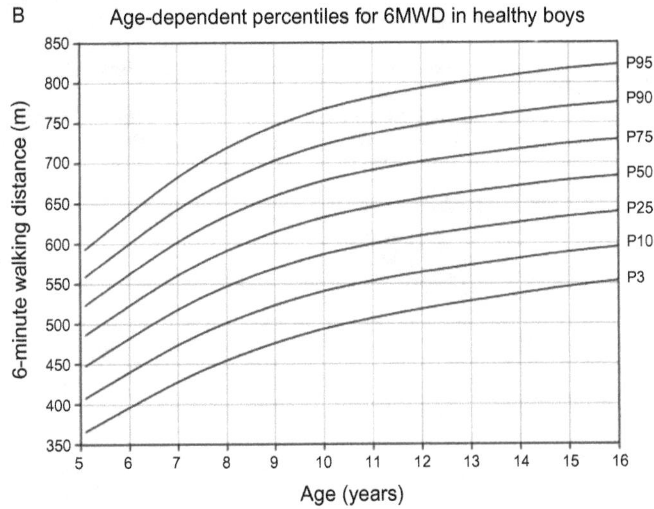

FIG. A.2

Reference percentile curves for 6-minute walking distance (6MWD) for girls and boys. (From Ulrich, S., Hildenbrand, F. F., Treder, U., et al. (2013). Reference values for the 6-minute walk test in healthy children and adolescents in Switzerland. *BMC Pulmonary Medicine, 13*(49)).

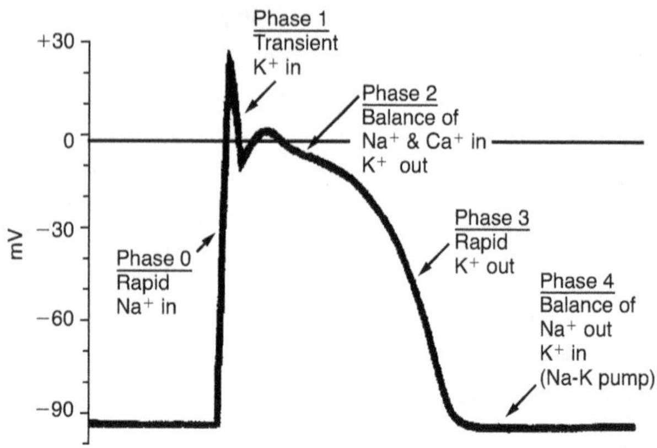

FIG. A.3

Action potential of human ventricular myocyte of subepicardial origin. **Phase 0** (rapid depolarization) is the result of sudden increase in membrane conductance to Na^+ iron. **Phase 1** (early rapid repolarization) is due to transient outward K^+ current. **Phase 2** (plateau) is maintained by the competition between outward current carried by K^+ and $Cl-$ ions and inward current carried by Ca^{2+} ions. **Phase 3** (final rapid repolarization) is due to activation of repolarizing outward K^+ current. **Phase 4** (the resting potential or diastolic depolarization) is due to the Na-K pump that maintains high K^+ concentration and low intracellular Na^+ concentration by pumping K^+ inward and Na^+ outward.

Appendix B

Blood Pressure Standards

TABLE B.1

BP LEVELS FOR BOYS BY AGE AND HEIGHT PERCENTILE (NHBPEP[a])

		SYSTOLIC BP (mm Hg)							DIASTOLIC BP (mm Hg)						
		PERCENTILE OF HEIGHT							PERCENTILE OF HEIGHT						
AGE (YR)	BP PERCENTILE	5TH	10TH	25TH	50TH	75TH	90TH	95TH	5TH	10TH	25TH	50TH	75TH	90TH	95TH
1	50th	80	81	83	85	87	88	89	34	35	36	37	38	39	39
	90th	94	95	97	99	100	102	103	49	50	51	52	53	53	54
	95th	98	99	101	103	104	106	106	54	54	55	56	57	58	58
	99th	105	106	108	110	112	113	114	61	62	63	64	65	66	66
2	50th	84	85	87	88	90	92	92	39	40	41	42	43	44	44
	90th	97	99	100	102	104	105	106	54	55	56	57	58	58	59
	95th	101	102	104	106	108	109	110	59	59	60	61	62	63	63
	99th	109	110	111	113	115	117	117	66	67	68	69	70	71	71
3	50th	86	87	89	91	93	94	95	44	44	45	46	47	48	48
	90th	100	101	103	105	107	108	109	59	59	60	61	62	63	63
	95th	104	105	107	109	110	112	113	63	63	64	65	66	67	67
	99th	111	112	114	116	118	119	120	71	71	72	73	74	75	75
4	50th	88	89	91	93	95	96	97	47	48	49	50	51	51	52
	90th	102	103	105	107	109	110	111	62	63	64	65	66	66	67
	95th	106	107	109	111	112	114	115	66	67	68	69	70	71	71
	99th	113	114	116	118	120	121	122	74	75	76	77	78	78	79

5	50th	90	91	93	95	96	98	98	50	51	52	53	54	55	55
	90th	104	105	106	108	110	111	112	65	66	67	68	69	69	70
	95th	108	109	110	112	114	115	116	69	70	71	72	73	74	74
	99th	115	116	118	120	121	123	123	77	78	79	80	81	81	82
6	50th	91	92	94	96	98	99	100	53	53	54	55	56	57	57
	90th	105	106	108	110	111	113	113	68	68	69	70	71	72	72
	95th	109	110	112	114	115	117	117	72	72	73	74	75	76	76
	99th	116	117	119	121	123	124	125	80	80	81	82	83	84	84
7	50th	92	94	95	97	99	100	101	55	55	56	57	58	59	59
	90th	106	107	109	111	113	114	115	70	70	71	72	73	74	74
	95th	110	111	113	115	117	118	119	74	74	75	76	77	78	78
	99th	117	118	120	122	124	125	126	82	82	83	84	85	86	86
8	50th	94	95	97	99	100	102	102	56	57	58	59	60	60	61
	90th	107	109	110	112	114	115	116	71	72	72	73	74	75	76
	95th	111	112	114	116	118	119	120	75	76	77	78	79	79	80
	99th	119	120	122	123	125	127	127	83	84	85	86	87	87	88
9	50th	95	96	98	100	102	103	104	57	58	59	60	61	61	62
	90th	109	110	112	114	115	117	118	72	73	74	75	76	76	77
	95th	113	114	116	118	119	121	121	76	77	78	79	80	81	81
	99th	120	121	123	125	127	128	129	84	85	86	87	88	88	89
10	50th	97	98	100	102	103	105	106	58	59	60	61	61	62	63
	90th	111	112	114	115	117	119	119	73	73	74	75	76	77	78
	95th	115	116	117	119	121	122	123	77	78	79	80	81	81	82
	99th	122	123	125	127	128	130	130	85	86	86	88	88	89	90

TABLE B.1 *(continued)*

BP LEVELS FOR BOYS BY AGE AND HEIGHT PERCENTILE (NHBPEP[a])

		SYSTOLIC BP (mm Hg)							DIASTOLIC BP (mm Hg)						
		PERCENTILE OF HEIGHT							PERCENTILE OF HEIGHT						
AGE (YR)	BP PERCENTILE	5TH	10TH	25TH	50TH	75TH	90TH	95TH	5TH	10TH	25TH	50TH	75TH	90TH	95TH
11	50th	99	100	102	104	105	107	107	59	59	60	61	62	63	63
	90th	113	114	115	117	119	120	121	74	74	75	76	77	78	78
	95th	117	118	119	121	123	124	125	78	78	79	80	81	82	82
	99th	124	125	127	129	130	132	132	86	86	87	88	89	90	90
12	50th	101	102	104	106	108	109	110	59	60	61	62	63	63	64
	90th	115	116	118	120	121	123	123	74	75	75	76	77	78	79
	95th	119	120	122	123	125	127	127	78	79	80	81	82	82	83
	99th	126	127	129	131	133	134	135	86	87	88	89	90	90	91
13	50th	104	105	106	108	110	111	112	60	60	61	62	63	64	64
	90th	117	118	120	122	124	125	126	75	75	76	77	78	79	79
	95th	121	122	124	126	128	129	130	79	79	80	81	82	83	83
	99th	128	130	131	133	135	136	137	87	87	88	89	90	91	91
14	50th	106	107	109	111	113	114	115	60	61	62	63	64	65	65
	90th	120	121	123	125	126	128	128	75	76	77	78	79	79	80
	95th	124	125	127	128	130	132	132	80	80	81	82	83	84	84
	99th	131	132	134	136	138	139	140	87	88	89	90	91	92	92

15	50th	109	110	112	113	115	117	117	61	62	63	64	65	66	66
	90th	122	124	125	127	129	130	131	76	77	78	79	80	80	81
	95th	126	127	129	131	133	134	135	81	81	82	83	84	85	85
	99th	134	135	136	138	140	142	142	88	89	90	91	92	93	93
16	50th	111	112	114	116	118	119	120	63	63	64	65	66	67	67
	90th	125	126	128	130	131	133	134	78	78	79	80	81	82	82
	95th	129	130	132	134	135	137	137	82	83	83	84	85	86	87
	99th	136	137	139	141	143	144	145	90	90	91	92	93	94	94
17	50th	114	115	116	118	120	121	122	65	66	66	67	68	69	70
	90th	127	128	130	132	134	135	136	80	80	81	82	83	84	84
	95th	131	132	134	136	138	139	140	84	85	86	87	87	88	89
	99th	139	140	141	143	145	146	147	92	93	93	94	95	96	97

[a]Based on the National High Blood Pressure Education Program.

From National High Blood Pressure Education Program Working Group on High Blood Pressure in Children and Adolescents. (2004). The fourth report on the diagnosis, evaluation, and treatment of high blood pressure in children and adolescents. *Pediatrics, 114*(suppl 4th Report), 555-5576.

TABLE B.2

BP LEVELS FOR GIRLS BY AGE AND HEIGHT PERCENTILE (NHBPEP[a])

		SYSTOLIC BP (mm Hg)							DIASTOLIC BP (mm Hg)						
		PERCENTILE OF HEIGHT							PERCENTILE OF HEIGHT						
AGE (YR)	BP PERCENTILE	5TH	10TH	25TH	50TH	75TH	90TH	95TH	5TH	10TH	25TH	50TH	75TH	90TH	95TH
1	50th	83	84	85	86	88	89	90	38	39	39	40	41	41	42
	90th	97	97	98	100	101	102	103	52	53	53	54	55	55	56
	95th	100	101	102	104	105	106	107	56	57	57	58	59	59	60
	99th	108	108	109	111	112	113	114	64	64	65	65	66	67	67
2	50th	85	85	87	88	89	91	91	43	44	44	45	46	46	47
	90th	98	99	100	101	103	104	105	57	58	58	59	60	61	61
	95th	102	103	104	105	107	108	109	61	62	62	63	64	65	65
	99th	109	110	111	112	114	115	116	69	69	70	70	71	72	72
3	50th	86	87	88	89	91	92	93	47	48	48	49	50	50	51
	90th	100	100	102	103	104	106	106	61	62	62	63	64	64	65
	95th	104	104	105	107	108	109	110	65	66	66	67	68	68	69
	99th	111	111	113	114	115	116	117	73	73	74	74	75	76	76
4	50th	88	88	90	91	92	94	94	50	50	51	52	52	53	54
	90th	101	102	103	104	106	107	108	64	64	65	66	67	67	68
	95th	105	106	107	108	110	111	112	68	68	69	70	71	71	72
	99th	112	113	114	115	117	118	119	76	76	76	77	78	79	79
5	50th	89	90	91	93	94	95	96	52	53	53	54	55	55	56
	90th	103	103	105	106	107	109	109	66	67	67	68	69	69	70
	95th	107	107	108	110	111	112	113	70	71	71	72	73	73	74
	99th	114	114	116	117	118	120	120	78	78	79	79	80	81	81

6	50th	91	92	93	94	96	97	98	54	54	55	56	56	57	58
	90th	104	105	106	108	109	110	111	68	68	69	70	70	71	72
	95th	108	109	110	111	113	114	115	72	72	73	74	74	75	76
	99th	115	116	117	119	120	121	122	80	80	81	81	82	83	83
7	50th	93	93	95	96	97	99	99	55	56	56	57	58	58	59
	90th	106	107	108	109	111	112	113	69	70	70	71	72	72	73
	95th	110	111	112	113	115	116	116	73	74	74	75	76	76	77
	99th	117	118	119	120	122	123	124	81	81	82	82	83	84	84
8	50th	95	95	96	98	99	100	101	57	57	57	58	59	60	60
	90th	108	109	110	111	113	114	114	71	71	71	72	73	74	74
	95th	112	112	114	115	116	118	118	75	75	75	76	77	78	78
	99th	119	120	121	122	123	125	125	82	82	83	83	84	85	86
9	50th	96	97	98	100	101	102	103	58	58	58	59	60	61	61
	90th	110	110	112	113	114	116	116	72	72	72	73	74	75	75
	95th	114	114	115	117	118	119	120	76	76	76	77	78	79	79
	99th	121	121	123	124	125	127	127	83	83	84	84	85	86	87
10	50th	98	99	100	102	103	104	105	59	59	59	60	61	62	62
	90th	112	112	114	115	116	118	118	73	73	73	74	75	76	76
	95th	116	116	117	119	120	121	122	77	77	77	78	79	80	80
	99th	123	123	125	126	127	129	129	84	84	85	86	86	87	88
11	50th	100	101	102	103	105	106	107	60	60	60	61	62	63	63
	90th	114	114	116	117	118	119	120	74	74	74	75	76	77	77
	95th	118	118	119	121	122	123	124	78	78	78	79	80	81	81
	99th	125	125	126	128	129	130	131	85	85	86	87	87	88	89
12	50th	102	103	104	105	107	108	109	61	61	61	62	63	64	64
	90th	116	116	117	119	120	121	122	75	75	75	76	77	78	78
	95th	119	120	121	123	124	125	126	79	79	79	80	81	82	82
	99th	127	127	128	130	131	132	133	86	86	87	88	88	89	90

TABLE B.2 *(continued)*

BP LEVELS FOR GIRLS BY AGE AND HEIGHT PERCENTILE (NHBPEP[a])

		SYSTOLIC BP (mm Hg)							DIASTOLIC BP (mm Hg)						
		PERCENTILE OF HEIGHT							PERCENTILE OF HEIGHT						
AGE (YR)	BP PERCENTILE	5TH	10TH	25TH	50TH	75TH	90TH	95TH	5TH	10TH	25TH	50TH	75TH	90TH	95TH
13	50th	104	105	106	107	109	110	110	62	62	62	63	64	65	65
	90th	117	118	119	121	122	123	124	76	76	76	77	78	79	79
	95th	121	122	123	124	126	127	128	80	80	80	81	82	83	83
	99th	128	129	130	132	133	134	135	87	87	88	89	89	90	91
14	50th	106	106	107	109	110	111	112	63	63	63	64	65	66	66
	90th	119	120	121	122	124	125	125	77	77	77	78	79	80	80
	95th	123	123	125	126	127	129	129	81	81	81	82	83	84	84
	99th	130	131	132	133	135	136	136	88	88	89	90	90	91	92
15	50th	107	108	109	110	111	113	113	64	64	64	65	66	67	67
	90th	120	121	122	123	125	126	127	78	78	78	79	80	81	81
	95th	124	125	126	127	129	130	131	82	82	82	83	84	85	85
	99th	131	132	133	134	136	137	138	89	89	90	91	91	92	93
16	50th	108	108	110	111	112	114	114	64	64	65	66	66	67	68
	90th	121	122	123	124	126	127	128	78	78	79	80	81	81	82
	95th	125	126	127	128	130	131	132	82	82	83	84	85	85	86
	99th	132	133	134	135	137	138	139	90	90	90	91	92	93	93
17	50th	108	109	110	111	113	114	115	64	65	65	66	67	67	68
	90th	122	122	123	125	126	127	128	78	79	79	80	81	81	82
	95th	125	126	127	129	130	131	132	82	83	83	84	85	85	86
	99th	133	133	134	136	137	138	139	90	90	91	91	92	93	93

[a]Based on the National High Blood Pressure Education Program.

From National High Blood Pressure Education Program Working Group on High Blood Pressure in Children and Adolescents. (2004). The fourth report on the diagnosis, evaluation, and treatment of high blood pressure in children and adolescents. *Pediatrics, 114*(suppl 4th Report), 555-5576.

TABLE B.3

AUSCULTATORY BLOOD PRESSURE VALUES FOR BOYS 5 TO 17 YEARS OLD (SAN ANTONIO CHILDREN'S BLOOD PRESSURE STUDY)

	PERCENTILES							
AGE (YR)	**5TH**	**10TH**	**25TH**	**MEAN**	**75TH**	**90TH**	**95TH**	**99TH[a]**
SYSTOLIC PRESSURE (mm Hg)								
5	78	81	87	92	98	103	106	112
6	81	84	89	95	100	105	108	114
7	82	85	90	96	102	107	110	116
8	83	86	92	97	103	108	111	117
9	85	88	93	99	104	109	113	118
10	86	89	95	100	106	111	114	120
11	88	91	97	102	108	113	116	122
12	91	94	99	105	111	116	119	125
13	94	97	102	108	113	118	122	127
14	96	99	105	110	116	121	122	130
15	99	102	107	113	118	124	127	132
16	100	103	108	114	120	125	128	134
17	100	103	109	114	120	125	128	134
DIASTOLIC PRESSURE (mm Hg) (Korotkoff phase 5)								
5	34	37	43	49	55	60	63	70
6	38	41	47	53	59	64	67	73
7	40	44	49	55	61	66	70	76
8	42	45	50	56	62	68	71	77
9	42	45	51	57	63	68	71	77
10	42	45	51	57	63	68	71	77
11	42	45	51	57	63	68	71	77
12	42	45	50	56	62	68	71	77
13	42	45	51	56	62	68	71	77
14	42	45	51	57	63	68	71	77
15	43	46	51	57	63	69	72	78
16	45	48	53	59	65	71	74	80
17	47	51	56	62	68	73	77	83

[a]The 99th percentile values were added after publication.

K5, Korotkoff phase 5.

Data presented in graphic form in Park, M.K., Menard, S.W., & Yuan, C. (2001). Comparison of blood pressure in children from three ethnic groups. *American Journal of Cardiology, 87*(1), 1305-1308.

TABLE B.4

AUSCULTATORY BLOOD PRESSURE VALUES FOR GIRLS 5 TO 17 YEARS OLD (SAN ANTONIO CHILDREN'S BLOOD PRESSURE STUDY)

	PERCENTILES							
AGE (YR)	5TH	10TH	25TH	MEAN	75TH	90TH	95TH	99TH[a]
SYSTOLIC PRESSURE (mm Hg)								
5	79	82	87	92	97	102	105	110
6	80	83	88	93	98	103	106	111
7	81	84	89	94	99	104	107	112
8	83	86	91	96	101	106	109	114
9	85	88	93	98	103	108	111	116
10	87	90	95	100	105	110	113	118
11	89	92	97	102	107	112	115	120
12	91	94	98	104	109	113	116	122
13	92	95	100	105	110	115	118	123
14	93	96	101	106	111	116	119	124
15	94	97	101	107	112	117	119	125
16	94	97	102	107	112	117	120	125
17	95	98	103	108	113	118	121	126
DIASTOLIC PRESSURE (mm Hg) (Korotkoff phase 5)								
5	35	38	44	49	55	60	63	69
6	38	41	47	52	58	63	66	72
7	40	41	49	54	60	65	68	74
8	42	45	50	56	61	67	70	75
9	43	46	51	56	62	67	70	76
10	43	46	51	57	63	68	71	77
11	43	46	51	57	63	68	71	77
12	43	46	52	57	63	68	71	77
13	43	47	52	57	63	68	71	77
14	44	47	52	58	63	68	72	77
15	44	47	52	58	64	69	72	78
16	45	48	53	59	64	69	73	78
17	46	49	54	59	65	70	73	79

[a]The 99th percentile values were added after publication.

K5, Korotkoff phase 5.

Data presented in graphic form in Park, M.K., Menard, S.W., & Yuan, C. (2001). Comparison of blood pressure in children from three ethnic groups. *American Journal of Cardiology, 87*(1), 1305-1308.

TABLE B.5

DINAMAP (MODEL 8100) BLOOD PRESSURE VALUES FOR BOYS 5 TO 17 YEARS OLD (SAN ANTONIO CHILDREN'S BLOOD PRESSURE STUDY)

	PERCENTILES							
AGE (YR)	5TH	10TH	25TH	MEAN	75TH	90TH	95TH	99TH[a]
SYSTOLIC PRESSURE (mm Hg)								
5	90	93	98	104	110	115	118	124
6	92	95	100	106	112	117	120	126
7	93	96	102	107	113	118	121	127
8	94	97	103	108	114	119	123	128
9	95	99	104	110	115	121	124	130
10	97	100	105	110	117	122	125	131
11	99	102	107	113	119	124	127	133
12	101	104	109	115	121	126	129	135
13	104	107	112	118	123	129	132	138
14	106	109	114	120	126	131	134	140
15	108	111	116	122	128	133	136	141
16	109	112	117	123	128	134	137	143
17	109	112	117	123	129	134	137	143
DIASTOLIC PRESSURE (mm Hg)								
5	46	49	53	58	63	68	71	76
6	47	49	54	59	64	68	71	76
7	47	50	54	59	64	69	72	77
8	48	51	55	60	65	70	72	78
9	49	51	56	61	66	70	73	78
10	49	52	56	61	66	71	74	79
11	49	52	57	62	67	71	74	79
12	50	52	57	62	67	71	74	79
13	50	52	57	62	67	71	74	79
14	50	52	57	62	67	72	74	79
15	50	52	57	62	67	72	74	79
16	50	53	57	62	67	72	74	80
17	50	53	57	62	67	72	75	80

[a]The 99th percentile values were added after submission of the manuscript.

From Park, M. K., Menard, S. W., & Schoolfield, J. (2005). Oscillometric blood pressure standards for children, *Pediatric Cardiology, 26*(5), 601-607.

TABLE B.6

DINAMAP (MODEL 8100) BLOOD PRESSURE VALUES FOR GIRLS 5 TO 17 YEARS OLD (SAN ANTONIO CHILDREN'S BLOOD PRESSURE STUDY)

	PERCENTILES							
AGE (YR)	**5TH**	**10TH**	**25TH**	**MEAN**	**75TH**	**90TH**	**95TH**	**99TH[a]**
SYSTOLIC PRESSURE (mm Hg)								
5	90	93	98	103	109	114	117	122
6	91	94	99	1043	110	115	118	123
7	92	95	100	106	111	116	119	125
8	94	97	102	107	113	118	121	126
9	95	98	103	109	114	119	122	128
10	97	100	105	110	116	121	124	129
11	98	101	106	112	117	122	125	131
12	100	103	107	113	118	123	126	132
13	101	104	109	114	120	125	128	133
14	102	104	109	115	120	125	128	134
15	102	105	110	115	121	126	129	134
16	102	105	110	115	121	126	129	134
17	102	105	110	115	121	126	129	134
DIASTOLIC PRESSURE (mm Hg)								
5	46	48	53	59	64	68	71	76
6	47	49	54	59	64	68	71	76
7	47	50	54	60	65	69	72	77
8	48	50	55	60	65	70	73	78
9	49	51	55	61	66	70	73	78
10	49	51	56	61	66	71	74	79
11	49	52	56	62	67	71	74	79
12	50	52	57	62	67	71	74	79
13	50	53	57	62	67	71	74	79
14	50	53	58	62	67	72	74	79
15	50	54	58	62	67	72	74	79
16	50	54	58	62	67	72	74	80
17	50	54	58	62	67	72	75	80

[a]The 99th percentile values were added after submission of the manuscript.

From Park, M. K., Menard, S. W., & Schoolfield, J. (2005). Oscillometric blood pressure standards for children, *Pediatric Cardiology, 26*(5), 601-607.

TABLE B.7

DINAMAP (MODEL 1846) BP PERCENTILES FOR NEONATES TO 5-YEAR-OLD CHILDREN

	PERCENTILES						
AGE	**5TH**	**10TH**	**25TH**	**MEAN**	**75TH**	**90TH**	**95TH**
SYSTOLIC PRESSURE (mm Hg)							
1-3 days	52	56	58	65	71	74	77
2-3 wk	62	66	71	78	84	89	92
1-5 mo	76	79	88	94	102	106	111
6-11 mo	79	84	88	94	99	104	109
1 yr	80	84	89	94	99	104	108
2 yr	82	85	91	95	101	106	109
3 yr	84	87	92	98	103	108	112
4 yr	86	90	95	100	105	110	114
5 yr	89	93	96	102	107	113	116
DIASTOLIC PRESSURE (mm Hg)							
1-3 days	31	33	37	41	45	50	52
2-3 wk	31	37	42	47	63	58	61
1-5 mo	45	48	53	59	64	71	75
6-11 mo	41	44	52	57	63	67	69
1 yr	44	48	52	57	73	67	69
2 yr	45	47	52	56	61	65	68
3 yr	44	47	52	56	61	65	69
4 yr	44	48	52	56	61	65	68
5 yr	44	48	53	57	62	66	68

Data presented in graphic form in Park, M., & Menard, S. M. (1989). Normative oscillometric BP values in the first 5 years in an office setting, *American Journal of Diseases of Children, 143*(7), 860-864.

TABLE B.8

NORMAL VALUES FOR AMBULATORY BLOOD PRESSURE FOR HEALTHY BOYS BY AGE

BP	AGE (YR)											
PERCENTILE	**5**	**6**	**7**	**8**	**9**	**10**	**11**	**12**	**13**	**14**	**15**	**16**
24-HOUR SBP												
50th	105	106	106	107	108	109	110	113	115	118	121	123
75th	109	110	111	112	113	114	116	118	121	124	127	129
90th	113	115	116	117	118	119	121	124	126	129	132	135
95th	116	118	119	120	121	123	125	127	130	133	136	138
99th	123	1241	125	127	128	129	131	134	137	140	142	145
DAYTIME SBP												
50th	111	112	112	112	113	113	1159	117	120	122	125	128
75th	116	116	117	117	118	119	1201	123	126	129	132	135
90th	120	121	122	122	123	124	126	128	131	134	137	140
95th	123	124	125	125	126	127	129	132	135	138	141	144
99th	129	130	131	132	132	134	136	139	142	144	147	150

NIGHTTIME SBP												
50th	95	96	96	97	97	98	99	101	103	106	108	111
75th	99	100	101	102	103	104	105	107	109	112	114	117
90th	103	105	106	108	109	110	111	113	115	118	120	123
95th	106	108	110	111	112	113	115	116	119	121	123	126
99th	112	115	117	118	120	121	122	123	126	128	130	132
24H DBP												
50th	65	66	66	66	67	67	67	67	67	68	68	69
75th	69	69	70	70	70	70	71	71	71	71	72	72
90th	72	73	73	73	73	73	74	74	74	75	75	76
95th	74	75	75	75	75	75	76	76	76	77	77	78
99th	79	79	79	79	79	79	79	80	80-	80	81	81
DAYTIME DBP												
50th	72	72	73	73	72	72	72	72	72	73	73	74
75th	76	76	76	76	76	76	76	76	76	77	77	78
90th	79	79	80	80	80	80	80	80	80	80	81	81
95th	81	81	82	82	82	82	82	82	82	82	83	84
99th	85	84	85	86	85	85	85	85	86	86	87	88

TABLE B.8 *(continued)*

NORMAL VALUES FOR AMBULATORY BLOOD PRESSURE FOR HEALTHY BOYS BY AGE

BP	AGE (YR)											
PERCENTILE	5	6	7	8	9	10	11	12	13	14	15	16
NIGHTTIME DBP												
50th	55	55	56	56	56	56	56	56	56	57	57	57
75th	59	59	60	60	60	60	60	60	60	61	61	61
90th	62	63	64	64	64	64	64	64	64	64	64	64
95th	65	66	67	67	67	67	67	67	67	67	66	66
99th	72	73	74	74	73	73	72	71	71	71	71	70
24-HOUR MAP												
50th	77	78	79	79	80	80	81	82	83	84	85	86
75th	81	82	83	83	84	84	85	86	86	88	89	91
90th	86	86	87	87	88	88	89	90	91	92	93	94
95th	88	89	90	90	90	91	91	92	93	94	95	96
99th	94	95	95	95	96	96	96	92	97	97	98	99

DAYTIME MAP												
50th	84	84	85	85	85	85	85	86	87	88	89	91
75th	88	88	89	89	89	90	90	91	92	93	94	96
90th	91	92	93	93	94	94	94	95	96	97	98	100
95th	94	95	95	96	96	96	97	97	98	99	101	102
99th	98	99	100	101	101	101	101	102	102	103	105	106
NIGHTTIME MAP												
50th	..67	68	69	69	70	70	71	71	72	73	74	75
75th	71	72	73	74	74	75	75	76	76	77	78	79
90th	75	76	77	78	79	79	79	80	80	81	81	82
95th	78	79	80	81	82	82	82	82	83	83	83	83
99th	84	86	86	88	88	88	87	87	87	87	87	86

DBP, Diastolic blood pressure; *MAP*, mean arterial pressure; *SBP*, systolic blood pressure.

Modified from Wühl E, Witte K, Soergel M, et al: Distribution of 24-h ambulatory blood pressure in children: normalized reference values and role of body dimension, *J Hypertens* 20:1995–2007, 2002.

TABLE B.9

NORMAL VALUES FOR AMBULATORY BLOOD PRESSURE FOR HEALTHY GIRLS BY AGE[a]

BP	AGE (YR)											
PERCENTILE	**5**	**6**	**7**	**8**	**9**	**10**	**11**	**12**	**13**	**14**	**15**	**16**
24-HOUR SBP												
50th	103	104	105	107	108	109	110	111	112	113	114	115
75th	108	109	110	112	113	114	115	116	117	118	118	119
90th	112	114	115	116	117	118	119	120	121	122	123	123
95th	114	116	118	119	120	121	122	123	124	125	125	126
99th	120	122	123	124	126	127	128	128	129	130	130	130
DAYTIME SBP												
50th	108.4	109.5	110.6	111.5	112.4	113.3	114.2	115.3	116.4	117.5	118.6	119.6
75th	113.8	114.9	115.9	116.8	117.6	118.5	119.5	120.6	121.7	122.6	123.5	124.3
90th	118.3	119.5	120.6	121.5	122.4	123.3	124.3	125.3	126.4	127.2	127.9	128.5
95th	120.9	122.2	123.3	124.3	125.2	126.2	127.2	128.2	129.2	129.9	130.4	130.9
99th	125.6	127.1	128.4	129.6	130.6	131.7	132.7	133.7	134.5	135.0	135.2	135.4

NIGHTTIME SBP												
50th	95	96	96	97	98	98	99	100	101	101	102	103
75th	100	101	102	103	103	104	105	105	106	106	107	107
90th	105	106	107	108	109	110	110	110	111	111	111	111
95th	108	110	111	112	112	113	114	114	114	114	114	114
99th	115	116	117	118	119	120	120	120	119	119	118	118
24-HOUR DBP												
50th	66	66	66	66	66	66	66	67	67	67	68	68
75th	69	69	69	69	70	70	70	70	71	71	71	71
90th	72	72	72	72	73	73	73	74	74	74	75	75
95th	74	74	74	74	74	75	75	76	76	76	77	77
99th	78	78	78	78	78	78	78	79	80	80	80	81
DAYTIME DBP												
50th	73	73	72	72	72	72	72	72	72	73	73	74
75th	77	77	76	76	76	76	76	76	77	77	77	77
90th	80	80	80	80	80	79	79	80	80	80	80	80
95th	82	82	82	82	82	81	81	82	82	82	82	82
99th	86	86	86	86	85	85	85	85	86	86	86	85

TABLE B.9 *(continued)*

NORMAL VALUES FOR AMBULATORY BLOOD PRESSURE FOR HEALTHY GIRLS BY AGE[a]

BP	AGE (YR)											
PERCENTILE	**5**	**6**	**7**	**8**	**9**	**10**	**11**	**12**	**13**	**14**	**15**	**16**
NIGHTTIME DBP												
50th	55	56	56	55	55	55	54	54	54	55	55	55
75th	61	61	60	60	59	59	59	59	59	59	59	59
90th	66	65	65	64	64	64	63	63	63	63	63	63
95th	69	68	67	67	67	67	66	65	66	65	65	65
99th	74	74	73	72	72	72	72	71	71	71	70	70
24H MAP												
50th	78	78	78	79	79	80	80	81	82	82	83	83
75th	81	82	82	83	83	83	84	85	85	86	87	87
90th	85	85	85	86	86	87	87	88	89	89	90	909
95th	87	87	87	88	88	88	89	90	91	91	92	92
99th	91	91	91	91	91	92	92	93	94	94	95	95

DAYTIME MAP												
50th	84	83	84	84	84	84	85	85	86	87	87	88
75th	88	88	88	88	88	89	89	89	90	91	91	92
90th	92	92	92	92	92	92	92	93	94	94	95	95
95th	95	95	94	94	94	94	94	95	96	96	97	97
99th	99	99	99	98	98	98	98	99	99	100	100	101
NIGHTTIME MAP												
50th	69	69	69	69	69	69	69	70	70	71	71	72
75th	73	73	73	73	73	74	74	74	75	75	75	76
90th	77	77	77	77	77	78	78	78	78	79	79	79
95th	79	79	80	80	80	80	80	80	81	81	81	81
99th	84	84	84	84	85	85	85	85	85	85	85	85

[a]Numbers have been rounded off to the nearest whole number.

DBP, Diastolic blood pressure; *MAP*, mean arterial pressure; *SBP*, systolic blood pressure.

Modified from Wühl E, Witte K, Soergel M, et al: Distribution of 24-h ambulatory blood pressure in children: normalized reference values and role of body dimension, *J Hypertens* 20:1995–2007, 2002.

Appendix C

Cardiovascular Risk Factors

TABLE C.1

ESTIMATED VALUE FOR PERCENTILE REGRESSION OF WAIST CIRCUMFERENCE FOR EUROPEAN-AMERICAN CHILDREN AND ADOLESCENTS ACCORDING TO SEX[a]

	PERCENTILE FOR BOYS					PERCENTILE FOR GIRLS				
AGE (YR)	10TH	25TH	50TH	75TH	90TH	10TH	25TH	50TH	75TH	90TH
2	42.9	46.9	47.1	48.6	50.6	43.1	45.1	47.4	49.6	52.5
3	44.7	48.8	49.2	51.2	54.0	44.7	46.8	49.3	51.9	55.4
4	46.5	50.6	51.3	53.8	57.4	46.3	48.5	51.2	54.2	58.2
5	48.3	52.5	53.3	56.5	60.8	47.9	50.2	53.1	56.5	61.1
6	50.1	54.3	55.4	59.1	64.2	49.5	51.8	55.0	58.8	64.0
7	46.5	50.6	51.3	53.8	57.4	46.3	48.5	51.2	54.2	58.2
8	48.3	52.5	53.3	56.5	60.8	47.9	50.2	53.1	56.5	61.1
9	50.1	54.3	55.4	59.1	64.2	49.5	51.8	55.0	58.8	64.0
10	46.5	50.6	51.3	53.8	57.4	46.3	48.5	51.2	54.2	58.2
11	59.1	63.6	65.8	72.2	81.1	57.5	60.2	64.4	70.3	78.3
12	60.9	65.5	67.9	74.9	84.5	59.1	61.9	66.3	72.6	81.2
13	62.7	67.4	70.0	77.5	87.9	60.7	63.6	68.2	74.9	84.1
14	64.5	69.2	72.1	80.1	91.3	62.3	65.3	70.1	77.2	86.9
15	66.3	71.1	74.1	82.8	94.7	63.9	67.0	72.0	79.5	89.8
16	68.1	72.9	76.2	85.4	98.1	65.5	68.6	73.9	81.8	92.7
17	69.9	74.8	78.3	88.0	101.5	67.1	70.3	75.8	84.1	95.5
18	71.7	76.7	80.4	90.6	104.9	68.7	72.0	77.7	86.4	98.4

[a]Waist circumference was measured with a tape at just above the uppermost lateral border of the right ileum at the end of normal expiration.
From Fernandez, J. R., Redden, D. T., Pietrobelli, A., & Allison, D. B. (2004). Waist circumference percentiles in nationally representative samples of African-American, European-American, and Mexican-American children and adolescents. *Journal of Pediatrics, 145*(4), 439-444.

TABLE C.2

ESTIMATED VALUE FOR PERCENTILE REGRESSION OF WAIST CIRCUMFERENCE FOR AFRICAN-AMERICAN CHILDREN AND ADOLESCENTS ACCORDING TO SEX[a]

	PERCENTILE FOR BOYS					PERCENTILE FOR GIRLS				
AGE (YR)	10TH	25TH	50TH	75TH	90TH	10TH	25TH	50TH	75TH	90TH
2	43.2	44.6	46.4	48.5	50.0	43.0	44.6	46.0	47.7	50.1
3	44.8	46.3	48.3	50.7	53.2	44.6	46.3	48.1	50.6	53.8
4	46.3	48.0	50.1	52.9	56.4	46.1	48.0	50.2	53.4	57.5
5	47.9	49.7	52.0	55.1	59.6	47.7	49.7	52.3	56.2	61.1
6	49.4	51.4	53.9	57.3	62.8	49.2	51.4	54.5	59.0	64.8
7	51.0	53.1	55.7	59.5	66.1	50.8	53.2	56.6	61.8	68.5
8	52.5	54.8	57.6	61.7	69.3	52.4	54.9	58.7	64.7	72.2
9	54.1	56.4	59.4	63.9	72.5	53.9	56.6	60.9	67.5	75.8
10	55.6	58.1	61.3	66.1	75.7	55.5	58.3	63.0	70.3	79.5
11	57.2	59.8	63.2	68.3	78.9	57.0	60.0	65.1	73.1	83.2
12	58.7	61.5	65.0	70.5	82.1	58.6	61.7	67.3	75.9	86.9
13	60.3	63.2	66.9	72.7	85.3	60.2	63.4	69.4	78.8	90.5
14	61.8	64.9	68.7	74.9	88.5	61.7	65.1	71.5	81.6	94.2
15	63.4	66.6	70.6	77.1	91.7	63.3	66.8	73.6	84.4	97.9
16	64.9	68.3	72.5	79.3	94.9	64.8	68.5	75.8	87.2	101.6
17	66.5	70.0	74.3	81.5	98.2	66.4	70.3	77.9	90.0	105.2
18	68.0	71.7	76.2	83.7	101.4	68.0	72.0	80.0	92.9	108.9

[a]Waist circumference was measured with a tape at just above the uppermost lateral border of the right ileum at the end of normal expiration.
From Fernandez, J. R., Redden, D. T., Pietrobelli, A., & Allison, D. B. (2004). Waist circumference percentiles in nationally representative samples of African-American, European-American, and Mexican-American children and adolescents. *Journal of Pediatrics, 145*(4), 439-444.

TABLE C.3

ESTIMATED VALUE FOR PERCENTILE REGRESSION OF WAIST CIRCUMFERENCE FOR MEXICAN-AMERICAN CHILDREN AND ADOLESCENTS ACCORDING TO SEX[a]

	PERCENTILE FOR BOYS					PERCENTILE FOR GIRLS				
AGE (YR)	10TH	25TH	50TH	75TH	90TH	10TH	25TH	50TH	75TH	90TH
2	44.4	45.6	47.6	49.8	53.2	44.5	45.7	48.0	50.0	53.5
3	46.1	47.5	49.8	52.5	56.7	46.0	47.4	50.1	52.6	56.7
4	47.8	49.4	52.0	55.3	60.2	47.5	49.2	52.2	55.2	59.9
5	49.5	51.3	54.2	58.0	63.6	49.0	51.0	54.2	57.8	63.0
6	51.2	53.2	56.3	60.7	67.1	50.5	52.7	56.3	60.4	66.2
7	52.9	55.1	58.5	63.4	70.6	52.0	54.5	58.4	63.0	69.4
8	54.6	57.0	60.7	66.2	74.1	53.5	56.3	60.4	65.6	72.6
9	56.3	58.9	62.9	68.9	77.6	55.0	58.0	62.5	68.2	75.8
10	58.0	60.8	65.1	71.6	81.0	56.5	59.8	64.6	70.8	78.9
11	59.7	62.7	67.2	74.4	84.5	58.1	61.6	66.6	73.4	82.1
12	61.4	64.6	69.4	77.1	88.0	59.6	63.4	68.7	76.0	85.3
13	63.1	66.5	71.6	79.8	91.5	61.1	65.1	70.8	78.6	88.5
14	64.8	68.4	73.8	82.6	95.0	62.6	66.9	72.9	81.2	91.7
15	66.5	70.3	76.0	85.3	98.4	64.1	68.7	74.9	83.8	94.8
16	68.2	72.2	78.1	88.0	101.9	65.6	70.4	77.0	86.4	98.0
17	69.9	74.1	80.3	90.7	105.4	67.1	72.2	79.1	89.0	101.2
18	71.6	76.0	82.5	93.5	108.9	68.6	74.0	81.1	91.6	104.4

[a]Waist circumference was measured with a tape at just above the uppermost lateral border of the right ileum at the end of normal expiration.
From Fernandez, J. R., Redden, D. T., Pietrobelli, A., & Allison, D. B. (2004). Waist circumference percentiles in nationally representative samples of African-American, European-American, and Mexican-American children and adolescents. *Journal of Pediatrics, 145*(4), 439-444.

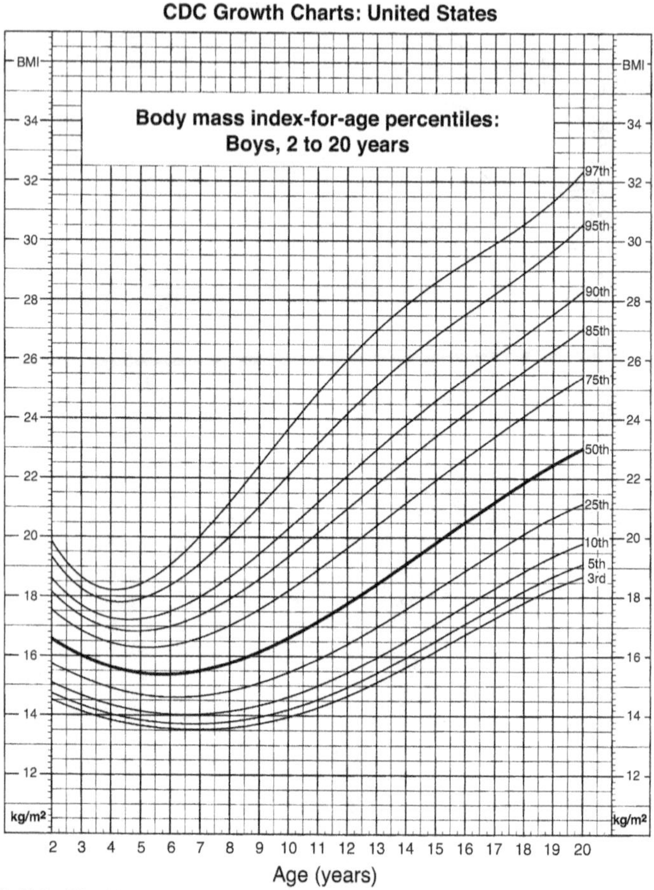

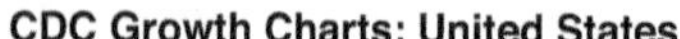

Published May 30, 2000.

Source: Developed by the National Center for Health Statistics in collaboration with the National Center for Chronic Disease Prevention and Health Promotion (2000).

FIG. C.1

Body mass index percentile curves for boys 2 to 20 years old.

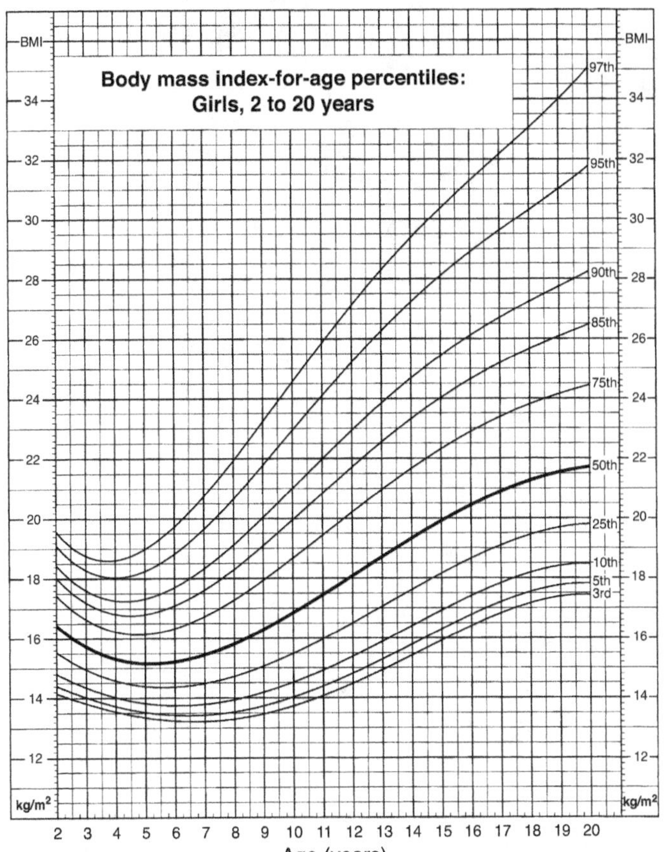

Published May 30, 2000.

Source: Developed by the National Center for Health Statistics in collaboration with the National Center for Chronic Disease Prevention and Health Promotion (2000).

FIG. C.2

Body mass index percentile curves for girls 2 to 20 years old.

Appendix D

Normal Echocardiographic Values

TABLE D.1

TWO-DIMENSIONAL ECHOCARDIOGRAPHY-DERIVED M-MODE MEASUREMENTS OF THE LV DIMENSION AND WALL THICKNESS: MEAN (−2 SD TO +2 SD) (IN MM)[a]

VIEWS	BSA	0.2	0.3	0.4	0.5	0.6	0.7	0.8	0.9	1.0	1.2	1.4	1.6	1.8	2.0	2.2
RV LV	LV EDD	19.5 (15.5-23.0)	23.0 (19.0-27.0)	26.0 (22.0-30.5)	29.5 (24.5-34.0)	31.5 (27.0-36.5)	33.5 (29.0-38.5)	35.5 (30.5-41.0)	37.5 (32.0-43.0)	39.5 (33.5-45.0)	42.0 (36.0-48.0)	45.0 (38.5-51.0)	47.0 (40.5-54.0)	49.5 (42.5-57.0)	51.5 (44.0-60.0)	53.5 (45.5-62.0)
	IVS (D)	4.5 (3.0-5.5)	5.0 (3.5-6.0)	5.0 (4.0-6.5)	5.5 (4.0-7.0)	6.0 (4.5-7.5)	6.0 (4.5-8.0)	6.5 (4.5-8.5)	7.0 (5.0-9.0)	7.0 (5.0-9.5)	8.0 (5.5-10.0)	8.5 (6.0-11.0)	9.0 (6.0-12.0)	9.5 (6.5-12.5)	10.5 (7.0-13.5)	11.0 (7.5-14.5)
	LVPW (D)	4.0 (3.0-5.0)	4.5 (3.0-5.5)	4.5 (3.5-6.0)	5.0 (3.5-6.5)	5.5 (4.0-7.0)	6.0 (4.0-7.5)	6.0 (4.5-8.0)	6.5 (4.5-8.0)	7.0 (5.0-8.5)	7.5 (5.5-9.5)	8.0 (5.5-10.0)	8.5 (6.0-11.0)	9.0 (6.5-11.5)	9.5 (7.0-12.0)	10.0 (7.5-13.0)
RV LV	LV ESD	12.0 (8.0-15.0)	15.0 (11.5-18.0)	17.0 (13.5-20.0)	18.5 (15.0-22.5)	20.0 (16.5-24.5)	21.5 (17.5-26.0)	23.0 (18.5-28.0)	24.0 (19.5-29.0)	25.5 (20.5-31.0)	28.0 (22.0-33.5)	29.5 (23.5-35.5)	31.5 (24.5-37.5)	33.0 (25.5-39.5)	34.5 (26.5-41.5)	36.0 (27.5-43.0)
	IVS (S)	6.5 (5.0-8.0)	7.0 (5.5-9.0)	7.5 (6.0-9.5)	8.0 (6.0-10.0)	8.5 (6.5-10.5)	9.0 (7.0-11.0)	9.5 (7.5-11.5)	9.5 (7.5-12.0)	10.0 (8.0-12.5)	10.5 (8.0-13.5)	11.5 (9.0-14.5)	12.0 (9.0-15.5)	12.5 (9.5-16.5)	13.5 (10.0-18.0)	14.0 (10.0-19.0)
	LVPW (S)	6.5 (5.5-8.0)	7.0 (6.0-8.5)	8.0 (6.5-9.5)	9.0 (7.0-10.5)	9.5 (7.5-11.0)	10.0 (8.0-12.0)	10.5 (8.5-12.5)	11.5 (9.0-13.5)	11.5 (9.0-14.0)	12.5 (10.0-15.0)	13.0 (10.5-16.0)	14.0 (11.0-17.5)	14.5 (11.0-18.5)	15.0 (11.5-19.5)	16.0 (12.0-20.0)

BSA, body surface area; *IVS (D)*, interventricular septal thickness, end-diastolic; *IVS (S)*, interventricular septal thickness, end-systolic; *LV*, left ventricular; *LVEDD*, LV end-diastolic dimension; *LVESD*, LV end-systolic dimension; *LVPW (D)*, LV posterior wall thickness, end-diastolic; *LVPW (S)*, LV posterior wall thickness, end-systolic; *SD*, standard deviation.

Values derived from graphic data of Appendix 1. In Lai, W. W., Mertens, L. L., Cohen, M. S., & Geva, T. (Eds.). (2010). *Echocardiography in pediatric and congenital heart disease*. Oxford, UK: Wiley-Blackwell.

[a]Values are rounded off to the nearest 0.5 mm.

TABLE D.2

STAND-ALONE M-MODE ECHOCARDIOGRAPHIC MEASUREMENTS: RIGHT VENTRICLE, AORTA, LEFT ATRIUM BY BODY SURFACE AREA: MEAN (90% TOLERANCE LIMITS) (IN MM)[a]

ECHO VIEWS	BSA	0.2	0.3	0.4	0.5	0.6	0.7	0.8	0.9	1.0	1.2	1.4	1.6	1.8	2.0
RV, LV	RV (diastolic)	7 (-16)	9.5 (0-17)	10 (0-17)	10 (2.5-18)	11 (3-19)	12 (3.5-21)	13 (4-22)	14 (4.5-23)	14 (5-24)	16 (6-26)	18 (6.5-29)	20 (7-32)	22 (7.5-35)	23 (8-42)
AV, AO, LA	Aorta (diastolic)	10 (6-14)	12 (7.5-16)	13 (9-17.5)	14 (9.5-19)	15 (10.5-21)	16 (11.5-22)	17 (12.5-24)	18 (13-24.5)	19 (13.5-25)	21 (14.5-27)	22 (15.5-29)	23 (16-30.5)	24 (16-32)	24 (16-33)
	LA (systolic)	13 (6-20)	16 (8-23)	18 (9-25)	19 (11-27)	20 (12-29)	22 (13-31)	23 (14-33)	24 (15-34)	26 (16-35)	27 (17-38)	28 (17-40)	29 (18-42)	29 (18-43)	30 (18-44)

BSA, body surface area; *LA*, left atrium; *RV*, right ventricle.
Values derived from graphic data of Rogé, C. L., Silverman, N, H., Hart, P. A., & Ray, R. M. (1978). Cardiac structure growth pattern determined by echocardiography. *Circulation, 57*(2), 285-290.
[a]Values rounded off to the nearest 0.5 mm or measurements <10 mm and to the nearest 1 mm for measurements ≥ 10 mm.

TABLE D.3

TWO-DIMENSIONAL ECHOCARDIOGRAPHIC MEASUREMENTS OF AORTIC ROOT AND AORTA: MEAN (−2 SD TO +2 SD) (IN MM)[a]

ECHO VIEWS	BSA	0.2	0.3	0.4	0.5	0.6	0.7	0.8	0.9	1.0	1.2	1.4	1.6	1.8	2.0	2.2
	Aortic annulus	17.0 (5.5-9.0)	8.5 (7.0-10.0)	10.0 (8.0-12.0)	11.0 (9.0-13.5)	12.0 (10.0-14.5)	13.5 (11.0-15.5)	14.0 (11.5-16.5)	15.0 (12.5-17.5)	15.5 (13.9-18.5)	17.5 (14.5-20.5)	18.5 (15.0-22.0)	20.0 (16.0-23.5)	21.0 (17.0-25.0)	22.0 (18.0-26.0)	23.0 (18.5-27.5)
	Sinus of Valsalva	9.5 (7.0-12.0)	11.5 (9.0-14.0)	13.0 (10.0-16.0)	14.5 (11.5-17.5)	16.0 (13.0-19.5)	17.5 (14.0-21.0)	18.5 (15.5-22.05)	19.5 (15.5-23.5)	20.5 (16-25.0)	22.0 (18.0-27.0)	24.0 (19.0-30.0)	25.5 (20.0-31.5)	27.0 (21.0-33.5)	28.5 (22.0-35.5)	30.5 (23.0-38.5)
	Sinotubular junction	8.0 (6.0-10.0)	10.0 (7.5-12.0)	11.0 (9.0-13.5)	12.5 (10.0-15.0)	14.0 (11.0-16.5)	15.0 (12.0-18.0)	16.0 (12.5-19.0)	16.5 (13.0-20.5)	17.5 (14.0-21.5)	19.5 (15.5-24.0)	21.0 (16.5-26.0)	22.0 (17.0-27.5)	24.0 (18.0-29.0)	25.0 (19.0-31.0)	26.0 (20.0-32.0)
	Ascending aorta	8.0 (5.5-11.0)	10.0 (7.0-13.0)	11.5 (8.5-15.0)	13.0 (10.0-16.0)	14.5 (11.0-17.5)	15.5 (12.0-19.0)	16.5 (13.0-20.5)	17.5 (14.0-21.5)	18.5 (14.5-23.0)	20.5 (15.5-25.5)	22.0 (16.5-27.5)	24.0 (18.0-29.5)	25.5 (19.0-31.0)	26.5 (20.0-33.0)	28.0 (21.0-35.0)
	Transverse aorta	6.5 (4.0-8.5)	8.0 (5.5-10.0)	9.5 (8.0-13.0)	10.5 (8.0-13.0)	11.5 (9.0-14.5)	12.5 (9.5-15.5)	13.0 (10.0-17.0)	14.0 (11.0-18.0)	15.0 (11.5-19.0)	17.0 (12.5-20.5)	18.0 (14.0-22.0)	19.5 (15.0-24.0)	20.5 (15.5-25.5)	21.5 (16.0-27.0)	22.5 (17.0-28.5)
	Aortic isthmus	5.5 (3.0-7.5)	6.5 (4.0-9.0)	7.5 (5.0-10.0)	8.5 (6.0-11.0)	9.5 (6.5-12.5)	10.5 (7.0-13.5)	11.0 (7.5-14.5)	12.0 (8.0-15.5)	12.5 (8.5-16.0)	13.5 (9.5-17.5)	15.0 (10.0-19.5)	16.0 (10.5-21.0)	17.0 (11.0-22.0)	17.5 (11.5-23.5)	18.0 (12.0-25.0)

BSA, body surface area; *SD*, standard deviation.

Values derived from graphic data of Appendix 1. In Lai, W. W., Mertens, L. L., Cohen, M. S., & Geva, T. (Eds.). (2010). *Echocardiography in pediatric and congenital heart disease*. Oxford, UK: Wiley-Blackwell.

[a]Values are rounded off to the nearest 0.5 mm.

TABLE D.4

TWO-DIMENSIONAL ECHOCARDIOGRAPHIC MEASUREMENTS OF THE PULMONARY VALVE AND PULMONARY ARTERIES: MEAN (−2 SD TO +2 SD) (IN MM)[a]

ECHO VIEWS	BSA	0.2	0.3	0.4	0.5	0.6	0.7	0.8	0.9	1.0	1.2	1.4	1.6	1.8	2.0	2.2
	Pulmonary annulus	8.5 (6.0-10.5)	10.0 (8.0-12.5)	11.5 (9.0-14.0)	13.0 (10.0-16.0)	14.0 (11.0-17.5)	15.5 (11.5-19.0)	16.5 (12.0-20.5)	17.5 (13.0-21.5)	18.5 (13.5-23.0)	20.0 (15.0-25.0)	22.0 (16.0-27.5)	23.5 (17.0-29.0)	25.0 (18.0-30.5)	26.0 (19.0-33.0)	27.0 (19.5-34.0)
	Main PA	7.5 (5.0-10.0)	9.0 (6.5-12.0)	10.5 (7.5-14.0)	12.0 (9.0-15.0)	13.0 (9.5-16.5)	14.0 (10.0-17.5)	15.0 (11.0-18.5)	16.0 (11.5-20.0)	17.0 (12.0-21.0)	18.5 (13.5-23.0)	20.0 (14.5-25.5)	21.0 (15.0-28.0)	22.5 (16.0-30.0)	24.0 (16.5-32.0)	25.0 (17.0-33.0)
	Right PA	5.0 (3.5-7.0)	6.0 (4.5-8.0)	7.0 (5.0-9.0)	8.0 (5.5-10.0)	9.0 (6.0-11.0)	9.5 (6.5-12.0)	10.0 (7.0-13.0)	10.5 (7.5-13.5)	11.0 (8.0-14.0)	12.5 (9.0-16.0)	13.0 (9.5-17.5)	14.0 (10.0-18.5)	15.0 (10.5-20.0)	15.5 (10.5-21.0)	16.5 (11.0-22.0)
	Left PA	4.5 (3.0-6.5)	5.5 (4.0-7.5)	6.5 (4.5-8.5)	7.5 (5.0-9.5)	8.0 (5.5-10.5)	9.0 (6.0-11.0)	9.5 (6.5-12.0)	10.0 (7.0-13.0)	10.5 (7.5-14.0)	11.5 (8.0-15.5)	12.5 (8.5-16.5)	13.5 (9.0-18.0)	14.0 (9.0-19.0)	15.0 (9.5-20.0)	15.5 (10.0-21.0)

BSA, body surface area; *PA*, pulmonary artery; *SD*, standard deviation.

Values derived from graphic data of Appendix 1. In Lai, W. W., Mertens, L. L., Cohen, M. S., & Geva, T. (Eds.). (2010). *Echocardiography in pediatric and congenital heart disease.* Oxford, UK: Wiley-Blackwell.

[a]Values are rounded off to the nearest 0.5 mm.

TABLE D.5

TWO-DIMENSIONAL ECHOCARDIOGRAPHIC MEASUREMENTS OF ATRIOVENTRICULAR VALVES: MEAN (−2 SD TO +2 SD) (IN MM)[a]

ECHO VIEWS	BSA	0.2	0.3	0.4	0.5	0.6	0.7	0.8	0.9	1.0	1.2	1.4	1.6	1.8	2.0	2.2
	Mitral (apical 4- chamber)	10.0 (8.0-12.0)	12.5 (9.5-15.0)	13.5 (10.5-17.5)	15.1 (12.0-19.0)	17.0 (12.5-21.0)	18.0 (13.5-22.5)	19.0 (14.5-24.0)	20.5 (15.0-25.5)	22.0 (15.5-27.5)	23.5 (16.5-30.5)	25.0 (17.5-33.0)	27.0 (18.0-35.5)	28.0 (18.5-37.5)	29.5 (19.0-40.0)	31.0 (19.0-42.0)
	Tricuspid (apical 4-chamber)	11.0 (7.5-14.0)	13.0 (8.5-17.0)	15.0 (10.5-18.5)	17.0 (12.0-20.5)	18.0 (13.0-22.5)	19.0 (14.0-23.5)	20.0 (15.0-25.0)	21.5 (16.0-27.5)	22.5 (17.0-28.0)	24.0 (18.0-30.5)	26.5 (19.0-33.0)	28.0 (20.5-35.0)	29.5 (21.5-37.5)	31.0 (22.5-39.5)	32.5 (23.5-42.0)
	Mitral (parasternal long)	10.0 (7.5-12.5)	11.5 (9.0-15.0)	13.0 (10.0-16.0)	14.5 (11.0-18.0)	16.0 (12.0-19.5)	17.0 (12.5-21.0)	18.0 (13.0-22.5)	19.0 (14.0-23.0)	20.0 (15.0-25.0)	22.0 (16.0-27.5)	23.0 (17.0-30.0)	25.0 (18.0-32.0)	26.0 (18.5-34.5)	28.0 (19.0-37.0)	29.0 (20.0-39.0)
	Tricuspid (RV inflow view)	10.5 (7.5-13.0)	12.5 (9.0-15.5)	14.5 (10.5-17.5)	15.5 (12.5-19.5)	17.5 (13.0-22.0)	18.5 (14.0-23.0)	20.0 (15.0-25.0)	21.5 (16.0-27.0)	22.0 (17.0-28.0)	23.5 (17.5-30.5)	25.5 (18.5-33.0)	27.5 (19.5-35.5)	29.0 (20.5-38.0)	30.5 (21.5-40.0)	32.5 (22.5-42.5)

BSA, body surface area; *RV*, right ventricular; *SD*, standard deviation.

Values derived from graphic data of Appendix 1. In Lai, W. W., Mertens, L. L., Cohen, M. S., & Geva, T. (Eds.). (2010). *Echocardiography in pediatric and congenital heart disease*. Oxford, UK: Wiley-Blackwell.

[a]Values are rounded off to the nearest 0.5 mm.

TABLE D.6

TWO-DIMENSIONAL ECHOCARDIOGRAPHIC MEASUREMENTS OF MEAN AND PREDICTION LIMITS FOR 2 AND 3 STANDARD DEVIATIONS FOR MAJOR CORONARY ARTERY SEGMENTS[a]

ECHO VIEWS	BSA		0.2	0.3	0.4	0.5	0.6	0.7	0.8	1.0	1.2	1.4	1.6	1.8	2.0
	Left anterior descending (LAD)	Mean	1.2	1.4	1.6	1.8	1.9	2.0	2.2	2.3	2.5	2.7	2.8	2.9	3.0
		Mean +2 SD	1.5	1.8	2.1	2.3	2.5	2.7	2.8	3.0	3.3	3.5	3.7	4.0	4.2
		Mean +3 SD	1.7	2.0	2.3	2.5	2.8	3.0	3.2	3.4	3.8	4.0	4.3	4.5	4.7
	Right coronary artery (RCA)	Mean	1.3	1.4	1.6	1.7	1.8	2.0	2.1	2.3	2.5	2.7	2.8	3.0	3.2
		Mean +2 SD	1.9	2.1	2.3	2.4	2.6	2.7	2.8	3.1	3.4	3.6	3.8	4.0	4.3
		Mean +3 SD	2.2	2.4	2.6	2.8	3.0	3.1	3.3	3.5	3.8	4.1	4.3	4.5	4.8
	Left main coronary artery (LMCA)	Mean	1.7	1.9	2.1	2.3	2.4	2.5	2.7	2.9	3.1	3.3	3.4	3.6	3.7
		Mean +2 SD	2.3	2.6	2.8	3.0	3.3	3.4	3.6	3.9	4.2	4.4	4.6	4.8	5.1
		Mean +3 SD	2.7	3.0	3.2	3.4	3.7	3.9	4.0	4.3	4.7	4.9	5.2	5.5	5.8

BSA, body surface area; *SD*, standard deviation.

Values from graphic data of Kurotobi, S., Nagai, T., Kawakami, N., & Sano, T. (2002). Coronary diameter in normal infants, children and patients with Kawasaki disease. *Pediatrics International, 44*(1):1-4.

[a]Measurements are made from inner edge to inner edge. Values are rounded off to the nearest 0.1 mm.

Appendix E

Dosages of Drugs Used in Pediatric Cardiology

TABLE E.1

DOSAGES OF DRUGS USED IN PEDIATRIC CARDIOLOGY

DRUG	ROUTE AND DOSAGE	TOXICITY OR SIDE EFFECTS	HOW SUPPLIED
Acetaminophen (Ofirmev, Tylenol)	***For PDA closure in premature infant (off-label):*** *Neonates* PO, IV: 15 mg/kg/dose q6 hr for 3-7 days	Hypersensitivity, anaphylaxis, edema, respiratory distress, rash, urticaria hepatotoxicity, Stevens-Johnson syndrome	Inj: 10 mg/mL Susp: 32 mg/mL
Acetylsalicylic acid (Aspirin)	*Children and adults:* ***Antiplatelet therapy:*** PO: 3-5 mg/kg, QD ***Antipyretic/analgesic:*** PO, PR: 10-15 mg/kg/dose, q4-6 hr (Max 4 g/24 hr) ***Antiinflammatory:*** PO: 80-100 mg/kg/24 hr, TID-QID	Rash, nausea, hepatotoxicity, GI bleeding, bronchospasm, GI distress, tinnitus Contraindications: hepatic failure, bleeding disorder, hypersensitivity, children <16 yr old with chickenpox or flu symptoms (due to the association with Reye syndrome)	Tab: 325, 500 mg Tab, enteric-coated: 81, 165, 325, 500, 650 mg Tab, chewable: 81 mg Supp: 60, 80, 120, 125, 200, 300, 325, 600, 650 mg, and 1.2 g
Adenosine (Adenocard) (Antiarrhythmic)	***For SVT:*** *Children and adults:* IV: 100-200 μg/kg Repeat q1-2 min, with increment of 50 μg/kg, to maximum of 250 μg/kg (Max single dose 12 mg)	Bronchospasm, chest pain, transient asystole, bradycardia and tachycardia Transient AV block in atrial flutter/fibrillation (±)	Inj: 3 mg/mL (2, 4 mL)
Amiodarone (Cordarone) (Class III antiarrhythmic)	*Children:* IV (in emergency situation): *Loading:* 5 mg/kg, slow infusion over 30 min, followed by infusion of 7 μg/kg/min (which is calculated to deliver 10 mg/kg/24 hr). Switch to oral maintenance dose as soon as clinical condition permits. PO: 10-20 mg/kg/24 hr (*infants*) or 10 mg/kg/24 hr (*children and adolescents*) in 2 doses for 5 to 14 days, followed by maintenance dose of 5-7 mg/kg once a day (*Therapeutic level:* 0.5-2.5 mg/L) *Adults:* PO: *Loading:* 800-1600 mg QD for 1-3 wk, then reduce to 600-800 mg QD for 1 mo *Maintenance:* 200-400 mg QD	Progressive dyspnea and cough (pulmonary fibrosis), worsening of arrhythmias, hepatotoxicity, nausea and vomiting, corneal microdeposits, hypotension, heart block, ataxia, hypo- or hyperthyroidism, photosensitivity Contraindications: AV block, sinus node dysfunction, sinus bradycardia	Tab: 200, 400 mg Susp: 5 mg/mL Inj: 50 mg/mL

Amlodipine (Norvasc) (Calcium channel blocker, antihypertensive)	***For hypertension:*** *Children:* PO: Initial 0.1 mg/kg/dose QD-BID; may be increased gradually to a max of 0.6 mg/kg/24 hr *Adults:* PO: 5-10 mg/dose QD (max 10 mg/24 hr)	Edema, dizziness, flushing, palpitation, headache, fatigue, nausea, abdominal pain, somnolence	Tab: 2.5, 5, 10 mg Susp: 1 mg/mL
Amrinone (Inocor) (Noncatecholamine inotropic agent with vasodilator effects)	*Children:* IV: *Loading:* 0.5 mg/Kg over 2-3 min in {1/2} NS (not D_5W) *Maintenance:* 5-20 μg/kg/min *Adults:* IV: *Loading:* 0.75 nmg/kg over 2-3 min *Maintenance:* 5-10 μg/kg/min	Thrombocytopenia, hypotension, tachyarrhythmia, hepatotoxicity, nausea and vomiting, fever	Inj: 5 mg/mL (20 mL)
Atenolol (Tenormin) (β_1-adrenoceptor blocker, antihypertensive, antiarrhythmic)	*Children:* PO: 1-2 mg/kg/dose, QD *Adults:* PO: 25-100 mg/dose, QD for 1-2 wk (alone or with diuretic for hypertension); may increase to 200 mg QD	CNS symptoms (dizziness, tiredness, depression), bradycardia, postural hypotension, nausea and vomiting, rash, blood dyscrasias (agranulocytosis, purpura)	Tab: 25, 50, 100 mg Susp: 2 mg/mL Inj: 0.5 mg/mL (10 mL)
Atorvastatin (Lipitor) (Antilipemic, "statin," HMG-CoA reductase inhibitor)	*Children:* PO: Starting dose 10 mg QD for 4-6 wk; increase to 20 mg QD and 40 mg QD as needed (Adult max dose: 80 mg/24 hr)	Headache, constipation, diarrhea, elevated liver enzymes, rhabdomyolysis, myopathy	Tab: 10, 20, 40, 80 mg

TABLE E.1 *(continued)*

DOSAGES OF DRUGS USED IN PEDIATRIC CARDIOLOGY

DRUG	ROUTE AND DOSAGE	TOXICITY OR SIDE EFFECTS	HOW SUPPLIED
Azathioprine (Imuran, Azasan) (Immuno-suppressant)	*Children:* IV, PO: *Initial:* 3-5 mg/kg/24 hr, QD *Maintenance:* 1-3 mg/kg/24 hr (to produce WBC count around 5000/mm^3); may be reduced if WBC count falls below 4000/mm^3	Bone marrow suppression (leukopenia, thrombocytopenia, anemia), GI symptoms (nausea and vomiting)	Tab: 25, 50, 75, 100 mg Susp: 50 mg/mL Inj: 100 mg powder for reconst
Bosentan (Tracleer) (Nonselective endothelin receptor blocker)	***For pulmonary hypertension:*** *Children:* PO: *< 20 kg*: 31.25 mg BID *20-40 kg*: 62.5 mg BID *> 40 kg*: 125 mg BID *Adults:* PO: 125 mg BID	Liver dysfunction, decrease in hemoglobin, fluid retention, heart failure, headache	Tab: 62.5, 125 mg
Bumetanide (Bumex) (Loop diuretic)	*Children:* PO, IM, IV: >6 mo: 0.015-0.1 mg/kg/dose, QD-QOD *Adults:* PO: 0.5-2 mg/dose, QD-BID IV: 0.5-1 mg over 1-2 min, q2-3 hr PRN (Max 10 mg/24 hr)	Hypotension, cramps, dizziness, headache, electrolyte losses (hypokalemia, hypocalcemia, hyponatremia, hypochloremia), metabolic alkalosis	Tab: 0.5, 1, 2 mg Inj: 0.25 mg/mL
Calcium glubionate (Neo-Calglucon 6.4% elemental calcium) (Calcium supplement)	***For neonatal hypocalcemia:*** PO: 1200 mg/kg/24 hr, q4-6 hr *Maintenance:* *Infants and children:* PO: 600-2000 mg/kg/24 hr, QID (Max 9 g/24 hr) *Adults:* PO: 6-18 g/24 hr, QID	GI irritation, diarrhea, dizziness, headache Best absorbed when given before meals.	Syrup: 1.8 g/5 mL (480 mL) (1.2 mEq Ca/mL)

Captopril (Capoten) (ACE inhibitor, antihypertensive, vasodilator)	*Neonates:* PO: 0.1-0.4 mg/kg/24 hr, TID-QID *Infants:* PO: Initially 0.15-0.3 mg/kg/dose, QD-QID; titrate upward if needed (Max 6 mg/kg/24 hr) *Children:* PO: Initially 0.3-0.5 mg/kg/dose, TID; titrate upward if needed (Max 6 mg/kg/24 hr, BID-QID) *Adolescents and Adults:* PO: Initially 12.5-25 mg/dose, BID-TID; increase weekly if needed by 25 mg/dose to max dose of 450 mg/24 hr (Adjust dose with renal failure)	Neutropenia/agranulocytosis, proteinuria, hypotension and tachycardia, rash, taste impairment, hyperkalemia Evidence of fetal risk if given during 2nd and 3rd trimesters (same with all other ACE inhibitors)	Tab: 12.5, 25, 50, 100 mg Susp: 0.75, 1 mg/mL
Carnitine (Carnitor)	*Children:* PO: 50-100 mg/kg/24 hr, BID-TID; increase slowly as needed (Max 3 g/24 hr) *Adults:* PO: 330 mg-1 g/dose, BID-TID IV (*child and adult*): 50 mg/kg as loading dose, then 50 mg/kg/24 hr, q4-6 hr	Nausea and vomiting, abdominal cramp, diarrhea, seizure	Tab: 330, 500 mg Caps: 250 mg Oral sol: 100 mg/mL (118 ml) Inj: 200 mg/mL (5 ml)
Carvedilol (Coreg, Coreg CR) (Nonselective α- and β-adrenergic blocker)	*Children:* PO: Initial 0.09 mg/kg/dose, BID; increase gradually to 0.36 and 0.75 mg/kg as tolerated to adult max dose of 50 mg/24 hr *Adults:* PO: 3.125 mg, BID for 2 wk; increase slowly to a max dose of 25 mg BID as needed (for heart failure) (Max 25 mg BID for <85kg; 50 mg BID for >85 kg)	Dizziness, hypotension, headache, diarrhea, rarely AV block	Tab: 3.125, 6.125, 12.5, 25 mg Tab, extended release: 10, 20, 40, 80 mg

TABLE E.1 *(continued)*

DOSAGES OF DRUGS USED IN PEDIATRIC CARDIOLOGY

DRUG	ROUTE AND DOSAGE	TOXICITY OR SIDE EFFECTS	HOW SUPPLIED
Chloral hydrate (Noctec, Aquachloral) (Sedative, hypnotic)	***As sedative:*** *Children:* PO, PR: 25-50 mg/kg/dose q6-8 hr Sedation for procedures: 25-100 mg (Max dose 2g) *Adults:* PO, PR: 250 mg/dose q8 hr ***As hypnotic:*** *Adults:* PO, PR: 500-2000 mg/dose	Mucous membrane irritation (laryngospasm if aspirated), GI irritation, excitement/ delirium, hypotension Contraindicated in hepatic and renal impairment	Caps: 500 mg Syrup: 250, 500 mg/5 mL Supp: 324, 500, 648 mg
Chlorothiazide (Diuril) (Diuretic)	*Children:* PO: 20-40 mg/kg/24 hr, BID IV: 2-8 mg/kg/24 hr, BID *Adults:* PO, IV: 250-2000 mg/dose QD-BID	Hypercalcemia, hyperbilirubinemia, hyperglycemia, hyperuricemia, hypochloremic alkalosis, hypokalemia, hyponatremia, prerenal azotemia, hyperlipidemia, rarely pancreatitis, blood dyscrasias, allergic reactions	Tab: 250, 500 mg Susp: 250 mg/5 mL (237 mL) Inj: 500 mg powder for reconst with 18 mL sterile water
Cholestyramine (Questran, Prevalite) (Antilipemic, bile acid sequestrant)	*Children:* PO: 250-1500 mg/kg/24 hr, BID-QID *Adults:* PO: *Starting:* 1 packet (or scoopful) of Questran powder or Questran Light 1 to 2 times/day *Maintenance:* 2 to 4 packets or scoopfuls/24 hr in 2 doses (or 1 to 6 doses) (Max 6 packets/24 hr)	Constipation and other GI symptoms, bleeding, hyperchloremic acidosis	Packet of 9-g Questran powder or 5-g Questran Light, each packet containing 4 g anhydrous cholestyramine resin
Clofibrate (Atromid-S) (Antilipemic, triglyceride-lowering agent)	*Children:* PO: 0.5-1.5 mg/24 hr, BID-TID *Adults:* PO: *Initial and maintenance:* 2 g/24 hr, BID-TID	Nausea and other GI symptoms (vomiting, diarrhea, flatulence), headache, dizziness, fatigue, rash, blood dyscrasias, myalgia, arthralgia, hepatic dysfunction	Caps: 500 mg

Drug	Dosage	Side Effects	How Supplied
Clopidogrel (Plavix) (Antiplatelet)	*Children:* PO: 1 mg/kg/24 hr to max (adult dose) of 75 mg/24 hr *Adults:* PO: 75 mg/dose, QD	Bleeding, especially when used with aspirin, neutropenia or agranulocytosis, abdominal pain, constipation, rash, syncope, palpitation	Tab: 75 mg
Colestipol (Colestid) (Antilipemic, bile acid sequestrant)	*Children:* PO: 300-1500 mg/24 hr in 2-4 doses *Adults:* PO: *Starting dose:* 5 g 1-2 times/24 hr; increment of 5 g q1-2 mo *Maintenance:* 5-30 g/24 hr, BID-QID (mix with 3-6 oz water or another fluid)	Constipation and other GI symptoms (abdominal distention, flatulence, nausea and vomiting, diarrhea), rarely rash, muscle and joint pain, headache, dizziness	Packet: 5 g
Cyclosporine, Cyclosporine microemulsion (Sandimmune, Gengraf, Neoral) (Immunosuppressant)	*Children:* PO: 15 mg/kg as a single dose given 4-12 hr pretransplant; give same daily dose for 1-2 wk posttransplant, then reduce by 5% per wk to 5-10 mg/kg/24 hr, QD-BID (*Therapeutic level:* 100-300 ng/mL) IV: 5-6 mg/kg as a single dose given 4-12 hr pretransplant; administer over 2-6 hr; give same dose posttransplant until patient able to tolerate oral form	Nephrotoxicity, tremor, hypertension, less commonly hepatotoxicity, hyperlipidemia, hirsutism, gum hypertrophy, rarely lymphoma, hypomagnesemia	Oral sol: 100 mg/mL (50 ml) Neoral sol: 100 mg/mL (50 mL) Caps: 25, 50, 100 mg Neoral caps: 25, 100 mg Inj: 50 mg/mL
Diazoxide (Hyperstat IV, Proglycem) (Antihypertensive, peripheral vasodilator)	***For hypertensive crisis:*** *Children and adults:* IV: 1-3 mg/kg (max 150 mg single dose); repeat q5-15 min; titrate to desired effect	Hypotension, transient hyperglycemia, nausea and vomiting, sodium retention (CHF ±)	Inj: 15 mg/mL

TABLE E.1 *(continued)*

DOSAGES OF DRUGS USED IN PEDIATRIC CARDIOLOGY

DRUG	ROUTE AND DOSAGE	TOXICITY OR SIDE EFFECTS	HOW SUPPLIED
Digoxin (Lanoxin, Digitek) (Cardiac glycoside, antiarrhythmic, inotrope)	*Children:* PO: *Total digitalizing dose:* Premature infant: 20 μg/kg; Full-term newborn: 30 μg/kg; Child 1 mo-2 yr: 40-50 μg/kg; Child >2-10 yr: 30-40 μg/kg; > 10 yr and <100 kg: 10-15 μg/kg PO: *Maintenance:* 25%-30% of TDD/24 hr BID IV: 75%-80% of PO dose *Adults:* PO: *Loading:* 8-12 μg/kg *Maintenance:* 0.10-0.25 mg/24 hr (*Therapeutic level:* 0.8-2 ng/mL)	AV conduction disturbances, arrhythmias, nausea and vomiting	Elixir: 50 μg/mL (60 mL) Tab: 125, 250, μg Caps: 50, 100, 200 μg Inj: 100, 250 μg/mL
Digoxin immune Fab (Digibind, Digifab) (Antidigoxin antibody)	*Infants and children:* IV: 1 vial (40 mg) dissolved in 4 mL H_2O, over 30 min *Adults:* IV: 4 vials (240 mg)	Allergic reaction (rare), hypokalemia, rapid AV conduction in atrial flutter	Inj: 38, 40 mg powder for reconst
Diltiazem (Cardizem, Cardizem SR, Cardizem CD, Dilacor XR, Tiazac) (Calcium channel blocker, antihypertensive)	*Children:* PO: 1.5-2 mg/kg/24 hr, TID-QID (Max 3.5 mg/kg/24 hr) *Adolescents:* Immediate release: PO: 30-120 mg/dose, TID-QID; usual range 180-360 mg/24 hr Extended release: PO: 120-300 mg/24 hr QD-BID (BID dosing with Cardizem SR; QD dosing with Cardizem CD, Dilacor XR, and Tiazac)	Dizziness, headache, edema, nausea and vomiting, heart block, arrhythmias Contraindicated in 2nd- and 3rd-degree AV block, sinus node dysfunction, acute MI with pulmonary congestion Maximum antihypertensive effect seen within 2 weeks	Tab: 30, 60, 90, 120 mg Tab, extended release: 120, 180, 240, 300, 360, 420 mg Caps, extended release: 60, 90, 120, 180, 240, 300, 360, 420 mg Inj: 5 mg/mL (5, 10 mL)

Drug	Dosage	Side effects	How supplied
Dipyridamole (Persantine) (Antiplatelet)	*Children:* PO: 2-6 mg/kg/24 hr, TID *Adults:* PO: 75-100 mg QID (As an adjunct to warfarin therapy. Not to use with aspirin)	Vasodilation, rarely dizziness, angina	Tab: 25, 50, 75 mg
Disopyramide (Norpace) (Class IA antiarrhythmic)	*Children:* PO: <1 yr: 10-30 mg/kg/24 hr, q6 hr; 1-4 yr: 10-20 mg/kg/24 hr, q6 hr; 4-12 yr: 10-15 mg/kg/24 hr, q6 hr; 12-18 yr: 6-15 mg/kg/24 hr, q6 hr (q4 hr dosing when using regular caps) *Adults:* PO: 150 mg/dose q6 hr or 300 mg (extended release) q12 hr (Max 1.6 g/24 hr) (*Therapeutic level:* 3-7 mg/L)	Heart failure or hypotension, anticholinergic effects (urinary retention, dry mouth, constipation), nausea and vomiting, hypoglycemia	Caps: 100, 150 mg Caps, CR: 100, 150 mg Susp: 1 mg/mL, 10 mg/mL
Dobutamine (Dobutrex) (β-adrenergic stimulator)	*Children:* IV infusion: 2.5-15 μg/kg/min in D_5W or NS (incompatible with alkali solution) (Max 40 μg/kg/min) *Adults:* IV infusion: 2.5-10 μg/kg/min (Max 40 μg/kg/min)	Tachyarrhythmias, hypertension, nausea and vomiting, headache Contraindicated in HOCM and atrial flutter/fibrillation	Inj: 12.5 mg/mL (20 mL)

TABLE E.1 *(continued)*

DOSAGES OF DRUGS USED IN PEDIATRIC CARDIOLOGY

DRUG	ROUTE AND DOSAGE	TOXICITY OR SIDE EFFECTS	HOW SUPPLIED
Dopamine (Intropin, Dopastat) (Natural catecholamine inotropic agent)	*Children:* IV: Effects are dose dependent: 2-5 μg/kg/min—increases RBF and urine output (minimum effects on heart rate and cardiac output) 5-15 μg/kg/min—increases heart rate, cardiac contractility, and cardiac output > 20 μg/kg/min—α-adrenergic effects with decreased RBF (±) (Incompatible with alkali solution)	Tachyarrhythmias, nausea and vomiting, hypotension or hypertension, extravasation (tissue necrosis [treat with local infiltration of phentolamine])	Inj: 40, 80, 160 mg/mL (5, 10, 20 mL)
Enalapril, Enalaprilat (Epaned, Vasotec) (ACE inhibitor, vasodilator)	*Children:* PO: 0.1 mg/kg/dose QD or BID Increase PRN over 2 wks (Max 0.5 mg/kg/24 hr) *Adults:* ***For CHF:*** PO: Start with 2.5 mg, QD or BID (Usual range 5-20 mg/24 hr) ***For hypertension:*** PO: Start with 5 mg, QD (Usual dose 10-40 mg/24 hr)	Hypotension, dizziness, fatigue, headache, rash, diminishing taste, neutropenia, hyperkalemia, chronic cough Evidence of fetal risk if given during 2nd and 3rd trimesters (same with all other ACE inhibitors)	Tab: 2.5, 5, 10, 20 mg (Enalapril) Oral susp: 1 mg/mL Inj: 1.25 mg/mL (Enalaprilat)

Enoxaparin (Lovenox) (Low-molecular-weight heparin, anticoagulant)	***For DVT treatment:*** *Infants <2 months:* SC: 1.5 mg/kg/dose, q12 hr *Infants ≥ 2 months to adults:* SC: 1 mg/kg/dose, q12 hr (Adjust dose to achieve target antifactor Xa levels of 0.5-1 units/mL) ***For DVT prophylaxis:*** *Infants <2 months:* SC: 1 mg/kg/dose, q12 hr *Infants ≥ 2 mo up to 18 yr:* SC: 0.5 mg/kg/dose, q12 hr *Adults:* SC: 30 mg, BID for 7-10 days	Bleeding Contraindicated in major bleeding and drug-induced thrombocytopenia Protamine sulfate is the antidote; 1 mg protamine sulfate neutralizes 1 mg enoxaparin	Inj: 100 mg/mL (3 mL)
Epinephrine (Adrenalin) (α-, β_1-, and β_2-adrenergic stimulator)	***For asystole and bradycardia:*** *Children:* IV/ET: 0.1-0.3 mL/kg of 1:10,000 sol (or 0.01-0.03 mg/kg) q3-5 min ***For circulatory shock or heart failure:*** *Children:* IV: 0.1-1 μg/kg/min; titrate to effect	Tachyarrhythmias, hypertension, nausea and vomiting, headache, tissue necrosis (±)	Inj: 0.1 mg/mL (1:10,000 sol, 10 mL prefilled syringe) 1 mg/mL (1:1000 sol, 1, 30 mL)

TABLE E.1 *(continued)*

DOSAGES OF DRUGS USED IN PEDIATRIC CARDIOLOGY

DRUG	ROUTE AND DOSAGE	TOXICITY OR SIDE EFFECTS	HOW SUPPLIED
Esmolol (Brevibloc) (β_1-selective adrenergic blocking agent, antihypertensive, class II antiarrhythmic)	*Children:* *Loading:* IV: 100-500 μg/kg over 1 min *Maintenance:* IV: 25-100 μg/kg/min; increase by 25-50 μg/kg to a maximum of 300 μg/kg/min (Usual maintenance dose 50-500 μg/kg/min)	Bronchospasm, CHF, hypotension, nausea and vomiting	Inj: 10, 20, 250 mg/mL
Ethacrynic acid (Edecrin) (Loop diuretic)	*Children:* PO: 1 mg/kg/dose, QD-TID (Max 3 mg/kg/24 hr) IV: 1 mg/kg/dose *Adults:* PO: 50-100 mg, QD (Max 400 mg) IV: 0.5-1 mg/kg/dose or 50 mg/dose	Dehydration, hypokalemia, prerenal azotemia, hyperuricemia, eighth cranial nerve damage (deafness), abnormal LFT, agranulocytosis or thrombocytopenia, GI irritation, rash	Tab: 25 mgInj: 50 mg vial for reconst with 50 mL D_5W
Flecainide (Tambocor) (Class IC antiarrhythmic)	***For sustained VT:*** *Children:* PO: *Initial:* 1-3 mg/kg/24 hr, q8 hr (Usual range: 3-6 g/kg/24 hr, q8 hr) Monitor serum level to adjust dose if needed *Adults:* PO: 100 mg/dose BID; may increase by 50 mg q12 hr every 4 days to max dose of 600 mg/24 hr (*Therapeutic level:* 0.2-1 mg/L)	Worsening of HF, bradycardia, AV block, dizziness, blurred vision, dyspnea, nausea, headache, increased PR and QRS duration	Tab: 50, 100, 150 mgSusp: 5, 20 mg/mL

Fludrocortisone acetate (Florinef) (Corticosteroid)	***For syncopal episodes:*** *Children:* PO: 0.1 mg/dose, QD *Adults:* PO: 0.2 mg/dose, QD	Hypertension, hypokalemia, acne, rash, bruising, headache, GI ulcers, growth suppression Weight gain (1-2 kg in 2-3 wk)	Tab: 0.1 mg
Furosemide (Lasix) (Loop diuretic)	*Children:* IV: 0.5-2 mg/kg/dose, BID-QID PO: 1-2 mg/kg/dose, QD-TID (Max 6 mg/kg/dose) *Adults:* IV, PO: 20-80 mg/24 hr, BID-QID	Hypokalemia, hyperuricemia, prerenal azotemia, ototoxicity, rarely bloody dyscrasias, rash	Oral liquid: 10 mg/mL, 40 mg/5 mLTab: 20, 40, 80 mgInj: 10 mg/mL
Heparin (Anticoagulant)	*Infants and children:* IV: *Initial:* 50 U/kg IV bolus *Maintenance:* 10-25 U/kg/hr or 50-100 U/kg q4 hr [Adjust dose to give APTT 1.5-2.5 times control, 6-8 hr after IV infusion (or 3.5-4 hr after intermittent injection)] *Adults:* IV: *Initial:* 10,000 U IV injection *Maintenance:* 5000-10,000 U q4-6 hr IV drip: *Initial dose:* 5000 U followed by 20,000-40,000 U/24 hr	Bleeding Antidote: protamine sulfate (1 mg per 100 U heparin in previous 4 hr)	Inj: 1000, 2000, 2500, 5000, 7500, 10,000, 20,000, 40,000 U/mL

TABLE E.1 *(continued)*

DOSAGES OF DRUGS USED IN PEDIATRIC CARDIOLOGY

DRUG	ROUTE AND DOSAGE	TOXICITY OR SIDE EFFECTS	HOW SUPPLIED
Hydralazine (Apresoline) (Peripheral vasodilator, antihypertensive)	***For hypertensive crisis:*** *Children:* IM, IV: 0.15-0.2 mg/kg/dose; may be repeated q4-6 hr (Max 20 mg/dose) *Adults:* IM, IV: 20-40 mg/dose; repeat q4-6 hr PRN ***For chronic hypertension:*** *Children:* PO: 0.75-3 mg/kg/24 hr, BID-QID *Adults:* PO: Start with 10 mg 4 times/24 hr for 3-4 days; increase to 25 mg/dose QID for 3-4 days; then up to 50 mg QID	Hypotension, tachycardia and palpitation, lupus-like syndrome with prolonged use (fever, arthralgia, splenomegaly, and positive LE-cell preparation), blood dyscrasias	Tab: 10, 25, 50, 100 mg Oral liquid: 1.25, 2, 4 mg/mL Inj: 20 mg/mL
Hydrochlorothiazide (Hydrodiuril, Esidrix, Hydro-Par, Oretic) (Thiazide diuretic)	*Children:* PO: 2-4 mg/kg/24 hr, BID (Max 100 mg/24 hr) *Adults:* PO: 25-100 mg/24 hr, QD-BID (Max 200 mg/24 hr)	Same as for chlorothiazide	Tab: 25, 50, 100 mgCaps: 12.5 mgSol: 10 mg/mL (500 mL)

Ibuprofen (NeoProfen) (Nonsteroidal antiinflammatory)	***For PDA closure in premature infants:*** *Neonates ≤ 32 weeks (500-1500 g):* IV: Initial dose 10 mg/kg, followed by 2 doses of 5 mg/kg after 24 and 48 hours (Hold 2nd and 3rd dose if urine output is <0.6 mL/kg/hr)	Sepsis, anemia, interventricular hemorrhage, apnea, GI disorders, renal impairment Contraindicated in interventricular hemorrhage, thrombocytopenia, necrotizing enterocolitis, significant renal dysfunction	Inj: 17.1 mg/mL ibuprofen lysine equivalent to 10 mg/mL of ibuprofen (2 mL)
Inamrinone (Inocor) (Phosphodiesterase type III inhibitor)	*Children:* IV: *Loading:* 0.75 mg/kg over 2-3 min *Maintenance:* 5-10 μg/kg/min *Adults:* IV: *Loading:* 0.75 mg/kg over 2-3 min *Maintenance:* 5-10 μg/kg/min	Thrombocytopenia, hypotension, tachyarrhythmias, hepatotoxicity, nausea and vomiting, fever	Inj: 5 mg/mL (20 mL)
Indomethacin (Indocin) (Nonsteroidal antiinflammatory, antipyretic agent, PG synthesis inhibitor)	***For PDA closure in premature infants:*** IV: *< 48 hr:* 0.2, 01, and 0.1 mg/kg/dose, q12-24 hr *2-7 days:* 0.2, 0.2, and 0.2 mg/kg/dose, q12-24 hr >7 days: 0.2, 0.25, and 0.25 mg/kg/dose, q12-24 hr	GI or other bleeding, GI disturbances, renal impairment, electrolyte disturbances (↓ Na, ↑ K levels)	Vial: 1 mg
Isoproterenol (Isuprel) (β_1- and β_2-adrenergic stimulator)	*Children:* IV: 0.1-2 μg/kg/min, titrated to desired effect *Adults:* IV: 2-20 μg/min, titrated to desired effect (incompatible with alkali solution)	Similar to epinephrine	Inj: 0.2 mg/mL (1: 5000 sol: 1, 5 mL)

TABLE E.1 *(continued)*

DOSAGES OF DRUGS USED IN PEDIATRIC CARDIOLOGY

DRUG	ROUTE AND DOSAGE	TOXICITY OR SIDE EFFECTS	HOW SUPPLIED
Ketamine (Ketalar) (General anesthetic)	***For cyanotic spells:*** *Infants:* IM: 2-3 mg/kg Repeat smaller doses q30 min PRN IV: 1-3 mg/kg/dose over 60 sec Repeat smaller doses q30 min PRN	Hypertension/tachycardia, respiratory depression or apnea, CNS symptoms (dreamlike state, confusion, agitation)	Inj: 10, 50, 100 mg/mL
Labetalol (Normodyne, Trandate) (α- and β-adrenergic antagonist)	*Children:* PO: *Initial:* 4 mg/kg/24 hr, BID (Max 40 mg/kg/24 hr) IV: (for hypertensive emergency) *Initial:* 0.2-1 mg/kg/dose q10 min PRN (Max 20 mg/dose)	Orthostatic hypotension, edema, CHF, bradycardiaContraindicated in asthma	Tab: 100, 200, 300 mg Susp: 10, 40 mg/mL Inj: 5 mg/mL (20, 40 mL)
Lidocaine (Xylocaine) (Class IB antiarrhythmic)	*Children:* IV: *Loading:* 1 mg/kg/dose slow IV, q5-10 min PRN *Maintenance:* 30 μg/kg/min (Range 20-50 μg/kg/min) *Adults:* IV: *Loading:* 1 mg/kg/dose q5 min *Maintenance:* 1-4 mg/min (*Therapeutic level:* 1.5-5 mg/L)	Seizure, respiratory depression, CNS symptoms (anxiety, euphoria, or drowsiness), arrhythmias, hypotension or shock	Inj: 0.5%, 1%, 1.5%, 2%, 4%, 10%, 20% (1% = 10 mg/mL)

Lisinopril (Zestril, Prinivil) (ACE inhibitor, antihypertensive)	***For hypertension:*** *Children ≥ 6 yr:* PO: *Initial:* 0.07 mg/kg/24 hr (max initial dose is 5 mg/24 hr), increase dose at 1-2 wk intervals (Max 0.6 mg/kg/day or 40 mg/24 hr) *Adults:* PO: *Initial:* 10 mg QD; may increase upward as needed to max dose of 80 mg/24 hr	Dry nonproductive cough, rash, hypotension, hyperkalemia, angioedema, rarely bone marrow depression Evidence of fetal risk if given during 2nd and 3rd trimesters (same with all other ACE inhibitors)	Tab: 2.5, 5, 10, 20, 30, 40 mg
Losartan (Cozaar) (Angiotensin II-receptor blocker)	***For hypertension:*** *Children ≥ 6 yr:* PO: 0.7 mg/kg/24 hr, QD-BID (Max 50 mg/24 hr) *Adults:* PO: *Initial:* 50 mg, QD (Max 100 mg QD)	Hypotension, dizziness, nasal congestion, muscle cramps Evidence of fetal risk if given during 2nd and 3rd trimesters	Tab: 25, 50, 100 mg
Lovastatin (Mevacor) (Antilipemic, HMG-CoA reductase inhibitor)	*Adolescents:* PO: Starting dose 10 mg/24 hr QD for 6-8 wk; increase to 20 mg/24 hr for 8 wk, and then increase to 40 mg/24 hr for 8 wk *Adults:* PO: Starting dose 20 mg/day, QD-BID (range 40-80 mg/24 hr) (Max dose with concurrent amiodarone or verapamil use is 40 mg/24 hr)	Mild GI symptoms, myositis syndrome, elevated transaminase levels, increased CK levels	Tab: 10, 20, 40 mg

TABLE E.1 *(continued)*

DOSAGES OF DRUGS USED IN PEDIATRIC CARDIOLOGY

DRUG	ROUTE AND DOSAGE	TOXICITY OR SIDE EFFECTS	HOW SUPPLIED
Methyldopa (Aldomet) (Antihypertensive)	***For hypertensive crisis:*** *Children:* IV: Start at 2-4 mg/kg/dose q6-8 hr (Max dose 65 mg/kg/24 hr or 3 g/24 hr, whichever is less) *Adults:* IV: 250-500 mg q6 hr (Max 1 g q6 hr) ***For hypertension:*** *Children:* PO: 10 mg/kg/24 hr, BID-QID May be increased or decreased (Max dose 65 mg/kg/24 hr or 3 g/24 hr, whichever is less) *Adults:* PO: 250 mg/dose, BID-TID for 2 days May be increased or decreased q2 days. (Usual dose: 0.5-2 g/24 hr, BID-QID) (Max 3 g/24 hr)	Sedation, orthostatic hypotension and bradycardia, lupus-like syndrome, Coombs (+) hemolytic anemia and leukopenia, hepatitis or cirrhosis, colitis, impotence	Inj: 50 mg/mL (5 mL) Susp: 50 mg/mL Tab: 250, 500 mg
Metoprolol (Lopressor) (β-adrenoceptor blocker)	*Children >2 yr:* PO: Initially 0.1-0.2 mg/kg/dose, BID; gradually increase to 1-3 mg/kg/24 hr *Adults:* PO: Initially 100 mg/24 hr, QD-TID May increase to 450 mg/24 hr, BID-TID (Usual dose 100-450 mg/24 hr) (Usually used with hydrochlorothiazide 25-100 mg/24 hr)	CNS symptoms (dizziness, tiredness, depression), bronchospasm, bradycardia, diarrhea, nausea and vomiting, abdominal pain	Tab: 25, 50, 100 mg Tab, extended release: 25, 50, 100, 200 mg

Metolazone (Zaroxolyn, Diulo, Mykrox) (Thiazide-like diuretic)	*Children:* PO: 0.2-0.4 mg/kg/24 hr, QD-BID *Adults:* PO: For hypertension: 2.5-5 mg QD For edema: 5-20 mg, QD	Electrolyte imbalance, GI disturbance, hyperglycemia, bone marrow depression, chills, hyperuricemia, hepatitis, rash May be more effective than thiazide diuretics in impaired renal function	Tab: 0.5 (Mykrox), 2.5, 5, 10 mg Susp: 1 mg/mL
Mexiletine (Mexitil) (Class IB antiarrhythmic)	*Children:* PO: 6-8 mg/kg/24 hr, BID-TID for 2-3 days; then 2-5 mg/kg/dose q6-8 hr Increase 1-2 mg/kg/dose q2-3 days until desired effect achieved (with food or antacid) *Adults:* PO: 200 mg q8 hr for 2-3 days Increase to 300-400 mg q8 hr (Usual dose 200-300 mg q8 hr) (*Therapeutic level:* 0.75-2 μg/mL)	Nausea and vomiting, CNS symptoms (headache, dizziness, tremor, paresthesia, mood changes), rash, hepatic dysfunction (±)	Caps: 150, 200, 250 mg
Milrinone (Primacor) (Phosphodiesterase type III inhibitor)	*Children:* IV: *Loading:* 10-50 μg/kg over 10 min; then 0.1-1 μg/kg/min *Adults:* IV: *Loading:* 50 μg/kg over 10 min 0.5 μg/kg/min (Range 0.375-0.75 μg/kg/min)	Arrhythmias, hypotension, hypokalemia, thrombocytopenia	Inj: 1 mg/mL (5, 10, 20 mL) Inj, premixed in D_5W: 200 μg/mL (100, 200 mL)

TABLE E.1 *(continued)*

DOSAGES OF DRUGS USED IN PEDIATRIC CARDIOLOGY

DRUG	ROUTE AND DOSAGE	TOXICITY OR SIDE EFFECTS	HOW SUPPLIED
Minoxidil (Loniten) (Peripheral vasodilator)	*Children <12 yr:* PO: 0.2 mg/kg/24 hr, QD-BID initially Increase 0.1-0.2 mg/kg/24 hr q3 days until desired effect achieved (Usual dose 0.25-1 mg/kg/24 hr, QD-BID; max 50 mg/24 hr) *Children >12 yr and Adults:* PO: 5 mg/dose, QD initially May be increased to 10, 20, 40 mg, QD-BID q3-day interval (Usual dose 10-40 mg/24 hr, QD-BID; max 100 mg/24 hr)	Reflex tachycardia and fluid retention (used with a β-blocker and diuretic), pericardial effusion, hypertrichosis, rarely blood dyscrasias (leukopenia, thrombocytopenia)	Tab: 2.5, 10 mg
Morphine sulfate (Narcotic, analgesic)	*Children:* SC, IM, IV: 0.1-0.2 mg/kg/dose q2-4 hr (Max 15 mg/dose) *Adults:* SC, IM, IV: 2.5-20 mg/dose q2-6 hr PRN	CNS depression, respiratory depression, nausea and vomiting, hypotension, bradycardia	Inj: 0.5, 1, 2, 4, 5, 8, 10, 15, 25, 50 mg/mL
Mycophenolate mofetil (CellCept) (Immunosuppressant)	*Children:* PO: 600 mg/m^2/dose, BID(Maximum 2000 mg/24 hr)(*Therapeutic level:* 5-7 ng/mL) *Adults:*PO/IV: 2000-3000 g/24 hr, BID	Headache, GI symptoms, hypertension, bone marrow suppression (anemia), fever, increased risk of developing lymphomas or other malignancies	Tab: 500 mg Caps: 250 mg Oral susp: 200 mg/ml Inj: 500 mg

Nifedipine (Procardia, Adalat) (Calcium channel blocker)	***For hypertrophic cardiomyopathy:*** *Children:* PO: 0.5-0.9 mg/kg/24 hr, TID-QID ***For hypertension:*** *Children:* PO: 0.25-0.5 mg/kg/24 hr, QD-BID (Max 3 mg/kg/24 hr up to 120 mg/24 hr) *Adults:* PO: Initially 10 mg/dose, TID Titrate up to 20 to 30 mg/dose, TID-QID over 7-14 days (Usual dose 10-20 mg TID; max dose 180 mg/24 hr)	Hypotension, peripheral edema, CNS symptoms (headache, dizziness, weakness), nausea	Caps: 10, 20 mg Tab, sustained release (Adalat CC, Procardia XL): 30, 60, 90 mg
Nitroglycerine (Nitro-Bid, Tridil, Nitrostat) (Peripheral vasodilator)	*Children:* IV: 0.5-1 μg/kg/min Increase 1 μg/kg/min q20 min to titrate to effect (Max 6 μg/kg/min) (Dilute in D_5W or NS with final concentration <400 μg/mL; light sensitive) *Adults:* IV: Initial dose: 5 μg/min through infusion pump Increase 5 μg/min q3-5 min until desired effect achieved	Hypotension, tachycardia, headache, nausea and vomiting	Inj: 0.5, 5 mg/mL Inj, premixed in D_5W: 100, 200, 400 μg/mL

TABLE E.1 *(continued)*

DOSAGES OF DRUGS USED IN PEDIATRIC CARDIOLOGY

DRUG	ROUTE AND DOSAGE	TOXICITY OR SIDE EFFECTS	HOW SUPPLIED
Nitroprusside (Nipride) (Peripheral vasodilator)	*Children:* IV: 0.3-0.5 μg/kg/min, titrate to effect with BP monitoring (Usual dose 3-4 μg/kg/min; max dose 10 μg/kg/min) (Dilute stock solution [50 mg] in 250-2000 mL D_5W; light sensitive)	Hypotension, palpitation, and cyanide toxicity (metabolic acidosis earliest and most reliable evidence) Monitor thiocyanate level when used >48 hr and in patients with renal or hepatic dysfunction. Thiocyanate level should be <50 mg/L; cyanate levels >2 μg/mL are toxic levels.	Inj: 25 mg/mL (2 mL) Inj: 50 mg for reconst with 2-3 mL D_5W
Norepinephrine (Levophed, levarterenol) (α_1- and β_1-adrenoceptor stimulant)	*Children:* IV: 0.1 μg/kg/min IV infusion initially; increase dose to attain desired effect (Max 2 μg/kg/min) *Adults:* IV: Start at 4 μg/min IV infusion; titrate to effect. (Usual dose range 8-12 μg/min)	Hypertension, bradycardia (reflex), arrhythmias, tissue necrosis (treat with phentolamine infiltration)	Inj: 1 mg/mL (4 mL)
Phentolamine (Regitine) (α-adrenoceptor blocker)	***For diagnosis of pheochromocytoma:*** *Children:* IM, IV: 0.05-0.1 mg/kg/dose; repeat q5 min until hypertension is controlled; then q2-4 hr PRN *Adults:* IM, IV: 2.5-5 mg/dose; repeat q5 min until hypertension is controlled; then q2-4 hr PRN ***For treatment of extravasated α-adrenergic drugs:*** SC: Make a solution of 0.5-1 μg/mL with NS. Inject 1-5 mL (in 5 divided doses) around the site of extravasation (Max 0.1-0.5 mg/kg or 5 mg total)	Hypotension, tachycardia or arrhythmias, nausea and vomiting	Inj: 5 mg powder for reconst

Phenylephrine (Neo-Synephrine) (α_1-adrenoceptor stimulant)	***For hypotension:*** *Children:* IM, SC: 0.1 mg/kg/dose q1-2 hr PRN (Max dose 5 mg) IV: 5-10 μg/kg/dose IV bolus q10-15 min or 0.1-0.5 μg/kg/min *Adults:* IM, SC: 2-5 mg/dose q1-2 hr PRN (Max dose 5 mg) IV: 0.1-0.5 mg/dose IV bolus q10-15 min PRN Start IV drip at 100-180 μg/min (Usual maintain dose 40-60 μg/min)	Arrhythmias, hypertension, angina	Inj: 10 mg/mL
Phenytoin (Dilantin) (Class IB antiarrhythmic, anticonvulsant)	*Children:* IV: 2-4 mg/kg/dose over 5-10 min followed by PO dose PO: 2-5 mg/kg/24 hr, BID-TID (*Therapeutic level:* 5-18 μg/mL for arrhythmias, 10-20 μg/mL for seizures) *Adults:* IV: 100 mg q5 min (total 500 mg) PO: 250 mg QID for 1 day, 250 mg/dose BID for 2 days, and 300-400 mg/24 hr, QD-QID	Rash, Stevens-Johnson syndrome, CNS symptoms (ataxia, dysarthria), lupus-like syndrome, blood dyscrasias, peripheral neuropathy, gingival hypertrophy	Susp: 125 mg/5 mL (240 mL) Tab, chewable: 50 mg (Infatab) Caps: 100 mg Caps, extended release: 30, 100, 200, 300 mg Inj: 50 mg/mL
Potassium chloride	***Supplement in diuretic therapy:*** *Children:* PO: 1-2 mEq/kg/24 hr, TID-QID (or 0.8-1.5 mL 10% potassium chloride/kg/24 hr, or 0.4-0.7 mL 20% potassium chloride/kg/24 hr, TID-QID)	GI disturbances, ulcerations, hyperkalemia	Oral sol: 10% (1.3 mEq/mL), 20% (2.7 mEq/mL) Caps, sustained release: 8, 10 mEq Tabs, sustained release: 8, 10, 15, 20 mEq
Potassium gluconate	***Supplement in diuretic therapy:*** *Children:* PO: 1-2 mEq/kg/24 hr TID-QID, or 0.8-1.5 mL/kg/24 hr TID-QID	Same as for potassium chloride	Elixir: 1.3 mEq/mL

TABLE E.1 *(continued)*

DOSAGES OF DRUGS USED IN PEDIATRIC CARDIOLOGY

DRUG	ROUTE AND DOSAGE	TOXICITY OR SIDE EFFECTS	HOW SUPPLIED
Pravastatin (Pravachol) (Antilipemic, HMG-CoA reductase inhibitor)	*Children (8-13 yr):* PO: Starting dose 10 mg QD for 4-6 wk Increase to 20 QD as needed. *Adolescents (14-18 yr):* PO: 40 mg QD (Adult max dose 40 mg/day)	Headache, constipation, diarrhea, elevated liver enzymes, rhabdomyolysis, myopathy	Tabs: 10, 20, 40, 80 mg
Prazosin (Minipress) (Postsynaptic α_1-adrenergic blocker, antihypertensive)	*Children:* PO: 5 μg/kg as a test dose; then 25-150 μg/kg/24 hr, QID *Adults:* PO: 1 mg/dose BID-TID initially Increase to 20 mg/24 hr, BID-QID (Usual dose 6-15 mg/24 hr)	CNS symptoms (dizziness, headache, drowsiness), palpitation, nausea	Caps: 1, 2, 5 mg
Procainamide (Procanbid, Pronestyl) (Class IA antiarrhythmic)	*Children:* IV: *Loading:* 2-6 mg/kg/dose over 5 min repeated q10-30 min (Max 100 mg) *Maintenance:* 20-80 μg/kg/min (Max 2 g/24 hr) PO: 15-50 mg/kg/24 hr q3-6 hr (Max 4 g/24 hr) *Adults:* IV: *Loading:* 50-100 mg/dose q5 min PRN *Maintenance:* 1-6 mg/min PO: Immediate release 250-500 mg/dose q3-6 hr (sustained release 500-1000 mg/dose q6 hr) (*Therapeutic level:* 4-10 μg/mL)	Nausea and vomiting, blood dyscrasias, rash, lupus-like syndrome, hypotension, confusion or disorientation	Tab, sustained release: 250, 500, 750, 1000 mg Caps: 250, 375, 500 mg Susp: 5, 50, 100 mg/mL Inj: 100, 500 mg/mL

Propranolol (Inderal) (β-adrenoceptor blocker, class II antiarrhythmic)	***For hypertension:*** *Children:* PO: 0.5-1 mg/kg/24 hr, BID-QID; may increase q3-5 days (Usual dose 2-4 mg/kg/24 hr; max dose 8 mg/kg/24 hr) ***For arrhythmias:*** *Children:* IV: 0.01-0.15 mg/kg/dose over 10 min; repeat q6-8 hr PRN (Max 1 mg/dose for infants; 3 mg/dose for children) PO: Start at 0.5-1 mg/kg/24 hr, TID-QID; increase dose q3-5 days PRN (Usual dose 2-4 mg/kg/24 hr; max dose 16 mg/kg/24 hr) *Adults:* IV: 1 mg/dose q5 min (maximum 5 mg) PO: 10-20 mg/dose TID-QID; increase PRN (Usual dose 40-320 mg/24 hr, TID-QID)	Hypotension, syncope, bronchospasm, nausea and vomiting, hypoglycemia, lethargy or depression, heart block	Tab: 10, 20, 40, 60, 80, 90 mg Caps, extended release: 60, 80, 120, 160 mg Oral sol: 20, 40 mg/5 mL Concentrated sol: 80 mg/mL Inj: 1 mg/mL
Prostaglandin E_1 or alprostadil (Prostin VR, PGE_1) (Vasodilator)	***For patency of ductus arteriosus:*** IV: Begin infusion at 0.05-0.1 μg/kg/min When desired effect achieved, reduce to 0.05, 0.025, and 0.01 μg/kg/min If unresponsive, dose may be increased to 0.4 μg/kg/min	Apnea, flushing, bradycardia, hypotension, fever	Inj: 500 μg/mL

TABLE E.1 *(continued)*

DOSAGES OF DRUGS USED IN PEDIATRIC CARDIOLOGY

DRUG	ROUTE AND DOSAGE	TOXICITY OR SIDE EFFECTS	HOW SUPPLIED
Protamine sulfate (Heparin antidote)	***Antidote to heparin overdose:*** IV: Each 1 mg protamine neutralizes approx 100 U heparin given in preceding 3-4 hr. Slow IV infusion at rate not exceeding 20 mg/min or 50 mg/10 min. (Check APTT)	Hypotension, bradycardia, dyspnea, flushing, coagulation problem	Inj: 10 mg/mL
Quinidine (Cardioquin, Quinidex, Quinaglute) (Class IA antiarrhythmic)	*Children:* Test dose for idiosyncrasy: 2 mg/kg once (PO as sulfate; IM/IV as gluconate) Therapeutic dose: IV (as gluconate): 2-10 mg/kg/dose, q3-6 hr PRN PO (as sulfate): 15-60 mg/kg/24 hr, q6 hr *Adults:* Test dose: 200 mg once PO/IM Therapeutic dose: PO (as sulfate, immediate release): 100-600 mg/dose q4-6 hr Begin at 200 mg/dose and titrate to desired effect, or PO (sulfate, sustained release): 300-600 mg/dose q8-12 hr PO (as gluconate): 324-972 mg q8-12 hr IM (as gluconate): 400 mg/dose q4-6 hr IV (as gluconate): 200-400 mg/dose, infused at a rate of ≤ 10 mg/min (*Therapeutic level:* 3-7 mg/L)	Nausea and vomiting, ventricular arrhythmias, prolonged QRS complex, depressed myocardial contractility, blood dyscrasias, symptoms of cinchonism	*Gluconate* (62% quinidine): Tab, slow-release: 324 mg Inj: 80 mg/mL *Sulfate* (83% quinidine): Tabs: 200, 300 mg Tab, slow-release: 300 mg Susp: 10 mg/mL

Sildenafil (Revatio, Viagra) (Phosphodiesterase type V inhibitor)	***For pulmonary hypertension:*** *Neonates:* PO: 0.25-1 mg/kg/dose, BID-QID *Infants and Children:* PO: 0.25-1 mg/kg/dose, q4-6 hr *Adults:* PO: 20 mg TID	Hypotension, tachycardia, flushing, headache, rash, nausea, diarrhea, priapism, platelet dysfunction, myalgia, paresthesia, blurred vision, epistaxis, dyspnea Contraindicated in concurrent use of organic nitrates	Tab: 20, 25, 50, 100 mg
Simvastatin (Zocor) (Antilipemic, HMG-CoA reductase inhibitor)	*Children:* PO: Starting dose 10 mg QD. Increment of 10 mg q6-8 wk to max dose of 40 mg QD as needed (Adult max 80 mg/24 hr)	Headache, constipation, diarrhea, elevated liver enzymes, rhabdomyolysis, myopathy	Tab: 5, 10, 20, 40, 80 mg
Sirolimus (Rapamune) (Immunosuppressant)	*Children:* PO: *Loading:* 3 mg/m^2 *Maintenance:* 1 mg/m^2/day QD *Adults:* PO: *Loading:* 6 mg *Maintenance:* 2 mg/day QD (*Therapeutic level:* 6-15 ng/mL)	Hypertension, peripheral edema, chest pain, fever, headache, acne, hirsutism, hypercholesterolemia, neurotoxicity, abdominal pain, anemia, pneumonitis	Tab: 1, 2 mg Oral sol: 1 mg/mL
Sodium polystyrene sulfonate (Kayexalate, Kionex) (Potassium-removing resin)	***For hyperkalemia*** (slowly effective, taking hours to days): *Children:* PO, NG: 1 g/kg/dose, q6 hr PR: 1 g/kg/dose, q2-6 hr *Adults:* PO, NG, PR: 15 g QD-QID (Cation exchange resin with practical exchange rates of 1 mEq potassium per 1 g resin) (NOTE: Delivers 1 mEq sodium for each mEq of potassium removed)	Nausea and vomiting, constipation, severe hypokalemia (muscle weakness, confusion [monitor serum potassium levels, ECG]), hypocalcemia or hypernatremia (edema)	Powder: 454, 480 g Susp: 15 g/60 mL

TABLE E.1 *(continued)*

DOSAGES OF DRUGS USED IN PEDIATRIC CARDIOLOGY

DRUG	ROUTE AND DOSAGE	TOXICITY OR SIDE EFFECTS	HOW SUPPLIED
Sotalol (Betapace) (Class II and III antiarrhythmic)	***For SVT and VT:*** PO: 80-120 mg/m²/24 hr, TID (*infants*) BID (*older children and adults*)	Chest pain, palpitation, hypoglycemia, hypotension, torsades de pointes, nausea and vomiting, abdominal pain, CNS symptoms (depression, weakness, dizziness), bronchospasm, heart block, bradycardia, negative inotropic effects, QT prolongation (Discontinue if QTc >550 msec)	Tab: 80, 120, 160, 240 mg Syrup: 5 mg/mL
Spironolactone (Aldactone) (Potassium-sparing diuretic, aldosterone antagonist)	*Children:* PO: 3 mg/kg/24 hr, BID-TID *Adults:* PO: 50-100 mg/24 hr, TID-QID (Max 200 mg/24 hr)	Hyperkalemia (when given with potassium supplements and ACE inhibitors), GI distress, rash, gynecomastia, agranulocytosis Contraindicated in renal failure	Tab: 25, 50, 100 mg Susp: 1, 2, 2.5, 5, 25 mg/mL
Streptokinase (Streptase, Kabikinase) (Thrombolytic enzyme)	***For thrombolysis:*** (Use in consultation with a hematologist) *Children:* IV: 3500-4000 U/kg over 30 min, followed by 1000-1500 U/kg/hr, or 2000 U/kg load over 30 min followed by 2000 U/kg/hr (Duration of infusion based on response but generally does not exceed 3 days. Obtain tests at baseline and q4 hr: APTT, TT, fibrinogen, PT, hematocrit, platelet count. APTT and TT should be <2 times control.)	Potential for allergic reaction with repeated use; premedicate with acetaminophen and antihistamine, and repeat q4-6hr	Inj: 250,000, 750,000, 1,500,000 IU powder for reconst

Drug	Dosage	Side Effects	How Supplied
Tacrolimus (Prograf) (Immunosuppressant)	*Children and adults:* PO: 0.15-0.4 mg/kg/day, BID IV: 0.03-0.15 mg/kg/day continuous infusion (*Therapeutic level:* 5-15 ng/mL)	Hypertension, hypotension, peripheral edema, myocardial hypertrophy, chest pain, fever, headache, encephalopathy, pruritus, hypercholesterolemia, electrolyte imbalance, neurotoxicity, nephrotoxicity, diarrhea, anemia, dyspnea	Caps: 0.5, 1, 5 mg Susp: 0.5 mg/mL Inj: 5 mg/mL (1 mL)
Tolazoline (Priscoline) (α-adrenoceptor blocker)	***For neonatal pulmonary hypertension:*** IV: *Loading:* 1-2 mg/kg over 10 min *Maintenance:* 1-2 mg/kg/hr	Hypotension and tachycardia, pulmonary hemorrhage, GI bleeding, arrhythmias, thrombocytopenia, leukopenia	Inj: 25 mg/mL
Triamterene (Dyrenium) (Potassium-sparing diuretic)	*Children:* PO: 2-4 mg/kg/24 hr, QD-BID. May increase up to max 6 mg/kg/24 hr or 300 mg/24 hr *Adults:* PO: 50-100 mg/24 hr, QD-BID (Max 300 mg/24 hr)	Nausea and vomiting, leg cramps, dizziness, hyperuricemia, rash, prerenal azotemia	Caps: 50, 100 mg

TABLE E.1 *(continued)*

DOSAGES OF DRUGS USED IN PEDIATRIC CARDIOLOGY

DRUG	ROUTE AND DOSAGE	TOXICITY OR SIDE EFFECTS	HOW SUPPLIED
Urokinase (Abbokinase) (Thrombolytic enzyme)	***For thrombolysis (in vein thrombosis or pulmonary embolism):*** (Should be used in consultation with a hematologist) *Children:* IV: *Loading:* 4400 U/kg over 10 min *Maintenance:* 4400 U/kg/hr for 6-12 hr. Some patients may require 12-72 hr of therapy (Monitor same laboratory tests as for streptokinase) ***For occluded IV catheter clearance:*** *Aspiration method:* Use 5000 U/mL concentrate. Instill into the catheter a volume equal to the internal volume of catheter over 1-2 min, leave in place for 1-4 hr, then aspirate. May repeat with 10,000 U/mL if no response. Do not infuse into the patient *IV infusion method:* 150-200 U/kg/hr in each lumen for 8-48 hr at a rate of at least 20 mL/hr *Adults:* ***For pulmonary embolism:*** IV: Priming dose: 4400 U/kg IV infusion: 4400 U/kg/hr for 12 hr by infusion pump	Bleeding, allergic reactions, rash, fever and chills, bronchospasm	Inj: 5000 U/mL

Verapamil (Isoptin, Calan) (Calcium channel blocker, class IV antiarrhythmic)	***For dysrhythmia (SVT):*** *Children:* IV: 1-15 yr (for SVT): 0.1-0.3 mg/kg over 2 min May repeat same dose in 15 min (Max dose 5 mg first dose; 10 mg second dose) *Adults:* IV: 5-10 mg, 10 mg second dose ***For hypertension:*** *Children:* PO: 4-8 mg/kg/24 hr, TID *Adults:* PO: 240-480 mg/24 hr, TID	Hypotension, bradycardia, cardiac depression	Tab: 40, 80, 120 mg Tab, extended release: 120, 180, 240 mg Caps, extended release: 100, 120, 180, 200, 240, 300, 360 mg Susp: 50 mg/mL Inj: 2.5 mg/mL
Vitamin K_1	***Antidote to dicumarol or warfarin:*** PO/IM/SC/IV: 2.5-10 mg/dose in 1 dose for correction of excessive PT from dicumarol or warfarin overdose		Tab: 5 mg Inj: 2, 10 mg/mL

TABLE E.1 *(continued)*

DOSAGES OF DRUGS USED IN PEDIATRIC CARDIOLOGY

DRUG	ROUTE AND DOSAGE	TOXICITY OR SIDE EFFECTS	HOW SUPPLIED
Warfarin (Coumadin, Sofarin) (Anticoagulant)	*Children:* PO: *Initial:* 0.1-0.2 mg/kg/dose QD in evening for 2 days (Max dose 10 mg/dose) (In liver dysfunction, 0.1 mg/kg/day, max 5 mg/dose) *Maintenance:* 0.1 mg/kg/24 hr QD (Monitor INR after 5-7 days of new dosage. Keep INR at 2.5-3.5 for mechanical prosthetic valve; 2-3 for prophylaxis of DVT, pulmonary emboli.) (Heparin preferred initially for rapid anticoagulation; warfarin may be started concomitantly with heparin or may be delayed 3-6 days.) *Adults:* PO: *Initial:* 5-15 mg/dose QD for 2-5 days *Maintenance:* 2-10 mg/day (Adjust dosage based on INR)	Bleeding (antidote: vitamin K or fresh frozen plasma) *Increased PT response:* salicylates, acetaminophen, alcohol, lipid-lowering agents, phenytoin, ibuprofen, some antibiotics *Decreased PT response:* antihistamines, barbiturates, oral contraceptives, vitamin C, diet high in vitamin K Onset of action: 36-72 hr, and full effects in 4-5 days. Mode of action: inhibits hepatic synthesis of vitamin K–dependent factors (I, VII, IX, X)	Tab: 1, 2, 2.5, 3, 4, 5, 6, 7.5, 10 mg Inj: 5 mg

ACE, angiotensin-converting enzyme; *approx.,* approximately; *APTT,* activated partial thromboplastin time; *AV,* atrioventricular; *BID,* two times a day; *BP,* blood pressure; *Caps,* capsule; *CHF,* congestive heart failure; *CK,* creatine kinase; *CNS,* central nervous system; *CR,* controlled release; *D_5W,* 5% dextrose in water; *DVT,* deep vein thrombosis; *ECG,* electrocardiogram; *ET,* endotracheal; *GI,* gastrointestinal; *HF,* heart failure; *HMG-CoA,* 3-hydroxy-3-methylglutaryl coenzyme A; *HOCM,* hypertrophic obstructive cardiomyopathy; *IM,* intramuscular; *Inj,* injection; *INR,* international normalized ratio; *IV,* intravenous; *LE,* lupus erythematosus; *LFT,* liver function test; *max,* maximum; *MI,* myocardial infarction; *NE,* norepinephrine; *NG,* nasogastric; *NS,* normal saline; *PDA,* patent ductus arteriosus; *PG,* prostaglandin; *PO,* by mouth; *PR,* per rectum; *PRN,* as necessary; *PT,* prothrombin time; *q,* every; *QD,* once a day; *QID,* 4 times a day; *QOD,* every other day; *RBF,* renal blood flow; *reconst,* reconstitution; *SC,* subcutaneous; *sol,* solution; *Supp,* suppository; *Susp,* suspension; *SVT,* supraventricular tachycardia; *Tab,* tablet; *TDD,* total digitalizing dose; *TID,* three times a day; *TT,* thrombin time; *U,* unit; *VT,* ventricular tachycardia; *WBC,* white blood cell; *(±),* may occur.

Index

Note: Page numbers followed by *f* refer to figures, by *t* to tables, and by *b* to boxes.

B

C

D

F

J

S